SALEM HEALTH
CANCER

SALEM HEALTH
CANCER

Volume IV

Sentinel lymph node (SLN) biopsy and mapping — Zollinger-Ellison syndrome
Appendixes
Indexes

Editor

Jeffrey A. Knight, Ph.D.
Mount Holyoke College

Medical Consultants

Laurie Jackson-Grusby, Ph.D.
Children's Hospital Boston, Harvard Medical School

Wendy White-Ryan, M.D., FAAP
Golisano Children's Hospital at Strong Memorial Hospital

SALEM PRESS, INC.
Pasadena, California   Hackensack, New Jersey

Editor in Chief: Dawn P. Dawson
Editorial Director: Christina J. Moose
Project Editors: Tracy Irons-Georges,
Rowena Wildin Dehanke
Editorial Assistant: Dana Garey

Production Editor: Joyce I. Buchea
Acquisitions Editor: Mark Rehn
Photo Editor: Cynthia Breslin Beres
Design and Graphics: James Hutson
Layout: William Zimmerman

Note to Readers

The material presented in *Salem Health: Cancer* is intended for broad informational and educational purposes. Readers who suspect that they or someone whom they know or provide caregiving for suffers from cancer or any other physical or psychological disorder, disease, or condition described in this set should contact a physician without delay; this work should not be used as a substitute for professional medical diagnosis or staging. Readers who are undergoing or about to undergo any treatment or procedure described in this set should refer to their physicians and other health care team members for guidance concerning preparation and possible effects. This set is not to be considered definitive on the covered topics, and readers should remember that the field of health care is characterized by a diversity of medical opinions and constant expansion in knowledge and understanding.

Library of Congress Cataloging-in-Publication Data

Salem health : cancer / Jeffrey A. Knight, Laurie Jackson-Grusby, Wendy White-Ryan.
  p. cm.
Includes bibliographical references and index.
  ISBN 978-1-58765-505-0 (set : alk. paper) — ISBN 978-1-58765-506-7 (vol. 1 : alk. paper) —
ISBN 978-1-58765-507-4 (vol. 2 : alk. paper) — ISBN 978-1-58765-508-1 (vol. 3 : alk. paper) —
ISBN 978-1-58765-509-8 (vol. 4 : alk. paper)
1. Cancer. I. Knight, Jeffrey A., 1948- II. Jackson-Grusby, Laurie. III. White-Ryan, Wendy.
RC265.S32 2008
616.99′4—dc22

                                                                                2008030861

First Printing

PRINTED IN THE UNITED STATES OF AMERICA

▶ Contents

► Complete List of Contents

VOLUME 1

VOLUME 2

Contents

VOLUME 3

VOLUME 4

Contents lxxvii
Complete List of Contents lxxix

SALEM HEALTH
CANCER

▶ Sentinel lymph node (SLN) biopsy and mapping

Category: Procedures

Definition: A sentinel lymph node (SLN) biopsy is a procedure in which the first lymph nodes to which cancer is likely to spread from the primary tumor are removed and examined to determine whether cancer cells are present. The process of identification of the SLNs is called SLN mapping.

Cancers diagnosed or treated: Mainly breast cancer and malignant melanoma; SLN is being studied for use with other cancer types

Why performed: Cancer cells spread first to one or several lymph nodes, called the sentinel lymph nodes (SLNs), before spreading to more distal lymph nodes and other sites in the body. Determining whether a SLN contains cancer cells provides the doctor with valuable information about whether the cancer has spread from its primary location.

Patient preparation: A small dose of a radioactive tracer compound and a blue dye are injected near the patient's tumor several hours before surgery to allow these chemicals time to travel from the tumor region to any SLNs.

Steps of the procedure: Once the radioactive tracer compound and dye have reached the lymph nodes, the surgeon scans the area with a small Geiger counter and removes the radioactive lymph nodes through a small incision, using the presence of the blue dye for additional visual confirmation. A pathologist performs a preliminary examination of the nodes under a microscope, and if cancerous cells are seen while the patient is still in surgery, additional lymph nodes may be removed at that time.

After the procedure: Pain or bruising at the biopsy site and temporary discoloration of urine or skin may occur. Some patients report postoperative nerve damage or swelling caused by lymph fluid accumulation in the area of the surgery. Rarely, a patient may be allergic to the blue dye used for sentinel node identification. Patients undergoing the procedure typically spend one day or less in the hospital.

Risks: A low percentage of SNL biopsies for breast cancer can turn out to be negative when other lymph nodes in the area do contain cancer.

Results: Doctors use SLN biopsy results to help determine the stage of cancer. A negative result implies that the cancer has not spread to the lymph nodes, and a positive result indicates that cancer is present in the SLN and therefore may be present in other lymph nodes. In this case, removal of other lymph nodes in the area may be performed.

Jill Ferguson, Ph.D.

See also Axillary dissection; Biopsy; Breast cancer in children and adolescents; Breast cancer in men; Breast cancer in pregnant women; Breast cancers; Lymphadenectomy; Lymphangiography; Lymphedema; Mastectomy; Melanomas; Merkel cell carcinomas (MCC); Penile cancer.

▶ Sertoli cell tumors

Category: Diseases, symptoms, and conditions
Also known as: Androblastomas, large-cell calcifying Sertoli cell tumors, sclerosing Sertoli cell tumors

Related conditions: Leydig cell tumors, Sertoli-Leydig cell tumors of the ovaries

Definition: Sertoli cell tumors are rare, typically benign tumors that form in the Sertoli cells of the testes, which nourish the sperm-producing germ cells.

Risk factors: Sertoli cell tumors are believed to arise from genetic abnormalities. Having a family history of testicular cancer may increase the risk. Sertoli cell tumors are often associated with Peutz-Jeghers syndrome (PJS), a rare inherited condition that causes many noncancerous growths to form in the stomach and intestines.

Etiology and the disease process: Sertoli cell tumors are thought to arise from chromosomal abnormalities. Benign tumors do not typically progress, but malignant tumors can spread to the lymph nodes, bone, liver, or lungs.

Incidence: Sertoli cell tumors account for only 1 to 3 percent of testicular tumors. These tumors are almost always benign in children but are cancerous in approximately 20 percent of the adults who have them.

Symptoms: Sertoli cell tumors are often painless and produce no symptoms, aside from a lump in the testicles. In rare cases, these types of tumors can release male or female hormones. Release of the female hormone, estrogen, can cause the patient to develop symptoms such as breast tenderness and enlargement, or loss of sexual desire. Release of the male hormone testosterone can cause boys to go into puberty prematurely.

Screening and diagnosis: The doctor will feel the testicles and abdomen to identify any lumps or masses. An ultrasound can be used to visualize the tumor. If the tumor is cancerous, the patient may have a computed tomography (CT) scan of the abdomen and pelvis, and a chest X ray to determine disease progression.

Treatment and therapy: Surgery to remove the testicles (orchiectomy) is the standard treatment for Sertoli cell tumors. In younger patients, the surgeon will attempt to spare the testes from significant damage. Cancerous tumors can be treated with chemotherapy, radiation, and surgery to remove the involved lymph nodes.

Prognosis, prevention, and outcomes: There is no way to prevent Sertoli cell tumors. The prognosis is good for children with nonmalignant tumors who have surgery to remove the tumor. Following surgery, patients may need to be monitored for several years to check for a recurrence.

Stephanie Watson, B.S.

See also Benign tumors; Cobalt 60 radiation; Computed tomography (CT) scan; Family history and risk assessment; Leydig cell tumors; Orchiectomy; Peutz-Jeghers syndrome (PJS); Testicular cancer; Ultrasound tests.

▶ Sexuality and cancer

Category: Social and personal issues

Definition: A substantial number of men and women with cancer report some negative effect of the disease or its treatment on their sexual lives. Some studies report that a majority of cancer patients experience long-term problems with sexual function.

Sexual response: Sexual response is often categorized into several components or dimensions, all of which can be affected by cancer and cancer treatment. Sexual desire refers to the experience of sexual thoughts, fantasies, daydreams, or desire for sexual activity. Sexual arousal comprises physiological and psychological events in preparation to engage in or continue sexual activity, including erection of the penis, lubrication of the vagina, and subjective feelings of excitement or anticipation. Orgasm is a peak of physiological and psychological arousal usually accompanied by rhythmic pelvic muscular contractions and intense pleasure, often (but not always) followed by resolution of sexual arousal and feelings of relaxation and well-being. In men, orgasm is usually accompanied by emission and ejaculation of semen.

Sexuality is not merely the sum of sexual responses but also comprises a person's self-concept as a sexual person, preferences for sexual partners and sexual activities, inter-actions with current and potential future partners, and experience within a sexual culture. Sexual values, ideals, and scripts are often rooted early in life and develop over a period of many years. In the face of serious illness, deeply held sexual beliefs can help or hinder recovery toward a satisfying sexual life.

Effects of cancer on sexuality: Generally, the effects of cancer on sexuality are both physical and psychological. The emotional distress of living with cancer can take an even larger toll when combined with the physical impact of the disease. Tumors of certain size and location can directly affect physical aspects of sexual function, particularly when they interfere with nerve and blood vessel pathways important to sexual function. More commonly, however, sexual function is affected by treatment-related side effects such as fatigue, nausea, changes to physical appearance, and pain. In advanced cancers, the discomfort and fatigue associated with disease are also likely to limit sexual expression.

Effects of treatment on sexuality: Although the effects of any cancer and its treatment can threaten to disrupt sexual function, certain types of cancers are especially high risk. Cancers of the reproductive organs (such as the cervix, ovary, uterus, vagina, prostate, testicle, penis) are associated with a high rate of sexual problems that often persist after treatment because of the potential for damage to nerves, blood vessels, and other tissues involved in sexual responses. Other cancers of the pelvic region and lower abdomen, such as bladder, colorectal, and anal cancers, may also affect sexual function due to the organs' proximity to and shared neurovascular environment with the reproductive system. In women, breast cancer may affect sexual function through negative effects on body image, particularly when the breasts are strongly connected with sexual attractiveness and femininity, and through posttreatment alteration of pleasurable breast sensations.

Chemotherapy: In addition to fatigue and other general physical symptoms, systemic chemotherapy can cause changes to testicular and ovarian function that decrease the production of sex hormones (testosterone and estrogen). These changes may result in decreased sexual desire and problems with sexual arousal, such as erectile dysfunction and poor vaginal lubrication. Although in men the hormonal effects of chemotherapy often reverse after treatment, women are susceptible to permanent loss of ovarian function. Other effects of chemotherapy include irritation of mucous membranes, including the lining of the vagina and the mouth, which can interfere with kissing, oral sex, and vaginal penetration.

Surgery: Surgical treatment of pelvic and lower abdominal cancers can damage nerves and occasionally blood vessels that are important to sexual arousal responses. Despite advances in surgical techniques to reduce pelvic nerve damage, erectile and ejaculatory dysfunctions remain common in men after procedures such as radical prostatectomy, radical cystectomy, and abdominoperineal resection. In women, sexual arousal problems, orgasm problems, and painful intercourse are common for a year or more after radical hysterectomy, though the effects of other abdominal surgeries on sexual function may be less severe than in men. Surgical menopause after removal of the ovaries may also affect short-term and long-term sexual function. Partial or complete removal of external genital tissue (such as vulvectomy or penectomy) perhaps poses the greatest threat to sexual function, though penile and vulvar cancers are rare.

Radiation: Radiation to the pelvic region can cause sexual difficulties by damaging nerves and blood vessels that control genital function and by affecting testicular and ovarian function, causing difficulties similar to those caused by other treatments. Furthermore, in women pelvic radiation can cause vaginal inflammation, sores, and scarring. This damage may lead to permanent shortening or collapse of the vaginal canal, limiting vaginal penetration because of pain and physical limitations. The severity of radiation side effects depends on the dose of radiation received and the extent of the irradiated region. Unlike surgery, the effects of radiation progress over a period of time.

Hormonal therapy: Adjuvant hormonal treatments, such as tamoxifen, for certain cancers have become more common. Effects are similar to those of other causes of decline in sex hormone levels and include changes in sexual interest and arousal.

Prognosis and treatment for sexual problems: Sexual problems often resolve over time or with treatment. The quality of sexual function before diagnosis and treatment is an important predictor of sexual recovery, as are age, general health status, and the partner's receptiveness to further sexual activity. When aggressive treatment causes significant physical damage, adjustment to long-term changes in sexual function is necessary.

It is important not to underestimate the effects of psychological and relationship factors on sexual function. Although physical changes resulting from disease or treatment can be devastating, psychological adaptation to these changes may be the ultimate limiting factor in recovery.

Ongoing problems with depression or anxiety can inhibit sexual desire and hinder efforts to resume sexual activity. Changes in appearance, health, fertility, or physical functioning may cause a sense of decreased self-worth, anxiety about recurrence, feelings of unattractiveness, and concern about a partner's rejection or abandonment. Sexual problems may also have origins in intimacy problems and conflict between sexual partners. Finally, rigid or unrealistic expectations of sexual activity or a lack of knowledge about sexuality can create barriers when recovery necessitates changes to the sexual repertoire. Individual, couple, or group therapy is helpful in addressing these issues. In many cases the resumption of a fulfilling sex life hinges on building confidence and intimacy between partners, re-evaluating beliefs about sexuality and sexual personhood, and orienting the patient and partner toward experiencing pleasure and satisfaction rather than achieving a specific goal (such as maintaining a full erection or always having an orgasm with sexual activity).

The use of sexual aids such as lubricants and vibrators can enhance sexual enjoyment in patients who have altered sexual function after cancer. Medical interventions for sexual problems are available, although it is inadvisable to pursue these options in lieu of counseling or psychotherapy. Medical treatment options are diverse and include local or systemic hormonal supplementation (although with some cancers hormonal treatment is contraindicated), the use of prescription medications for erectile dysfunction (such as Viagra, or sildenafil; Cialis, or tadalafil; Levitra, or vardenafil), penile injection therapy, and penile and clitoral vacuum devices. Invasive surgical options are less common. Reconstructive surgery, when possible, may improve body image. Penile prosthesis surgery can partially restore erectile function when other treatments have failed or are unacceptable. Although reparative surgery may address neurological or vascular causes of sexual dysfunction, current evidence to support this approach is limited.

Sexuality is increasingly viewed as an important element of quality of life, but more often than not, health care providers are hesitant to discuss sexual issues with their patients. Referral to a provider with special expertise in sexual problems can be helpful. Although there is no recognized medical specialty in sexual medicine, physicians with expertise in sexual problems are represented in several fields, including urology, gynecology, psychiatry, and endocrinology. The American Association of Sex Educators, Counselors, and Therapists (AASECT) also provides referrals and certification for mental health professionals with special expertise in human sexuality.

Andrea Bradford, M.A.

▶ **For Further Information**

Katz, Anne. *Breaking the Silence on Cancer and Sexuality: A Handbook for Healthcare Providers.* Pittsburgh: Oncology Nursing Society, 2007.

Leiblum, Sandra R., ed. *Principles and Practice of Sex Therapy.* 4th ed. New York: Guilford Press, 2007.

Owens, Annette F., and Mitchell S. Tepper, eds. *Sexual Health.* Westport, Conn.: Praeger, 2007.

Schover, Leslie R. *Sexuality and Fertility After Cancer.* New York: Wiley, 1997.

▶ **Other Resources**

American Association of Sex Counselors, Educators, and Therapists
http://www.aasect.org

American Cancer Society
Sexuality for Men and Their Partners
http://www.cancer.org/docroot/MIT/
MIT_7_1x_SexualityforMenandTheirPartners.asp

American Cancer Society
Sexuality for Women and Their Partners
http://www.cancer.org/docroot/MIT/
MIT_7_1x_SexualityforWomenandTheirPartners.asp

National Cancer Institute
Sexuality and Reproductive Issues
http://www.cancer.gov/cancertopics/pdq/
supportivecare/sexuality

Sexual Health Network
http://www.sexualhealth.com

See also Anxiety; Depression; Elderly and cancer; Fatigue; Fertility issues; Living with cancer; Nausea and vomiting; Pregnancy and cancer; Psychosocial aspects of cancer; Relationships; Self-image and body image; Sterility; Stress management; Young adult cancers.

▶ **Sézary syndrome**

Category: Diseases, symptoms, and conditions
Also known as: Baccaredda-Sézary syndrome, cutaneous T-cell lymphoma, T-cell erythroderma, Sézary-Baccaredda syndrome, Sézary-Bouvrain syndrome, Sézary's disease, Sézary erythroderma

Related conditions: Mycosis fungoides; some experts consider Sézary syndrome to be an advanced form of mycosis fungoides, while others consider it a separate disease.

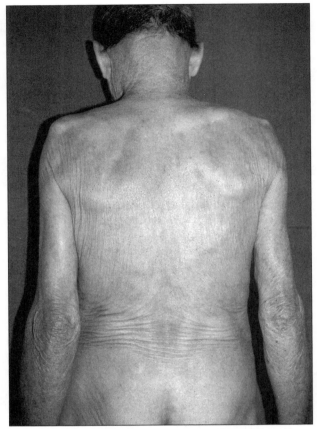

The back of a man with Sézary syndrome. (©ISM/Phototake—All rights reserved)

Definition: Sézary syndrome is a variant of cutaneous T-cell lymphoma. In this disease, T lymphocytes (the cells that help the immune system by killing bacteria in the body) become cancerous, affecting the skin and blood. After these cancerous cells enter the bloodstream, the disease may spread to other organs. It is named for Albert Sézary, A. Baccaredda, and Yves Bouvrain, who first described it in 1938.

Risk factors: There are no known risk factors for Sézary syndrome. Exposure to certain chemicals or viruses has been thought to increase risk, but these ideas have not been proven.

Etiology and the disease process: Sézary syndrome develops slowly, usually over years. In early stages, the skin itches and forms dry, dark patches. Then tumors, called mycosis fungoides, form on the skin, and the skin may become infected. When many tumor cells appear in the blood and travel throughout the body, this disease has progressed into Sézary syndrome. The disease may then spread to the lymph nodes or other organs such as the lungs, liver, or spleen.

Incidence: Sézary syndrome affects only about 1 out of 1 million people. Most cases appear in people who are over the age of fifty. Men get this disease more often than women, and African Americans develop it more often than members of other ethnicities.

Symptoms: Symptoms include itching; a dry, red skin rash; skin tumors; and enlarged lymph nodes.

Screening and diagnosis: A physical exam is the general screening tool for this disease. If Sézary syndrome is suspected, blood tests or skin biopsies may be used to confirm the diagnosis. Other tests, such as X rays, computed tomography (CT) scans, magnetic resonance imaging (MRI), or lymph node biopsies, may be used to see if the disease has spread to other parts of the body.

Sézary syndrome involves these stages:

• Stage I: Only parts of the skin are affected with a red, scaly rash. There are no tumors, and lymph nodes are normal.

• Stage II: Either lymph nodes are normal or enlarged but have no cancerous cells and the skin has a red, scaly rash but no tumors or the lymph nodes are normal or enlarged but do not contain cancerous cells although the skin has tumors.

• Stage III: Most of the skin is affected by a red, scaly rash, but the lymph nodes, either normal or enlarged, do not contain cancerous cells.

• Stage IV: In addition to the skin rash, either cancer cells are in the lymph nodes or cancer cells have spread to other organs.

• Recurrent: The cancer has been previously treated but has returned, either where it began or in another area of the body.

Treatment and therapy: The three treatments generally used for Sézary syndrome are radiation therapy, chemotherapy, and phototherapy.

In radiation therapy for this disease, a special type of radiation that only penetrates the outer layers of the skin (total skin electron beam radiation) may be directed to the entire body to kill cancer cells in the skin. Another method is to direct radiation only to small areas of skin that are highly affected.

Chemotherapy for this disease may involve traditional systemic chemotherapy (putting chemicals that kill cancer cells into the bloodstream by mouth or intravenously) or a topical cream that contains chemicals that kill cancer cells.

With one type of phototherapy for this cancer (PUVA therapy, psoralen plus ultraviolet light A), patients are given certain drugs that make cancer cells sensitive to light; then a laser light is shone on the skin to kill the cancer cells. In another type of phototherapy (extracorporeal photochemotherapy), patients are given certain drugs; then some of the blood cells are taken out of the body, exposed to a special light, then reinserted into the body. Sometimes patients who are treated with phototherapy need to avoid sunlight.

Other treatments, such as steroid creams, may be used to ease the itching and swelling of the skin with this disease.

Clinical trials testing biological therapy (using the body's own immune system) and bone marrow transplants to fight this type of cancer are ongoing.

Prognosis, prevention, and outcomes: Sézary syndrome is difficult to cure and no way of preventing it is known, but treatments can relieve symptoms. Patients who are diagnosed with Sézary syndrome at Stage I of the disease have a survival rate of twenty or more years and generally do not die of causes related to this disease. However, 50 percent of those whose disease progresses into Stage IV eventually die of causes related to this disease within five years.

Marianne M. Madsen, M.S.

Relative Survival Rates for Sézary Syndrome, 1988-2001

Years	Survival Rate (%)
1	97.1
2	95.1
3	92.4
5	88.4
8	84.5
10	82.6

Source: Data from L. A. G. Ries et al., eds., *Cancer Survival Among Adults: U.S. SEER Program, 1988-2001—Patient and Tumor Characteristics*, NIH Pub. No. 07-6215 (Bethesda, Md.: National Cancer Institute, 2007)

▶ **For Further Information**

Foss, F. "Mycosis Fungoides and the Sézary Syndrome." *Current Opinion in Oncology* 16, no. 5 (September, 2004): 421-428.

Siegel, Richard S., et al. "Primary Cutaneous T-Cell Lymphoma: Review and Current Concepts." *Journal of Clinical Oncology* 18, no. 15 (August, 2000): 2908-2925.

Zackheim, Herschel S., ed. *Cutaneous T-Cell Lymphoma: Mycosis Fungoides and Sézary Syndrome*. New York: Informa Healthcare, 2004.

▶ **Other Resources**

Cutaneous Lymphoma Foundation
http://www.clfoundation.org

National Cancer Institute
Mycosis Fungoides and the Sézary Syndrome
http://www.cancer.gov/cancertopics/pdq/treatment/
mycosisfungoides/Patient

See also Cutaneous T-cell lymphoma (CTCL); Itching;
Lymphomas; Mycosis fungoides.

▶ Side effects

Category: Diseases, symptoms, and conditions
Also known as: Concomitant events, adverse events
 (AEs), adverse effects, adverse drug reactions
 (ADRs), complications

Definition: Side effects include any unintended action,
reaction, effect, or change in a person's condition that
occurs as a result of medical treatment in addition to the
intended action, effect, or change in condition. It can be
caused by medication, drug interactions, an unintentional
overdosage, a drug allergy, a vaccination, or any other
procedure, therapy, or treatment. Side effects may also be
associated with diseases and conditions, nutritional or
herbal supplements, comorbid conditions (those existing
simultaneously with another condition), lifestyle behaviors, and medications unrelated to the condition being
treated.

General side effects from drugs: All drugs, whether prescription or over-the-counter (OTC), can cause side effects ranging in duration from acute (transient) to chronic
(long-term) and in intensity from mild to life-threatening.
Whether or not a person experiences drug-related side effects depends on a number of factors, including individual
differences in physiologic makeup. All prescription and
OTC drugs have known, documented (labeled) side effects. Those of prescription drugs are listed on each medication's package insert (PI). The PI for each marketed
drug must be approved by the U.S. Food and Drug Administration (FDA) and must include comprehensive efficacy
data, pharmacokinetic and pharmacodynamic data (information on the way the body absorbs, distributes, and me-
tabolizes the drug), dosage and administration data, and
safety data including contraindications (a listing of known
conditions that may preclude safe usage), warnings (a listing of serious side effects), precautions (a listing of poten-

tial concerns involving drug interactions, laboratory test
interactions, carcinogenesis, mutagenesis, impairment of
fertility, pregnancy, teratogenicity, use by nursing mothers, pediatric use, geriatric use, adverse reactions, and an
assessment of potential for drug abuse and dependence),
signs and symptoms indicative of overdose, and treatment
recommendations in the event of overdose.

 In general, the most commonly experienced drug-related
side effects involve the gastrointestinal system (including
anorexia, constipation, diarrhea, nausea, and vomiting).
Other commonly experienced side effects involve the nervous system (including fatigue, headache, and insomnia).
The *Physicians' Desk Reference* (PDR), a commercially
published, annually updated reference book, is a compen-
dium of PIs. It is available to the public in original format,
in layterm format, and in CD-ROM format. An online version is also available to medical professionals.

Drug interactions: Drug-related side effects may occur
due to any of the following types of interaction: one medication with another medication (a "drug-drug interaction"), one therapy with another therapy (a "concurrent
therapy interaction"), and a medication with a certain food
type (a "drug-food interaction").

 Drug-drug interactions. Concomitant use of certain
medications can result in either a reduction of or an increase in the effects of either or both drugs, thereby increasing the incidence or severity of side effects. For example, antidiarrheal drugs taken with tranquilizers can
increase the sedative effect; anticoagulants with antacids
can decrease absorption of the anticoagulant and increase
bleeding; diuretics with decongestants can increase hypertension; and antihistamines with antitussives (cough medications) can increase drowsiness.

 Concurrent therapy interactions. Concurrent therapy
interactions can occur when two or more different types of
treatments are used simultaneously for the same indication
(to treat the same symptom). For example, combined treatment with chemotherapy and radiation therapy, as is administered for many types of cancer, can result in a decrease in neutrophils (white blood cells) as well as other
types of blood cells. When administered to those with diabetes, the resultant decrease in cell count could increase
the risk of infection.

 In addition to adverse drug interactions, however, the
possibility exists that a drug-drug interaction may have a
positive synergistic effect. In such cases, either the efficacy of the concomitant drugs is greater than that of each
drug individually or the side effects associated with the
concomitant drugs are fewer or less severe than those associated with either drug individually.

Drug-food interactions. The presence in the gut of certain types of foods may affect the bioavailability and safety profiles of an orally administered drug by interfering with its ADMET profile. ADMET stands for the following properties:

- absorption into the circulatory system
- distribution to organs and tissues
- metabolism of the parent compound into metabolites
- excretion of the parent compound and metabolites, usually via urine and feces
- toxicity (harmfulness) of the parent compound and metabolites

For example, an enzyme present in grapefruit may inhibit drug metabolism, resulting in the presence of more parent compound in the circulatory system than would otherwise be there. This could increase in the incidence or severity of side effects caused by drugs in the following drug classes: analgesics, antiarrhythmics, antibiotics, anticoagulants, anticonvulsants, antidepressants, antihypertensives, antitussives, and chemotherapy agents. Certain foods may also block drug absorption if taken within a certain interval before or after a drug dose. For example, ingestion of a dairy product shortly before or after taking the antibiotic tetracycline can result in the drug's reduced efficacy.

Obversely, the systemic presence of certain types of drugs may affect nutrient absorption, nutrient metabolism, or appetite. The magnitude of a drug-food effect, however, is dependent upon such variables as drug dosage and route of administration; duration of the interval between medication ingestion and food ingestion; and the age, weight, gender, and health status of the person taking the medication.

Unintentional overdosage. Toxicity can occur as the result of an unintentional overdose either from taking more than the correct dose at any one time or from taking the correct dose more often than prescribed or recommended. Side effects of acute toxicity include blurred vision, dizziness, headache, loss of muscle coordination, nausea, and vomiting. For certain antihypertensive drugs, dosages only slightly higher than the recommended therapeutic dose can cause bradycardia (slow heartbeat), hypotension, or vomiting.

Since the route of excretion for most drugs is renal (through kidney metabolism), hepatic (through liver metabolism), or both, overdosage can result in renal or hepatic toxicity. An overdosage of analgesics (painkillers) is the most prevalent cause of acute hepatoxicity (liver failure) in the United States.

Toxicity can result not only from drug exposure but also from radiation exposure. Such toxicity can be minimized by limiting the volume of tissue irradiated.

Drug allergies: Certain drugs can cause allergic reactions, whereby the immune system launches a histamine response to rid the body of the drug. The resultant adverse events can range in intensity from life-threatening to mild and include anaphylactic symptoms (apnea, bronchoconstriction, cyanosis, and loss of consciousness), anxiety, confusion, diarrhea, dizziness, hives and itching, lung congestion, mouth and throat edema, nausea, rash, and tachycardia (rapid heartbeat).

The most common trigger for allergic reactions is antibiotics in the penicillin family. Others include anticonvulsants, barbiturates, insulin, iodine (present in radiographic contrast dyes), and sulfa drugs.

Photoallergies and phototoxicities: Photoallergy and phototoxicity are two types of photosensitivity that can be caused by prescription or over-the-counter drugs. Occurrences can be either acute and isolated, or chronic.

Photoallergies can occur following the topical administration of certain medications that undergo structural change when exposed to the ultraviolet wavelengths of sunlight, resulting in the production of antibodies that cause the photosensitivity. Symptoms include incidence of an eczema-type rash a few days after treatment.

Phototoxicity can occur following topical, oral, or injected administration of certain medications. These medications absorb ultraviolet wavelengths of sunlight and then distribute them transdermally (through absorption by the skin), resulting in cell death. Symptoms occur a few days after treatment and can last up to twenty years after the treatment's cessation.

Drugs that cause photosensitivity can exacerbate existing skin conditions and may precipitate or exacerbate certain autoimmune disorders, such as lupus. Drugs that most commonly cause photosensitivity are in the following drug classes: antianxiety medications, antibiotics, anticholesterol medications, antidepressants, antiepileptic medications, antifungals, antihistamines, antihypertensives, diuretics, neuroleptic medications, nonsteroidal anti-inflammatories (NSAIDs), and vaccinations.

Side effects of chemotherapy: Chemotherapy drugs are often among the most toxic, given that their function is to destroy or otherwise mitigate tumor tissue. Hence, these agents often have strong side effects that are managed by other drugs. Among the side effects of chemotherapy are alopecia (hair loss), anemia, anorexia, anxiety disorders, bradycardia, congestive heart failure, constipation, decreased fertility, depression, diarrhea, dyspnea (shortness of breath), fatigue, febrile neutropenia, heart arrhythmias, hypertension, incontinence, insomnia, lymphedema, mucositis (mouth sores), nausea, peripheral neuropathy (nerve damage), pulmonary infections due to a compromised immune system, renal (kidney) damage (sometimes requiring dialysis), skin and nail changes, and vomiting.

Other procedures, therapies, and treatments: Diagnostic procedures, and non-drug-related therapies or treatments, such as surgery and radiation therapy, can also cause side effects.

Diagnostic procedures. Imaging procedures are among the most common diagnostic procedures. For example, a patient undergoing computed tomography (CT) scan with ingestion or injection of contrast medium may undergo a reaction to the contrast dye. Magnetic resonance imaging (MRI) may induce headache or nausea resulting from the noise of the machine or, in cases where contrast is used, injection site pain. Nuclear scans, including positron emission tomography (PET) and single photon emission computed tomography (SPECT) scans, may cause fever or (rarely) tissue damage.

Nonpharmaceutic therapies or treatments. Side effects may also result from non-drug-related therapies or treatments, including acupuncture, blood product transfusions, hyperbaric oxygen therapy, metabolic therapy, plasmapheresis (for prevention of potential side effects), radiation therapy, surgery (including bone marrow, organ, or peripheral blood stem cell transplantation), and whole-body heat therapy. For cancer patients, toxic side effects may occur from radiation exposure, but risk is minimized by limiting the volume of tissue irradiated.

Nutritional supplements. All vitamins and other nutritional supplements can cause side effects. Hypervitaminosis, or toxicity due to the cellular storage of an overabundance of fat-soluble vitamins (A, D, E, K), is the primary cause of nutritionally related side effects. For example, acute vitamin A toxicity can cause alopecia, blurry vision, bone calcification or inflammation. Symptoms of chronic vitamin A toxicity include alopecia, fatigue, dizziness, drowsiness, nausea, kidney damage, liver damage, elevated cholesterol, and prostate cancer. Toxic doses of mineral supplements can occur with excessive amounts of iron and zinc. Herbal supplements can cause side effects as well; dimethyl sulfoxide (DMSO), valerian, and yohimbe are only a few examples of herbals that can have toxic and sometimes life-threatening side effects. Herbal supplements can also negatively interact with prescription preparations like anesthesia, anticoagulants, and beta- blockers.

One reason that nutritional supplements can be particularly dangerous concerns the way they are regulated: Manufacturers of supplements are not required to test those supplements for either safety or efficacy prior to market-

ing them. Unless a manufacturer makes specific claims that a supplement can treat, cure, or prevent a specific disease, that manufacturer does not need to prove to the FDA that those claims are true, provide quality assurance that the supplement actually contains what the label states that it contains, or provide quality control to ensure that the supplement is contaminant-free.

Diseases and conditions: Having a specific disease or condition may predispose an individual to experience side effects. Moreover, disease-related physiologic changes may cause pharmacodynamic anomalies and resultant reduction in drug efficacy or increase in incidence of drug-related adverse events.

Cancer's side effects include bone metastasis, resulting in pain, fracture, and resultant hypercalcemia due to calcium from damaged bone being released into the bloodstream. Chronic lymphocytic leukemia causes alterations in the immune system, resulting lysis (dissolution) of red blood cells. Retinoblastoma results in glaucoma, eye pain, and vision loss.

A comorbid condition—a concurrent condition that is unrelated to the primary disease—may also predispose an individual to experience side effects and precipitate disease-related physiologic changes that may cause pharmacodynamic anomalies and resultant reduction in drug efficacy or increase in incidence of drug-related adverse events. In the case of cancer, a variety of comorbidities have side effects that mitigate treatment.

Some comorbid conditions may predate the primary disease, while others develop after onset of the primary disease. For example, cancer treatment may be compromised by comorbidities such as compromised cardiac or lung function (which makes the patient a poor surgical risk and a poor risk for concomitant chemotherapy and radiation therapy); Alzheimer's disease (which makes the patient a poor risk for brain irradiation to counteract brain metastasis); and diabetes, hypertension, renal problems, or congestive heart failure (all of which interfere with the healing process). Cancers that affect comorbid conditions, on the other hand, include small-cell lung cancer (SCLC), which may cause Lambert-Eaton syndrome (LEMS) and resultant muscle weakness.

Special populations: Drug therapy used by those in certain subpopulations—geriatric, pediatric, and adult females—requires increased vigilance given the possibility of increased incidence of drug side effects at dosages that would otherwise be considered therapeutic.

Geriatric populations. Clinically significant age-associated differences in a drug's efficacy profile or safety profile can occur in the elderly, who tend to take more medications, which increases the potential for drug reactions and drug-drug interactions. The elderly also have a decreased metabolic rate, which increases both a drug's mean residence time in the body and the resultant potential for toxicity. Often, these drug-related side effects—which can include fatigue, weight loss, and loss of balance—are attributed to natural aging changes, signs or symptoms of underlying diseases, and an existing or newly acquired medical condition rather than to the drugs themselves. Therefore, dosing both by body weight and by metabolic rate is an important consideration in the elderly population.

Pediatric populations. Drug-related side effects are of great concern regarding those in the pediatric population, in which drugs can have a significant impact on growth, development, and maturation at many levels: behavioral, cognitive, immunological, physiological (organ systems), physical, sexual, and skeletomuscular.

Additional concerns include the possibility of teratogenicity (genetic mutations) or of reductions in body weight gain. Also of concern is the possibility that, because of differences in developing systems as opposed to mature, adult systems, drug-related adverse events or drug interactions may not be immediately identifiable but rather may be manifested at a later state of growth, development, or maturation.

Women. The risk of drug-related side effects is sometimes gender-dependent. Hormonal differences, including cyclic hormonal variations as well as physiologic differences, may cause women to be at greater risk for side effects than men. The tendency for women both to weigh less and to have a higher percentage of body fat also predisposes them to the possibility of additional side effects related to toxicity. With respect to body fat, a certain amount of drug is often stored in adipose tissue for later release, thereby resulting in an amount of drug present systemically that exceeds the intended therapeutic dose, given the cumulative effect of the administered dose combined with release of previously stored drug. Another concern for women is the possibility of impairment of fertility and the possibility of maternal or fetal risk during pregnancy. Therefore, dosing by body weight is an important consideration in managing a drug's safety margin for women.

Lifestyle: Lifestyle choices can either increase or decrease the likelihood of the incidence of adverse events. Certain lifestyle choices, moreover, are associated with both negative and positive side effects. An example of the latter is caffeine consumption (via chocolate, certain soda drinks, coffee, tea): Positive effects include bronchodilation (an effective asthma treatment), decreased fatigue, and increased alertness; negative effects can include dizziness, impairment of fine motor control, increased excretion of calcium (contributing to osteoporosis), increased respiratory rate, insomnia, and tachycardia.

Negative lifestyle choices include smoking and alcohol or narcotic consumption. The negative side effects associated with smoking include cardiopulmonary adverse events, increased incidence of certain forms of cancer, and increased incidence of complications following breast reconstruction surgery. The negative side effects associated with alcohol or narcotic consumption include hypertension and hepatic adverse events, including an increased risk of acute liver failure resulting from acetaminophen hepatotoxicity.

Positive lifestyle choices include healthy eating habits, optimal weight maintenance, and regular exercise. The positive side effects of these choices may include an overall improvement in general health, a decrease in blood pressure, a decrease in cholesterol levels (LDL and triglycerides), a reduction in heart attack risk, and a reduction in stroke risk.

Beneficial side effects: Although the term "side effects" has an inherently negative connotation, not all side effects are undesirable, unwanted, or deleterious to one's health. In certain instances, a side effect can actually be desirable. In addition to beneficial side effects from positive lifestyle choices, unintended beneficial side effects have been associated with certain drugs. This often results in their off-label (unindicated) use for their efficacy in treating conditions for which they were not originally developed. Examples include aspirin, which in addition to being used as an analgesic has a beneficial side effect as an anticoagulant in helping to prevent heart attacks. Similarly, DMSO (approved for treatment of interstitial cystitis) can improve the efficacy of certain chemotherapy drugs, and tamoxifen (used to treat breast cancer) may be useful in preventing breast cancer and also decreases blood cholesterol levels. It should be noted, however, that these drugs can be associated with negative side effects as well.

Cynthia L. De Vine, B.A.

▶ **For Further Information**

Cukier, Daniel, et al. *Coping with Chemotherapy and Radiation Therapy.* 4th ed. New York: McGraw-Hill, 2004.

Galloway, D. "Treating Patients with Cancer Requires Looking Beyond the Tumor." *OncoLog* 49, nos. 7/8 (July/August, 2004).

Kelvin, Joanne, and Leslie Tyson. *One Hundred Questions and Answers About Cancer Symptoms and Cancer Treatment Side Effects.* Sudbury, Mass.: Jones and Bartlett, 2004.

Physician's Desk Reference, 2008. 62d ed. Montvale, N.J.: Thomson Healthcare, 2007.

▶ Other Resources

American Cancer Center of the University of Pennsylvania
OncoLink
    http://www.oncolink.com/coping/

American Cancer Society
    http://www.cancer.org

See also Anemia; Anxiety; Appetite loss; Chemotherapy; Chronic lymphocytic leukemia (CLL); Cobalt 60 radiation; Depression; Diarrhea; Fatigue; Fever; Infection and sepsis; Nausea and vomiting; Nutrition and cancer prevention; Nutrition and cancer treatment; Weight loss.

▶ Sigmoidoscopy

Category: Procedures
Also known as: Proctosigmoidoscopy

Definition: Sigmoidoscopy is the insertion of a slender, lighted tube (sigmoidoscope) through the anus to examine the lining of the rectum and lower colon. Sigmoidoscopes vary in insertion tube design (such as size, flexibility, and viewing angle), viewing technology (lens, fiber-optic, or electronic), and procedural capabilities (sample, destroy, remove, or treat abnormalities).

Cancers diagnosed: Sigmoid colon cancer, rectal cancer

Why performed: For cancer, sigmoidoscopy may be performed as a screening procedure to detect abnormalities in the rectum and lower colon; as a diagnostic procedure to determine the cause of symptoms, confirm other findings, or plan treatment; or as a follow-up procedure to verify that tissues healed properly after surgery.

Patient preparation: A few days before the procedure, the patient may need to stop certain medications (such as

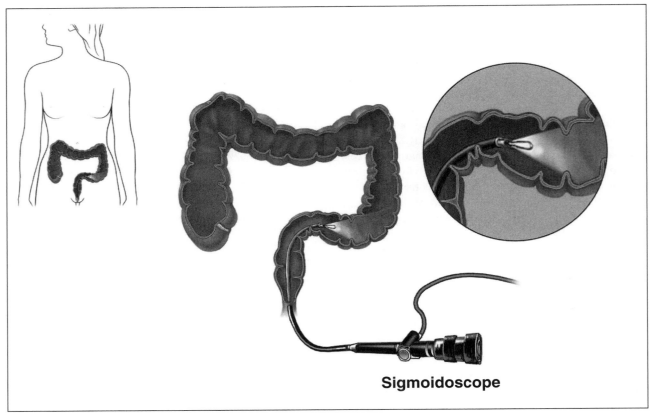

Sigmoidoscope

The lower colon is inspected with a sigmoidoscope. (©Visuals Unlimited/Corbis)

aspirin products and blood thinners). The day of the procedure, the patient cleans his or her rectum and lower colon (such as with an enema).

Steps of the procedure: Sigmoidoscopy is scheduled in a physician's office or other outpatient setting. The patient wears a gown and lies on the side, awake; if needed, sedation or local anesthetic may be given. First, the physician performs a digital rectal exam. The sigmoidoscope (.25 to .5 inch wide, 10 to 26 inches long) is lubricated and carefully inserted through the anus. Puffs of air gently expand the rectum and lower colon as the physician advances the sigmoidoscope, steering around bends until the sigmoidoscope is fully inserted. The physician slowly withdraws the sigmoidoscope, carefully viewing the lining for abnormalities. When an abnormality is found, its location and characteristics are recorded. Depending on the abnormality, it may be sampled (biopsied), destroyed (ablated), removed (excised and retrieved), or otherwise treated. All biopsy samples and excised tissues are taken to the laboratory for histopathologic evaluation.

After the procedure: The patient leaves and resumes normal activities, unless sedation or anesthetic was needed. The patient may feel bloated and have cramps until the extra air passes.

Risks: Sigmoidoscopy is relatively safe, with a small risk for these side effects: perforation, bleeding, infection, irritation, and discharge.

Results: A normal bowel has smooth folds lining the muscular wall, with an even distribution of blood vessels. Abnormalities include inflammation, stricture, vascular changes, anatomic distortions, and abnormal growths, such as mucosal growths, polypoid lesions (polyps), and cancer. Histopathologic evaluation determines whether an abnormal growth is or is not likely to become cancerous and, if the abnormal growth was removed, whether the diseased tissue was completely removed. Additional treatment, follow-up examinations, or both may be recommended.

Patricia Boone, Ph.D.

See also Adenomatous polyps; Anal cancer; Colon polyps; Colorectal cancer; Colorectal cancer screening; Diarrhea; Digital rectal exam (DRE); Endoscopy; Enterostomal therapy; Fecal occult blood test (FOBT); Gastrointestinal complications of cancer treatment; Hemorrhoids; Hereditary polyposis syndromes; Medicare and cancer; Peutz-Jeghers syndrome (PJS); Polypectomy; Polyps; Premalignancies; Primary care physician; Rectal cancer; Screening for cancer.

▶ Silica, crystalline

Category: Carcinogens and suspected carcinogens
RoC status: Reasonably anticipated human carcinogen since 1991; known human carcinogen since 2000
Also known as: Quartz, cristobalite, tridymite, sand

Related cancers: Lung cancer is related to exposure to respirable quartz and cristobalite but not to amorphous silica.

Definition: Respirable crystalline silica, primarily quartz dusts occurring in industrial and occupational settings, is known to be a human carcinogen, based on studies in humans indicating a causal relationship between exposure to respirable crystalline silica and increased lung cancer rates in workers. Respirable crystalline silica was first listed in the *Sixth Report on Carcinogens* (RoC), published in 1991 by the National Toxicology Program of the U.S. Department of Health and Human Services, as "reasonably anticipated to be a human carcinogen" based on evidence of carcinogenicity in experimental animals; however, the listing was revised to "known to be a human carcinogen" in the *Ninth Report on Carcinogens* in 2000.

Exposure route: Inhalation

Where found: Silica sand has been used in the manufacture of glass and ceramics and in foundry castings and has been used as an abrasive in sandpaper and grinding and polishing agents. It is also found in sandblasting materials, in oil and natural gas recovery, in quarries, in water filtration for sewage treatment plants, and in the production of silicon. Cristobalite is a major component of refractory silica bricks. Extremely fine grades of silica sand known as flours may be used in toothpaste, scouring powders, metal polishes, paints, rubber, paper, plastics, wood fillers, cements, road-surfacing materials, and foundry applications. Crystalline silica is also found in tobacco products.

At risk: Quarry and granite workers as well as workers involved in the ceramic, pottery, refractory brick, and diatomaceous earth industries are most at risk.

Etiology and symptoms of associated cancers: Marked and persistent inflammation, specifically inflammatory cell-derived oxidants, may provide a mechanism by which respirable crystalline silica exposure can result in lung cancer.

History: Crystalline silica is composed of silicon and oxygen. The mineral is ubiquitous in both nature and people's daily lives. Scientists have known for decades that prolonged excessive exposure to crystalline silica dust in mining environments can cause silicosis, a lung disease. During the 1980's, studies were conducted that suggested that crystalline silica also was a carcinogen. As a result of these findings, crystalline silica has been regulated under the Occupational Safety and Health Administration's Hazard Communication Standard (HCS).

Debra B. Kessler, M.D., Ph.D.

See also Asbestos; Bronchial adenomas; Carcinogens, known; Carcinogens, reasonably anticipated; Chewing tobacco; Lung cancers; Mesothelioma; Occupational exposures and cancer; Prevention; Tobacco-related cancers.

▶ Simian virus 40

Category: Carcinogens and suspected carcinogens
Also known as: Simian vacuolating virus 40, SV40

Related cancers: Malignant mesothelioma, osteosarcoma, choroid plexus tumors, ependymomas, non-Hodgkin lymphoma

Definition: Simian virus 40 is a polyomavirus of the family Papovaviridae and is found in several species of monkeys.

Exposure routes: The actual route of exposure of simian virus 40 in humans is under investigation. There is speculation that millions of Americans were exposed to the virus between 1955 and 1963 during the mass immunizations with the original Salk (injectable) and Sabin (oral) polio vaccines. However, some people too young to have received the original polio vaccines have tested positive for exposure to the virus. Therefore, other routes of exposure, such as person to person, may be possible.

Where found: As a latent infection in several species of macaque monkeys; also in biomedical research labs to transform human cells or be inoculated into laboratory animals for oncology studies

At risk: People who were vaccinated with the Sabin and Salk polio vaccines between 1955 and 1963; about one hundred army camp men who were inoculated with adenovirus vaccines contaminated with simian virus 40 in the 1950's and 1960's; lab researchers working with the virus

Etiology and symptoms of associated cancers: Carcinogenesis may be induced by inactivation of cellular tumor-suppressor proteins (TP53 and RB1).

History: The virus was discovered in 1960 in the rhesus macaque kidney cells used to amplify the polio virus for the original Salk and Sabin polio vaccines. In 1961, after learning that inoculated simian virus 40 caused cancer in laboratory animals, the U.S. federal government required that new stocks of polio vaccine be free of the virus. Since then, the Salk and Sabin vaccine stocks have been produced using human or African green monkey cell lines extensively screened for viral contaminants.

The National Cancer Institute has reported that forty years of epidemiological studies in the United States and Europe have not shown increased cancer risk in people who may have been exposed to simian virus 40. However, polymerase chain reaction (PCR) testing has revealed traces of simian virus 40 in many malignant mesothelioma tumors and (in one study) 42 percent of non-Hodgkin lymphomas, among others. However, association does not mean causation, and PCR testing techniques for simian virus 40 have not been standardized. Lab contamination could also be a problem. The linkage between simian virus 40 exposure and cancer in humans is still being actively investigated.

Lisa J. Shientag, V.M.D.

See also Adenoviruses; Carcinogens, known; Carcinogens, reasonably anticipated; Ependymomas; Hodgkin disease; Human T-cell leukemia virus (HTLV); Lymphomas; Medical oncology; Mesothelioma; Non-Hodgkin lymphoma; Oncogenes; *RB1* gene; TP53 protein; Tumor-suppressor genes.

▶ Singlehood and cancer

Category: Social and personal issues

Definition: The development and outcome of all kinds of cancer are influenced by a variety of risk factors, such as ethnicity, genetic disposition, preventive health behavior, and socioeconomic or sociodemographic factors. The impact of singlehood as a sociodemographic factor on cancer is rather complex but seems to show a trend toward a statistically unsalutary outcome of this chronic disease.

Description of the population: Singlehood defines the marital status of individuals who never married or are separated, divorced, or widowed.

Incidence, death, and survival statistics: The impact of singlehood on the incidence, death, or survival of cancer patients is very complex, because the studies and surveys conducted on this topic are often differently designed, investigating only one specific kind and stage of cancer in a specific population group. Therefore, the survival or death percentages in the individual studies cannot be generalized for all cancers and population groups.

However, studies suggest that there may be a trend toward a generally less beneficial impact of singlehood on cancer survival or mortality, as well as on the quality of life of cancer patients. Studies also suggest that the evolution of cancer and therefore cancer incidence may not be affected by marital status per se; however, several surveys indicate that single individuals may be less willing to participate in specific screening programs, such as breast, prostate, or colorectal screenings, to help diagnose and subsequently remove the cancer at an earlier stage or before it becomes inoperable.

The most attractive model of the generally more salutary effect of marriage on cancer survival and quality of life relies on social support, such as access to appropriate health care, and mood. Some investigators have found an interaction between mood and the body's immune function, which may affect cancer survival.

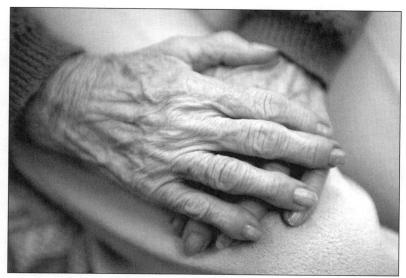

Some studies suggest a link between a person's marital status, and cancer mortality and quality of life after diagnosis. (PhotoDisc)

Risk statistics: Only a few analytical studies have been conducted to assess the direct relationship between singlehood (or marital status in general) and the etiology of cancer. There is one analysis from an Italian databank containing data (collected between 1983 and 2001) from almost 18,000 incident cancer cases, assessing the relationship between marital status and the development of cancer at different sites such as oral cavity and pharynx, esophagus, stomach, colon, rectum, liver, gallbladder, pancreas, larynx, breast, endometrium, ovary, prostate, bladder, kidney, and thyroid, as well as Hodgkin disease, multiple myelomas, and sarcomas. The analysis, published in 2004, indicated that never-married individuals, but not divorced or widowed individuals, were at a significantly increased risk of oral cavity and pharyngeal cancers but at a reduced risk of cancer of the colon, liver, bladder, kidney, and thyroid. Overall, the study suggested that marital status is not materially associated with cancer risk.

However, because there is the not uncommon belief that cancer may be associated with psychological distress that may, for example, arise from major life events such as becoming a widow or widower, many studies have focused on the relationship between psychological factors and cancer risk. In 2002, the Danish Cancer Society published the results of a review of several prospective and retrospective studies about the relationship between major life events, depression, personality factors, and the risk of cancer. The outcome failed to support the hypothesis that psychological factors are risk factors of cancer. These results are in agreement with numerous other studies that failed to find an association between depression and cancer deaths.

Other studies and surveys have investigated the relationship between several sociodemographic factors, such as marital status, and preventive health behaviors, for example, participating in screening programs to detect cancer at early stages. In 2004, the U.S. Centers of Disease Control and Prevention (CDC) published data from the 1999 Behavioral Risk Factor Surveillance System. These data showed that not having a mammogram within the past two years to detect breast cancer in women over the age of forty was associated with, among other factors, not being currently married. Other studies support this finding that being single may be associated with fewer positive intentions and lower attendance rates at screening programs.

Perspective and prospects: Studies and surveys have shown that marital status, such as singlehood, may play a role in cancer mortality, the quality of life after cancer diagnosis, and the overall adjustment to the disease, although it does not directly affect the evolution of human cancer. Therefore, health care professionals should take sociodemographic characteristics into consideration in addition to ordinary clinical health care when treating cancer patients, such as providing social and psychological support, as needed, to improve quality of life or adjustment to the disease. They should also be more aware of properly identifying those having trouble coping with cancer. Future studies should particularly pay attention to determining whether an increased risk from cancer may be introduced by the very medications used to treat depression or other psychological distress that may arise from specific sociodemographic factors, such as being single through death or divorce.

Silke Haidekker, Ph.D.

▶ **For Further Information**

Coughlin, S. S., et al. "Nonadherence to Breast and Cervical Cancer Screening: What Are the Linkages to Chronic Disease Risk?" *Preventing Chronic Disease* 1, no. 1 (January, 2004): A04.

Kravdal, O. "The Impact of Marital Status on Cancer Survival." *Social Science and Medicine* 52, no. 3 (February, 2001): 357-368.

Randi, Giorgia, et al. "Marital Status and Cancer Risk in Italy." *Preventive Medicine* 38, no. 5 (May, 2004): 523-528.

▶ **Other Resources**

American Cancer Society
The Single Woman and Cancer
    http://www.cancer.org/docroot/MIT/content/
    MIT_7_2X_The_Single_Woman_and_Cancer
    .asp?sitearea=MIT

Breastcancer.org
Single Women: Finding Your Way
    http://www.breastcancer.org/tips/intimacy/single.jsp

See also Aging and cancer; Depression; Ethnicity and cancer; Personality and cancer; Psychosocial aspects of cancer; Relationships; Statistics of cancer; Stress management.

▶ Sjögren syndrome

Category: Diseases, symptoms, and conditions
Also known as: Sicca syndrome, Sjögren disease, Sjögren's syndrome, SS

Related conditions: Lymphoma, rheumatoid arthritis, scleroderma, systemic lupus erythematosus (SLE)

Definition: Named after Swedish ophthalmologist Henrik Sjögren, Sjögren syndrome is a chronic disorder in which the body's immune system attacks and destroys the glands that make lubricating fluids, such as tears and saliva. It is commonly associated with inflammatory disorders, such

as rheumatoid arthritis and systemic lupus erythematosus. Patients with this syndrome have been found to have a higher incidence of lymphoma than the general population.

Risk factors: Risk factors for Sjögren syndrome include a history of rheumatic disease, gender, age, and a family history of the disease.

Etiology and the disease process: The etiology of Sjögren syndrome is unknown. Given the prevalence of this disorder among women, hormones are suspected to play a role. Genetic, viral, and neuroendocrine causes have also been investigated. In primary Sjögren syndrome (50 percent of cases), the disorder occurs alone. In the secondary form of the syndrome, it is accompanied by an underlying autoimmune connective tissue disorder, such as rheumatoid arthritis, polymyositis, scleroderma, or systemic lupus erythematosus.

Incidence: Although Sjögren syndrome occurs in both sexes and all age groups, 90 percent of patients are women, and the average age of onset is the late forties. As many as 4 million people in the United States are affected. Sjögren syndrome is one of the most prevalent autoimmune disorders but is commonly misdiagnosed or underdiagnosed because of its generalized symptoms. The syndrome is rare in children.

Symptoms: The hallmark symptoms of Sjögren syndrome are dry mouth (xerostomia) and dry eyes (keratoconjunctivitis sicca, or KCS). Other oral symptoms include a sore, cracked tongue and lips; difficulty chewing, speaking, or swallowing; salivary gland enlargement; and tooth decay. Other eye-related symptoms include a gritty sensation in the eyes (especially in the morning); itching, burning, or redness of the eyes; intolerance to light (photosensitivity); and an inability to tear.

Other symptoms include fever; fatigue; muscle and joint pain; dry, itchy skin; digestive problems; and vaginal dryness. These symptoms may be associated with involvement of other organs (such as the lungs, kidneys, intestines, stomach, and blood vessels) or with lymphoma.

In women, symptom onset commonly coincides with the onset of menopause.

Screening and diagnosis: Because many symptoms of Sjögren syndrome are generalized and symptoms may be treated individually, Sjögren commonly goes undiagnosed or misdiagnosed. The average time from onset of symptoms to diagnosis is more than six years. Diagnosis is commonly made when the complex syndrome of symptoms has been noted.

No single test confirms the diagnosis. Diagnostic testing includes blood tests for the presence of certain antibodies, such as rheumatoid factor, antinuclear antibodies (ANAs), and the extractable nuclear antigen antibodies SSA and SSB. Differing antinuclear antibody profiles help to distinguish between the primary and secondary forms of Sjögren syndrome.

Nonspecific laboratory abnormalities commonly noted in Sjögren syndrome include increased erythrocyte sedimentation rate, mild anemia, elevated immunoglobulin levels, and a low albumin level.

Ophthalmologic tests include a Schirmer test to measure the production of tears and a Rose-Bengal staining test to detect corneal inflammation and dryness on the surface of the eye.

Dental tests include salivary flow rates to determine the presence of decreased saliva production, biopsy of the lip or salivary gland, and salivary scintigraphy.

Treatment and therapy: Sjögren syndrome has no known cure. Treatment is lifelong and generally focuses on controlling and relieving symptoms (by increasing lubrication and moisturization of affected tissues), limiting organ involvement, and helping improve quality of life. Moisture replacement therapies, such as artificial tears, are used to ease dry eye symptoms. Chronic dry eye may be treated with prescription cyclosporin (Restasis) or punctal occlusion, in which the tear-draining ducts of the eyes are plugged to help maintain moisture. Prescription drugs (cevimeline, pilocarpine) are also used to stimulate salivary flow. For many patients, fluid intake is necessary with and between meals because of dry mouth. Patients should avoid medications that are known to dry secretions, including antihistamines and decongestants.

Other treatments vary depending on the involved organ, severity of symptoms, and presence of any coexisting autoimmune disorders. Medications such as nonsteroidal anti-inflammatory drugs and corticosteroids (such as prednisone) may be prescribed to reduce autoimmune effects and treat musculoskeletal symptoms. Hydroxychloroquine, an antimalarial drug, may be used to treat fatigue and joint pain associated with primary Sjögren syndrome or to decrease antibody levels or sedimentation rate. Cytotoxic agents should be used cautiously because they can increase the risk of lymphoma.

Prognosis, prevention, and outcomes: Prognosis varies with the type and severity of disease, although Sjögren syndrome generally is not fatal if diagnosed and treated early. Some people experience only very mild symptoms; others suffer from periods of severe disease. Symptoms can remain stable, go into remission, or worsen over the course of the disease. Individuals with secondary Sjögren syndrome typically have milder disease than those with primary Sjögren syndrome. Debilitating joint pain and fatigue can affect quality of life. Lymphoma develops in approximately 6 percent of people with Sjögren syndrome who have systemic disease.

Although Sjögren syndrome has no known preventive measures, early diagnosis and treatment are extremely important for preventing major organ damage and other complications.

Jaime Stockslager Buss, M.S.P.H., ELS

▶ **For Further Information**

Fremes, R., and N. Carteron. *A Body Out of Balance: Understanding and Treating Sjögren's Syndrome.* New York: Avery, 2003.

Rumpf, T. P., and K. M. Hammitt. *The Sjögren's Syndrome Survival Guide.* Oakland, Calif.: New Harbinger, 2003.

Smedby, K., et al. "Autoimmune and Chronic Inflammatory Disorders and Risk of Non-Hodgkin Lymphoma by Subtype." *Journal of the National Cancer Institute* 98 (2006): 51-60.

Wallace, D. J., ed. *The New Sjögren's Syndrome Handbook.* 3d ed. New York: Oxford University Press, 2004.

Zintzaras, E., M. Voulgarelis, and H. M. Moutsopoulos. "The Risk of Lymphoma Development in Autoimmune Diseases: A Meta-Analysis." *Archives of Internal Medicine* 165 (2005): 2337-2344.

▶ **Other Resources**

National Institute of Neurological Disorders and Stroke
Sjögren's Syndrome Information Page
http://www.ninds.nih.gov/disorders/sjogrens/sjogrens.htm

Sjögren's Syndrome Foundation
http://www.sjogrens.org

See also Dry mouth; Family history and risk assessment; Lymphomas; Non-Hodgkin lymphoma; Primary central nervous system lymphomas; Salivary gland cancer.

▶ Skin cancers

Category: Diseases, symptoms, and conditions
Also known as: Basal cell carcinomas, squamous cell carcinomas, melanomas

Related conditions: Actinic keratosis, Bowen disease

Definition: Skin cancers are the result of uncontrolled mitosis (cell division) in the epidermal cells of the skin. The three most common skin cancers are basal cell carcinomas (BCCs), squamous cell carcinomas (SCCs), and melanomas. Each is named for the cell type (basal cell, squamous cell, or melanocyte) that gives rise to the cluster of cells dividing uncontrollably. This cluster of cells is a skin cancer.

Risk factors: Exposure to sunlight and other sources of ultraviolet (UV) radiation is the overwhelmingly predominant risk factor in all the common skin cancers. Ozone in the stratosphere absorbs UV radiation so that it does not reach the earth, so the destruction and thinning of the stratospheric ozone layer constitute a secondary risk factor.

Etiology and the disease process: The epidermis, the outermost layer of the skin, sits on a deeper layer, the dermis. Cells in the bottom layer of the epidermis, called the basal cell layer, divide to form keratinocytes, or squamous cells, which move to the surface of the skin to form a protective cover for the organism. As the keratinocytes move to the surface, they become packed with the protective protein keratin, take on variable amounts of the pigment melanin, flatten, attach firmly to neighboring keratinocytes, and die. These cells form a layer of dead, protective cells that are continually being sloughed off and must be replaced by new keratinocytes derived from mitosis in cells of the basal cell layer. In the basal cell carcinomas, one of the cells from the basal cell layer escapes the cellular control mechanisms and divides repeatedly to form a mass of cells no longer coordinated with the rest of the organism. In the squamous cell carcinomas it is one of the keratinocytes (squamous cells) in which control of cell division is lost. The basal cell layer also contains cells called melanocytes that produce the melanin that gives skin its color. Normally, the melanin is passed from the melanocytes to the keratinocytes as the latter move to the surface of the

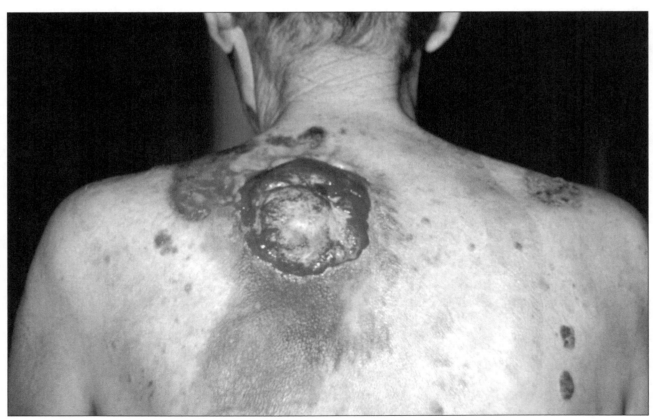

A metastatic basal cell epithelioma on a person's back. (©Lester V. Bergman/Corbis)

epidermis. Control of a melanocyte's mitosis may also be lost, resulting in a melanoma.

All the skin cancers are most commonly triggered by UV radiation from the sun or some other source such as a tanning lamp. The UV light damages deoxyribonucleic acid (DNA), the material that forms the cell's genes. As a result, the damaged gene no longer performs its function. If that function was to control mitosis, the organism may lose control over that cell's division process. The cell divides, forming a mass of cells growing out of control, a tumor.

The tumor itself is minimally harmful, though it may be unsightly. However, if the cancerous cells move into the lymphatic and circulatory systems, they may be carried to other sites in the body, where they may lodge and produce other tumors. This process of spreading the cancer throughout the body is called metastasis and, untreated, will normally end in death. The skin carcinomas do not normally metastasize, but melanomas often do.

Incidence: Skin cancers are the most common cancers in the United States, with more than 1 million cases diagnosed annually. Basal cell carcinoma makes up about 75 percent of skin cancer cases, squamous cell carcinoma about 20 percent, and melanoma only 3 percent. The remaining 2 percent are produced by other, far less common, types of skin cancer. Skin cancer is more frequent in men than in women, in light-complexioned people than in dark-skinned ones, in people who spend a lot of time outdoors than those who spend more time indoors, and in older people than in younger ones.

Symptoms: Most skin cancer lesions are on the skin of the arms, face, and legs, the body parts most often exposed to the sun. The lesions differ depending on the cells involved. Basal cell and squamous cell carcinomas often begin as red or other colored spots on the skin. Unlike other skin lesions, the spots do not heal or, if they do go away, they reappear. These spots are often rough to the touch. Melanomas are often brown, appearing much like a mole. If the molelike spot is round and smooth edged, contrasts sharply with the surrounding skin, and does not change, it is probably a harmless mole. If it is asymmetric and rough-edged, fades into the surrounding skin, and grows in size, it is probably a melanoma.

Screening and diagnosis: Individuals can screen themselves by periodically checking their skin for indications of these cancers and for precursors of skin cancer. Actinic

---

Skin Cancer Prevention Tips from the Skin Cancer Foundation

- Avoid sunburns.
- Do not try to get a tan, and stay out of tanning parlors.
- Head for shade, especially between 10 A.M. and 4 P.M.
- Use a sunscreen with a sun protection factor (SPF) of 15 or greater.
- Use a sunscreen that blocks UVA and UVB rays.
- Thirty minutes before going out, apply 1 ounce of sunscreen to all exposed areas. Reapply every two hours or more often if swimming or sweating.
- Remember to apply sunscreen to commonly overlooked areas such as ears, lips, around the eyes, neck, hands, feet, and scalp (especially if hair is thinning).
- Wear protective clothing, including long-sleeved shirts and long pants in darker colors.
- Wear UV-blocking sunglasses and a broad-brimmed hat.
- Keep newborns out of the sun.
- Use sunscreen on babies the age of six months and up.

---

keratosis and Bowen disease are two of the most common precursors of skin cancer. Both begin as colored or rough spots or bumps on the skin that do not respond to treatment with ointments. They should be watched carefully, as should moles. If any of these skin abnormalities change in size, shape, or color, they should be shown to a dermatologist.

Regular examination by a dermatologist is one way to screen for potential skin cancers. If upon examination, skin cancer is suspected, a biopsy will probably be the next step. The dermatologist will cut out all or part of the suspect skin and send it to a laboratory for a microscopic examination of the cells in the sample. Four of the most common types of biopsy are the shave biopsy, in which a thin layer of the troublesome skin is shaved off and submitted to the laboratory; the punch biopsy, in which a small cylinder samples the lesion through its entirety; the incision biopsy, in which a part of the suspicious patch of skin is cut out; and the excision biopsy, in which the entire patch of troublesome skin is removed.

Biopsies of nearby lymph nodes are carried out if the cancer is thought to have spread beyond the lesion itself. Fine needle biopsy of a lymph node consists of inserting a very slender needle into a lymph node adjacent to the lesion and drawing some cells from the lymph node into the needle for examination. A second type of lymph node biopsy removes an entire lymph node for examination. If microscopic examination of the cells submitted in the biopsy reveals that some of the cells are cancer cells, further diagnosis is often combined with treatment.

Based on the observation of one or more dermatologists, on the results of the biopsy, and on any other information available, the cancer is staged. Staging determines and reports how far the cancer has spread. Basal cell and squamous cell carcinomas are often not staged because they spread so infrequently, although squamous cell carcinoma spreads and is staged more frequently than basal cell carcinoma. When these two types of skin cancers are staged, the system used is similar to the one for melanomas.

The staging systems used for melanomas are based on the size of the melanoma (how far it has spread laterally in the skin), its depth into the skin (a measure of spread downward), and whether it has spread into the lymph or elsewhere beyond the skin. To give the general idea of such a staging system, here is a simplified version.

• Stage 0: Only the top layer of the skin is involved (for all subsequent stages, deeper skin layers are involved).
• Stage I: The lesion is less than 2 millimeters (mm) thick (or deep into the skin).
• Stage II: The lesion is more than 2 mm thick (deep).
• Stage III: The cancer has spread into the lymph, cartilage, muscle, or bone nearby.
• Stage IV: The cancer has spread through the blood and lymph to distant sites in the body.

Treatment and therapy: Surgery is usually the treatment of choice for skin cancer or for its precursors. Cryosurgery, freezing the skin with liquid nitrogen, is often used to remove precancers such as actinic keratoses. Excision biopsy itself is a minor surgery and may be designed to remove the entire cancerous lesion. If it fails to do so, or if the biopsy was a scrape, punch, or incision biopsy, a more extensive surgery may attempt removal of the entire lesion. The excised tissue is examined to see whether all the cancer cells were removed. Lymph nodes in the affected area are examined and removed if their invasion is suspected.

If the surgery is extensive, a skin graft may be required to cover the wound. The skin is taken from another part of the patient's body, usually some part that is normally covered by clothing. Often, the excision to remove the cancer is small enough to be covered by stretching skin in the area of the surgery and no graft is needed. This is a good argument for careful screening to catch the cancer early.

A treatment system called curettage and electrodesiccation combines cutting out the cancerous skin with an instrument called a curette, a small surgical device with a handle attached to a sharpened spoon or ring. The size used is determined by the size of the skin lesion. Curettage is followed by insertion of electrical probes and application of electrical stimuli to the area to kill cancer cells left behind. This is the electrodesiccation part of the process.

Mohs surgery consists of a series of scrapes from the diseased area. Each layer scraped off is tested for cancer cells. The scraping continues until no cancer cells are found in the last layer scraped, an indication that the outermost cancer cells in the lesion were removed by the previous scrape.

As an alternative to surgery, chemicals may be applied to the lesion to destroy it. Often surgery is followed by a chemical application to kill any cancer cells missed by the surgery. Chemotherapy may be topical, with the chemical applied to the skin lesion, or systemic, with the chemical taken by mouth.

Radiation is used to kill cancer cells and, in skin cancers that have not metastasized, can be applied directly to the cancerous spot. However, radiation is capable of causing cancer in healthy cells, as high-energy radiation (UV radiation) is the primary cause of skin cancers. Therefore, the side effects of radiation treatment may include problems, even cancers, later in life.

Prognosis, prevention, and outcomes: Caught early, skin cancers are almost always curable, so good screening practices are essential defenses against the diseases. Minimizing exposure to sunlight and other sources of UV light (tanning salons) is an excellent preventive measure. With these simple measures applied consistently, skin cancers need not be a scourge. However, they are the most common cancers contracted by the people of the United States today. This may be because when skin cancer patients received the damaging sun exposure early in their lives, the preventive measures were not known or practiced. As this knowledge has become widespread, skin cancers may decline in the future.

Protecting the stratospheric ozone layer, which absorbs UV radiation before it reaches the earth, would also help to minimize the occurrence of skin cancers. Such global action requires international cooperation and may not be as important as individuals' efforts to protect themselves. Nonetheless, it would be an important contribution to the control of skin cancers.

Carl W. Hoagstrom, Ph.D.

▶ **For Further Information**
Colver, Graham. *Skin Cancer: A Practical Guide to Management.* London: Martin Dunitz, 2002.
Hill, David, J. Mark Elwood, and Dallas R. English, eds. *Prevention of Skin Cancer.* Boston: Kluwer Academic, 2004.
McClay, Edward F., Mary-Eileen T. McClay, and Jodie

Smith. *One Hundred Questions and Answers About Melanoma and Other Skin Cancers.* Sudbury, Mass.: Jones and Bartlett, 2004.

Rigel, Darrell S., et al., eds. *Cancer of the Skin.* Philadelphia: Elsevier, 2005.

▶ Other Resources

American Cancer Society
http://www.cancer.org

MedlinePlus
Skin Cancer
http://www.nlm.nih.gov/medlineplus/skincancer.html

Skin Cancer Foundation
http://www.skincancer.org

See also Basal cell carcinomas; Bowen disease; Carcinomas; Core needle biopsy; Dermatofibrosarcoma protuberans (DFSP); Dermatology oncology; Itching; Keratosis; Melanomas; Merkel cell carcinomas (MCC); Metastasis; Moles; Needle biopsies; Squamous cell carcinomas; Sunscreens.

▶ Small intestine cancer

Category: Diseases, symptoms, and conditions

Also known as: Small bowel cancer, small bowel neoplasm, small intestine adenocarcinoma

Related conditions: Familial adenomatous polyposis

Definition: Small intestine cancer is a primary cancer that arises in the small intestine (small bowel), the part of the digestive system that connects the stomach and the colon.

Risk factors: Small intestine cancer is between fifteen and one hundred times more likely to occur in individuals who have Crohn disease or celiac disease. Individuals who have the genetic conditions familiar adenomatous polyposis (FAP), nonpolyposis colorectal cancer, and Peutz-Jeghers syndrome also have a higher risk of developing small intestine cancer. Tobacco and alcohol use and a diet heavy in animal fats have been found to increase small intestine cancer in some, but not all, studies.

Etiology and the disease process: There are five kinds of small intestine cancer: adenocarcinoma, sarcoma, car-

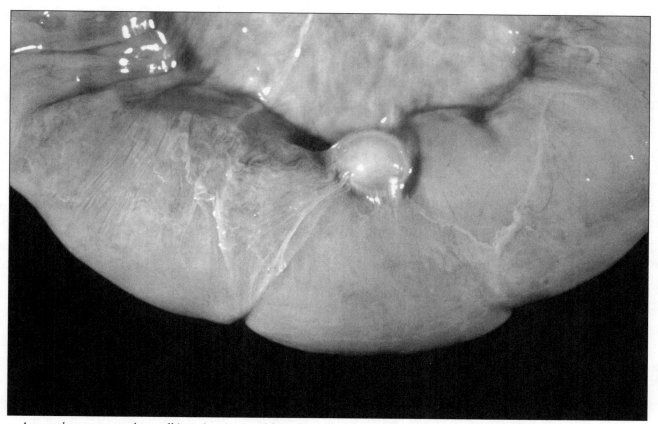

A secondary tumor on the small intestine; it spread from the primary site on the sigmoid colon. (CNRI/Photo Researchers, Inc.)

Relative Survival Rates for Small Intestine Cancer, 1988-2001

Cancer Type	Survival Rates (%)					
	1-Year	*2-Year*	*3-Year*	*5-Year*	*8-Year*	*10-Year*
All types, excluding carcinoids	55.1	37.3	32.6	27.5	24.8	24.3
Carcinoids	89.9	87.5	84.8	76.5	67.1	61.5

Source: Data from L. A. G. Ries et al., eds., *Cancer Survival Among Adults: U.S. SEER Program, 1988-2001—Patient and Tumor Characteristics*, NIH Pub. No. 07-6215 (Bethesda, Md.: National Cancer Institute, 2007)

cinoid tumors, gastrointestinal stromal tumors (GIST), and lymphoma. These cancers arise from different cell types. Adenocarcinoma is the most common type of small intestine cancer, making up about half of all diagnosed cases.

The development of small intestine cancer is thought to be similar to the development of colorectal cancer. Like colorectal cancer, it begins as a benign (noncancerous) polyp (growth) on the wall of the intestine. Adenocarcinoma, for example, develops from glandular, fluid-secreting cells. Over time, changes occur in the cells in the polyp that cause it to become cancerous. Most small intestine cancer develops in the duodenum, which is the part of the small intestine closest to the stomach. In time the polyps may grow to block the intestine.

Incidence: Small intestine cancer is rare. It accounts for only 1 to 2 percent of all cancers of the gastrointestinal system. The American Cancer Society estimates that in 2006 about 6,200 new cases were diagnosed in the United States and that about 1,100 people died from the disease. This cancer is slightly more common in men than in women and in blacks than in whites. The average age at diagnosis is sixty. Internationally, small intestine cancer is more common in the United States and Western Europe and less common in Asia.

Symptoms: In its early stages, small intestine cancer causes few signs. In later stages, possible signs include unexplained weight loss, abdominal cramps or pain, a lump in the abdomen, or blood in the stool. These symptoms are general and may be caused by many other diseases and conditions.

Screening and diagnosis: Because of the rarity of small intestine cancer, routine screening is not done. Because symptoms are general, diagnosis requires an extensive se-

ries of tests. These include a physical examination, blood work, liver function tests, and a fecal occult blood test to test for blood in the stool. Imaging studies may include abdominal X rays, an upper gastrointestinal endoscopy, a barium enema and lower gastrointestinal X rays, and a computed tomography (CT) scan. Definitive diagnosis comes from a biopsy of polyps in the intestine.

To stage the cancer, a laparotomy may be performed. In this surgical procedure, the abdomen is opened and samples are taken to determine how far the cancer has spread. Likewise, a lymph node biopsy may also be done to determine how far the cancer has spread.

Staging is done based on the degree of invasiveness of the tumor, how far the cancer has spread, and whether it can be completely removed with surgery:
- Stage I: The tumor is localized and has invaded the intestinal wall only to a limited degree.
- Stage II: The cancer has grown through the intestinal wall but has not spread to the surrounding lymph nodes.
- Stage III: The cancer has spread to the lymph nodes.
- Stage IV: The tumor has spread to distant organs such as the lung or liver.

Treatment and therapy: The preferred treatment for all small intestine cancer is surgical removal of the diseased portion of the bowel. This is usually followed by chemotherapy, radiation therapy, or both. When the cancer cannot be removed, palliative care includes surgery to bypass any portions of the small bowel that are blocked by polyp growth.

Prognosis, prevention, and outcomes: Small intestine cancer is difficult to treat successfully because it is rarely diagnosed at an early stage. The American Cancer Society estimates the five-year survival rate for people with small intestine cancers diagnosed in each stage as 65 percent for Stage I, 48 percent for Stage II, 30 percent for Stage III, and 9 percent for Stage IV.

Martiscia Davidson, A.M.

▶ **For Further Information**

Icon Health. *The Official Patient's Sourcebook on Small Intestine Cancer: Directory for the Internet Age.* San Diego, Calif.: Author, 2004.

Keane, Maureen, and Daniella Chace. *What to Eat If You Have Cancer.* 2d ed. New York: McGraw-Hill, 2007.

Zeh, H. "Cancer of the Small Intestine." In *Cancer: Principles and Practice of Oncology*, edited by Vincent T. DeVita, Jr., Samuel Hellman, and Steven A. Rosenberg. 7th ed. Philadelphia: Lippincott Williams & Wilkins, 2005.

▶ **Other Resources**

American Cancer Society
Detailed Guide: Small Intestine Cancer
http://www.cancer.org/docroot/CRI/
CRI_2_3x.asp?dt=86

National Cancer Institute
Small Intestine Cancer Treatment
http://www.cancer.gov/cancertopics/pdq/treatment/
smallintestine/patient

See also Barium swallow; Bile duct cancer; Crohn disease; Duodenal carcinomas; Enteritis; Esophagectomy; Fiber; Gastrointestinal cancers; Hereditary polyposis syndromes; Leiomyosarcomas; Ovarian epithelial cancer; Upper gastrointestinal (GI) endoscopy; Zollinger-Ellison syndrome

▶ **Smoking cessation**

Category: Lifestyle and prevention

Definition: Smoking cessation is the stopping of the smoking of cigarettes, cigars, or pipes. Most smokers are physically addicted to nicotine and psychologically addicted to the habit.

The depth of the problem: About 21 percent of adults in the United States (45.1 million people) are smokers. In 2006, the number of cigarettes consumed totaled 371 billion. The use of tobacco products varies with gender, age, and ethnic background. According to the Centers for Disease Control, in 2006 more men smoked (23.9 percent) than women (18.0 percent). Smoking was more common among adults between the ages of eighteen and forty-four (23.7 percent) and forty-five to sixty-four (21.8 percent) than among those age sixty-five and older (10.2 percent). Overall smoking rates are highest among American Indians and Alaska Natives (32 percent), non-Hispanic whites (21.9 percent), and those identifying as black (23 percent).

Each year, an estimated 438,000 people in the United States die prematurely from smoking or exposure to secondhand smoke, and another 8.6 million suffer from serious smoking-related illnesses, including cancer, heart disease, and lung disease. Cancer was among the first diseases causally linked to smoking, and cigarette smoking is the primary cause of cancer mortality in the United States (responsible for at least 30 percent of all cancer deaths). Smoking is the leading risk factor for lung cancer.

Smoking cessation is a difficult challenge that involves overcoming both physical and psychological dependence. Most smokers are addicted to nicotine, a psychoactive drug naturally found in tobacco products that produces dependence and makes quitting difficult. In addition, smoking becomes a routine or habit that can be hard to break, especially when it is as a coping mechanism for stress or anxiety. Cessation is difficult and may require multiple attempts. Users commonly relapse because of withdrawal symptoms and mental dependence. Cigarette cravings are usually the worst during the first two to three days of smoking cessation.

Quit and relapse rates: An estimated 46.5 million American adults are former smokers, and more than half of all living adults who ever smoked have quit. In addition, approximately 70 percent of current U.S. adult smokers and 62 percent of high school age smokers report that they

---

How to Quit Smoking

Get ready.
- Set a date to quit smoking.
- Get rid of all tobacco products, ashtrays, and lighters at home, in your car, and at work.
- Do not let people smoke around you.

Get medicine.
- Talk to a doctor or pharmacist.
- Choose nonprescription aids such as nicotine gum, patches, or lozenges.
- Or choose prescription aids such as a nicotine inhaler or nasal spray, buproprion hydrochloride, or varenicline tartrate.

Get help.
- Tell your friends and family that you are quitting and enlist their support.
- Ask a health care provider, such as a doctor or nurse, for help.
- Get help from your state's quitline or other supportive group.

Stay quit.
- If you start smoking again, set a new quit date.
- Avoid alcohol and smokers.
- Eat a balanced, healthful diet, and exercise.
- Stay positive that you can quit.

Sources: Agency for Healthcare Research and Quality; U.S. Department of Health and Human Services

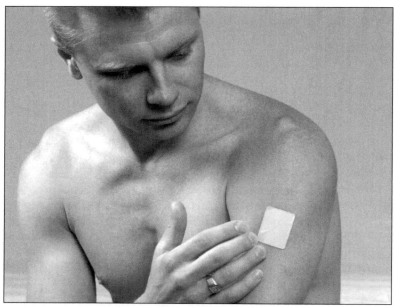

A nicotine patch is one way to stop smoking and lessen the risk of developing cancer. (Digital Stock)

In the long term, the health benefits of smoking cessation can be substantial. Smoking cessation greatly reduces the risk of premature death by reducing the risk of smoking-related diseases. Even former smokers live longer than those who continue to smoke. Smoking cessation lowers the risk of developing and dying from lung cancer, other types of cancer, and other diseases (such as heart disease, stroke, and emphysema). The risk of developing cancer declines with the number of years of smoking cessation. For example, about ten years after quitting, a former smoker's risk of dying from lung cancer is 30 to 50 percent less than the risk faced by those who continue to smoke. Additional benefits include an improved sense of taste and smell and increased lung funtion. Women who stop smoking before or during pregnancy reduce their risk of having miscarriages and having babies that are small or have low birth weights.

Although cessation is beneficial at all ages, the earlier a person stops smoking, the greater the health benefits.

would like to quit. In 2005, an estimated 42.5 percent of adult smokers and 54.6 percent of high school students had attempted to quit smoking during the preceding twelve months.

However, not all smokers are successful in their attempts to stop smoking, and many try several times before they are able to quit. Less than 10 percent of smokers who attempt to quit on their own have long-term success. The majority of smokers cite symptoms of withdrawal and cravings as the main reasons for smoking relapse. Most relapses occur within three months of quitting. Smoking-cessation aids can increase the chances of success.

Although research findings conflict, some studies suggest that women are less successful than men in their attempts to quit smoking. Success in quitting seems to increase with higher levels of education. Motivation to quit smoking also increases success rates.

Health benefits of cessation: Smoking cessation leads to almost immediate health benefits for people with and without smoking-related diseases. For example, almost immediately after quitting, people experience improved circulation, decreased blood pressure and pulse rates, and increased body temperature in the hands and feet. In addition, cessation also leads to an almost immediate improvement in such respiratory symptoms as coughing, wheezing, and shortness of breath. Carbon monoxide and nicotine levels in the body rapidly decrease.

Smoking cessation methods: Smoking cessation is a two-step process that includes overcoming the physical dependence on nicotine and breaking the smoking habit. Methods used to increase smoking cessation rates include medications, counseling, support groups, behavioral therapies, and alternative therapies such as hypnotism and acupuncture.

Medications that have proven to be effective in treating tobacco dependence include nicotine replacement therapies (NRTs) and non-nicotine treatments, such as bupropion hydrochloride (Zyban) and varenicline tartrate (Chantrix). NRTs are designed to provide users with small amounts of nicotine that help reduce the craving for cigarettes and relieve the withdrawal symptoms associated with smoking cessation, making it easier to quit. Some are available over the counter without a doctor's prescription. Although they contain some nicotine, NRTs are not as bad as smoking because they do not contain the toxins and carcinogens found in tobacco products. Types of NRTs include gums, inhalers, nasal sprays, lozenges, and patches. Although these treatments have been shown to be safe and effective when used as directed, smokers should talk with their health care providers before beginning any smoking cessation medication.

Nicotine gum (such as Nicorette) was the first pharmacologic smoking cessation aid approved by the U.S. Food and Drug Association (FDA). First approved in 1984, it is available over the counter. The recommended treatment is typically ten to fifteen pieces of gum per day for twelve weeks.

Available only by prescription, the nicotine inhaler (Nicotrol) is a plastic cylinder that looks like a cigarette and has a cartridge that delivers nicotine. Each cartridge delivers up to four hundred puffs. The maximum recommended dosage is sixteen cartridges a day for up to twelve weeks. Side effects include mouth and throat irritation.

Nicotine nasal sprays are dispensed from pumps similar to over-the-counter decongestant sprays. The nicotine is rapidly absorbed through the nasal membranes and quickly reaches the bloodstream. A usual dose is two sprays, one in each nostril. The maximum recommended dosage is forty total doses per day. Side effects include nose and throat irritation.

Nicotine patches (such as Nicoderm) release a constant amount of nicotine into the body throughout the day. Most patches are replaced daily, and treatment periods typically range from six to ten weeks. They come in different shapes and sizes and are available over the counter or by prescription. Side effects of nicotine patches include skin irritation, dizziness, headache, and nausea and vomiting.

In 2002, the first and only over-the-counter nicotine lozenge was introduced to the market. It comes in the form of a hard candy and slowly releases nicotine as it dissolves in the mouth. Treatment typically consists of up to twenty lozenges per day for twelve weeks. The most common side effects are sore teeth and gums, indigestion, and throat irritation.

Available only by prescription, bupropion hydrochloride (Zyban) was approved by the FDA as a smoking cessation aid in 1997. Unlike with NRTs, treatment with bupropion begins while the user is still smoking—specifically, one week before the quit date—and continues for seven to twelve weeks. Length of treatment is individualized. Common side effects include insomnia, dry mouth, and dizziness.

The prescription drug varenicline tartrate (Chantrix) was approved in 2006 for smoking cessation. Typically, this nicotine-free tablet is taken twice daily for twelve weeks. Common side effects include headache, nausea and vomiting, gas, insomnia, and change in taste perception.

Symptoms of smoking withdrawal: Smokers who try to quit may face physical and psychological symptoms of withdrawal. Physically, the body reacts to the absence of nicotine. Symptoms of withdrawal include dizziness, de-

pression, irritability, anxiety, sleep disturbances, headaches, difficulty concentrating, drowsiness, and increased appetite. They typically start within a few hours of the last cigarette and peak about two to three days later. Mentally, the smoker must break the habit of coping with stress by smoking.

Jaime Stockslager Buss, M.S.P.H., ELS

▶ **For Further Information**

Aldrich, Matthew. *Stop Smoking*. Chicago: Contemporary Books, 2006.

Centers for Disease Control and Prevention. *Targeting Tobacco Use: The Nation's Leading Cause of Death, 2005*. Bethesda, Md.: Author, 2005.

DeNelsky, Garland Y. *Stop Smoking Now! The Rewarding Journey to a Smoke-Free Life*. Cleveland, Ohio: Cleveland Clinic Press, 2007.

Perkins, Kenneth A., Cynthia A. Conklin, and Michele D. Levine. *Cognitive-Behavioral Therapy for Smoking Cessation: A Practical Guidebook to the Most Effective Treatments*. New York: Routledge, 2008.

U.S. Department of Health and Human Services. *The Health Benefits of Smoking Cessation: A Report of the Surgeon General*. Washington, D.C.: Author, 1990.

▶ **Other Resources**

American Cancer Society
Tobacco and Cancer
    http://www.cancer.org/docroot/PED/PED_10.asp

American Lung Association
Quit Smoking
    http://www.lungusa.org/site/c.dvLUK9O0E/b.33484/

Nicotine Anonymous
    http://www.nicotine-anonymous.org

Smokefree.gov
    http://www.smokefree.gov

See also American Cancer Society (ACS); Chewing tobacco; Cigarettes and cigars; Coughing; Dry mouth; Family history and risk assessment; Geography and cancer; Medical marijuana; Occupational exposures and cancer; Personality and cancer; Pneumonia; Pregnancy and cancer; Prevent Cancer Foundation; Prevention; Psycho-oncology; Psychosocial aspects of cancer; Statistics of cancer; Tobacco-related cancers.

► Social Security Disability Insurance (SSDI)

Category: Social and personal issues
Also known as: DI, Title II

Definition: Social Security Disability Insurance (SSDI) is a U.S. government income replacement program for persons who have paid taxes mandated by the Federal Insurance Contributions Act (FICA) and meet the guidelines for serious disabilities.

History: SSDI can be traced to the Social Security Act of 1935, which established a retirement plan for older adults. At that time disability coverage was not included. In 1950 Congress passed a bill designating restrictive grants to the states to support lower-income disabled workers. In 1955 a disability program was proposed by the Social Security Administration (SSA). Politicians disagreed about this plan but made compromises to get the program passed. Many of the stipulations from that early program still exist today in SSDI.

Cancer and SSDI: The cancer patient seeking SSDI must qualify for disability benefits like any other person with a disability. There is a basic five-step process to qualify:

• Determine if the cancer patient is "working (engaging in a substantial gainful activity)" to meet the SSA guideline.

• The cancer disability has to be severe enough that the patient cannot do most jobs.

• The cancer disability either meets or equals the medical listing under neoplastic (malignant) diseases. The four factors of consideration are origin of the malignancy; extent of cancer involvement; response and duration of antineoplastic therapy, such as surgery, immunotherapy, bone marrow or stem cell transplantation, radiation, or chemotherapy; and the effects or magnitude of post-therapeutic residuals (lasting impact after cancer therapy).

• The person cannot be able to do work he or she has done in the past.

• SSA uses vocational guidelines on age, education, physical/mental ability, and past work experience to decide if the patient can perform any work.

Experienced consultants recommend that cancer patients apply for SSDI as soon as possible, as the process takes time. The disability must be severe enough to be terminal (end in death) or to be continuous for at least twelve months. SSA acts on the assumption that cancer treatment will not meet the twelve-month duration guideline. However, patients can have unique responses to cancer therapies and treatments that would meet the twelve-month requirement.

By law anyone who qualifies for Society Security benefits can file a claim, but the process is lengthy and difficult. An estimated 35 to 40 percent of all SSDI applications are approved when first filed. If benefits are denied, the applicant can appeal the decision by filing a Request for Reconsideration and try again. About 20 percent of appeals are successful. Some people hire an attorney to represent them to decrease the stress and increase the likelihood of an award. At the least, severely disabled cancer patients will need consistent support and assistance from family or friends to complete the application process and make appeals.

If the cancer patient is successful in making a SSDI claim, there is a waiting period between the date the person stopped working and the date benefits are received. After twenty-four months on SSDI, the patient qualifies for Medicare A and B regardless of the person's age.

Tips for successful filing of application: Cancer patients should make application for SSDI benefits as soon as they can no longer work because of their illness and can establish that they will not be able to work for at least the next twelve months. Patients are responsible for assembling all information necessary to file for SSDI. With all documentation complete, the initial claims process may take up to six months to process, and an appeal can take longer. Collecting necessary documentation before applying may help move the process along.

Patients are advised to purchase a portable file organizer and label the tabs for each category of information needed. Separate folders hold the following information:

• Copies of social security card and a certified birth certificate

• List of health care providers, such as doctors, hospitals, or clinics, with phone numbers and addresses

• Copies of medical records from each health care provider

• Copies of lab test results

• List of current medications and known allergies

• Copy of the last W-2 form or tax return

• List of the names of spouses and dependents (from all marriages)

• List of previous employment companies with dates of employment and explanation of the type of work done at each

• Copies of applications or communications with any disability programs or workers' compensation

Alternative insurance should be maintained until the decision on the claim is final. COBRA health insurance (mandated by the Consolidated Omnibus Budget Reconciliation Act) is available to employees after they are terminated from the company's health plan. An application to the patient's state Medicaid plan should be made in addition to the application for SSDI. If this process is too burdensome, patients should consider a disability lawyer to handle their claim. Otherwise, they can seek the counsel of a family or a trustworthy friend.

Marylane Wade Koch, M.S.N., R.N.

▶ For Further Information

Morton, David. *Nolo's Guide to Social Security Disability: Getting and Keeping Your Benefits.* 2d ed. Berkeley, Calif.: Nolo Press, 2003.

Pfeiffer, David. "Social Security's Disability Insurance Program: A History." *Ragged Edge* 23, nos. 2/3 (2002).

▶ Other Resources

American Cancer Society
Making End of Life Decisions
  http://www.cancer.org/docroot/MLT/content/
  MLT_5_1x_Making_End_of_Life_Decisions
  .asp?sitearea=MLT

Social Security Administration
Benefits for People with Disabilities
  http://www.ssa.gov/disability

See also Health maintenance organizations (HMOs); Hospice care; Insurance; Managed care; Medicare and cancer; Oncology social worker; Preferred provider organizations (PPOs).

▶ Soots

Category: Carcinogens and suspected carcinogens
RoC status: Known human carcinogen since 1980
Also known as: Lampblack, carbon black

Related cancers: Scrotal and other skin cancers, lung cancer, leukemia, esophageal cancer, lymphatic and hematopoietic cancers, bladder cancer

Definition: Soots are dark, powdery deposits formed by the incomplete combustion of carbon-rich organic fuels, including gasoline and diesel fuel, coal, wood, fuel oil, paper, plastics, and household refuse. They are complex and variable mixtures of chemical compounds and differ depending on their source; soots from the same source can also differ depending on the conditions of their formation. Soots are composed primarily of elemental carbon; however, particles may also contain sulfates, ammonium, nitrates, condensed organic compounds, and reactive gases and heavy metals such as arsenic, selenium, cadmium, and zinc.

Exposure routes: Inhalation, ingestion, dermal contact

Where found: Particulate emissions from any combustion source, including emissions from fireplaces and furnaces, and exhaust from gasoline and diesel engines; chemical products such as pigments in paints and inks, and in toners for xerography and laser printers; in the vulcanization process for rubber tires, imparting their typical black color

At risk: Workers cleaning home and industrial chimneys and boilers, brick masons, building demolition personnel, insulators, firefighters, metallurgical workers, horticulturists, people exposed to gasoline or diesel engine exhaust, and anyone who is present where organic material is burned

Etiology and symptoms of associated cancers: Compounds extracted from a number of soots cause mutations in standardized mutagenicity assays. Studies with laboratory animals demonstrated that soot from the same source produced skin tumors after dermal application and lung tumors when directed to the lungs. Soots are of concern when inhaled because their small size allows them to migrate deep into the lungs.

History: Scrotal cancer was identified in chimney sweeps in 1775. More recently, studies in Sweden, Denmark, Germany, and the United Kingdom demonstrated a significantly increased risk of lung cancer among chimney sweeps. Research is ongoing to determine which components of soots and other small particles are responsible for their carcinogenicity and other health effects such as respiratory illnesses.

Soots are in the general category of airborne particulate matter (PM). PM is classified as a criteria pollutant by the U.S. Environmental Protection Agency (EPA), meaning that it is an air pollutant for which the EPA has established a national ambient air-quality standard. These pollutants are measured in air-quality-control regions to determine whether the area meets federal air-quality standards.

Bernard Jacobson, Ph.D.

See also Air pollution; Arsenic compounds; Bronchial adenomas; Cadmium and cadmium compounds; Carcinogens, known; Carcinogens, reasonably anticipated; Esophageal cancer; Leukemias; Lung cancers; Lymphedema; Occupational exposures and cancer; Polycyclic aromatic hydrocarbons; Skin cancers.

▶ Soy foods

Category: Lifestyle and prevention

Definition: Soy foods or foods made from soybeans include tofu, tempeh, edamame, miso, and soymilk. Soy foods are an excellent source of protein and contain a number of substances that are being studied for the prevention of cancer.

Background: Since the late 1990's, researchers have conducted thousands of studies on the links between diet and cancer. Epidemiological studies (studies of population-wide patterns of disease) show that many cancers are less common in Asian than in Western countries. The Japanese breast cancer mortality rate, for instance, is only one-fourth that of the women with breast cancer in the United States. Unfortunately, these types of studies are hard to interpret because they cannot account for many potential confounding factors. For example, the average person in Asia may have a more active lifestyle than a typical Westerner.

Although it is not completely clear what factors are responsible for the lower rates of cancer in these countries, many researchers have focused on the potential influence of diet on cancer risks and outcomes. There are many differences between a traditional Asian diet and a modern Western diet, such as the amount of vegetables and fruits, processed foods, meat, fish, and whole grains consumed. However, one thing that is very common in traditional Asian cuisine and historically absent from the typical Western diet is soy foods. However, this may be changing—in the year 2000, more than 25 percent of Americans reported consuming soy products at least once a week. In addition, high-dose soy protein and isoflavone supplements are being marketed in the United States to healthy people to prevent cancer.

How these compounds work: Soy products contain a number of anticarcinogenic (anticancer) compounds, including phytosterols and isoflavones. The two primary isoflavones in soybeans are genistein and daidzein. The National Cancer Institute classifies genistein (the main soybean isoflavone) as a key anticancer agent. Isoflavones act as weak estrogens, with less than 0.1 percent of the activity of estradiol (the main naturally occurring form of estrogen in humans). Isoflavones may act like antiestrogens in the body, because they can bind with the body's estrogen receptors and block some of the body's own estrogens. For cancers that have a hormonal basis, such as breast and prostate, this estrogen blocking could help reduce a person's cancer risk.

Research issues: About six hundred soy-related studies a year are published in the medical literature. There are three basic kinds of studies that have been conducted on the link between soy and cancer: population, animal, and laboratory. With population studies, there are always concerns about the accuracy of the methods used. For instance, food frequency questionnaires depend on study participants to remember what they ate over days, weeks, or even months. In addition, many of these studies have been conducted in small groups of people, so even when there is an apparent association, the link is often not statistically significant.

Animal studies have shown many potential benefits (and some risks) of soy consumption, but there is controversy over how applicable these results are to humans, be-

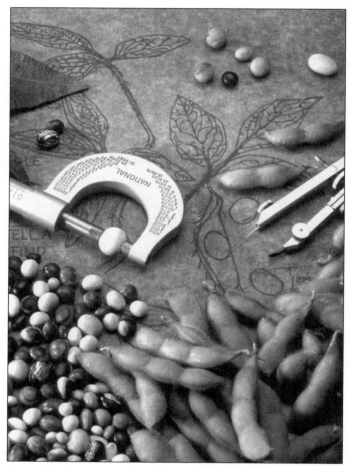

Genistein, the main isoflavone in soybeans, is classified as a key anticancer agent by the National Cancer Institute. (U.S. Department of Agriculture)

cause animal biology, anatomy, and physiology are not the same as those of humans. Laboratory studies, such as those that use cultured human cells to investigate the biochemical response of specific human tissues to elements found in soy, can be similarly controversial because they cannot take into account the complexity of the whole human body and its systems.

Possible risks: Although there have been more than one hundred published studies that suggest possible harm from eating soy, most are lab and animal studies, and this research represents only about 1 to 2 percent of all soy research published. One of the more prominently reported studies dealt with the interaction between soy compounds and drugs to treat breast cancer. One soy compound (genistein) was shown to decrease the effects of tamoxifen, a common breast cancer treatment, while another compound (daidzein) was shown to enhance tamoxifen's effects. There is currently no consensus on whether high levels of soy foods are appropriate for current or former breast cancer patients. In addition, animal studies have found that soy (in supplement form or highly processed isolated proteins) can promote tumor growth under some circumstances, and one study showed that high levels of soy food intake are associated with an increased risk of bladder cancer, although this was based on sixty-one cases and depended on a food-frequency questionnaire.

Possible benefits: Soy foods have been shown in many human and animal studies to be associated with statistically significant reductions in prostate, colorectal, breast, endometrial, and stomach cancer risk. Soy seems to have a particularly strong protective effect against prostate cancer. In fact, on a calorie-for-calorie basis, soy foods protect against prostate cancer at least four times more than any other dietary factor.

The best estimate is that those who eat the most soy have a 30 percent lower risk of developing colorectal cancer than those who eat the least. Regarding stomach cancer, intake of at least 10 grams per day of unfermented soy foods such as tofu may result in lower risk, but there is some question about whether these results reflect other factors, such as fruit and vegetable consumption.

As for breast cancer, modest reductions in risk have been shown for some groups of women, but most of the medical research suggests that soy intake protects against breast cancer mainly if consumed in childhood and adolescence. Postmenopausal women seem to receive little, if any, reduction in breast cancer risk. More research is needed for the effects of soy foods on cancer risk to be fully understood.

Lisa M. Lines, M.P.H.

▶ **For Further Information**

Badger, T. M., M. J. Ronis, R. C. Simmen, and F. A. Simmen. "Soy Protein Isolate and Protection Against Cancer." *Journal of the American College of Nutrition* 24, no. 2 (April, 2005): 146S-149S.

Sun, C. L., et al. "Dietary Soy and Increased Risk of Bladder Cancer: The Singapore Chinese Health Study." *Cancer Epidemiology: Biomarkers and Prevention* 11, no. 12 (December, 2002): 1674-1677.

Trock, B. J., L. Hilakivi-Clarke, and R. Clarke. "Meta-analysis of Soy Intake and Breast Cancer Risk." *Journal of the National Cancer Institute* 98, no. 7 (April 5, 2006): 459-471.

Wu, A. H., D. Yang, and M. C. Pike. "A Meta-analysis of Soyfoods and Risk of Stomach Cancer: The Problem of Potential Confounders." *Cancer Epidemiology: Biomarkers and Prevention* 9, no. 10 (October, 2000): 1051-1058.

Yan, L., and E. L. Spitznagel. "Meta-analysis of Soy Food and Risk of Prostate Cancer in Men." *International Journal of Cancer* 117, no. 4 (November 20, 2005): 667-669.

▶ **Other Resources**

American Cancer Society
Soybean page
http://www.cancer.org/docroot/ETO/content/
ETO_5_3X_Soybean.asp?sitearea=ETO

Memorial Sloan-Kettering Cancer Center
Soy
http://www.mskcc.org/mskcc/html/69383.cfm

See also Antiestrogens; Breast cancer in children and adolescents; Breast cancer in men; Breast cancer in pregnant women; Breast cancers; Carcinogens, known; Carcinogens, reasonably anticipated; Childhood cancers; Epidemiology of cancer; Fruits; Isoflavones; Nutrition and cancer prevention; Nutrition and cancer treatment; Omega-3 fatty acids; Phytoestrogens; Prevention; Prostate cancer; Rectal cancer; Risks for cancer.

▶ **Spermatocytomas**

Category: Diseases, symptoms, and conditions
Also known as: Spermatocytic seminomas

Related conditions: Germ-cell tumors, seminomas

Definition: Spermatocytomas are a type of rare, germ-cell-derived testicular cancer.

Risk factors: No definitive genetic mutations or lifestyle habits have been identified that correlate with increased risk for developing spermatocytoma. Cryptorchidism, failure of the testes to descend by the time a boy reaches school age, is associated with increased risk of testicular cancer, as is a family history of testicular cancer. There is some suggestion that the presence of environmental estrogens may be related to an increased incidence of testicular pathologies, including spermatocytoma, but there is no definitive evidence for this hypothesis.

Etiology and the disease process: The etiology is unknown. Spermatocytomas do not appear to arise from the same precursor cells as other germ-cell-derived testicular cancers. Some data indicate that spermatogonia (early sperm precursor cells) may be the cells from which spermatocytoma is derived. Spermatocytoma has a soft gray appearance on gross examination, with cystic areas in the tumor that do not show any hemorrhaged or necrotic areas. Microscopically, the tumor consists of tubular clusters of round cells that are highly variable in size. These cells are characterized by small, intermediate, and large nuclear regions. These are extremely slow-growing tumors, and metastasis of these tumors has been reported only anecdotally.

Incidence: Spermatocytomas represent 2 to 3 percent of all testicular tumors, and approximately 10 percent occur in both testicles. They occur in older men, age forty-five to eighty. One retrospective study of 200 cases reported a single metastasis.

Symptoms: These tumors generally manifest as a painless swelling in one testicle, although there are some reports of tenderness associated with the tumors.

Screening and diagnosis: This cancer is diagnosed by physical exam. Spermatocytoma is most often confined to one or both testes (Stage I). In Stage II, the cancer has spread to lymph nodes, and in Stage III, it has metastasized. There are no specific chromosomal aberrations of the germ line or genetic mutation linked to this cancer. There are no specific blood markers for these tumors, although high expression of the tumor-suppressor gene *TP53* has been reported.

Treatment and therapy: Spermatocytoma is rarely metastatic and is usually contained within the testicle. Most often it is treated surgically by removing the affected testicle (orchidectomy).

Prognosis, prevention, and outcomes: Since spermatocytoma is slow growing and rarely metastatic, the prognosis is positive, with five-year survival rates of 80 to 100 percent reported after surgical treatment.

Michele Arduengo, Ph.D., ELS

See also Cancer clusters; Family history and risk assessment; Germ-cell tumors; Metastasis; Survival rates; Testicular cancer; TP53 protein; Tubular carcinomas; Tumor-suppressor genes.

▶ Spinal axis tumors

Category: Diseases, symptoms, and conditions
Also known as: Spinal tumors, osteoid osteomas, osteoblastomas, osteochondromas, giant cell tumors, chondroblastomas, vertebral hemangiomas, aneurysmal bone cysts, multiple myeloma, solitary plasmacytomas, osteosarcomas, Ewing sarcoma, soft-tissue sarcomas, chordomas, chondrosarcomas, central nervous system tumors

Related condition: Central nervous system metastasis

Definition: Spinal axis tumors are rare cancers of the spinal cord, an integral component of the central nervous system (CNS). Spinal tumors constitute between 10 and 19 percent of all primary neoplasms (tumors) in the central nervous system. The most common primary spinal axis tumors, which are usually benign, are schwannomas and meningiomas. The majority of spinal tumors are metastases from primary neoplasms elsewhere in the body, most commonly, the breast, prostate, and lung. Spinal cord tumors can be classified according to their location in the spinal column: Extradural tumors are those that occur outside the dura mater lining. Intradural tumors occur within the dural matrix, and intramedullary tumors occur inside the spinal cord.

Risk factors: Vinyl chloride (also known as vinyl chloride monomer, or VCM, and cholorethene in International Union of Pure and Applied Chemistry literature) has been implicated in the development of gliomas. VCM is an industrial chemical chiefly used to produce its polymer, polyvinyl chloride (PVC). VCM is a toxic, colorless gas at room temperature with a sickly sweet odor. Once polymerized, it is stable and nonhazardous. Billions of pounds of PVC are produced per year and used in products such as PVC pipes (used in construction) and bottles. VCM was used as an anesthetic until its toxic effects were uncovered.

Etiology and the disease process: Considerable advances have been made in the last several decades with regard to genetic and environmental factors involved in tumors in general; however, information pertaining to spinal tumors is still scant. Spinal tumors have been found to contain abnormal genes, but the causes of the genetic alterations remain unclear. Some of the better established hereditary (familial) models include neurofibromatosis 2 and von Hippel-Lindau (VHL) disease.

Incidence: Spinal tumors are generally rare, with incidence ranging between 10 to 20 per 1 million people. However, incidence depends on age, with bimodal distribution. The first peak occurs among children age four and younger, and the second peak rises gradually from about age twenty-four and plateaus between the ages of sixty-five and seventy-nine. The incidence for each type of spinal tumor is also age dependent. Low-grade astrocytomas (primary intracranial tumors derived from astrocyte cells of the brain) are common among children. Gliomas (tumors that arise from glial brain cells) tend to afflict adults, particularly those between the ages of forty and sixty. Certain spinal tumors are more common in one gender than the other. For example, the ratio of spinal meningioma is 10:1, women to men; for ependymoma it is 1.8:1, men to women.

Symptoms: Clinical signs and symptoms reflect sequelae of spinal cord compression: Back pain in the middle and lower back, incontinence, and decreased sensitivity in the buttocks are warning signs of spinal nerve compression. The pain may spread beyond the aforementioned regions to the hips, legs, feet, or arms and may continue to worsen even with treatment. Depending on the location and type of tumor, other symptoms—loss of sensation including pain and temperature sensation, muscle weakness, difficulty with locomotion, and scoliosis (spinal deformity)—may develop.

Screening and diagnosis: Spinal tumors are often overlooked because of their rarity and because their associated symptoms resemble more common conditions. Spinal magnetic resonance imaging (MRI) is commonly used for diagnostic purposes. Less commonly, computed tomography (CT) scans, either alone or in combination with contrast dyes as well as myelograms, are used. Biopsies (small tissue sampling technique) are conducted to determine the malignancy and grade (aggressiveness) of the tumor. In patients with known metastasis, particularly those with back pain, bone scans are used to confirm or exclude spinal metastasis.

Treatment and therapy: Surgery is usually the recommended treatment. Radiotherapy or chemotherapy is used in cases in which the tumor is incompletely resected or when malignant lesions are discovered. Although corticosteroids do not affect the tumors themselves, they are commonly administered to reduce inflammation following surgery or during radiation treatments. They are usually used for short durations to minimize the risk of osteoporosis, high blood pressure, diabetes, and infection.

Prognosis, prevention, and outcomes: Prognosis varies depending on the type of tumor, extent of invasion, and how much of the tumor can be resected. For example, the prognoses for meningiomas and schwannomas are good, moderate for gangliomas, and poor for glioblastoma multi-

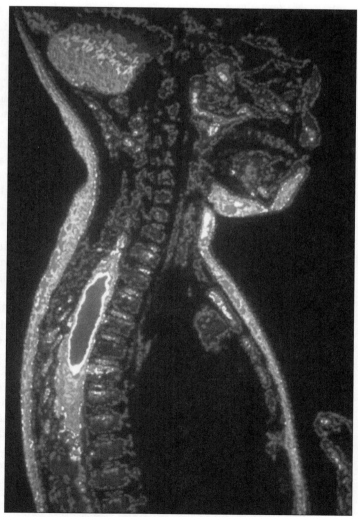

A scan reveals a tumor in this patient's spine. (©Howard Sochurek/ Corbis)

Relative Survival Rates for Spinal Cancers, 1988-2001

Years	Survival Rate (%)
1	92.1
2	87.9
3	83.5
5	78.8
8	74.8
10	73.0

Source: Data from L. A. G. Ries et al., eds., *Cancer Survival Among Adults: U.S. SEER Program, 1988-2001—Patient and Tumor Characteristics*, NIH Pub. No. 07-6215 (Bethesda, Md.: National Cancer Institute, 2007)

Note: Cancers of the spine made up 53.9 percent of the central nervous system cancers.

forme. A spinal tumor can impinge on nerves and cause pain, edema, ischemia, infarction, motor and sensory deficits including paralysis (below the level of the tumor), and death.

Rena C. Tabata, M.Sc.

▶ For Further Information

Hackney, D. B. "Neoplasms and Related Disorders." *Topics in Magnetic Resonance Imaging* 4 (1992): 37-61.

Pascual Castroviejo, I. *Spinal Tumors in Children and Adolescents.* New York: Raven Press, 1990.

Rossi, A., C. Gandolfo, G. Morana, and P. Tortori-Donati. "Tumors of the Spine in Children." *Neuroimaging Clinics of North America* 17 (2007): 17-35.

Sansur, C. A., et al. "Spinal-Cord Neoplasms: Primary Tumours of the Bony Spine and Adjacent Soft Tissue." *The Lancet Oncology* 8 (2007): 137-147.

Van Goethem, J. W., et al. "Spinal Tumors." *European Journal of Radiology* 50 (2004): 159-176.

▶ Other Resources

Cord Foundation
http://www.cordfoundation.org/

Spinal Cord Tumor Association
http://www.spinalcordtumor.homestead.com/

See also Bone cancers; Bone scan; Computed tomography (CT) scan; Meningiomas; Metastasis; Schwannoma tumors; Spinal cord compression; Surgical biopsies; Symptoms and cancer; X-ray tests.

▶ Spinal cord compression

Category: Diseases, symptoms, and conditions
Also known as: Nerve root compression, spinal column compression

Related conditions: Primary spinal cord tumors, metastatic tumors

Definition: Spinal cord compression occurs as a result of tumor invasion of the spinal canal or vertebrae, or from a primary tumor of the spinal cord pressing on the spinal cord and nerve roots. Occasionally, a malignant lymph node may grow to a size that can press on the cord. Metastasis, or spread of cancer cells from the primary tumor site, accounts for 85 percent of the cases of spinal cord compression. The spinal cord controls motor, sensory, and other functions, including walking, breathing, and bowel and bladder control. Compression may occur anywhere along the spinal cord from the neck to the lower back.

Risk factors: The most significant risk factors are tumors that are in a higher stage, such as Stage III or Stage IV, because metastasis may already be present at diagnosis, or cancers that do not respond well to treatment, leading to metastases. Breast, lung, prostate, and renal cancers tend to have a greater risk of metastasis to the spinal cord. Gynecologic cancers tend to spread to the lower spine, and metastasizing breast and lung cancers affect higher areas in the spinal column. Primary tumors located in the spinal column, such as gliomas, pose a significant risk of cord compression.

Etiology and the disease process: The cause of spinal cord compression is generally mechanical in nature, with a tumor pushing against the spinal cord's thecal sac. The thecal sac surrounds the nerve roots and contains spinal fluid. When compression occurs, edema, inflammation, and nerve and circulation damage can result. Primary tumors of the spinal cord may originate inside the spinal column and cause pressure on the cord as the tumor expands. The vertebrae can be destroyed as the mass grows. Compression of the spinal cord begins with pain and weakness. If untreated, damage to the cord causes significant and permanent neurologic problems such as paralysis and an inability to control the bowel and bladder. If the compression is in the cervical area, where nerves control breathing, death can occur if a mechanical respirator is not employed until the compression is relieved.

Incidence: Spinal cord compression may occur in up to 30 percent of cancer patients and in 12 to 15 percent of patients with primary central nervous system tumors. Men tend to have a slightly higher incidence of cord compression from primary tumors. Older patients, usually age fifty and up, are more likely to experience cord compression from a metastatic tumor. Primary tumors affecting the spinal cord are seen more often in children and people between the ages of thirty and fifty.

Symptoms: Symptoms often depend on the level of the spinal cord compression, but back pain is the main symptom regardless of site in 95 percent of patients. The pain can be local or radiating. As the tumor grows, progressive symptoms occur, including tenderness to touch, muscle weakness, tingling or numbness, inability to feel hot and cold, loss of bladder and bowel control, difficulty breathing, and paralysis.

Screening and diagnosis: Patients at risk for spinal cord compression should be screened at each doctor's visit for symptoms that indicate spinal cord compression. Educating the patient about symptoms that need to be reported to the doctor is critical to early intervention. Diagnosis is based on a careful history and physical examination to differentiate cord compression from other causes of symptoms. Back pain that does not get better with rest or lying down is diagnostic in nature. Laboratory tests are not usually helpful. Radiology studies, such as X rays to look for bone destruction and magnetic resonance imaging (MRI) to look at the entire spine, are more useful in identifying the site of damage. Staging is not used with spinal cord compression.

Treatment and therapy: The goals of treatment are to relieve pain, restore nerve function, support the spine, and control or reduce the size of the tumor. Treatment includes dexamethasone, a corticosteroid, given intravenously over several days to reduce edema. Radiation therapy is the standard treatment when spinal cord compression is caused by tumor involvement. Treatments may range from five days to four weeks. Pain may be relieved in hours, but a return of spinal cord nerve function may take several weeks to months. Surgery may be used to stabilize the spine in a small group of patients, but recovery and healing are difficult, especially after radiation. If the tumor is sensitive to chemotherapy, drugs may be used to support other treatments. If the patient fails to respond to therapy, palliative care or hospice referral to include pain management and supportive care may be the only option.

Prognosis, prevention, and outcomes: Because disease progression is the cause of spinal cord compression in 85 percent of cases, the prognosis for the patient is not good. Reversal of symptoms from spinal cord compression can occur with prompt intervention, leading to an improved quality of life. Prevention is based on disease control when metastatic disease is involved. There is no prevention of a primary tumor. Outcomes depend directly on controlling the underlying cancer and early intervention to relieve spinal cord compression and alleviate symptoms.

Patricia Stanfill Edens, R.N., Ph.D., FACHE

▶ **For Further Information**

Abrahm, J. L. "Assessment and Treatment of Patients with Malignant Spinal Cord Compression." *Journal of Supportive Oncology* 2, no. 5 (2004): 377-388, 391.

National Cancer Institute. *Pain Control: A Guide for People with Cancer and Their Families.* NIH Publication 03-4746. Bethesda, Md.: Author, 2003.

Osowski, M. J. "Spinal Cord Compression: An Obstructive Oncologic Emergency." *Topics in Advanced Practice Nursing eJournal* 2, no. 4 (2002).

▶ **Other Resources**

American Cancer Society
http://www.cancer.org

Merck Manuals Online Medical Library
Compression of the Spinal Cord
http://www.merck.com/mmhe/sec06/ch093/
ch093c.html

See also Brain and central nervous system cancers; External beam radiation therapy (EBRT); Non-Hodgkin lymphoma; Radiation therapies; Spinal axis tumors.

▶ **Splenectomy**

Category: Procedures
Also known as: Spleen removal

Definition: A splenectomy is the surgical removal of the spleen. The spleen is located in the upper-left portion of the abdominal cavity. The function of the spleen is to filter the blood, removing old or damaged blood cells from the circulation and eliminating bacteria, parasites, and other organisms that can cause infection. The spleen also produces and stores blood.

Cancers diagnosed or treated: Hodgkin disease (staging), non-Hodgkin lymphoma, chronic myelogenous leukemia, chronic B-cell leukemias (hairy cell leukemia and prolymphocytic leukemia)

Why performed: A splenectomy is most commonly performed on a ruptured spleen, which, if not immediately

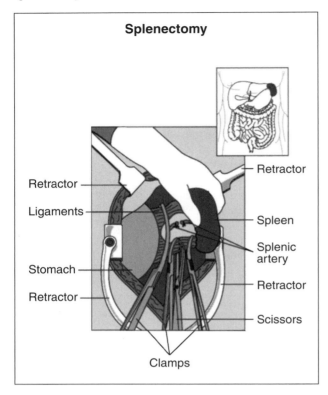

Splenectomy

Retractor

Ligaments

Stomach

Retractor

Retractor

Spleen

Splenic artery

Retractor

Scissors

Clamps

treated, can cause life-threatening bleeding into the abdominal cavity. Splenectomies are also performed in patients with Hodgkin disease for staging the extent of disease; with non-Hodgkin lymphoma, leukemias, and splenomegaly for symptom control; or for correction of cytopenias (low blood cell counts) in patients with immune-mediated destruction of one or more blood elements.

Patient preparation: A few days before the procedure, blood and urine tests and X rays of the abdomen are performed. Immunizations against pneumococcal and meningococcal infections are administered, preferably a couple of weeks before the procedure (frequently this is not possible, particularly in the case of a ruptured spleen as a result of trauma or injury). If blood counts (red blood cells or platelets) are low, then a transfusion may be necessary before the procedure can be performed.

Steps of the procedure: A splenectomy may be performed by the classic, open incision method or by laparoscopy. Before the procedure, anesthesia is administered and an airway tube is placed in the windpipe.

In the classic surgery method, one incision is made in the abdomen over the spleen, and the blood vessels to and around the spleen are cut and tied off. This detaches the

spleen from the rest of the body, and no further exchange of blood between the spleen and the rest of the body can occur. The spleen is then removed. If bleeding occurs, then it may be controlled with a cautery, which burns the tissue, or by tying the blood vessels. The incision is cleaned and closed with stitches or staples, which are generally removed approximately one week after surgery.

During a laparoscopy, three to four small incisions are made in the abdomen. A laparoscope (a lighted tube with a small camera that projects a view of the internal structures to a video monitor) is inserted through one of these incisions. Specialized instruments are inserted through the two to three additional incisions for the doctor to perform the procedure. To provide more room for the doctor to work, carbon dioxide gas is pumped into the abdomen to inflate the abdomen. As with the classic surgery, blood vessels to the spleen are cut and tied off and the spleen is removed. The incisions are closed with stitches and covered with surgical tape.

After the procedure: Blood tests and a pathology exam of the removed spleen may be performed. If necessary, a blood transfusion may be administered.

Risks: Factors that may increase the risk for complications during the procedure include obesity, smoking, poor nutrition, recent or chronic illness, diabetes, advanced age, or a preexisting heart or lung disease. Complications that may be associated with a splenectomy include an increased risk for infection and, though rare, injury to surrounding organs (pancreas, stomach, or colon). Possible complications of any surgery include infection and excess bleeding. Additional complications that may occur with any surgery involving anesthesia include a collapsed lung, deep-vein blood clots, or thromboembolism (blockage of a blood vessel caused by a blood clot), especially in older adults.

Results: Recovery time can vary depending on the underlying disease or condition. In general, however, complete healing from the procedure occurs in about four to six weeks. The results of splenectomy also vary according to the reason for the procedure:

• Ruptured spleen: Once a ruptured spleen is removed, the risk of life-threatening bleeding is eliminated.

• Splenomegaly: Pain and discomfort are effectively reduced if the patient was experiencing symptoms attributable to splenomegaly.

• Chronic myelogenous leukemia: A splenectomy significantly improves symptoms and simplifies management (by reducing transfusion requirements) in patients with chronic myelogenous leukemia.

- Chronic B cell leukemia: A splenectomy may also be an effective secondary treatment for hairy cell leukemia and prolymphocytic leukemia, significantly reducing the tumor.
- Cytopenias: Splenectomy has been shown to correct cytopenias in a large proportion of patients with immune-mediated destruction of one or more cellular blood elements.

Anita P. Kuan, Ph.D.

▶ For Further Information

Bridget, S. Wilkins, and Dennis H. Wright. *Illustrated Pathology of the Spleen*. New York: Cambridge University Press, 2000.

"Guidelines for the Prevention and Treatment of Infection in Patients with an Absent or Dysfunctional Spleen." *BMJ* 312 (1996): 430-434. Also available at http://www.bmj.com.

Hiatt, Jonathan R., Edward H. Phillips, and Leon Morgenstern, eds. *Surgical Diseases of the Spleen*. New York: Springer, 1997.

Townsend, Courtney M., Jr., et al., eds. *Sabiston Textbook of Surgery*. 17th ed. Philadelphia: Elsevier Saunders, 2005.

"Updated Guidelines: The Prevention and Treatment of Infection in Patients with an Absent or Dysfunctional Spleen." British Committee for Standards in Haematology. *BMJ*, June 2, 2001. Also available at http://www.bmj.com.

Uranus, S. *Current Spleen Surgery*. Munich: Zuckschwerdt, 1995.

▶ Other Resources

Cleveland Clinic
http://www.clevelandclinic.org

Familydoctor.org
Splenectomy
http://familydoctor.org/online/famdocen/home/articles/655.html

Lymphoma Research Foundation
http://www.lymphoma.org

National Institutes of Health
http://www.nih.gov

See also Chronic lymphocytic leukemia (CLL); Hairy cell leukemia; Hodgkin disease; Laparoscopy and laparoscopic surgery; Leukemias; Lymphomas; Myelofibrosis; Myeloproliferative disorders; Non-Hodgkin lymphoma.

▶ Sputum cytology

Category: Procedures

Definition: Sputum cytology is a screening for the presence of abnormal cells in sputum (saliva).

Cancers diagnosed: Lung cancer

Why performed: If a tumor is centrally located and has invaded the airways, then this procedure may allow visualization of tumor cells for diagnosis. It is a risk-free and inexpensive procedure.

Patient preparation: A sputum sample may be collected from coughed-up mucus (sometimes induced by an inhaled saline mist) or by bronchoscopy, which uses a bronchoscope to examine the throat and airways.

No special preparation is required if the sputum sample is to be collected by coughing with or without a saline mist at home or in the doctor's office. If a sputum sample is to be obtained by bronchoscopy, then the patient may not eat or drink for eight to ten hours before the procedure. The patient may be given medications to dry the secretions in the mouth and airways. A chest X ray may also be done before bronchoscopy.

Steps of the procedure: For simple coughing procedures, three sputum samples are usually collected over three days in a container with fixative to preserve the sample.

Bronchoscopy is performed with a flexible or a rigid bronchoscope. Rigid bronchoscopy requires general anesthesia. In either case, the patient must sign a consent form.

After the procedure: There are no requirements following sputum collection by coughing. A second chest X ray is taken after bronchoscopy, and the patient should be driven home. Patients should call immediately if they cough up more than two tablespoons of blood, have difficulty breathing, or have a fever for more than twenty-four hours.

Risks: There is no risk in collecting sputum samples by coughing procedures. Bronchoscopy is usually a safe procedure, and complications are rare. Complications that may occur include spasms of the bronchial tubes, irregular heart rhythms, infections, hoarseness, and bubbles under the skin.

Results: The most common screening tests for lung cancer are a chest X ray and sputum cytology. According to a 2007 report by the United States National Cancer Institute, the results of many studies have shown no evidence that screening for lung cancer using sputum cytology or chest X ray reduces lung cancer mortality. The institute also concludes that screening could lead to false positive tests and unnecessary, invasive diagnostic procedures and treatments. Hence, these tests are not used for routine screening of healthy individuals but only when symptons indicate their use.

Bernard Jacobson, Ph.D.

See also Bronchial adenomas; Bronchoalveolar lung cancer; Carcinoid tumors and carcinoid syndrome; Coughing; Head and neck cancers; Hemoptysis; Infection and sepsis; Lung cancers; Mesothelioma; Pneumonia; Radon; Screening for cancer.

▶ Squamous cell carcinomas

Category: Diseases, symptoms, and conditions
Also known as: Skin cancer, SCC

Related condition: Basal cell carcinomas

Definition: Squamous cell carcinomas are malignant tumors that begin in the squamous cells that form the outer layer, or epidermis, of the skin.

Risk factors: Risk factors for squamous cell carcinomas include exposure to sunlight and ultraviolet radiation, age above fifty years, male gender, light-colored skin that burns easily, blue or green eyes, blond or red hair, residence in a geographical area that receives high sun exposure, exposure to chemical carcinogens such as arsenic and tar, history of a large number of X rays, history of prior nonmelanoma skin cancer, and chronic immunosuppression.

Etiology and the disease process: Cumulative lifetime sun exposure is the main cause of squamous cell carcinoma. The shorter-wavelength portion of the ultraviolet spectrum (known as UVB) is believed to be about one thousandfold more active in inducing skin cancer than the longer-wavelength portion (known as UVA). Squamous cell carcinoma spreads faster than basal cell carcinoma (skin cancer that originates from basal keratinocytes in the top layer of the skin, the epidermis) but still may be relatively slow growing. A subset of high-risk squamous cell carcinoma is capable of infiltrating the local area and metastasizing to regional lymph nodes as well as to distant locations and internal organs, most often to the lungs. This subset accounts for most of the morbidity and mortality associated with squamous cell carcinoma. The overall risk of metastasis for squamous cell carcinoma is 2 to 6 percent and as high as 47 percent for certain high-risk lesions.

Five-year survival rates as high as 73 percent have been reported for patients with squamous cell carcinoma that has metastasized to the lymph nodes and has been treated with surgery and radiation therapy.

Incidence: The annual incidence of squamous cell carcinoma in the United States is estimated to be 107 cases per 100,000 people in the general population. Because health registries often exclude squamous cell carcinoma from their databases and the rate of this cancer varies based on geographical location, this number is difficult to determine with accuracy.

Squamous cell carcinoma is the second most common form of skin cancer after basal cell carcinoma in whites. In people of African and Asian descent, squamous cell carcinoma, although relatively rare, is the most common form of skin cancer. Squamous cell carcinoma carries a higher mortality rate in blacks than in whites, probably because of delayed diagnosis, and occurs at a two to three times higher frequency in men than in women, presumably because of a higher cumulative exposure to sunlight.

There has been an apparent dramatic increase in the incidence of squamous cell carcinoma over the past several decades in the United States. This has been attributed to an increase in sun exposure in the general population, the advancing age of the population, and earlier diagnosis because of increased public awareness of skin cancer.

Symptoms: Squamous cell carcinoma may manifest as a variety of primary morphologies. The main symptom is a growing bump that may have a rough, scaly surface and flat, reddish patches. A sore that does not heal can be a sign of squamous cell carcinoma. Squamous cell carcinomas typically occur on portions of the skin that have been exposed to sunlight over a period of years; approximately 70 percent of lesions occur on the head and neck, and about 15 percent occur on the arms and hands. Histologically, a squamous cell carcinoma lesion involves the full thickness of the epidermis, the outer layer of the skin, but without involvement of the dermis, the deep vascular inner layer of the skin.

Screening and diagnosis: Screening for squamous cell carcinoma involves regular skin examinations for new lesions or changes in an existing lesion. Suspicious changes in an existing lesion include a change in appearance, color, size, or texture; pain; inflammation; bleeding; or itching. A lesion that is asymmetrical, has irregular or diffuse borders, has multiple colors, or is larger than six millimeters (mm) in diameter should be examined by a doctor.

The appearance of a skin lesion may indicate a squamous cell carcinoma, but a skin biopsy is required for a definitive diagnosis. The common types of biopsy are shave biopsy, punch biopsy, incisional biopsy (removes only a portion of the suspicious tissue), and excisional biopsy (removes the entire suspicious region). A biopsy for squamous cell carcinoma is normally done in the doctor's office after the patient is given a local anesthetic. Biopsy samples must be deep enough to reach the mid-dermis to allow for determination of the presence or absence of invasive disease. For high-risk lesions, a larger tissue sample may be taken to assess the extent of invasion into nerves and to look for other features that would indicate a greater risk of metastasis.

Squamous cell carcinoma is staged according to the TNM (tumor/lymph node/metastasis) classification system. Because most squamous cell carcinomas are not metastatic at the time of diagnosis, the stage (T1-T4) is based on the size and characteristics of the lesion.

Treatment and therapy: Most squamous cell carcinomas are treated in the doctor's office by cryotherapy, electrodesiccation and curettage, excision with conventional margins, or Mohs micrographic surgery. It is important to remove the lesion completely in the first treatment because it can recur, metastasize, and cause death. More advanced or more invasive squamous cell carcinomas may require more aggressive treatment, including surgical management, radiation therapy, or both.

Cryotherapy with liquid nitrogen is a safe and low-cost procedure. For appropriate lesions and with good technique, the five-year cure rate for squamous cell carcinoma is 95 percent. Electrodesiccation and curettage, which may be used to treat squamous cell carcinoma on the trunk and extremities, is a simple procedure involving scraping and burning the tissue in the lesion. Its effectiveness is considered to be very dependent on technique; cure rates improve with a doctor's experience. Excision with conventional margins (4 mm for lower-risk lesions is recommended) is highly effective for many squamous cell carcinomas, with a five-year cure rate of 92 percent for primary squamous cell carcinoma and 77 percent for recurrent squamous cell carcinoma. This technique commonly involves removal of a greater amount of normal tissue than is necessary for complete tumor removal. Mohs surgery, performed by dermatologic surgeons, has the highest cure rate for squamous cell carcinoma (94 to 99 percent) and is the procedure of choice when it is desirable to remove as little tissue as possible (such as on the face) and for high-risk squamous cell carcinoma. Unlike with simple excision, Mohs surgery allows for examination of the entire surgical margin during the procedure and the removal of the tumor in a step-wise procedure until clear margins are

obtained. Mohs surgery is routinely performed as an outpatient procedure with the patient under local anesthesia and is widely available in the United States.

Nonsurgical treatment options for squamous cell carcinoma include topical chemotherapy and immune response modifiers (generally used for premalignant lesions), photo-

---

A Few Facts About Ultraviolet Light

Ultraviolet light is part of the invisible spectrum of sunlight. It has a wavelength shorter than visible light and longer than that of X rays. It can be divided into three wavelengths: UVA, UVB, and UVC.

- UVA, with a wavelength of 320-400 nanometers (nm), has the least energy of the three. It penetrates glass and clouds. It is responsible for long-term skin damage and aging of the skin and decreases the amount of vitamin A in the skin. Because it produces indirect damage to deoxyribonucleic acid (DNA), it also plays a role in causing cancer.
- UVB, with a wavelength of 290-320 nm, causes sunburns. It directly damages DNA and therefore results in skin cancers. It decreases the amount of vitamin A in the skin and can damage the eye and lead to cataracts. On the positive side, it causes the body to produce vitamin D and is an important source of this vitamin. It also is used to treat some skin conditions such as psoriasis.
- UVC, with a wavelength of 200-290 nm, has the most energy of the three types. Although UVC is the most carcinogenic, it generally does not penetrate the atmosphere as it is absorbed by the ozone layer.

Exposure to ultraviolet light is believed to alter people's immune response and make them more susceptible to infection as well as to activate certain viruses, including the human immunodeficiency virus (HIV).

The levels of ultraviolet light radiation vary by time of day, peaking at the solar noon, when the sun reaches its highest point in the sky, and by time of year, peaking in the Northern Hemisphere in June and ebbing in December. Geography also plays a part in people's exposure to ultraviolet light. The nearer the equator, the higher the levels, as the sunlight passes through less atmosphere, and people who live in places such as Australia and Arizona, where there are many days of sunshine, are exposed to more ultraviolet rays. Because of the thinner air, the higher the elevation, the higher the intensity of the ultraviolet light, rising 4 percent with every 1,000 feet of elevation. Proximity to reflective surfaces—fresh snow, water, sand, and pavement—also increases the intensity, while air pollution and a thick cloud layer decrease the intensity.

Sources: Skin Cancer Foundation, Ohio State University Extension Fact Sheet CDFD-199-07

dynamic therapy, radiation therapy (generally used in patients for whom surgery is not feasible and as an adjuvant therapy for patients with metastatic or high-risk squamous cell carcinoma), and systemic chemotherapy (for patients with metastatic disease).

Prognosis, prevention, and outcomes: Localized squamous cell carcinoma of the skin has a high cure rate if treated early. The overall three-year survival rate is estimated to be 85 percent. For patients with no high-risk factors, this rate approaches 100 percent, and for patients with at least one high-risk factor, it decreases to 70 percent. Risk factors associated with higher rates of recurrence and metastasis include tumors on the lips or ears; tumor size greater than 2 centimeters; an invasive, poorly differentiated, or recurrent tumor; nerve involvement; being an organ transplant recipient; having received chronic immunosuppressive therapy; and being infected with the human immunodeficiency virus (HIV) or having acquired immunodeficiency syndrome (AIDS).

Patients who develop one squamous cell carcinoma have a 40 percent risk of developing additional squamous cell carcinomas within the next two years and therefore should receive a complete skin examination every six to twelve months. Patients with high-risk tumors should receive complete skin and lymph node examinations every three to six months for at least two years.

The most important preventive measure is limiting exposure to sunlight. Skin should be protected by wearing protective clothing such as hats, long-sleeved shirts, long skirts, or pants. A high-quality broad-spectrum sunscreen that blocks UVA and UVB light should be applied at least thirty minutes before going outside and reapplied frequently. Exposure to the sunlight at midday when the sun is most intense should be limited.

Jill Ferguson, Ph.D.

▶ For Further Information

Aboutalebi, S., and F. M. Strickland. "Immune Protection, Natural Products, and Skin Cancer: Is There Anything New Under the Sun?" *Journal of Drugs in Dermatology* 5 (2006): 512-517.

Alam, M., and D. Ratner. "Cutaneous Squamous-Cell Carcinoma." *New England Journal of Medicine* 344 (2001): 975-983.

Clayman, G. L., et al. "Mortality Risk from Squamous Cell Skin Cancer." *Journal of Clinical Oncology* 23 (2005): 759-765.

Green, A., and R. Marks. "Squamous Cell Carcinoma of the Skin (Non-Metastatic)." *Clinical Evidence* 14 (2005): 2086-2090.

Takata, M., and T. Saida. "Early Cancers of the Skin: Clinical, Histopathological, and Molecular Characteristics." *International Journal of Clinical Oncology* 10 (2005): 391-397.

▶ Other Resources

National Cancer Institute
Squamous Cell Carcinoma of the Skin
    http://www.cancer.gov/cancertopics/pdq/treatment/
    skin/HealthProfessional/page6

Skin Cancer Foundation
Squamous Cell Carcinoma
    http://www.skincancer.org/squamous/index.php

See also Basal cell carcinomas; Carcinomas; Dermatology oncology; Epidermoid cancers of mucous membranes; Eye cancers; Eyelid cancer; Geography and cancer; Itching; Lip cancers; Melanomas; Moles; Recurrence; Skin cancers; Sunlamps; Sunscreens; Ultraviolet radiation and related exposures.

▶ Staging of cancer

Category: Procedures
Also known as: Clinical staging, pathological staging, restaging

Definition: Staging is the process in which the location, extent, and degree of metastasis (spread) of a primary, or original, cancerous tumor is determined.

Cancers diagnosed or treated: Essentially all solid tumor cancer diagnoses are staged similarly. Nonlocalized leukemias are staged in unique ways according to the specific diagnosis. The diagnostic processes used to stage a specific case vary somewhat according to cancer type and location.

Why performed: Cancer staging plays an integral role in determining overall disease prognosis as well as influencing treatment modality choices. Stage assessment also plays an important role in assuring effective communication among the patient's medical team and accurate disease surveillance and epidemiology efforts.

Patient preparation: Patient preparation will vary according to the technique, or supporting procedures, used to help stage the cancer. These procedures range from physical examination and imaging—X rays, ultra sounds, computed tomography (CT), magnetic resonance imaging (MRI) scans—to laboratory tests, biopsies, and surgical excisions with subsequent pathological examination of the tumor. Any preparation normally required of these supporting procedures will apply to the process.

Steps of the procedure: Cancer staging is composed of three distinct phases: clinical staging, pathological staging, and restaging. Clinical staging is accomplished by nonpathologic means based on physical examination and imaging technology such as X ray, MRI, and CT, as well as immunologic and molecular blood tests to detect and measure cancer markers where applicable.

Pathological staging is accomplished following tissue removal by biopsy in which surgical tumor excision is assessed as a sound treatment option. The biopsied tissue and/or removed tumor, surrounding tissue, and nearby lymph nodes are examined microscopically and histologically to determine the type and extent of the cancer from a pathologic perspective. Because treatment considerations and survival statistics are based on the stage of a patient's cancer, the initial stage assessment remains static throughout the course of the disease regardless of progression and/or response to treatment.

Should a cancer patient enter remission but subsequently present with a recurrence, restaging may be accomplished if additional treatment is planned. The restaging process is identical to the original one, including both clinical and pathological staging, but is now designated with a lowercase *r*. For example, a restaged Stage IV grouping would be recorded as Stage rIV.

In order to maintain terminology consistency, a limited number of classification systems are utilized, and efforts toward additional interpretive continuity are ongoing. Although the type of cancer dictates which specific categorization is applied, common elements include tumor location, size and number, lymph node involvement, and degree of metastasis (spread). The most prevalent systems used include tumor-node-metastasis (TNM) and overall group staging.

The tumor-node-metastasis (TNM) classification is adapted by the American Joint Committee on Cancer (AJCC) and the Union Internationale Contre le Cancer/International Union Against Cancer (UICC).

The category T, for tumor, provides information about the original tumor such as measurement (in millimeters, centimeters) at the site of origin and its degree of invasion into nearby tissues and organs.
- TX: Cannot be measured/evaluated
- T0: No evidence of primary tumor
- Tis: In situ tumor (tumor limited to cell layers of the original site)

Beyond Tis, numerical tumor categorization offers a relative degree of severity, with higher numbers reflecting a larger tumor and/or more aggressive invasion.
- T1: Smaller tumor, least aggressive
- T2
- T3
- T4: Larger tumor, most aggressive

The tumor grade is the degree of abnormality (amount of differentiation from normal cells) and is determined pathologically—by microscopic analysis. Typically, well-differentiated, or low-grade, tumors are considered the least aggressive and are associated with the best outcomes overall.
- GX: Cannot be determined
- G1: Tumor cells well differentiated from surrounding tissue
- G2: Tumor cells moderately well differentiated from surrounding tissue

G3: Tumor cells poorly differentiated from surrounding tissue

G4: Tumor cells undifferentiated from surrounding tissue

Special cases are prostate cancer and central nervous system (CNS) cancers. The most common approach to classification of prostate cancer is the Gleason system, which is based on the degree of glandular change, including size, shape, and pathologic differentiation. The Gleason Score or Sum (GS) represents the sum of the primary and secondary grade of the prostate tumor. Based on a ranking from G2 (least aggressive, best prognosis) to G10 (most aggressive, poorest prognosis), the higher the sum is, the more severe is the disease. There are several, similar classification systems used to grade CNS/brain cancers: World Health Organization (WHO), Kernohan, or Ringertz. Rather than tumor size, grading is based on tissue differentiation and degree of vascularity and necrosis. Classification is made based on a three- or four-grade system, with the higher number associated with more aggressive cancer.

The category N, for node, describes the degree that lymph nodes have been affected by cancer. This is typically accomplished by a process termed "sentinal node biopsy." The (nearby) sentinal node or nodes are detected by injection of a radioactive or colored dye solution at the tumor site. The indicator solution will travel a path within the lymph system that circulating cancer cells would be expected to follow. The area is then scanned to detect the presence of the indicator solution in nearby, or sentinal, lymph nodes. One or more lymph nodes are then removed and examined pathologically for the presence of cancer cells. Positive findings will typically result in further removal and testing of nearby lymph nodes to determine extent.

- NX: Cannot be measured/evaluated
- N0: Nearby lymph nodes are clear of cancer

Beyond N0, numerical categorization describes the size, location, and number of lymph nodes affected. The higher the number, the more lymph nodes are involved.

- N1: Fewer lymph nodes affected
- N2
- N3: More lymph nodes affected

The M category, for metastasis, describes the degree to which the primary tumor has spread (metastasized) into surrounding tissues and/or organs.

- MX: Cannot be measured/evaluated
- M0: No cancer metastasis detected
- M1: Cancer metastasis detected

Although the TNM metrics are relatively universal, each cancer type has a customized version of this classification system. In some instances, there may be many additional subcategories to refine tumor classification and offer additional prognostic information to the provider. In other cases, the staging classification may be simplified by means of truncated categorization.

Based on the established TNM categories, an overall cancer group stage is determined. Although criteria for stage assignment varies somewhat according to cancer type, the following provides a top-level overview of stage groupings:

- Stage 0: Carcinoma in situ (cancer is limited to the site of origin)

Stages I through III classify cancer where higher numbers indicate more extensive and aggressive disease. Some cancers types utilize subcategories in staging to provide more specific information about type, behavior, and prognosis.

- Stage IV: Distant metastatic cancer (cancer has spread to another, distant organ)

Special cases are female reproductive cancers, Hodgkin disease/lymphoma, colorectal cancer, and leukemia. Female reproductive cancers are stage according to the International Federation of Gynecologists and Obstetricians (FIGO). Although FIGO staging classification guidelines generally follow the general TNM/group staging approach, many of the female reproductive cancers, including those of the breast, cervix, and uterus, are subclassified in great detail.

Hodgkin disease and other cancers of the lymphoid system are staged using the Ann Arbor classification system. Stages I through IV are defined by the anatomical location of affected lymph nodes. The higher the stage number, the more lymph nodes are affected and the more aggressive is the disease. Each stage assignment is then subclassified as either "A" (asymptomatic) or "B" (symptomatic).

Colorectal cancer uses the Dukes' staging classification, an older system that corresponds closely to group staging. Dukes' A through D colorectal cancer stages effectively translate to group Stages I through IV.

Because leukemia involves the bone marrow and has often affected many organs, including the liver, spleen, and lymph nodes, staging is based primarily on the patient's survival outlook according to disease progression. Although not all forms of leukemia utilize a formal staging system, each form that does has a dedicated staging classification system. For example, chronic myelogenous leukemia (CML) is classified into three phases (as opposed to stages):

- Chronic: Fewer than 5 percent immature cells in circulation/bone marrow; mildly symptomatic, readily responsive to treatment
- Accelerated: 5 to 30 percent immature cells in circulation/bone marrow; more symptomatic, less responsive to treatment
- Acute/blast phase: Less than 30 percent immature cells in circulation/bone marrow; very aggressive, acute disease

Additional staging classifications, such as Rai (Stages 0-IV; U.S. predominant) and Binet (Stages A, B, and C; European predominant), are used for chronic lymphocytic leukemia (CLL). Still other systems are applied to different leukemia types such as the Stage 1 through Stage 3 classification based on level of anemia and spleen size for hairy cell leukemia (HCL).

In addition to providing information on the size, extent, and prognostic status of each cancer case, staging plays a vital role in epidemiology and treatment studies. The National Cancer Institute Surveillance, Epidemiology, and End Results (SEER) program and other cancer registries such as the National Program of Cancer Registries (NPCR) use summary staging classification in their surveillance and epidemiology efforts. For these purposes, all cancers are grouped into one of the following five summary categories:

- In situ: Early-stage cancer, present only in the cell layers where first detected
- Localized: Cancer localized to tissue/organ where first detected; no evidence of metastasis
- Regional: Cancer metastasized to nearby lymph nodes, tissues, organs
- Distant: Cancer metastasized to distant lymph nodes, tissues, organs
- Unknown: Insufficient data available to classify

Data collected are made available to clinical and research professionals so that they may better understand and address the cancer burden according to a variety of demographics and metrics, including cancer stage.

Results: Cancer staging is a vital component of the diagnostic process. Accurate stage assessment will guide the medical team in making optimal treatment recommendations for patient care according to prognostic expectations. Because the epidemiologic value of the original stage is significant, the classification remains constant throughout the course of disease. Restaging occurs only if treatment is planned following a recurrence.

Pam Conboy, B.S.

▶ **For Further Information**

Benedet, J. L., et al. "FIGO Staging Classifications and Clinical Practice Guidelines in the Management of Gynecologic Cancers." *International Journal of Gynecology and Obstetrics* 70 (2000): 209-262.

Greene, F. L. "Updates to Staging System Reflect Advances in Imaging, Understanding." *Journal of the National Cancer Institute* 22 (2002): 1664-1666.

_____. "Updating the Strategies in Cancer Staging." *American College of Surgeons Bulletin* 87 (2002): 13-15.

Greene, F. L., et al., eds. *American Joint Committee on Cancer Staging Manual.* 6th ed. New York: Springer, 2002.

O'Dowd, G. J., et al. "The Gleason Score: A Significant Biologic Manifestation of Prostate Cancer Aggressiveness on Biopsy." *PCRI Insights* 4, no. 1 (January, 2001).

Wittekind, C., et al. "TNM Residual Tumor Classification Revisited." *Cancer* 94 (2002): 2511-2516.

▶ **Other Resources**

American Cancer Society
http://www.cancer.org

American Joint Committee on Cancer (AJCC)
http://www.cancerstaging.org/

CancerCare
http://www.cancercare.org

Centers for Disease Control and Prevention (CDC) National Program of Cancer Registries (NPCR)
http://www.cdc.gov/cancer/npcr/

CureSearch
http://www.curesearch.org

International Federation of Gynecologists and Obstetricians (FIGO)
http://www.figo.org

International Union Against Cancer
http://www.uicc.org/

Lung Cancer Online Foundation
http://www.lungcanceronline.org

National Cancer Institute
http://www.cancer.gov

See also Biopsy; Cancer care team; Carcinomas; Chemotherapy; Childhood cancers; Dukes' classification; Epidemiology of cancer; Gleason grading system; Leukemias; Lymphomas; Medical oncology; Metastasis; National Cancer Institute (NCI); Oncology; Sentinel lymph node (SLN) biopsy and mapping; Statistics of cancer; TNM staging.

▶ **Statistics of cancer**

Category: Social and personal issues

Definition: Cancer statistics are numerical values regarding aspects of cancer that characterize the population or sample from which the data was taken.

Common statistics: Statistics provide a good estimate of the impact of cancer on the general population. The most common way to show this impact is to report the incidence, death or mortality, and survival rates. Incidence is the number of newly diagnosed, or found, cancer cases in a given time period. Mortality is the number of deaths from cancer during a certain time period. Incidence and death rates are reported as a specific number for every 100,000 people in the general population, per year. Survival looks at the length of time patients live after their cancer is diagnosed. Relative survival compares cancer patients still living after a certain period of time (for example, five years) to a similar group of people in age, sex, and race without diagnosed cancer. Relative survival rates are useful for group predictions but not individual survival predictions, because this rate does not account for an individual's medical condition, such as other medical illnesses. Some rates will be age-adjusted to give a more accurate statistic, which is often done when comparing populations where the age distributions are very different. Data used for the general population come from the U.S. Census.

Description of the population: Cancer statistics take a look at cancer's impact by dividing the population by sex, age, and race and ethnicity. The U.S. Census divides race into five groups. White is any person whose origin can be traced to Europe, the Middle East, or North Africa. Black or African American is any person whose origin can be traced to the black groups of Africa. American Indian and Alaska Native refer to any person whose origins can be traced to the native peoples of North, South, and Central

America and who remains affiliated with the tribe or community. Asian is any person with origins in the Far East, Southeast Asia, or the Indian subcontinent. Native Hawaiian and other Pacific Islander refer to any person whose origins can be traced back to Hawaii, Guam, Samoa, or another Pacific island.

Incidence, death, and survival statistics: In 2007 the American Cancer Society estimated that about 1,444,920 Americans would be diagnosed with an invasive cancer (called incidence), and 559,650 would die from an invasive cancer. Invasive means the cancer has spread beyond the site where it developed. An example of an invasive cancer would be a breast tumor that has spread to surrounding tissue or lymph nodes. Cancer is the second leading cause of death after heart disease.

A person's risk, or chance, of developing cancer increases as he or she ages; about 77 percent of all cancer diagnoses occur in persons fifty-five years and older. According to the Surveillance Epidemiology and End Results (SEER) Cancer Statistics Review, the average age of diagnosis for all cancer sites per year between 2000 and 2004 was sixty-seven years. Broken down into age ranges, about 10 percent were under age forty-four; 35 percent were between forty-five and sixty-four; 48 percent were between sixty-five and eighty-four; and 7 percent were eighty-five years or older. The average age at death for all cancer sites for 2000 to 2004 was seventy-three years of age. By age ranges, about 4 percent were under age forty-four; 26 percent were between forty-five and sixty-four; 56 percent were between sixty-five and eighty-four; and 14 percent were eighty-five years of age or older.

The American Cancer Society reported the following age-adjusted rates for men and women per year between 1999 and 2003 (numbers in parentheses are per 100,000 people from the general population). Men had a higher incidence of cancer (562) and death from cancer (244) than women (415 incidence; 164 deaths). The major cancers diagnosed among men were prostate (165), lung and bronchial area (90), colon and rectum (64), urinary bladder (38), and non-Hodgkin lymphoma (23). The highest incidence of cancer in women occurred as breast cancer (128), lung and bronchial area cancer (55), colon and rectum cancer (47), non-Hodgkin lymphoma (16), and urinary bladder cancer (10). Men died most often from lung and bronchial cancers (75), prostate cancer (29), colon and rectum cancers (24), pancreatic cancer (12), and non-Hodgkin lymphoma (10). Women died most often from lung and bronchial cancers (41), breast cancer (26), colon and rectum cancers (17), pancreatic cancer (9), and non-Hodgkin lymphoma (6).

By race and ethnicity for the same time period, age-adjusted cancer incidence for all sites per 100,000 people was highest among African Americans (1,024), followed by whites (976), Hispanics and Latinos (771), Asian Americans and Pacific Islanders (689), and finally American Indians and Alaska Natives (665). Cancer incidence among African Americans occurred most often in the prostate (243), lung and bronchial area (161), colon and rectum (124), female breast (112), kidney and renal pelvis (28), and stomach (26). Cancer incidence among whites occurred most often in the prostate (156), lung and bronchial area (145), female breast (131), colon and rectum (110), kidney and renal pelvis (27), and stomach (14). Cancer incidence among Asian Americans and Pacific Islanders occurred most often in the prostate (104), female breast (91), colon and rectum (91), lung and bronchial area (85), stomach (31), and liver and bile duct (30). Cancer incidence among American Indians and Alaska Natives occurred most often in the colon and rectum (95), lung and bronchial area (89), female breast (74), prostate (71), stomach (34), and kidney and renal pelvis (31). Cancer incidence among Hispanics and Latinos occurred most often in the prostate (141), female breast (93), colon and rectum (90), lung and bronchial area (79), kidney and renal pelvis (26), and stomach (25).

African Americans were at the top of the list relative to deaths from cancer (523), followed by whites (403), Hispanics and Latinos (275), American Indians and Alaska Natives (265), and finally Asian Americans and Pacific Islanders (244). By racial group, and six cancer sites with highest rates, cancer deaths among African Americans occurred in the lung and bronchial area (138), prostate (65), colon and rectum (57), female breast (34), stomach (18), and liver and bile duct (13). Cancer deaths among whites occurred in the lung and bronchial area (116), colon and rectum (40), prostate (27), female breast (25), liver and bile duct (9), and kidney and renal pelvis (9). Cancer deaths among Asian Americans and Pacific Islanders occurred in the lung and bronchial area (58), colon and rectum (26), liver and bile duct (22), stomach (18), female breast (13), and prostate (12). Cancer deaths among American Indians and Alaska Natives occurred in the lung and bronchial area (70), colon and rectum (27), prostate (18), female breast (14), liver and bile duct (12), and stomach (11). Cancer deaths among Hispanics and Latinos occurred in the lung and bronchial area (52), colon and rectum (29), prostate (22), female breast (16), liver and bile duct (16), and stomach (14).

In comparing race and ethnic groups, African American men had a 38 percent higher death rate and African American women a 17 percent higher death rate than whites from colorectal, lung (male), breast (women), and prostate cancers. In addition, African Americans had higher incidence for all cancers except for female breast cancer when compared with whites. Hispanics had a higher incidence of uterine cervix, liver, and stomach cancers than whites. Asian Americans and Pacific Islanders had the highest incidence and death rates from stomach and liver cancers when compared with all racial and ethnic groups, with the exception of death rates from stomach cancer in men of this minority group. Within the Asian American and Pacific Islander group, Vietnamese women were four times more likely to be diagnosed with cervical cancer than other women in this minority group. Finally, American Indians and Alaska Natives appear to have the highest incidence and death rate from kidney cancer. As available data for American Indians and Alaska Natives are limited, this last statement should be viewed as a rough estimate.

The SEER Program looked at trends in five-year relative survival rates for several time periods using data from nine regions of the United States. The five-year relative survival rate for all cancers diagnosed per year between 1996 and 2002 for all races was 66 percent, which increased from 51 percent for the years 1975 to 1977. Comparing the two largest race populations, whites had a higher five-year relative survival rate for all cancers (68 percent) than African Americans (57 percent) between 1996 and 2002. By cancer sites for 1996 and 2002, prostate cancer had the highest five-year relative survival rate (100 percent) and pancreatic cancer the lowest survival rate (5 percent). Finally, the five-year relative survival rates for some of the more familiar cancers were breast, 89 percent; lung and bronchial area, 16 percent; and skin cancer, 92 percent.

Risk statistics: The major risk factors for developing cancer among all populations are tobacco use, obesity or overweight, physical inactivity, poor nutrition, infectious agents (for example, human immunodeficiency virus, or HIV, and human papillomavirus, or HPV), sun exposure, irregular or no cancer screenings, carcinogens (for example, asbestos and pollution), inherited genes, and age. Of the 559,650 cancer deaths expected in 2007, about 30 percent were estimated to be tobacco-related, and 33 percent related to poor diet, overweight or obesity, and no exercise. More than 1 million skin cancer diagnoses were expected in 2007; most of these could be prevented with proper sunscreen use. Occupational and environmental exposure to carcinogens account for about 6 percent of cancer deaths. Only about 5 percent of cancers are hereditary (meaning an altered gene that conveys a significant chance of developing cancer is passed from parent to child). Age is a main risk factor for cancer in general and closely associated with breast cancer (age fifty and older), prostate cancer (65 percent of cases diagnosed after age sixty-five), and colorectal cancer (age fifty and older).

In addition, poverty, lack of health insurance, geographic location, and cultural and language barriers are some of the main factors that prevent minorities from accessing health care services. Some 12 percent of whites, 18 percent of African Americans, and 35 percent of Hispanics and Latinos have no health insurance. In addition, 24 percent of African Americans and 23 percent of Hispanics and Latinos live below the poverty line compared with 11 percent of whites.

Perspective and prospects: The five-year relative survival rate for all races and all cancer sites increased 16 percent between 1977 and 1996. Improvements in prevention, earlier detection of cancer, and advances in cancer treatments helped lower incidence and deaths from cancer. Screenings are available for breast, cervix, colon, rectum, prostate, mouth, and skin cancers. About half of newly diagnosed cancer cases are found through a screening; the five-year relative survival rate for these cancers is about 86 percent. For example, breast cancer is the most frequently diagnosed cancer among women, but death rates have steadily decreased since 1990 largely because of earlier detection and improved treatments.

However, cancer is still the second leading cause of death, with 75 to 80 percent of cancer cases and deaths caused by lifestyles and behaviors, such as smoking and not exercising. Lung and bronchial cancer is the number-one cause of cancer death among all Americans. Men have the highest incidence and death rates from cancer, as do African American men and women. The American Cancer Society attributes higher death rates for minorities to lower socioeconomic status and poorer-quality health care than whites. Issues to address in the future to reduce the incidence of cancer and deaths from cancer are smoking cessation, eating right, exercising, and improved health care for all Americans.

Christine G. Holzmueller, B.L.A.

▶ **For Further Information**

American Cancer Society. *Cancer Facts and Figures 2008*. Atlanta: Author, 2008.

National Cancer Institute. *SEER Cancer Statistics Review, 1975-2004*. Bethesda, Md.: Author, 2006.

U.S. Department of Commerce. U.S. Census Bureau. *Profiles of General Demographic Characteristics: 2000 Census of Population and Housing*. Washington, D.C.: Author, 2001.

See also African Americans and cancer; Africans and cancer; Aging and cancer; Alcohol, alcoholism, and cancer; Ashkenazi Jews and cancer; Asian Americans and cancer; Cancer clusters; Developing nations and cancer; Elderly and cancer; Epidemiology of cancer; Ethnicity and cancer; Genetics of cancer; Insurance; Latinos/Hispanics and cancer; Native North Americans and cancer; Poverty and cancer; Psycho-oncology; Risks for cancer; Survival rates.

▶ Stem cell transplantation

Category: Procedures
Also known as: Bone marrow transplantation (BMT), peripheral blood stem cell transplantation (PBSCT), umbilical cord blood stem cell transplant

Definition: A stem cell transplant is the infusion of healthy stem cells into the body. Stem cells are early blood-forming cells, also referred to as hematopoietic cells, that grow and mature in the bone marrow but can circulate in blood as well. Hematopoietic cells are immature cells capable of dividing and developing into all blood cell types, including cells of the immune system. Stem cell transplantation involves replenishing hematopoietic cells following high-dose chemotherapy and radiation by infusing stem cells into the patient's body.

Stem cell transplants are classified based on the source of stem cells, including where they are collected. Stem cells may be collected from the bone marrow, peripheral blood, or umbilical cord. To represent the source of stem cells, the terms "bone marrow transplantation," "peripheral blood stem cell transplantation," and "umbilical cord transplantation" are utilized. There are important advantages and disadvantages associated with using stem cells from these different sources.

Stem cell transplants are also classified by who donates them. If stem cells come from the patient, they are termed autologous. They may also come from an identical twin, called syngeneic, or from someone other than the patient,

called allogeneic. Allogeneic stem cells are then further classified by whether the individual donating the stem cells is related or unrelated to the patient.

The best-known stem cell therapy is bone marrow transplantation (BMT). While most blood stem cells reside in bone marrow, a small number are present in the blood. These multipotent peripheral blood stem cells (PBSCs) can be used similarly to bone marrow stem cells to treat leukemia and other cancers. PBSC transplants are less invasive than BMT because PBSCs can be collected from blood, although the difficulty arises in collecting sufficient numbers to perform a transplant.

Stem cells from umbilical cords can also be used in stem cell transplants. Newborns no longer need umbilical cords, a tissue that has traditionally been discarded during birth. Recently it was realized that umbilical cord blood is rich in multipotent stem cells and thus useful against health problems similar to those treated with bone marrow and peripheral blood stem cells. An important advantage of umbilical cord stem cell transplants is reduced rejection, probably because the cells have not yet developed features that can be recognized by the recipient's immune system. Similarly, because umbilical cord blood lacks well-developed immune cells, there is less chance that transplanted cells will attack the recipient's body, a problem called graft-versus-host disease (GVHD).

Bone marrow or PBSC transplants can be either autologous or allogeneic. An autologous transplant requires infusion of the patient's own hematopoietic cells to restore the body's ability to make blood cells. In an autologous stem cell transplant, stem cells are collected from the patient's bone marrow or blood before high-dose chemotherapy is administered. An allogeneic stem cell transplant combines high-dose therapy with immunotherapy. High-dose therapy is administered to treat the cancer as in autologous transplants but is followed by an infusion of stem cells from a donor's blood or bone marrow. The donor cells supply the patient with new blood cells as well as a new immune system, which helps eliminate any residual disease, a process called immunotherapy. Allogeneic transplants can vary based on intensity. A stem cell transplant that utilizes high-dose chemotherapy combined with radiation to stop bone marrow function to allow donor cells to engraft, or grow, is referred to as myeloablative. A non-myeloablative transplant, sometimes called a minitransplant, uses lower radiation and chemotherapy doses to allow the bone marrow to function until donor cells replace the patient's marrow.

Cancers treated: Hematological (blood) malignancies such as chronic leukemias, lymphomas, and myelomas;

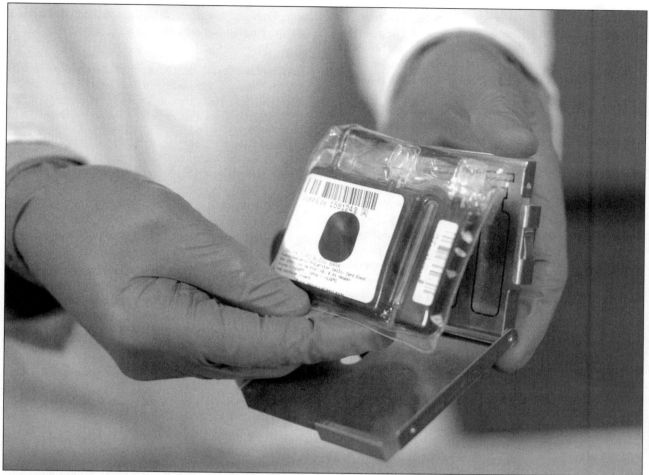

This sample of stem cells from a donated umbilical cord is to be used in research on cancers and blood diseases. (Tek Image/Photo Researchers, Inc.)

also cancers such as neuroblastoma and selected solid tumors

Why performed: High-dose chemotherapy is the best treatment for certain types of cancers. One of the major side effects of high-dose chemotherapy is the destruction of bone marrow stem cells. Stem cell transplants can help restore or replace these cells. Using stem cell transplants in cancer treatment makes it possible for patients to receive very high doses of chemotherapy and/or radiation therapy. In addition, immune factors in the transplanted cells may help destroy any cancer cells remaining in the bone marrow.

Patient preparation: Usually, patients remain at home until the time that the transplant is scheduled. During this time, the patient is often encouraged to build strength and maintain a healthy diet. An important part of patient preparation is researching insurance coverage in order to maxi-

mize care. If not nearby, the patient should make arrangements to stay closer to the hospital. It is also necessary to make arrangements for caregiving for up to four months. Caregiving will be needed for help with household chores, grocery shopping, food preparation, medications, central venous catheter care, monitoring of food and fluid intake, companionship, and transportation.

Steps of the procedure: Once donor stem cells become available, many tests and procedures are conducted to ensure that the patient is healthy enough to receive the transplant. A catheter, called a central line, is inserted intravenously in the chest area near the neck. The central line remains in place for duration of the treatment and will be used for the infusion of stem cells. The central line is also used to collect blood samples, administer chemotherapy, and provide blood transfusions and nutrition.

The next step in the procedure is called conditioning and occurs the week before the transplant. During conditioning, the patient undergoes chemotherapy and possibly radiation in order to destroy cancer cells and suppress the immune system to prevent the patient's body from rejecting transplanted stem cells. Conditioning may be conducted in the hospital or on an outpatient basis. Even if it is conducted as an outpatient, hospitalization for side effects may be required. Numerous side effects may occur, including nausea and vomiting, diarrhea, hair loss, mouth sores or ulcers, infections, bleeding, infertility, sterility, premature menopause, anemia, fatigue, cataracts, organ failure, and secondary cancers. Medications may help reduce side effects.

After the patient is treated with high-dose anticancer drugs and/or radiation during the conditioning process, stem cells are introduced into the patient's bloodstream intravenously. If the transplant is successful, then the stem cells will migrate into the patient's bone marrow and begin producing healthy cells.

After the procedure: After entering the bloodstream, stem cells travel to the bone marrow, where they produce new white blood cells, red blood cells, and platelets. This process occurs within about two to four weeks and is known as engraftment. Until the new stem cells begin functioning, transplant recipients will be at risk for complications such as infections and bleeding. Complete recovery of immune function can take several months for autologous transplant recipients and up to two years for patients receiving allogeneic or syngeneic transplants. Doctors conduct various tests to confirm that cancer cells have been eliminated and new blood cells are being produced. Bone marrow aspiration, the removal of a small sample of bone marrow, may be conducted to determine whether the transplant is working. Some patients can leave the hospital within three to five weeks, but others may require longer hospitalization.

Risks: Stem cell transplants are associated with many risks and complications, some potentially fatal. Complications that can arise include stem cell failure, organ and blood vessel damage, cataracts, secondary cancers, and death. Other major risks associated with stem cell transplants are increased susceptibility to infection and bleeding. Stem cell transplant recipients may experience short-term side effects such as nausea, vomiting, fatigue, loss of appetite, mouth sores, hair loss, and skin reactions.

A very serious complication known as graft-versus-host disease (GVHD) may occur when immune cells from the donor attack the patient's cells. Generally, the most commonly damaged organs in a GVHD response are the skin, liver, and intestines. GVHD is treated with steroids or other immunosuppressive agents.

Results: Stem cell transplants can extend the lives of transplant recipients and cause some cancers to go into remission. Many transplant recipients enjoy a good quality of life and are able to resume their normal activities. Side effects and transplant success vary among recipients, with some patients experiencing very few complications, while others experience numerous problems.

C. J. Walsh, Ph.D.

▶ **For Further Information**

Cant, A. J. *Practical Hematopoietic Stem Cell Transplantation.* New York: John Wiley & Sons, 2007.

Stewart, Susan K. *Bone Marrow and Blood Stem Cell Transplants: A Guide for Patients.* Highland Park, Ill.: BMT Newsletter, 2002.

_____. *Bone Marrow Transplants: A Book of Basics.* Highland Park, Ill.: BMT Newsletter, 1995.

▶ **Other Resources**

Cancer Backup
http://www.cancerbackup.org.uk

Mayo Clinic
http://www.mayoclinic.com

National Cancer Institute
http://www.cancer.gov

See also Blood cancers; Bone marrow aspiration and biopsy; Bone marrow transplantation (BMT); Childhood cancers; Graft-versus-host disease (GVHD); Hematologic oncology; Leukemias; Lymphomas; Multiple myeloma; Myeloma; Umbilical cord blood transplantation; Young adult cancers.

▶ # Stent therapy

Category: Procedures

Definition: Stent therapy is the placement of a rigid plastic or expandable metal tube to open a blocked airway, a stenosed blood vessel, the colon, or the esophagus.

Cancers treated: Lung cancer, esophageal cancer, colon cancer, gastric carcinoma, vena cava syndrome

Why performed: When cancerous growth constricts or occludes an airway or major blood vessel, a stent can be an important option if removal of tissue alone is not effective.

Stents can be used to strengthen a weakened airway or blood vessel.

Stents made by the Schneider company are used as an entro-endo prosthesis for colonic stenting and also for gastroduodenal stenting. Such stents are used for two purposes: preoperative relief of obstruction and palliative treatment. Stricture formation can be a major problem among patients who have an anastomosis between the esophagus and stomach or jejunum following subtotal or total gastrectomy.

Although first used as a simple adjunct to radiotherapy, stenting of the superior vena cava can be an effective first-line procedure for immediate relief in patients with malignancy. Growth of malignant lesions surrounding the vena cava often causes stenosis or obstruction of the vena cava and symptoms of venous congestion result, the so-called vena cava syndrome. Stent therapy can be effective to treat such cases and to improve quality of life for patients with advanced malignant disease.

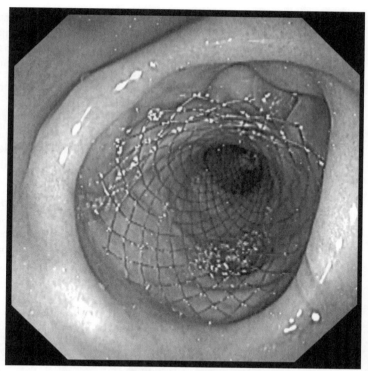

This metallic mesh stent holds open the duodenum of a woman with a pancreatic carcinoma. (David M. Martin, M.D./Photo Researchers, Inc.)

Patient preparation: Patients diagnosed with superior vena cava (SVC) syndrome caused by severe stenosis secondary to mediastinal malignancy may be referred for stent insertion. Most cases of SVC syndrome are attributable to an underlying primary thoracic malignancy, lymphoma, or metastatic tumor. Symptoms include venous congestion and edema in the upper half of the body. These symptoms are associated with dyspnea, dysphagia, and cognitive dysfunction as a result of cerebral venous hypertension. In these cases, patients must decide along with their doctors whether to undergo stent therapy or instead proceed with radiotherapy and chemotherapy.

Prior to SVC stent therapy, patients undergo a bilateral arm venography to determine the site and degree of stenosis. Patients in which the SVC is severely stenosed and the obstruction involves confluence of the brachiocephalic veins may be candidates for stent therapy. Patients with very extensive total occlusions involving both SVC and subclavin veins may be referred to other therapy. Short occlusions can also be treated with thrombolysis and then stented.

Steps of the procedure: For preoperative relief of colon obstruction, the stent is placed across the acute obstruction, with the intent of decompressing and cleaning the colon, which may allow a single-stage procedure. In studies of stent treatment of colon cancer, successful stent placement is usually achieved in lesions of the sigmoidal colon, descending colon, and transverse colon. The stent delivery system is quite flexible and can be maneuvered into the transverse colon if necessary.

Effective symptom relief can be achieved with an expandable stent. The rigid plastic tube stent, on the other hand, is shoved through the distal tumor with the use of a pusher-tube device. The newest type of stent treatment is the self-expanding metal stent, which was first modified for esophageal use in 1991. One example is the Schneider Wallstent, which can be mounted onto a delivery catheter where it is held in check with a sheath.

Percutaneous access can be achieved via the right common femoral vein for SVC stent insertion. An angled guidewire is inserted, dilatation is achieved with a small balloon, and a self-expanding stent (such as produced by Boston Scientific) is inserted.

After the procedure: The duration of palliative stent therapy, when placed properly, averages seventeen weeks and can extend as long as sixty-four weeks. Stent insertion is successful for most patients receiving treatment for SVC syndrome, with patients experiencing symptomatic relief within a few hours of the procedure. Few major complications are reported, and most patients are able to start radiotherapy the next day after stenting. During the procedure, heparin is administered to prevent clotting.

Risks: Insertion of a self-expanding metallic stent into an esophagojejunal anastomotic stricture can be a successful and uncomplicated therapy. The risks of palliative stent therapy for treatment of colon cancer include migration in the colon with colonic motility. Especially when the stent is placed at an anatomical curve such as the splenic flexure, these stents are much more likely to migrate. Migration in the treatment of colon cancer occurs in about 20 percent of cases. Perforation can occur, although this outcome is often the result of balloon dilation performed before the stent is placed.

Results: Stent therapy to treat SVC syndrome usually results in patients being able to undertake an ideal radiotherapy course, which maximizes the quality and length of their lives.

Michael R. King, Ph.D.

▶ **For Further Information**

Altman, Arnold J., ed. *Supportive Care of Children with Cancer: Current Therapy and Guidelines from the Children's Oncology Group.* Boston: Johns Hopkins University Press, 2004.

Boyiadzis, Michael, et al. *Hematology-Oncology Therapy.* New York: McGraw-Hill, 2006.

Talamonti, Mark S., and Sam G. Pappas, eds. *Liver-Directed Therapy for Primary and Metastatic Liver Tumors.* New York: Springer, 2001.

▶ **Other Resources**

Library of the National Medical Society
http://www.medical-library.org

See also Colorectal cancer; Esophageal cancer; Gastrointestinal cancers; Lung cancers; Palliative treatment; Superior vena cava syndrome.

▶ Stereotactic needle biopsy

Category: Procedures
Also known as: Breast biopsy, image-guided biopsy

Definition: Stereotactic needle biopsy is an outpatient procedure, usually performed by a radiologist or breast surgeon, in which a biopsy is obtained following imaging of a breast lesion using X rays. A stereo pair of the breast to be biopsied is generated using an X-ray tube at two slightly different positions and the images are combined with a computer, much the way the eyes capture the same object with two slightly different images that the brain then unites to form the final three-dimensional image.

Cancer diagnosed: Breast cancer

Why performed: Stereotactic needle biopsy is used to determine whether a suspicious lesion is cancer.

Patient preparation: Before stereotactic needle biopsy, sterile technique is observed, and a topical anesthetic is administered.

Steps of the procedure: The doctor obtains the informed consent of the patient and verifies the correct breast to be biopsied. A stereotable is used, whereby the patient is prone with the affected breast hanging down through an opening in the table. A stereo pair of the breast is generated and the relative shift in the lesion's position between the two X-ray pictures, called parallax shift, allows the computer to determine the exact location of the lesion in three dimensions.

The skin surface of the breast to be biopsied is cleaned with antiseptic and local anesthetic is given. The needle is inserted into the breast lesion through a tiny nick in the skin under computer guidance. Several samples of the lesion are then obtained. Adhesive skin closures (Steri-Strips) are applied to close the nick in the skin, and a sterile dressing is then applied. The samples are labeled and sent to pathology.

After the procedure: The patient is given discharge instructions, including to avoid the use of aspirin or ibuprofen and to instead take acetaminophen (Tylenol) for pain, to apply cold compresses over the biopsy site that evening to reduce swelling, to avoid exercise for seventy-two hours, and to monitor for any sign of fever or infection.

Risks: The risks of this procedure, although minimal, include infection, bleeding at the biopsy site, and bruising and/or scarring.

Results: The pathology results are usually available within forty-eight hours postprocedure, and if the lesion is benign, then no further workup is usually necessary. If the lesion is cancer, however, an open surgical biopsy may then be necessary to ensure complete removal.

Debra B. Kessler, M.D., Ph.D.

See also Acoustic neuromas; Astrocytomas; Biopsy; Cordotomy; Core needle biopsy; Craniopharyngiomas; Gamma Knife; Medulloblastomas; Microcalcifications; Needle biopsies; Needle localization; Radiation oncology; Stereotactic radiosurgery (SRS); Surgical biopsies.

▶ Stereotactic radiosurgery (SRS)

Category: Procedures
Also known as: Fractionated stereotactic radiosurgery

Definition: Stereotactic radiosurgery (SRS) is a noninvasive procedure that uses multiple beams of radiation to treat a selected target, such as a brain tumor or a difficult-to-reach tumor in the chest or abdomen. The radiation comes from either cobalt or a linear accelerator.

Cancers treated: Benign and malignant brain tumors, acoustic neuroma, metastases, head and neck cancers, lung cancer, pancreatic cancer, gynecological cancers, liver cancer, spinal cancer, other cancers that are difficult to reach

Why performed: SRS is the most precise in tumor targeting of the radiation therapy interventions. While stereotactic radiosurgery is noninvasive and similar to radiation therapy, it is so accurate that it is considered surgical in nature. Most often, SRS is used to reach tumors that are not candidates for surgery or near structures that could be damaged by a surgical approach. SRS provides the option for an outpatient procedure rather than a traditional surgery that may require several days or weeks of hospitalization. In some instances, SRS may be used when patients have had previous radiation.

Patient preparation: Stereotactic radiosurgery preparation depends on the site of the tumor and the type of equipment used. The traditional approach to SRS in the head uses a lightweight halo frame attached to the skull with four small screws and cobalt radiation beams for treatment. Another option for SRS is a robotically controlled linear accelerator that delivers multiple beams and uses a variety of techniques to hold the patient still. A facial mask or a body frame is fitted for each patient when the robotically controlled linear accelerator is used. Since treatments may last thirty minutes to two hours, positioning devices help the patient lie still during the treatment.

A computed tomography (CT) scan with contrast dye, a magnetic resonance imaging (MRI) scan, or an angiogram, all very accurate radiology procedures, may be done

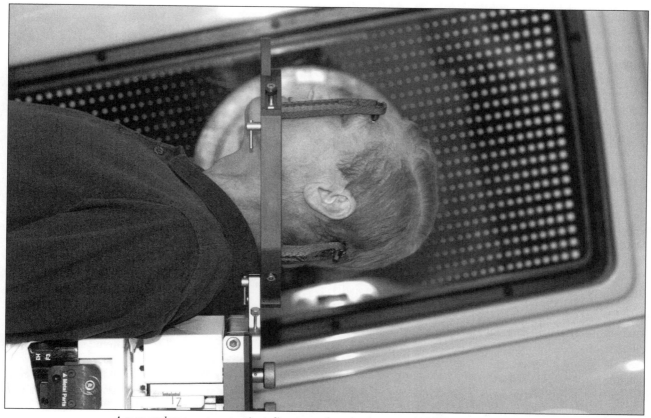

A man undergoes stereotactic radiosurgery for a brain tumor. (AP/Wide World Photos)

to determine the size and location of the tumor or blood vessels to be treated. If treatment is in the head, then a neurosurgeon will work with a radiation oncologist to review the images and other patient data to determine the site to be treated. Other physician specialists may be involved in planning the SRS treatment for other body sites along with the radiation oncologist. Information is loaded into a treatment-planning computer that calculates how much radiation the patient is to receive and precisely where to direct the beams. The patient may receive a mild drug to be more comfortable during the treatment.

Steps of the procedure: For a stereotactic radiosurgery treatment of the head using a cobalt radiation source, the patient lies down on the treatment table and the halo head frame is attached to the equipment, securing the position of the head to prevent movement that might cause the radiation beams to stray onto normal tissue. Up to 201 separate beams may be used to shape the treatment area. The treatment may last two to forty-five minutes during the session. There is no pain during the treatment.

For a stereotactic radiosurgery treatment using a robotically controlled linear accelerator, the patient lies down on the treatment table and the premade positioning devices are adjusted to hold the patient in one position for the treatment. One beam of radiation is used as the linear accelerator moves around the patient in a circle to shape the treatment area. A single treatment or a daily treatment of one or two sessions for five or more days may be used.

Regardless of equipment, the patient is awake and can talk with the radiation therapy staff using an intercom. The staff watches the patient on closed-circuit television. The patient may hear noises from the equipment as adjustments of the beam are made to move around the tumor.

After the procedure: If a head frame was used, then it is removed. Depending on the procedure and the site treated, the patient may be able to go home in just a few hours or may stay overnight in the hospital. The patient may need to lie still for a while after the procedure. The doctor will provide information about when the patient may resume normal activities, but it is usually in just a few days. It is safe for patients to be around others, including children and pregnant women, because no radiation is in the body.

Risks: Side effects depend on the site treated but may include headache, swelling as the tumor cells die, minor swelling where the head frame was attached to the skin, nausea, skin irritation, diarrhea, or bladder problems. There is a slight chance of paralysis or other deficits, such as weakness or difficulty with speech or hearing, when the brain or spine receives radiation.

Results: Stereotactic radiosurgery does not work immediately but causes cell death over time. The tumor decreases in size over time based on the type of tumor and its growth rate before treatment. Malignant tumors and metastatic tumors usually respond more rapidly because their growth rate is faster. The patient sees the physician frequently to monitor the tumor destruction and to be sure that side effects are not developing as the cells die.

Patricia Stanfill Edens, R.N., Ph.D., FACHE

▶ **For Further Information**

Le, Q. T., B. W. Loo, A. Ho, et al. "Results of a Phase I Dose-Escalation Study Using Single-Fraction Stereotactic Radiotherapy for Lung Tumors." *Journal of Thoracic Oncology* 1, no. 8 (October, 2006): 802-809.

National Cancer Institute. *Radiation Therapy and You: A Guide to Self-Help During Cancer Treatment.* NIH Publication 01-2227. Bethesda, Md.: National Institutes of Health, 2001. Also available at http://www.cancer.gov.

Slotman, B. J., T. D. Solberg, and D. Verellen. *Extracranial Stereotactic Radiotherapy and Radiosurgery.* New York: Taylor and Francis, 2006.

▶ **Other Resources**

American Cancer Society
http://www.cancer.org

International Radiosurgery Association
http://www.irsa.org

See also Acoustic neuromas; Afterloading radiation therapy; Astrocytomas; Cobalt 60 radiation; Craniopharyngiomas; Gamma Knife; Linear accelerator; Medulloblastomas; Radiation oncology; Radiation therapies; Stereotactic needle biopsy.

▶ Sterility

Category: Diseases, symptoms, and conditions
Also known as: Intractable infertility, azoospermia, menopause

Related condition: Infertility

Definition: Sterility is the inability to achieve pregnancy due to the absence of viable sperm in the testicles (azoospermia) or an absence of mature, viable eggs in the ovaries (menopause). Sterility is often diagnosed when conception does not occur even after assisted reproductive technology treatments. Sterility can be caused by some cancer treatments.

Risk factors: The risk of sterility depends on the type of cancer and its location, the specific cancer treatment, and the use of any fertility-preservation or -sparing procedures before or during treatment. The risk of sterility is also affected by the person's age, general health, and pretreatment fertility status.

Etiology and the disease process: Sterility can be caused by chemotherapy, especially alkylating agents; high doses of radiation to the entire body, cranium, abdomen, or pelvis; and surgical treatments that remove or damage reproductive structures.

Incidence: The occurrence of sterility is highly variable based on patient- and treatment-related factors. The frequency of sterility across all cancer patients is unknown.

Symptoms: Sterility is not often detected until a person attempts to conceive. Azoospermia is not evident without medical screening, but the inability to ejaculate or produce semen during ejaculation may be a symptom of sterility. The absence or cessation of menstruation is symptomatic of menopause.

Screening and diagnosis: Male sterility is diagnosed through semen analysis and sometimes testicular biopsy to assess the presence of sperm. Female sterility is diagnosed by assessing hormone levels and an ultrasound examination for ovulation, usually after ovulation induction with fertility medications.

Treatment and therapy: There are no known treatments for sterility due to azoospermia or menopause. Sterility related to cancer treatments, such as surgery and chemotherapy, is often of less concern than addressing the cancer itself.

Prognosis, prevention, and outcomes: It is advised that cancer patients consider fertility-preservation or -sparing options before treatment and consult a fertility specialist. Before treatment, men can have healthy sperm frozen for future use. Researchers are testing whether frozen testicular tissue or sperm stem cells transplanted back into the testicles can restore sperm production. Women can have their eggs collected and fertilized in the laboratory, with the resulting embryos frozen for future use. The possibility of freezing unfertilized eggs for later use or ovarian tissue for transplantation is being researched. Patients may benefit from fertility-sparing options during treatment, which include protecting reproductive organs from radiation, using conservative surgery when possible, and engaging in experimental hormonal therapy.

Amanda McQuade, Ph.D.

See also Alkylating agents in chemotherapy; Amenorrhea; Chemotherapy; Fertility issues; Infertility and cancer; Klinefelter syndrome and cancer; Pregnancy and cancer; Self-image and body image.

▶ Stomach cancers

Category: Diseases, symptoms, and conditions
Also known as: Gastric cancer, esophageal cancer, adenocarcinoma

Related conditions: Peptic ulcers, gastritis, *Helicobacter pylori* infection, lymphoma, adenomatous polyps, pernicious anemia

Definition: Stomach cancers are malignant tumors of the stomach, about 95 percent of which are adenocarcinomas that develop from the glandular epithelial cells of the innermost lining of the stomach (mucosa). Others are stomach lymphoma (about 4 percent of stomach cancers), carcinoid tumors of the hormone-producing cells (3 percent), and rare gastrointestinal stromal tumors (GISTs) of the interstitial cells of Cajal (part of the autonomic nervous system controlling stomach muscle movement).

Risk factors: Long-term infection with the bacterium *Helicobacter pylori* causes inflammation that can cause precancerous changes in the stomach lining. Age and gender are also risk factors, because most people who develop stomach cancer are older than the age of fifty, and men develop stomach cancers at double the rate of women. Familial cancer syndromes, inherited disorders, and having a parent or sibling with the disease increase the risk of stomach cancer. Pernicious anemia (inability to absorb vitamin B_{12}), obesity, and having type A blood are also risk factors.

Rates of stomach cancer, especially at the esophagus-stomach junction, are doubled in cigarette smokers. High alcohol intake contributes to increased risk. A diet high in foods preserved by smoking, salting, or pickling; large amounts of red meat, particularly if barbecued or well-done; and foods that contain nitrites and nitrates (that can form N-nitroso carcinogens), such as bacon, ham, hot dogs, and processed meats, increase the risk.

People with part of their stomach and pyloric valve removed as a treatment for peptic ulcers also are at increased risk. After stomach surgery, bile or pancreatic juices can accumulate, causing gastritis. The amount of protective stomach acid also decreases while nitrite-producing bacteria may increase, leading to stomach cancer. The risk is greatest for the first twenty years after the initial surgery.

Small growths (polyps) in the stomach lining, especially adenomatous polyps, may also be precancerous.

Etiology and the disease process: Most stomach cancers start in the innermost mucosal layer of the stomach, where stomach acid and digestive enzymes are made, and develop slowly over many years. Before a true cancer develops, precancerous changes occur in the lining of the stomach, such as atrophic gastritis, a condition in which the acid-producing glands are slowly destroyed. Low acid levels prevent cancer-causing toxins from being properly broken down or flushed out of the stomach. Stomach cancers can spread in different ways: through the wall of the stomach to invade nearby organs; through the bloodstream to the lungs, bones, and ovaries; or to the lymph vessels and lymph nodes slowly or aggressively. Carcinoid tumors grow less quickly and metastasize less frequently.

Incidence: In the United States, about 21, 260 people were expected to be diagnosed with stomach cancer in 2007, and 11,210 were expected to die of it. The rate of incidence

of stomach cancer is higher in men older than the age of forty. Hispanics, Native Americans, Asian Americans, and African Americans are roughly twice as likely to develop gastric cancer as whites. The incidence of stomach cancer has declined by 50 percent in the United States and Western Europe since the 1930's, probably because of better, more balanced diets; the frequent use of antibiotics that reduce *H. pylori* and childhood infections; and refrigeration, which reduces nitrate-producing bacteria in food.

The disease remains a serious problem in many parts of the world, however, because of infection with *H. pylori* and diets high in meat or smoked, cured, heavily salted, or pickled foods. Stomach cancer is therefore more common in Japan, Korea, parts of Eastern Europe, and Latin America. Stomach cancer incidence rates decrease in Chinese who have immigrated to the United States, but not if they maintain their traditional diet. Gastric cancer affects all races, but unexplained geographic and cultural differences in incidence occur, with higher mortality in Japan, Chile, Austria, and Iceland.

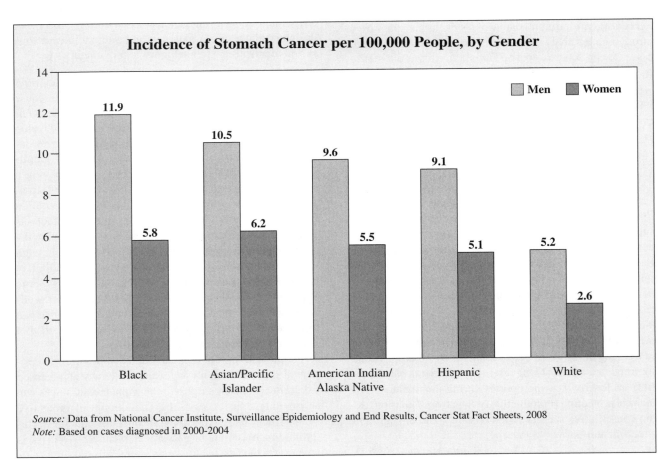

Incidence of Stomach Cancer per 100,000 People, by Gender

	Men	Women
Black	11.9	5.8
Asian/Pacific Islander	10.5	6.2
American Indian/Alaska Native	9.6	5.5
Hispanic	9.1	5.1
White	5.2	2.6

Source: Data from National Cancer Institute, Surveillance Epidemiology and End Results, Cancer Stat Fact Sheets, 2008
Note: Based on cases diagnosed in 2000-2004

Symptoms: Stomach cancer rarely produces initial symptoms and is usually detected in advanced stages. Depending on their location in the stomach, cancers may have different symptoms and outcomes. One early sign is microscopic internal bleeding, which is detected only by tests that check the stool for blood. Other early symptoms are heartburn and abdominal pain, which can be mistaken for other common problems such as peptic ulcers.

Advanced cases produce discomfort in the upper or middle region of the abdomen that may not be relieved by food or antacids; abdominal discomfort aggravated by eating; chronic abdominal pain; swelling; black, tarry stools; indigestion; nausea; vomiting blood; vomiting after meals; weakness and fatigue; unintended weight loss; and a full feeling after meals, even when eating less than normal.

Screening and diagnosis: Early diagnosis of stomach cancer is hindered by its initial vague symptoms; the disease can easily be mistaken for less serious problems such as a stomach virus or heartburn. Diagnosis includes a complete medical history and physical examination, barium X rays of the gastrointestinal tract with fluoroscopy showing changes, gastroscopy with fiber-optic endoscopy that helps rule out other diffuse gastric mucosal abnormalities, photography with a fiber-optic endoscope that provides a permanent record of gastric lesions, and biopsy for microscopic examination to confirm cancer when abnormal cells are discovered.

Screening of serum sample glycoprotein antigens produced by cancer cells reveals undetected cancer and monitors established cancer.

Polymerase chain reaction (PCR) kits, which amplify and detect altered deoxyribonucleic acid (DNA) base sequences in minute samples of cells, facilitate the diagnosis of cancer types that are difficult to categorize by conventional pathology.

Treatment and therapy: Stomach cancer is treatable if caught early. Less than one in five stomach cancers are diagnosed before spreading outside the stomach. Pain is often relieved by food or acid-buffering medications in the early stages. The kind of treatment for stomach cancer depends on the location of the cancer, how advanced it is, and the patient's overall health and personal preferences. The most common treatment for stomach cancer is surgery.

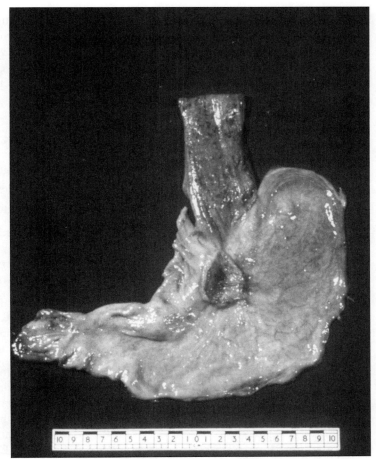

A section of a stomach showing a cancerous tumor (triangular shaped area). (St. Bartholomew's Hospital/Photo Researchers, Inc.)

Depending on the extent of the cancer, the doctor may remove part of the stomach (via subtotal, or partial, gastrectomy) or all of the stomach (via total gastrectomy) as well as surrounding tissue and lymph nodes. After subtotal gastrectomy, the remaining part of the stomach is connected to the esophagus and small intestine. For total gastrectomy, the esophagus is connected directly to the small intestine.

Prognosis and treatment for stomach lymphoma depend on the extent of aggressiveness. Individuals who have *H. pylori*-associated gastric lymphomas may be cured by antibiotic therapy that eliminates the bacteria. In some advanced cases, a laser beam directed through an endoscope can vaporize most of the tumor without an operation.

Radiation therapy, chemotherapy, or a combination of both is used to completely destroy all remaining cancer cells after surgery.

Prognosis, prevention, and outcomes: The prognosis for stomach cancer depends on the stage of the disease at the time of diagnosis and is dim if the cancer has grown deeper into layers of the stomach or has spread to the lymph nodes. The general five-year survival rate for stomach cancer is about 20 percent because it is often detected at an advanced stage but rises to 60 percent when the disease is diagnosed early. A 2006 study suggested that chemotherapy before and after surgery improves outcomes for some people.

It is estimated that diet could prevent 70 percent of stomach cancers in 1 million global instances of the disease. To help prevent cancer, people should eat plenty of fresh fruits and vegetables with antioxidant vitamins and polyphenols, especially those high in vitamin C and beta-carotene and those that are red, deep green, orange, or deep yellow—such as mango, cantaloupe, strawberries, carrots, tomatoes, red bell peppers, Swiss chard, bok choy, spinach, acorn and butternut squash, and sweet potatoes—and vegetables from the cabbage family, including broccoli, brussels sprouts, and cauliflower. People following the diet should avoid nitrites and nitrates in processed and cured meats; consume more fish or poultry instead of red meat; limit smoked, pickled, and heavily salted foods; avoid smoking; and limit or avoid alcohol consumption.

Samuel V. A. Kisseadoo, Ph.D.

▶ **For Further Information**

Beers, Mark H., ed. *The Merck Manual of Medical Information.* 2d home ed. Whitehouse Station, N.J.: Merck Research Laboratories, 2003.

King, R. J. B. *Cancer Biology.* 2d ed. New York: Prentice Hall, 2000.

Shah, Manish A. Dx/Rx. *Upper Gastrointestinal Malignancies: Cancers of the Stomach and Esophagus.* Sudbury, Mass.: Jones and Bartlett, 2006.

▶ **Other Resources**

American Cancer Society
Detailed Guide: Stomach Cancer
    http://www.cancer.org/docroot/CRI/content/
    CRI_2_4_1X_What_is_stomach_cancer_40.asp

National Cancer Institute
Stomach (Gastric) Cancer
    http://www.cancer.gov/cancertopics/types/stomach/

See also Achlorhydria; Adenocarcinomas; Adenomatous polyps; Bacteria as causes of cancer; Barium swallow; Carcinomatous meningitis; Colon polyps; Diarrhea; Elderly and cancer; Esophageal cancer; Fiber; Fruits; Gas-

trointestinal cancers; Gastrointestinal complications of cancer treatment; Gastrointestinal stromal tumors (GISTs); *Helicobacter pylori*; Hereditary diffuse gastric cancer; Krukenberg tumors; Nausea and vomiting; Obesity-associated cancers; Polyps; Small intestine cancer.

▶ **Stomatitis**

Category: Diseases, symptoms, and conditions
Also known as: Mucositis

Related condition: Esophagitis

Definition: Stomatitis is a general term used to describe injury or inflammation to the tissues of the mouth such as the gums, tongue, roof or floor of the mouth, lips, and cheeks.

Risk factors: This inflammation can be caused by many things, such as poor oral hygiene, medications, infections, or poorly fitted dentures. Many cancer treatments, such as chemotherapy drugs and radiation, can cause stomatitis.

Etiology and the disease process: Chemotherapy and radiation treatments stop the growth of cancer cells and all other rapidly dividing cells. As the cells in the lining of the mouth also divide rapidly, some of the treatments for cancer make it difficult for the lining of the mouth to repair itself. Cancer treatments can also weaken the immune system and make it easier for a person to develop an infection.

Incidence: Stomatitis occurs in approximately 40 percent of the patients receiving chemotherapy and cancer treatments, such as radiation to the head and neck. Stomatitis can affect a patient's cancer treatment and quality of life.

Symptoms: The symptoms of stomatitis can vary depending on the causes. Generally, redness, swelling, and pain in the mouth are common. Ulcers can develop and make eating and drinking difficult. This can lead to dehydration and weight loss. Bleeding in the mouth, fever, and irritability can also occur.

Screening and diagnosis: Stomatitis can be diagnosed by a careful examination of the patient's mouth, tongue, and lips. A blood test may be done to detect infection. Sometimes a scraping of the lining of the mouth may be sent to the laboratory to identify a specific organism causing the infection.

Treatment and therapy: Treatment is also based on the cause of stomatitis. The most important part of treatment is to keep the mouth and teeth clean. A soft toothbrush and mild toothpaste can be used, brushing carefully to prevent any further damage to the gums. Patients should consume soft foods and liquids and avoid acidic foods and alcohol-based mouthwashes. Pain medicine in the form of a topical anesthetic such as lidocaine gel, systemic inflammatory or narcotic pain medications, or both may also be used.

Prognosis, prevention, and outcomes: One way to prevent or lessen the severity of stomatitis is to find and treat oral problems before cancer treatment begins. In addition, eating a well-balanced diet can help the body tolerate the stress of treatment and fight infection. Keeping the mouth and teeth clean and having regular dental checkups are also important.

Michelle Kasprzak, R.N., B.S.N., O.C.N.

See also Chemotherapy; Cobalt 60 radiation; Dry mouth; Esophagitis; Fever; Herpes simplex virus; Infection and sepsis; Mucositis; Side effects; Stress management; Weight loss.

▶ Stress management

Category: Social and personal issues

Definition: Stress management reduces and controls tensions rising from emotional and physical stress. Emotional stress can occur in response to situations that seem out of control or difficult to manage, such as a diagnosis of or treatment for cancer. Physical stress, such as nausea, vomiting, and hair loss occurring as side effects of chemotherapy, can lead to emotional distress.

Physiology: The physiology of stress is oftened referred to as the "fight-or-flight response." Faced with an immediate physical threat, the body gears up for physical confrontation or rapid retreat with the following physiological responses:
- Neurotransmitters are released by the sympathetic nervous system
- Catecholamines and epinephrine surge, increasing body metabolism
- Heart and breathing rates increase
- Blood pressure rises
- Blood-clotting increases
- Digestive activities are suspended

Stress hormones: Catecholamines, epinephrine, and cortisol—the "stress hormones"—prepare the heart to beat harder and faster, cause the lungs to inhale more oxygen, and tense muscles in preparation for fight or flight. The

blood levels of these hormones remain elevated for hours and have lingering effects on the body. Cortisol, a steroid hormone, stays at high levels for several hours and is particularly troublesome. One effect of this hormone is to reduce the immune response (which is why hydrocortisone creams can address the itchy symptoms of skin rashes and inflammations; hence, it is important not to use these creams on infections, which may become worse in the presence of cortisol). People who are chronically or often stressed therefore are likely to have suppressed immune systems, resulting in more infections like colds or sinus infections.

Chronic stress: Problems arise when the stress response occurs in reaction to emotional problems, such as concerns over chronic illnesses, financial difficulties, criticism, traffic jams, or deadlines. Repetitive and prolonged stress leads to physical problems, including immune system dysfunction, digestive tract problems such as diarrhea or constipation, and cardiovascular difficulties including palpitations (heart pounding) or irregular heartbeats. Sleep disturbances such as insomnia or lack of restful sleep can occur. Increased blood clotting contributes to heart attacks and strokes. Hence, stress feeds on itself, creating problems that in turn place more stress on human physiology.

One of the greatest stressors human beings face is that of a chronic illness, such as cancer. Not only does the diagnosis of cancer increase stress, but also the ongoing decisions, treatments, medical bills, insurance paperwork, and the simple coping with normal stresses of daily life escalate in the face of a cancer diagnosis and treatment. Moreover, the plethora of treatment options for different types of cancer has made it possible to live with many types of cancer for months or years. The ability of medical pharmacology and technology to increase the life span, while positive overall, also prolongs the period of time patients must cope with their disease, in turn increasing stress.

Stress reduction: Any chronic and repetitive stress must be recognized and met with stress reduction methods. Managing stress is as important for healthy people as it is for those facing cancer: Most people think of calming situations such as watching the sun set, curling up with an interesting book, or meditating. Although these relaxing situations may be good for some, others may need a thrilling situation, like a vigorous aerobic workout or a competitive game of tennis.

Sometimes seeking balance is a good approach. A job that requires a great deal of thinking, decision making, and problem solving may be counterweighted by physical activity, such as a walking to work or a basketball game after work. Those with physical jobs, on the other hand, may re-

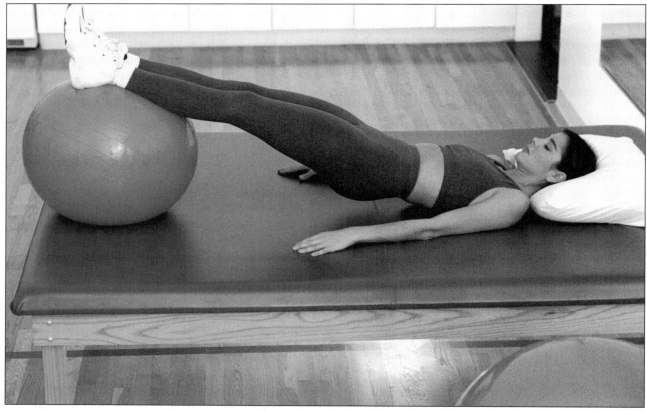

Exercise may help some people reduce stress. (PhotoDisc)

duce their stress by engaging in more intellectual pursuits, such as playing cards or learning a foreign language. Managing stress improves not only the immune system but also one's quality of life and may well help protect against the physiological vulnerabilities that open the door to precancerous and cancerous conditions.

For those diagnosed with cancer, stress management is equally if not more important: Social support systems, like meeting with friends or associating with groups that have interests similar to one's own, can help reduce stress and anxiety. Helpful support groups are usually available in most communities. Patients are also advised to seek advice from their personal health care provider, who is in the best position to offer it.

In one study, volunteers who wrote about "the most stressful event they had ever undergone" for twenty minutes on three consecutive days showed significant improvement compared with those who spent the same amount of time writing about neutral topics. Researchers theorize that writing may help patients make sense of what has happened to them and come to terms with its impact, thus reducing stress.

Making an effort to maintain a healthy diet can also reduce stress. Although some medical situations, such as postchemotherapy nausea and vomiting, may require vitamin supplementation and management with other medications, the best way to obtain necessary minerals and vitamins during most stressful episodes is via fresh, whole fruits and vegetables. Minerals and vitamins in this natural state are more bioavailable, meaning they are more readily absorbed and utilized by the body than supplements in pill or powder forms.

Fortunately, a number of medications can relieve pain, alleviate nausea, and lessen anxiety. Music, deep breathing, caring for pets, and allowing oneself to engage in enjoyable activities with family and friends are some other well-known stress relievers. Many cancer patients report that they discover a new appreciation for life and do not delay activities they find rewarding. Among the best stress relievers for cancer patients is the sense of well-being and purpose friends and family can bring by simply visiting and reminding patients of their value as a friend and human being.

Richard P. Capriccioso, M.D.

► For Further Information

Hales, D. *An Invitation to Health.* 10th ed. Belmont, Calif.: Wadsworth/Thomson Learning, 2003.

Sobel, D. S., and R. E. Ornstein. *The Healthy Mind, Healthy Body Handbook.* New York: Time Life Medical-Time Warner, 1996.

Whitney, E., and F. Sizer. *Nutrition: Concepts and Controversies.* 9th ed. St. Paul, Minn.: West, 2003.

► Other Resources

American Institute of Stress
http://www.stress.org

MedlinePlus
Stress Management
http://www.nlm.nih.gov/medlineplus/ency/article/001942.htm

See also Aids and devices for cancer patients; Anxiety; Caregivers and caregiving; Complementary and alternative therapies; Counseling for cancer patients and survivors; Depression; Diarrhea; Exercise and cancer; Financial issues; Infection and sepsis; Insurance; Journaling; Living with cancer; Nausea and vomiting; Nutrition and cancer prevention; Nutrition and cancer treatment; Personality and cancer; Prayer and cancer support; Psychooncology; Relationships; Self-image and body image; Support groups.

► Sunlamps

Category: Carcinogens and suspected carcinogens
RoC status: Known human carcinogen since 2000
Also known as: Ultraviolet radiation (UVR), ultraviolet A (UVA), ultraviolet B (UVB), artificial ultraviolet radiation, nonsolar ultraviolet radiation

Related cancers: Skin cancer, squamous cell carcinoma, basal cell carcinoma, nonmalignant melanoma, malignant melanoma, intraocular melanoma

Definition: Sunlamps are lamps that produce ultraviolet radiation.

Exposure routes: Through skin

Where found: Sunlamps, sunbeds, tanning salons, tanning booths, home tanning lamps

At risk: People who use artificial sources of ultraviolet radiation such as sunlamps or tanning salons

Etiology and symptoms of associated cancers: Sunlamps or other artificial sources of ultraviolet radiation are used primarily for cosmetic reasons, such as to obtain a suntan, as well as for treatment of certain medical conditions. Approximately 25 million people in the United States use sunbeds each year, with 1 to 2 million people visiting tanning facilities as often as one hundred times a year. Teenagers and young adults, usually female, use sunlamps most often.

Epidemiological studies report that exposure to sunlamps increases the risk of skin cancer. A person's risk of skin cancer is related to lifetime exposure to ultraviolet (UV) radiation, with greater incidence observed with increasing duration of exposure, especially in those using sunlamps before the age of thirty and in those who readily sunburn. Ultraviolet radiation from sunlamps can affect all skin types, but people with fair skin that freckles or burns easily, a skin type generally associated with red or blond hair and light-colored eyes, are at greater risk.

Sunlamps increase the risk of skin cancer because they involve exposure to ultraviolet radiation. Although ultraviolet radiation emissions vary substantially according to the device, the radiation exposure can be similar to or greater than that from the sun. Depending on the frequency of use, commonly used sunlamps deliver several times the annual ultraviolet A dose. Newer indoor tanning units may emit ultraviolet A and ultraviolet B radiation at levels as much as fifteen times greater than solar ultraviolet radiation. Ultraviolet radiation damages deoxyribonucleic acid (DNA) in skin cells, which can lead to skin cancer.

Skin cancers that have been associated with use of a sunlamp include basal and squamous cell carcinomas as well as melanoma. Most basal cell and squamous cell skin cancers can be cured if found and treated early. Both basal and squamous cell skin cancers occur on parts of the skin frequently exposed to the sun, such as the face. Basal cell carcinoma grows slowly and rarely spreads to other parts of the body. Squamous cell carcinoma is more aggressive and sometimes spreads to lymph nodes and organs inside the body.

Although much less prevalent than other types of skin cancer, melanoma is the most serious. Melanoma occurs in pigment cells in the skin called melanocytes. When melanoma becomes cancerous, it can become invasive and spread to other parts of the body. When melanoma starts in the skin, it is called cutaneous melanoma. Melanoma may also occur in the eye and is then called ocular melanoma or intraocular melanoma.

Not all skin cancers look the same, but a change on the skin is the most common sign of skin cancer. Some skin changes that may occur include a new growth, a sore that does not heal, a change in an existing growth, or red or brown spots that are rough, dry, and scaly. Melanoma usually begins in a mole, with the first symptom typically a change in size, shape, or color of an existing mole or the appearance of a new mole. Melanomas vary in their appearance, but most melanomas have a black or blue-black area and usually appear abnormal or "ugly looking."

History: Sunlamps have been used for many years to treat a range of skin conditions, vitamin D deficiency, and neonatal jaundice. Sunlamps have also been used increasingly for cosmetic tanning in commercial salons or at home. Ultraviolet emissions from artificial tanning devices have changed over time. Before the mid-1970's, sunlamps were primarily used in the home, except for medical use, and mostly emitted ultraviolet B and with a small amount of ultraviolet C. In the early 1980's sunlamps that emitted ultraviolet A radiation were developed and used mainly at commercial tanning salons. Sunlamps in use in the twenty-first century emit mostly ultrlaviolet A radiation and some ultraviolet B radiation.

The U.S. Food and Drug Administration (FDA) Center for Devices and Radiological Health developed regulations concerning ultraviolet lamps in sunlamps that specify requirements for performance, protective eyewear, and labeling, and require tanning salons to post warnings about the dangers associated with exposure to artificial ultraviolet radiation. The American Medical Association, the American Academy of Dermatologists, and the Centers for Disease Control and Prevention have all issued statements discouraging the use of sunlamps for nonmedical purposes.

Catherine J. Walsh, Ph.D.

▶ For Further Information

Chen, Y. T., et al. "Sunlamp Use and the Risk of Cutaneous Malignant Melanoma: A Population-Based Case-Control Study in Connecticut, USA." *International Journal of Epidemiology* 27 (1998): 759-765.

Gallagher, R. P., J. J. Spinelli, and T. K. Lee. "Tanning Beds, Sunlamps, and Risk of Cutaneous Malignant Melanoma." *Cancer Epidemiology Biomarkers and Prevention* 14, no. 3 (2005): 562-566.

Swerdlow, A. J., et al. "Fluorescent Lights, Ultraviolet Lamps, and Risk of Cutaneous Melanoma." *British Medical Journal* 297 (1988): 647-650.

U.S. Department of Health and Human Services, Public Health Service, National Toxicology Program. *Eleventh Report on Carcinogens*. Research Triangle Park, N.C.: Author, 2005.

▶ Other Resources

American Academy of Dermatology
http://www.aad.org

Centers for Disease Control and Prevention
Skin Cancer
http://www.cdc.gov/cancer/skin/

National Cancer Institute
What You Need to Know About Skin Cancer
http://www.cancer.gov/cancertopics/wyntk/skin

National Toxicology Program
FDA Radiological Health Program
http://www.fda.gov/cdrh/radhealth/products/
sunlamps.html

See also Basal cell carcinomas; Electromagnetic radiation; Melanomas; Moles; Skin cancers; Squamous cell carcinomas; Ultraviolet radiation and related exposures; Young adult cancers.

▶ Sun's soup

Category: Lifestyle and prevention; complementary and alternative therapies
Also known as: Selected Vegetables (SV)

Definition: Sun's soup is a nutritional supplement consisting of plant nutrients containing phytochemicals believed to enhance immune properties and disease prevention.

Cancers treated or prevented: Cancerous tumors; effectiveness not scientifically verified

Delivery routes: Oral by diet

How this agent works: Sun's soup is believed to boost the immune system, although how it works and whether it is effective are considered unverified scientifically.

In the late 1980's, Dr. Alexander Shihkaung Sun (1939-2006), a Taiwanese American biochemist with a Ph.D. from the University of California, Berkeley, investigated the use of specific foodstuffs, mainly shiitake mushrooms, mung beans, and Chinese herbs associated with reinforcing immune systems, to aid his mother after she became ill with lung cancer. Affiliated professionally with Mount Sinai Medical Center and the Yale University School of Medicine, Sun chose ingredients with phytochemicals that Asian physicians had incorporated into treatments.

Sun freeze-dried his concoction, which he initially called Selected Vegetables (SV), as a supplement to medical treatments to extend the life spans of patients with cancerous tumors. In the early 1990's, he conducted trials with mice to assess the impact of SV on tumors. He then tested SV in humans, focusing on patients diagnosed with non-small-cell lung cancer, who orally consumed one ounce of hydrated SV powder daily and a control group who did not ingest SV. Everyone in the trial simultaneously received chemotherapy, radiation, or surgery. Sun revised his recipe for a frozen version, which included soy and legumes, and conducted a second clinical study for sixty months in which patients ate ten ounces of Sun's soup every day.

Applying for a U.S. patent, Sun sought protection of his recipe to mitigate cancerous conditions and received a patent on August 1, 1995. Sun, who established the Connecticut Institute for Aging and Cancer, summarized his results with colleagues in two *Nutrition and Cancer* articles published in 1999 and 2001. He hypothesized that some aspect of SV battled cancer and extended lives but did not address or control for the impact of chemotherapy. Sun's testing was flawed because of the limited number of subjects, most of whom volunteered, knowing about his soup's anticancer possibilities and not representing a random test group. Also, the freeze-dried powder and frozen soup thawed for consumption in the two trials differed chemically. Researchers acknowledged that Sun's soup needed more scientific trials before definitive results regarding its ability to impede cancer could be determined.

Sun stated that his mother was free of cancerous growths fifteen years after he created his first soup, crediting it for her health. Founding Sun Farm Soup Company at Milford, Connecticut, Sun oversaw the production of Sun's soup for commercial sale.

The anticancer benefits of Sun's soup remain scientifically unproven. The U.S. Food and Drug Administration (FDA) does not endorse Sun's soup because it is advertised as a supplement, and by law the FDA does not regulate supplements in the stringent way that it does drugs.

Side effects: There are no known side effects to ingesting Sun's soup, other than a bloated sensation felt by those who participated in Sun's early studies. Later study participants who ingested a frozen, rather than the earlier freeze-dried, formulation of SV did not report bloating.

Elizabeth D. Schafer, Ph.D.

See also Bronchial adenomas; Cancell; Chemotherapy; Cobalt 60 radiation; Complementary and alternative therapies; Herbs as antioxidants; Lung cancers; Nutrition and cancer prevention; Nutrition and cancer treatment.

▶ Sunscreens

Category: Lifestyle and prevention
Also known as: Avobenzone, oxybenzone, mexoryl, zinc oxide, titanium dioxide

Definition: Sunscreens are lotions or sprays that, when applied correctly, can help prevent sunburn and other kinds of skin damage from the sun's ultraviolet (UV) rays. Using sunscreen can lower a person's risk for skin cancer.

Cancers treated or prevented: Skin cancers

Delivery routes: Topical via lotions and creams

How these agents work: There are two types of UV light from the sun, UVA and UVB. UVA rays damage the skin with long-term effects such as premature wrinkles and skin aging because they penetrate deep into the skin. UVB radiation causes sunburns and most likely contributes to skin cancers. Most sunscreens do not block UVA as well as they do UVB rays. It is recommended that a broad-spectrum sunscreen be used to protect against both types of UV rays.

Sunscreens contain both organic and inorganic ingredients such as avobenzone, oxybenzone, mexoryl, zinc oxide, and titanium dioxide. They work by absorbing, reflecting, or scattering UVA and UVB rays from the sun. Most sunscreens contain a combination of these ingredients, which work together to have a synergistic effect in protecting the skin. The newest Food and Drug Administration (FDA)-approved ingredient is mexoryl, which has proven to be more photostable than other ingredients and therefore retains its stability when exposed to sunlight.

Sunscreens have a sun protection factor (SPF) number that refers to how long the sunscreen is effective on the skin. The higher the SPF, the more sun protection the sunscreen offers. This number is only an estimate, however, because many additional factors—such as how much and how often the sunscreen is applied, how much sunscreen is absorbed, and the person's activity (for example, sleeping in the sun, swimming, or exercising)—affect how the sunscreen works.

Sunscreen works best when applied fifteen to thirty minutes before sun exposure, followed by a reapplication fifteen to thirty minutes after being out in the sun. Sunscreen then needs to be applied every two to three hours to remain effective. Most people do not apply enough sunscreen. Studies have shown that 1 ounce or 2 tablespoons is needed to cover the average body adequately.

In reality, no matter what sunscreen is used, some UV still gets through to the skin. A total program is needed to decrease the sun's harmful effects:

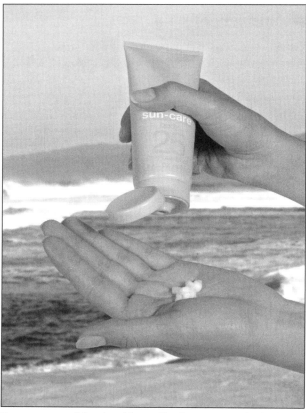

Sunscreens work by absorbing, reflecting, or scattering UVA and UVB rays from the Sun. (©Stephen Coburn/Dreamstime.com)

- Use sunscreen with an SPF of 15 or higher every day, even on cloudy days
- Avoid the sun during the hours of 10:00 A.M. to 4:00 P.M.
- Wear a hat, sunglasses, and long-sleeved protective clothing when out in the sun
- Select a sunscreen that contains some combination of avobenzone, oxybenzone, mexoryl, zinc oxide, and titanium dioxide—products that also provide UVA protection

Side effects: Occasionally, some people develop a mild to moderate allergic reaction or rash in reaction to some of the active ingredients in sunscreens. Discontinuing that sunscreen and switching to another type usually corrects this problem.

Michelle Kasprzak, R.N., B.S.N., O.C.N.

See also Basal cell carcinomas; Bowen disease; Carcinomas; Eyelid cancer; Lip cancers; Melanomas; Premalignancies; Prevention; Skin cancers; Squamous cell carcinomas; Sunlamps; Ultraviolet radiation and related exposures; Young adult cancers.

► Superior vena cava syndrome

Category: Diseases, symptoms, and conditions
Also known as: Superior vena cava (SVC) obstruction

Related conditions: Fibrosing mediastinitis, lung cancer

Definition: Superior vena cava syndrome is puffiness of the face, swelling of the eyelids and arms, and enlargement of the neck that results from obstruction of the superior vena cava (the vein connecting the upper half of the body and right atrium of the heart, formed by brachiocephalic veins) from any number of causes, including malignancy, infection, or an iatrogenic cause (inadvertently caused during the course of medical treatment).

Risk factors: The most common cancer that causes superior vena cava syndrome is bronchogenic carcinoma, responsible for 65 to 80 percent of cases. Other types of cancers that can cause this syndrome include small-cell lung cancer, primary mediastinal neoplasms such as thymoma and lymphoma, and metastases, especially from breast carcinoma. The most common infectious cause is histoplasmosis-induced fibrosing mediastinitis, most often seen in the midwestern part of the United States. This syndrome can also be caused by idiopathic fibrosing mediastinitis. Central venous catheters are the most common iatrogenic cause, followed by pacemaker electrodes and hyperalimentation lines.

Etiology and the disease process: When the superior vena cava is obstructed, there is an increase in venous pressure to between 20 and 50 millimeters of mercury (mmHg), which is diagnostic. In about 40 percent of patients, the obstruction occurs above the azygous vein and is responsible for the most disabling symptoms. Obstruction between the azygous vein and the right atrium is less serious, as the azygous vein can provide collateral venous decompression.

Incidence: Although superior vena cava syndrome is considered a rare disease, affecting less than 200,000 people in the U.S. population, the incidence of superior vena cava syndrome due to iatrogenic causes has been reported in 2 per 1,000 implantation procedures for pacemakers and defibrillators, and it is a well-described complication of both device implantation and central venous catheter placement.

Symptoms: The symptoms of superior vena cava syndrome vary depending on the degree of increase in venous pressure that develops, as well as the level of obstruction, the rate at which it developed, and the cause. If extrinsic compression of the superior vena cava is caused by a benign process such as fibrosing mediastinitis, the obstruction is gradual, allowing time for collateral circulation to develop, and therefore the symptoms are milder. With mild obstruction, symptoms include headache, puffiness of the face, and swelling of the eyelids or neck. Patients quickly find that severity is related to posture, with symptoms often worsening when they lie down or bend over.

If invasion of the superior vena cava or thrombosis occurs, the obstruction develops rapidly, and the symptoms are more acute. If acute obstruction occurs because of hemorrhage into a rapidly growing neoplasm, cerebral edema with blurring of vision and drowsiness occur. As the majority of cases are caused by rapidly growing bronchogenic lung cancer, pulmonary symptoms such as shortness of breath, orthopnea, cough, hemoptysis, and chest pain predominate. Other symptoms include hoarseness, stridor, and laryngeal edema from laryngeal obstruction.

Screening and diagnosis: In the past, superior vena cava syndrome was diagnosed by upper extremity venography; however, with the advent of contrast computed tomography (CT), helical CT scanning is now the most common modality used for diagnosis. CT scanning can show not just the extent of the obstruction but also the likely cause, a distinct advantage over venography. Direct CT signs of superior vena cava obstruction include nonopacification of the superior vena cava with or without intraluminal filling defects or encasement, or extrinsic compression of the superior vena cava by tumor. Indirect signs of superior vena cava obstruction include opacification of venous collateral circulation. The five major routes of collateral circulation include internal mammary veins, azygous or hemiazygous veins, paravertebral veins or Batson's plexus, anterior jugular veins, and lateral thoracic and thoracoepigastric veins. Additional collaterals include the superior intercostal veins, parascapular veins, superficial thoracoabdominal and epigastric veins, and the vertebral veins. The location and extent of the obstruction determine the collaterals that opacify during the contrast CT exam. Sometimes marked focal enhancement of the liver is seen in cases of superior vena cava obstruction and is thought to represent low-resistance collateral flow from the superior vena cava through the liver to the inferior vena cava. In patients with contraindications to CT intravenous contrast, magnetic resonance imaging (MRI) can be performed; however, MRI occasionally fails to differentiate complete obstruction from incomplete obstruction because of marked narrowing and slow flow. An advantage of MRI over CT involves the ability to clear up confusion regarding flow-related artifacts seen on CT because of the mixing of opacified and unopacified blood.

Treatment and therapy: Because most cases involve a malignant process that precludes surgical resection, standard therapy includes radiation therapy (often in combination with diuretics and corticosteroids to reduce cerebral edema) and chemotherapy. Some 80 to 90 percent of patients are relieved of superior vena cava syndrome; however, approximately 50 percent of patients relapse, even in benign disease because, although collaterals develop, thrombosis will continue to propagate and occlude even these collaterals over time. Thrombolytic therapy has been used for selected cases of acute thrombosis. Superior vena cava bypass with composite autogenous vein grafts has also been used for patients with a benign process in whom collateral circulation is inadequate to relieve symptoms.

Prognosis, prevention, and outcomes: With benign causes, symptoms will improve or subside as collateral circulation develops. With malignant causes, an improvement in symptoms varies with the type of tumor involved but most patients improve rapidly within a few weeks from the decrease in edema after the intensive radiation therapy, steroids, diuretics, and chemotherapy. Death from the cancer within the next several months is inevitable, however, with rare survivors beyond two years.

Debra B. Kessler, M.D., Ph.D.

▶ **For Further Information**

Abner, A. "Approach to the Patient Who Presents with Superior Vena Cava Obstruction." *Chest* 103 (1993): 394S-397S.

Hagga, John R., and Charles F. Lanzieri. *Computed Tomography and Magnetic Resonance Imaging of the Whole Body.* 4th ed. St. Louis: Mosby, 2003.

Schwartz, Seymour I. *Principles of Surgery.* New York: McGraw-Hill, 1984.

▶ **Other Resources**

American Society of Clinical Oncology
http://opl.asco.org

Cancer.Net
http://www.cancer.net/portal/site/patient

National Cancer Institute
Cardiopulmonary Syndromes
http://www.cancer.gov/cancertopics/pdq/
supportivecare/cardiopulmonary/Patient/page5

See also Lung cancers; Risks for cancer; Stent therapy; Thymomas.

► Support groups

Category: Social and personal issues

Definition: Cancer support groups are designed to provide comfort, information, and education within a confidential group setting. They are intended to provide a safe place for individuals with common cancer-related concerns to experience mutually provided emotional support.

The need for support: At critical points in the course of cancer, such as designation of high-risk status, diagnosis, initiation or cessation of treatment, and recurrence, patients face challenges that can be overwhelming. They may find that their usual ways of coping are ineffective and find it difficult to talk to family and friends. Commonly, patients want to protect their family and friends from their pain or are reluctant to admit how scared they feel.

Support groups can help patients feel less isolated, improve their coping skills, and afford the opportunity to express concerns to others who share similar problems. The group format provides multiple perspectives on many issues; thus, participants can acquire new information, learn new skills, and observe, firsthand, better ways to manage problems that they would not have thought of on their own.

Cancer support groups can also assist with managing practical aspects of cancer, such as providing patients with knowledge of innovative ways to manage treatment effects or tips about returning to work after treatment. In the United States, there are more than 450 cancer-related patient support and advocacy groups, and many have been instrumental in providing assistance to people affected by cancer.

Goals of groups: General goals of cancer support groups include the following:

- Provision of support among homogeneous groups affected by cancer
- Improvement of morale and self-esteem
- Enhancement of coping skills, personal control, and problem-solving abilities
- Reduction of emotional distress
- Provision of education regarding cancer and treatment-specific issues
- Clarification of medical information that may be missed in other settings because of anxiety
- Clarification of misconceptions and misinformation regarding cancer and its treatment
- Normalizing emotional reactions that occur throughout the course of the patient's cancer

Attainment of group goals is often enhanced by the disease-specific or role-specific membership of cancer support groups and the nonmedical environment in which they meet.

Types of groups and therapeutic approaches: Cancer support groups employ a variety of psychotherapeutic approaches. They vary widely in structure, focus, and activities. Some are time limited with specific content and goals, or teach a specific skill targeted to improving quality of life. In general the these types are called psycho-educational groups.

Other cancer groups may be ongoing, patient-centered, and focused on general expression of fears and concerns that may be too painful for patients to reveal to family and friends. These groups are called psychotherapy groups. Psychotherapy groups should be run by a professional with special training in both mental health and group intervention modalities relevant to patients with cancer.

Some cancer support groups include a combination of education, group interaction, support, and behavioral training. Behavioral training teaches new skills such as progressive muscle relaxation, meditation, or biofeedback, which can be effective in reducing stress and minimizing treatment side effects. The fact that behavioral skills are learned and self-administered is of benefit in improving symptom management, self-efficacy, and quality of life.

Cancer-specific versus general support groups: General psychotherapy groups tend to explore a range of life experiences, often promote confrontation among members in an effort to identify and eradicate maladaptive communication styles and relationship patterns, and may focus on past rather that current experiences to examine the origin of destructive relationship patterns. However, groups specifically for people with cancer typically maintain a focus on the cancer diagnosis, including its meaning and implications, and offer education and support specific to cancer-related topics. They are usually time limited and use a brief therapy, supportive, or crisis-intervention model. Normalizing emotional distress, providing realistic reassurance, bolstering strengths and positive coping skills, and gently suggesting behavioral alternatives to replace destructive methods of coping are essential components of the cancer support group's process and goals. Cancer support groups offer participants a range of perspectives about cancer-specific topics within the context of guidance, protection, and boundaries provided by a knowledgeable leader. Confrontational communication, exploration of past trauma, and problems not directly relevant to current issues are usually not addressed. Obviously, the rationale for this approach is based on the goal of enhancing coping skills and keeping stress within manageable limits.

Group composition: Cancer support groups exist for a range of individuals affected by cancer. Usually membership is limited to individuals with similar characteristics and problems. For example, new genetic technologies have given rise to groups for those at risk but not yet diagnosed with cancer. These groups offer multiple perspectives and education about issues such as genetic testing, risks and benefits of testing, and various prevention and screening practices. Membership may be centered on characteristics including cancer site, point in the course of cancer, and relationship to patient (for example, parents with an affected child, children with an affected parent). The benefit of a homogeneous group is the focus on similar content and themes that are relevant to all participants; thus members are protected from painful experiences that do not pertain to them and could overwhelm and undermine rather that enhance their coping skills.

Groups for cancer caregivers: Family and friends may benefit from participating in a cancer support group, especially if they love, depend on, or take care of the affected person. Family members may need help in dealing with stresses such as family disruptions, financial worries, and changing roles.

To help meet these needs, some support groups are designed just for family members of cancer patients. There has been an increase in the number of groups designed for family cancer caregivers that combine education, support, and links to community services, although far more caregiver resources are needed. This rapidly growing need is based on changes in health care financing and delivery and resultant trends that have displaced a large burden of cancer care onto family members. Patients are discharged from hospitals while still needing some care; they often require highly technical, complex care that at one time was performed by professionals in a clinical setting.

For example, it has become common practice for a breast cancer patient to be discharged from the hospital on

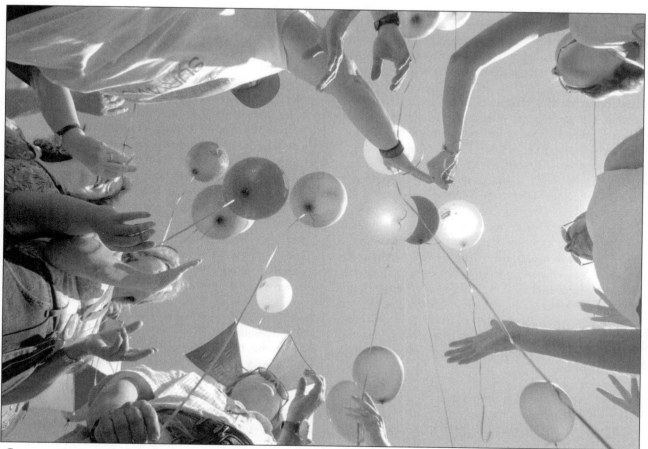

Cancer survivors can find comfort by participating in support groups and events such as this cancer walk. (AP/Wide World Photos)

the day of a mastectomy. Drains are still in place, pain management and risk for infection are primary concerns, and the need for monitoring, direct care, functional assistance, and support is constant. Coupled with dramatic reductions in third-party reimbursement for home health services, the burden of this complex care falls to family and friends who typically are not equipped, from an educational or emotional standpoint, to manage it. Stress may be compounded among caregivers who work and depend on maintenance of their income, have others who depend on them such as children or other ill or elderly family members, have limited finances or people available to provide assistance and respite, are ill themselves, or are experiencing countless other issues.

Caregiver burden and the need for additional services promise to be critical well into the future. The practical and emotional needs of family caregivers and the far-reaching impact of these issues on the social and economic welfare of the United States and its citizens are immense. There are support groups specific to the needs of professional caregivers, although more resources are needed in this area. Professional caregiver support groups are valuable for countless reasons, not the least of which are validation of the stressful nature of the work and stress management in the service of maintaining professional morale and promoting and maintaining high-quality oncology care.

Research regarding efficacy: One of the most important predictors regarding the efficacy of any behavioral or group technique is whether the person receiving the treatment believes it will be helpful. That is a major limitation to studies examining efficacy of cancer support group treatments. Although several studies have demonstrated positive outcomes, from increased survival time to improved quality of life among support group members, subjects are largely self-selected, meaning that they participate in the support group because they start out with the belief that it will benefit them. The consensus among researchers is that cancer support groups enhance quality of life by providing information, reducing isolation and helplessness, and normalizing emotions. Studies have shown that participation in cancer support groups promotes positive coping; reduces symptoms such as tension, anxiety, fatigue, and confusion; and improves compliance with cancer treatment.

One of the most widely publicized studies regarding efficacy of cancer support group treatment was a 1989 clinical trial of women with metastatic breast cancer conducted by physician David Spiegel. Study findings suggested that women who participated in a cancer support group lived eighteen months longer than a control group of women who did not participate. The study was later criticized because average rather than median survival was the statistic used to compare group survival differences. Averages can be dramatically skewed in one direction or another by just one early death or long-term survivor in a particular group; therefore it was concluded that study findings were misleading. A subsequent clinical trial that followed a sample of women with breast cancer found no survival differences between support group participants and nonparticipants, and yet another study reported that patients with malignant melanoma who had taken part in a psycho-educational cancer group lived longer than those who did not take part.

A 2005 review of four studies of women with breast cancer found no relationship between support group participation and survival other than that reported in Spiegel's study. Limitations of studies that have examined the link between support group participation and survival include the self-selective nature of research samples and the group's impact on treatment compliance, which directly impacted survival. One study at the Ontario Cancer Institute found that women with breast cancer who lacked support from their families and friends were helped the most by support groups; therefore there may be factors that predispose some patients to benefit from participation in support groups. Finally some data link cancer support group participation with negative consequences.

At this point, there is insufficient evidence to support the efficacy of cancer support group interventions. Nonetheless there is abundant anecdotal evidence to support the benefits of attending if participants believe the experience will help and are not unduly stressed by exposure to the feelings and problems of others, and their needs are met by the group's content, goals, and activities.

Internet-based groups: Recent years have seen an explosion of Internet sites designed to provide information, support, and education for individuals affected by cancer. They usually involve interaction in real time among individuals who communicate via computer in chat rooms. Other sites are informational in nature. Questions can be posed and answers received at a future time, or individuals may be directed to a number of question-specific predetermined resources.

Internet-based groups vary widely in content, process, and quality. Some are led by moderators; others are not moderated or monitored at all. At present, there is scant empirical evidence supporting the efficacy of Internet-based cancer support. Even more problematic is that there are no quality control measures to ensure accuracy of information, nor are there procedures to screen or assist those who may be upset or otherwise harmed by content.

Tension between patient advocacy groups, clinicians, and groups devoted to freedom of information has prevented the limitation of the content of Internet sites or access to sites by specific vulnerable populations. Although many cancer-related sites provided by respected institutions and organizations such as the American Cancer Society and the National Cancer Institute are of excellent quality and aim to assist patients in every way, the Internet has provided a breeding ground for unscrupulous practices. Vulnerable patients—especially those with progressive illness or those not faring well with conventional treatment—can fall prey to false hope and financial as well as psychological exploitation, whether visiting an unmonitored support group or other Web site. The virtual explosion of technology, Web sites, unclear laws, and the ability of Internet sites to disappear and emerge overnight under new names makes their regulaton difficult. Further, the technological expertise of unscrupulous Web site administrators often surpasses that of law enforcement, although that gap is closing. Therefore, the safety, accuracy, and ethics of Internet support groups and the validity of their informational content will remain a formidable challenge.

Jeannie V. Pasacreta, Ph.D., A.P.R.N.

▶ For Further Information

Breitbart, W. "Spirituality and Meaning in Supportive Care: Spirituality- and Meaning-Centered Group Psychotherapy Interventions in Advanced Cancer." *Journal of Supportive Care in Cancer* 10, no. 4 (2002): 272-280.

Cunningham, A. J., et al. "A Randomized Controlled Trial of the Effects of Group Psychological Therapy on Survival in Women with Metastatic Breast Cancer." *Psychooncology* 7 (1998): 508-517.

Edmonds, C. V., G. A. Lockwood, and A. J. Cunningham. "Psychological Response to Long-Term Group Therapy: A Randomized Trial with Metastatic Breast Cancer Patients." *Psycho-oncology* 8 (1999): 74-91.

Fawzy, F. I., N. W. Fawzy, L. A. Arndt, and R. O. Pasnau. "Critical Review of Psychosocial Interventions in Cancer Care." *Archives of General Psychiatry* 52 (1995): 100-113.

Goodwin, Pamela J. "Support Groups in Advanced Breast Cancer." *Cancer* 104, suppl. 11 (December 1, 2005): 2596-2601.

_____. "Support Groups in Breast Cancer: When a Negative Result Is Positive." *Journal of Clinical Oncology* 22, no. 21 (November 1, 2004): 4244-4246.

Zabalegui, A., S. Sanchez, P. D. Sanchez, and C. Juando. "Nursing and Cancer Support Groups." *Journal of Advanced Nursing* 51, no. 4 (2005): 369-381.

▶ Other Resources

Association of Cancer Online Resources
http://www.acor.org

National Cancer Institute
Cancer Support Groups: Questions and Answers
http://www.cancer.gov/cancertopics/factsheet/
Support/support-groups

The Wellness Community
http://www.thewellnesscommunity.org/

See also Anxiety; Caregivers and caregiving; Case management; Complementary and alternative therapies; Counseling for cancer patients and survivors; Long-distance caregiving; Oncology social worker; Prayer and cancer support; Psychosocial aspects of cancer; Relationships; Self-image and body image; Stress management; Young adult cancers.

▶ Surgical biopsies

Category: Procedures
Also known as: Tissue sampling, incisional biopsy, excisional biopsy, endoscopic or laparoscopic biopsy, open biopsy, transvenous biopsy

Definition: A surgical biopsy is the removal of tissue through an incision during an open or laparoscopic surgical procedure. A pathologist examines the tissue sample in the laboratory to detect the presence of cancer cells and determine the grade of the tumor.

There are several types of surgical biopsy procedures. The one performed is dependent on the type of suspected cancer and the area of the body being examined.

In incisional biopsy, a scalpel or similar instrument is used to remove a portion of the suspected cancerous tissue through an incision made in the skin. Incisional biopsies are most commonly used to remove soft tissue, such as skin, connective tissue, breast tissue, muscle, and fat. For skin lesions, an incisional biopsy may be performed with a hollow, circular-shaped instrument (punch biopsy), or a razor may be used (shave biopsy). Depending on the type of procedure, general or local anesthesia may be used.

In excisional biopsy, a whole lump, tumor, or organ and a margin of normal tissue around it are removed. Some open surgical biopsy procedures include laparotomy, thoracotomy, or mediastinotomy. General anesthesia is used for excisional and open biopsy procedures.

In endoscopic or laparoscopic biopsy, an endoscope (small camera on a thin tube) is used to view an internal area and identify the tissue for removal. The endoscope transmits magnified images of the area onto a video monitor to guide the physician during the procedure. The endoscope can be inserted through a natural body opening (endoscopy), such as the throat to remove esophageal tissue, or through a small abdominal incision (laparoscopy). When the laparoscope is used to view the inside of the chest cavity, the procedure is called a thoracoscopy and the scope is called a thoracoscope. When the laparoscope is used to view the mediastinum (space between and in front of the lungs), the procedure is called a mediastinoscopy, and the scope is called a mediastinoscope.

Surgical instruments attached to the endoscope or inserted through other small incisions are used to remove the tissue. Laparoscopic biopsy procedures are the most common type of biopsies and are often used when a tissue sample is needed from more than one area or when a larger tissue sample is needed. Depending on the biopsy site, the patient may be under general or local anesthesia.

Cancers diagnosed or treated: Various, including breast cancer, bone cancer, carcinoid tumors, germ-cell tumors, liver cancer, lung cancer, sarcoidosis, Hodgkin disease, myasthenia gravis, neurogenic tumors, thymic cancer and thymomas, malignant mesothelioma, mediastinal tumors, pericardial tumors, lymphoma, skin cancer, and thyroid cancer

Why performed: Surgical biopsies are performed to diagnose a variety of conditions and to assess the degree of organ damage (disease staging). Surgical biopsies may be performed when abnormalities are found during other tests such as an ultrasound, computed tomography (CT) scan, magnetic resonance imaging (MRI), or a nuclear scan. Surgical biopsies also may be performed to determine the cause of unexplained symptoms or to match organ tissue before a transplant.

An excisional biopsy may be used to remove some types of tumors or suspected cancers that need to be entirely removed for an accurate diagnosis, such as the removal of lymph nodes to accurately diagnose lymphoma. A surgical biopsy procedure also may be recommended when other, less invasive biopsy procedures do not provide conclusive results for an accurate diagnosis to be made.

Patient preparation: Preprocedure tests may include a chest X ray, electrocardiogram (EKG), CT, MRI, and other imaging tests. Urine tests and blood tests are performed before the procedure to evaluate the patient's blood count, platelet count, and blood clotting ability. Depending on the type of surgical biopsy procedure to be performed, additional tests may be required.

The patient preparation for a biopsy procedure varies, depending on the type of procedure and biopsy location. One week before the procedure, patients must stop taking aspirin and products containing aspirin, ibuprofen, and anticoagulants, as directed by the physician. Other anticoagulant medications may be prescribed as needed. In most cases, the patient must not eat or drink for eight to twelve hours beforehand. The patient will receive specific preparation instructions from the health care team.

Patients at most health care facilities must sign a form stating their willingness to permit diagnosis and medical treatment, a process called informed consent.

Steps of the procedure: An intravenous (IV) line is inserted into a vein in the patient's arm to deliver medications. For some surgical biopsy procedures, such as liver biopsy and some laparoscopic procedures, the patient is given a sedative and the procedure is performed under conscious sedation. With conscious sedation, the patient is awake but relaxed and able to respond to the physician's instructions during the procedure. The majority of surgical biopsy procedures, however, are performed while the patient is under general anesthesia.

The biopsy site is cleansed, and sterile drapes may be placed around the area. A local anesthetic is injected into the area. In some cases, such as with sentinel node biopsy, a radioactive substance or dye is injected into the tumor, and a scanner is used to locate the lymph node or tissue containing the radioactive substance or stained with the dye.

During a laparoscopic biopsy, a laparoscope is inserted into a small abdominal incision. The laparoscope transmits magnified images onto a video monitor to guide the physician as laparoscopic instruments are inserted through additional small abdominal incisions to remove tissue samples. Ultrasound or CT guidance may be used to aid the surgeon during the procedure.

Transvenous biopsy is a technique used to remove a tissue sample via a catheter inserted into a vein in the neck. This technique is not common, but it may be used for certain high-risk patients, including those who have a blood-clotting disorder, fluid in the abdomen, or liver failure or who are morbidly obese.

During an incisional biopsy, the surgeon uses a scalpel to remove a sample of tissue from the area. During an excisional biopsy, the lesion and surrounding margin of normal tissue are removed. During an open surgical biopsy, an incision is made in the abdomen (laparotomy), upper chest (thoracotomy or mediastinoscopy), or breast, allowing visualization of the area. The location and size of the tumor are identified, and a tissue sample or lymph nodes can be removed for analysis. Ultrasound or CT guidance may be used to aid the surgeon during the procedure.

After the tissue has been removed, a pathologist sends it to a laboratory for microscopic analysis to determine how much the tissue sample differs from normal tissue. A variety of methods can be used to process tissue samples. Histologic sections involve preparing stained, thin "slices" of tissue mounted on slides. The histologic method may take up to forty-eight hours to produce results. With this method, the tissue sample is placed in a machine that replaces all water in the sample with paraffin wax. The sample is embedded into a larger block of paraffin and is then sliced into very thin sections and stained with dye to aid microscopic analysis. Frozen tissue analysis involves freezing the tissue, slicing it into thin sections, and staining the sections to aid analysis. Smears are tissue samples that are spread onto a slide for examination. The results of smears can usually be obtained very quickly, although the smear technique cannot be used on all types of biopsy samples.

After the procedure: The length of a patient's recovery and the steps for recovery vary depending on the type of biopsy procedure, biopsy location, and type of anesthesia. The patient may stay in an intensive care unit (ICU) or recovery room for a certain amount of time after the procedure. The incision is closed with sutures, and the biopsy site is usually covered with a bandage or dressing. A catheter may remain after surgery to drain urine. Drains or chest tubes may remain in place at the incision site to remove fluid or air that may have accumulated during the procedure. Pain medication is prescribed as needed for relief of pain, which may include discomfort at the biopsy site or muscle pain. The patient usually stays in the hospital overnight but may need to recover in the hospital three to four days, depending on the biopsy site, type of procedure, and type of anesthesia given during the procedure.

Specific instructions for driving, activity, incision care, medications, nutrition, and managing emergencies and a follow-up care schedule are provided to the patient, as applicable. In most cases, the patient is not permitted to drive home after the procedure, and driving or operating machinery may be limited for a certain amount of time. Depending on the physician's instructions, the patient may be required to stay on bed rest at home for a certain amount of time after the procedure.

The patient should avoid vigorous physical activity and heavy lifting after the procedure, as directed by the physician. For one week after the procedure, the patient should avoid aspirin and products containing aspirin, ibuprofen, and anticoagulants, as these medications decrease blood clotting, which is necessary for healing. Other anticoagulant medications may be prescribed if necessary after the procedure. The patient may take acetaminophen (Tylenol) to relieve pain as needed.

Risks: The risks of biopsy procedures are dependent on the type of procedure performed and the biopsy location. Possible risks of all surgical biopsy procedures include allergic reaction to the anesthetic, bleeding, infection, and scarring, and these risks are greater with open surgical biopsy procedures.

The risk of death associated with biopsy procedures is generally very low. The physician can discuss specific mortality rates and risks with the patient, depending on the type of procedure performed.

Results: Biopsy results are available either right away or within twenty-four to forty-eight hours after the tissue removal, depending on the type of biopsy analysis that is being performed. The tissue sample removed during the procedure is either normal, which means it is benign or noncancerous, or abnormal, which means it has unusual characteristics and may be malignant or cancerous. The grade of tumor may also be determined from the biopsy sample, indicating how quickly the tumor is likely to grow and spread. Surgical biopsy procedures remove a larger tissue sample than other biopsy methods, increasing the accuracy of a diagnosis. The type of cancerous cells and extent of disease will help guide the patient's treatment.

Angela M. Costello, B.S.

▶ **For Further Information**

DeVita, Vincent, Jr., Samuel Hellman, Steven A. Rosenberg, et al., eds. *Cancer: Principles and Practice of Oncology.* 7th ed. Philadelphia: Lippincott Williams & Wilkins, 2005.

McPhee, Stephen J., Maxine A. Papadakis, and Lawrence M. Tierney, eds. *Current Medical Diagnosis and Treatment 2008.* New York: McGraw-Hill Medical, 2007.

Ota, D. M. "What's New in General Surgery: Surgical Oncology." *Journal of the American College of Surgeons* 196, no. 6 (2003): 926-932.

Skandalakis, John E., Panajiotis N. Skandalakis, and Lee John Skandalakis. *Surgical Anatomy and Technique: A Pocket Manual.* 2d ed. New York: Springer, 2000.

▶ **Other Resources**

American Cancer Society
http://www.cancer.org

American Pathology Foundation
http://www.apfconnect.org

College of American Pathologists
http://www.cap.org

National Cancer Institute
http://www.cancer.gov

Radiology Info, provided by the American College of Radiology and the Radiological Society of North America
http://www.radiologyinfo.org

Society of Interventional Radiology
http://www.sirweb.org

Society for Hematopathology
http://socforheme.org

See also Biopsy; Liver biopsy; Needle biopsies; Needle localization; Stereotactic needle biopsy.

▶ Surgical oncology

Category: Medical specialties

Definition: Surgical oncologists are doctors who have been trained in general surgery techniques and practices and then completed additional training in surgical techniques specific to cancer treatment. They may perform various diagnostic surgeries, such as removing a lymph node to see if skin cancer has spread, or may perform treatment surgeries such as the removal of tumors and surrounding cancerous tissues. Surgical oncologists work closely with other allied health professionals to ensure that the patient receives the best possible care.

Subspecialties: Surgical oncologists generally specialize in cancers that occur in certain areas of the body. Some specializations include breast, lung, kidney, skin, gastrointestinal tract, and colorectal, and endocrine system cancers. Surgical oncologists may also specialize in either patient treatment or research.

Research specialists do treat patients, but instead of consulting with patients and doing surgeries during the majority of their time, they spend a significant portion of their time working to develop new and better diagnostic procedures and treatments. Improved procedures are generally intended to improve positive patient outcomes or reduce the number of side effects generally experienced.

Cancers treated: Nearly all forms of cancer

Training and certification: After completing medical school, surgical oncologists must successfully complete a five-year residency in surgery. After completing the residency, they must then complete a fellowship in surgical oncology. These fellowships generally last from two to four years and must be completed at one of the fourteen schools accredited by the Society of Surgical Oncology. There is no board certification for surgical oncology, but upon completion of the fellowship, a certificate is usually awarded.

During their training, surgical oncologists generally receive instruction in both commonly accepted, frequently performed surgeries, such as a lumpectomy for breast cancer, and very new or experimental procedures, such as cryosurgery, a treatment procedure that involves killing the cancerous cells through freezing them with liquid nitrogen or argon gas, or isolated limb perfusion, a treatment for cancers involving the limbs that is considered an alternative to amputation in some cases.

Research techniques can also be an important part of the training received by surgical oncologists. Many are involved in research and the development of new procedures and techniques for diagnosis and treatment. Often the development of new procedures focuses on techniques to treat rare or unusual forms of cancer or those believed to provide a better outcome or have a lower incidence of side effects. Doctors trained in research techniques can participate in research or be better equipped to recommend clinical trials or experimental procedures to their patients if appropriate.

Services and procedures performed: Surgical oncologists perform many different diagnostic procedures as well as procedures intended to remove or otherwise treat the cancer. Depending on the location of the cancer, a surgical oncologist may be required to take a sample from the area in which cancer is suspected or some cells from a tumor that is believed to be malignant. For this type of procedure, the surgeon will often insert a small instrument into the patient, guided by X ray or other images, and remove tissue from the area in question.

An important procedure that surgical oncologists commonly perform is the removal of tumors. During this type of procedure, the surgeon makes the smallest incision possible to allow access to the tumor and the area around the tumor. Then the tumor is removed, along with adjoining tissue that is also believed to be cancerous. This type of treatment may be used alone, or it may be used along with other treatment options. Radiation and chemotherapy may actually be delivered during the surgery, when the cancerous area is exposed and it is possible to apply radiation or chemotherapeutic agents very accurately to the cancerous area.

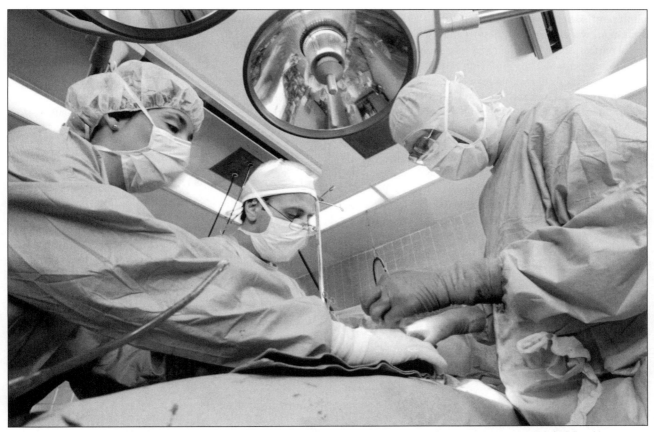

Surgical oncologists specialize in both the therapeutic and palliative removal of cancerous tumors. (Digital Stock)

Surgery can also be performed for reasons that are not directly intended to cure the cancer, such as to reduce the size of the tumor or to remove it from a specific area where it is causing damage. It is not always possible to completely surgically remove a tumor, because it may have invaded areas that are necessary for the body to function. In this case, surgery may be performed to remove as much of the tumor as possible, with the hope that radiation therapy or chemotherapy will be able to combat what remains.

Palliative surgery may also be performed by a surgical oncologist. This type of surgery is done when the cancer has metastasized extensively, and the surgery is not expected to provide a cure. If a tumor is causing the patient pain, some or all of the tumor may be surgically removed to provide pain relief and improve the patient's quality of life.

Related specialties and subspecialties: The surgical oncologist works closely with many different members of the health professions. The surgical oncologist may have a patient referred by a primary physician, gynecologist, der-matologist, or other doctor, and will work closely with the referring physician throughout the cancer treatment process. During the process of diagnosis, the surgical oncologist may perform surgery to take a sample from the area where cancer is suspected and send it to a pathologist for evaluation. The pathologist can then determine if cancer is in fact present, and if it is, which type of cancer is present. The surgical oncologist will also work closely with nurses, medical technologists, and members of the office or hospital staff.

During cancer treatment, the surgical oncologist will work with various other health professionals depending on the type and extent of the cancer being treated and the treatment option chosen. During surgery, nurses and medical technologists will assist the surgical oncologist by providing various services such as patient and equipment monitoring. Nurses will prepare the patient for surgery by communicating necessary information and instructions and administering any medications necessary preoperatively. The anesthesiologist is present at surgery to ensure that the patient is fully and safely anesthetized using the minimum level of anesthesia. Depending on the type of treatment, the surgical oncologist may work with additional professionals during surgery. For example, if targeted chemotherapeutic agents are being introduced to treat residual cancer cells during surgery, a chemotherapy expert will be present to oversee and administer the chemotherapeutic treatment.

After surgery, another set of health care professionals will work with the surgical oncologist. Nurses will provide aftercare for the incision or wound site; administer pain, anti-inflammatory, and other medications; and communicate information to the patient about self-care. Physical or occupational therapists may be necessary to assist patients in recovering skills and mobility lost through surgery. A prosthetist may be required to make a prosthetic for any body part removed during the surgery, and a plastic or reconstructive surgeon may be necessary to repair damage or scarring caused by the surgery or the cancer itself. A psychological counselor or therapist may help the patient with any emotions brought about by the surgery or the cancer itself. Throughout the process, the surgical oncologist may also work closely with a case manager who oversees and organizes the patient's care and treatment.

Helen Davidson, B.A.

▶ **For Further Information**
Damron, Timothy A., ed. *Oncology and Basic Science.* Philadelphia: Lippincott Williams & Wilkins, 2008.
Lyons, Lyman. *Diagnosis and Treatment of Cancer.* New York: Chelsea House, 2007.
Sabel, Michael S., Vernon K. Sondak, and Jeffrey J. Sussman, eds. *Surgical Foundations: Essentials of Surgical Oncology.* Philadelphia: Mosby Elsevier, 2007.
Stroszczynski, E., ed. *Minimally Invasive Tumor Therapies.* New York: Springer, 2006.
Wrightson, William R., ed. *Current Concepts in General Surgery: A Resident Review.* Georgetown, Tex.: Landes Bioscience, 2006.

▶ **Organizations and Professional Societies**

American Society of Clinical Oncology
http://www.asco.org
1900 Duke Street, Suite 200
Alexandria, VA 22314

Society of Surgical Oncology
http://www.surgonc.org
85 West Algonquin Road, Suite 550
Arlington Heights, IL 60005

▶ **Other Resources**

American Cancer Society
http://www.cancer.org

MayoClinic.com
Cancer Surgery: Physically Removing Cancer
http://www.mayoclinic.com/health/cancer-surgery/CA00033

See also Bilobectomy; Biopsy; Cholecystectomy; Colectomy; Cordectomy; Cordotomy; Core needle biopsy; Electrosurgery; Esophagectomy; Glossectomy; Hysterectomy; Hystero-oophorectomy; Laparoscopy and laparoscopic surgery; Laryngectomy; Lobectomy; Loop electrosurgical excisional procedure (LEEP); Lumbar puncture; Lumpectomy; Lymphadenectomy; Mastectomy; Mohs surgery; Oophorectomy; Oral and maxillofacial surgery; Orchiectomy; Pancreatectomy; Pneumonectomy; Polypectomy; Prostatectomy; Salpingectomy and salpingo-oophorectomy; Splenectomy; Stereotactic radiosurgery (SRS); Surgical biopsies; Vasectomy and cancer.

▶ Survival rates

Category: Social and personal issues
Also known as: Mortality rates

Definition: Survival rate is a statistic that states the percentage of people with a disease who live a specified length of time after diagnosis (such as one year, five years, or ten years).

Types of survival rates: The overall or observed survival is the percentage of a group of people diagnosed with a disease who are alive after a specified time period, often five years. Overall survival rates do not distinguish between different causes of death—deaths from cancer and car accidents are both included. The net survival filters out deaths from causes other than the disease of interest, by calculating either relative survival or cancer-specific survival. Relative survival compares the overall survival rate of a group of people after diagnosis with a disease to the survival rate of a similar (age- and sex-matched) group without the disease. Cancer-specific survival includes only deaths by cancer, usually determined using death certificates.

Overall and relative survival rates do not always give a clear picture. For example, there is no way to tell whether cancer survivors are still undergoing treatment at five years or if they have gone into remission. Two other types of survival rates can give more information: progression-free survival and disease-free survival. The progression-free survival rate is the percentage of people who survive without their cancer spreading, such as the proportion of people who have had partial treatment success—their diseases are not in remission, but the tumors are not growing. Disease-free survival represents the proportion of patients during a specified time period who achieve remission or are completely cancer-free.

One of the newer methods of calculating survival is period survival, which uses only the most recent information available. This method is believed to take newer treatment regimens and modalities into account more effectively than other methods. However, restricting the analysis to a relatively short, recent time period (such as the most recent calendar year for which cancer registry data are available) results in a loss of precision in the estimate.

Although surviving is the opposite of dying, mortality rates are not always the inverse of survival rates. The mortality rate is often defined as the proportion of the entire population that died from a disease in a specified period, often reported as deaths per 1,000 or 100,000 (for example, 89 per 100,000 persons rather than 0.089 percent). Population-based mortality rates do not help to measure advances in treating cancers because they reflect changes in incidence. For example, death rates from lung cancer have declined since 1990, but that is more related to the reduction in tobacco use over the past forty years than to any improvement in treatments for lung cancer. When the mortality rate is defined as the proportion of people diagnosed with a disease who died from that disease during a specific period, then its value is simply the inverse of the survival rate.

How survival rates are used: Survival rates are important in determining prognosis, or the prediction of the course of the disease. Survival rate estimates are used in health services research for studying trends over time, such as the effect of a new therapy or the effect of stage at diagnosis or socioeconomic status. Survival statistics are also important in clinical research to measure the efficacy of treatments for cancer. On an individual patient level, survival rates can give patients a better understanding of their disease and help them evaluate different treatment plans in consultation with their medical providers.

How survival rates are calculated and reported: Cancer survival rates are usually calculated based on observations of hundreds or thousands of people, often using cancer registries or other databases. Survival rates can be reported in simple percentages, or in life tables, survival curves, or Kaplan-Meier survival curves. Life tables show the actual observed survival over time, and although they are one of the oldest techniques in biostatistics, they are no

longer seen much outside of government reports. Survival curves are graphical presentations of the probabilities for surviving different lengths of time, often derived from life tables. In the actuarial method, they present the probabilities of surviving to set, specific intervals, such as one year or one month.

Kaplan-Meier survival curves also graphically represent survival probabilities, but unlike the actuarial survival curve, the Kaplan-Meier method (named for its originators) identifies the exact point in time when each death occurred and uses those timepoints as the intervals. The goal is to produce the most accurate survival curve possible, taking into account all the information available. The Kaplan-Meier method allows researchers to analyze complex data, such as data from a study in which patients have been diagnosed or started treatment at different times and have varying lengths of follow-up. The Kaplan-Meier method is so widely used and so well known that, more often than not, research papers will refer to survival curves as Kaplan-Meier curves.

Limitations of survival rate statistics: It is well known that statistics can be both accurate in general and completely wrong in particular. Survival rates are no different from other statistics in this regard. Statistics cannot predict the course of an individual's disease. Because statistics are based on many different people and every person is different, they cannot give the exact chances of remission or progression in a particular case. Even when survival rates can be calculated for smaller groups—even very specific groups, such as fifty-five- to sixty-four-year-old white women in Texas with Stage II breast cancer—the differences between people in that subpopulation in genetics, body type, lifestyle, and socioeconomic factors means that the survival rates can vary considerably. It is always important to remember that survival rates represent an average and cannot reflect a person's individual experience. Because of this limitation, many cancer patients choose to disregard survival rate statistics.

In addition, survival rates usually do not reflect the latest treatment options. Because there is a lag between when cancer patients die and when this information is reported, the data are usually at least several years old. In other words, the effects of new treatments are not seen in the statistics for a number of years after the treatment becomes commonplace.

Another limitation of survival rates has to do with improvements in screening. When screening is widespread, a higher five-year survival rate may be observed not because people live longer but only because an earlier diagnosis has been made.

Age-Adjusted Five-Year Relative Survival Rates in the United States, 1996-2003

Site	Total	Men	Women
All Sites	64.9	64.6	65.2
Prostate	98.4	98.4	–
Thyroid	96.7	93.9	97.5
Testis	95.4	95.4	–
Melanoma of the skin	91.1	89.1	93.5
Breast	88.6	85.0	88.6
Hodgkin disease	84.9	83.0	87.0
Corpus uteri	83.9	–	83.9
Urinary bladder	79.5	80.9	75.3
Cervix uteri	71.6	–	71.6
Kidney and renal pelvis	65.5	65.1	66.3
Rectum	65.0	64.1	66.2
Colon	63.5	64.0	63.1
Non-Hodgkin lymphoma	63.4	60.8	66.4
Larynx	62.9	64.1	58.3
Oral cavity and pharynx	59.1	57.6	62.6
Kaposi sarcoma	56.3	55.8	63.7
Leukemia	49.6	49.7	49.4
Ovary	44.9	–	44.9
Brain and nervous system	33.9	32.2	36.0
Myeloma	33.7	35.5	31.7
Stomach	24.3	22.6	26.9
Esophagus	15.6	15.3	16.8
Lung and bronchus	15.0	13.0	17.4
Liver and bile duct	10.8	10.4	11.7
Mesothelioma	8.4	6.8	13.8
Pancreas	5.0	4.9	5.1

Source: Data from L. A. G. Ries et al., *SEER Cancer Statistics Review, 1975-2004* (Bethesda, Md.: National Cancer Institute, 2007)

Survival rate trends: The five-year survival rate is commonly used to report progress in the so-called war against cancer. Experts disagree as to whether cancer patients are living longer than cancer patients did in the past. Although survival rates have increased for many cancers since the 1970's, this could be because of a number of different factors (or combinations of factors), including improvements in surgical treatment or chemotherapy, changes in definitions of diseases, diagnoses of cases that would have been undetectable in years past, improvements in access to care, and earlier diagnoses through advances in screening.

Many cases of cancer are diagnosed earlier than they would have been even in the late 1990's because of improvements in imaging technology, advancements in genetic screening, and increasing awareness among patients and physicians. However, earlier diagnosis does not necessarily imply longer survival. If one person is diagnosed when symptoms appear in 2005 and survives until 2007, while another is diagnosed while still asymptomatic in 2003 and survives until 2007, the survival statistics will seem to be improved even though both people died at the same time. From the point of view of the cancer patient, there may even be negative consequences of earlier diagnosis—the patient's emotional well-being may worsen or there may be longer exposure to the side effects of treatment.

Survival rates by cancer site and stage: The most up-to-date survival rates for different cancers are available through the National Cancer Institute. Among different types of cancer, the highest relative five-year survival rate is seen in prostate cancer, at 98.4 percent, while the lowest is seen in cancer of the pancreas, at 5.0 percent.

Survival rates can vary greatly based on how early the cancer is diagnosed. For example, for patients diagnosed with Stage I (local) lung cancer, the five-year relative survival rate is 56 percent, while the rate is only 2 percent for those with Stage IV disease. Only 12 percent of lung cancers are diagnosed at Stage I, and the overall relative survival rate is very low. Even so, it is unlikely that the survival rate would increase significantly if all lung cancer were diagnosed at Stage I or II, since treatment options are limited and the disease spreads rapidly. Such is not the case for cancers that can be cured relatively easily with surgery if caught early, such as melanoma. Prostate cancer, on the other hand, has a high survival rate because it is generally a very slow form of cancer, and most men with prostate cancer will die of other causes before the cancer has a chance to spread.

Survival rates in different populations: Survival rates can vary greatly between different groups of people. For instance, women have better relative survival rates than men, both overall and in most of the major types of cancer, although these differences are generally not large. In addition, age at diagnosis has been shown to influence survival rate, since older people are less likely to be treated aggressively. This may be related to their perceived or actual lowered capability of withstanding severe side effects from treatment, or it may be an example of age-related bias on the part of medical providers.

Compared with non-Hispanic whites, African Americans, and American Indians, Hispanic whites have poorer survival rates both overall and for nearly every type of cancer. This is attributed to the fact that they are more likely to be diagnosed with advanced cancer, as a result of disparities in access to and receipt of health care services. In breast cancer, it has been shown that American women of Japanese and Chinese descent have better survival rates and Hawaiians have worse survival rates relative to non-Hispanic whites. Some studies suggest that most of these racial and ethnic disparities are actually socioeconomic disparities, and that when nonwhite people receive cancer treatment and medical care similar to that received by whites, their survival rates also are similar. This is supported by the fact that higher income has been shown to be a predictor of better survival.

Lisa M. Lines, M.P.H.

▶ For Further Information

Dickman, P. W., and H. O. Adami. "Interpreting Trends in Cancer Patient Survival." *Journal of Internal Medicine* 260, no. 2 (August, 2006): 103-117.

Gordis, L. *Epidemiology.* Philadelphia: Elsevier/Saunders, 2004.

Jemal, A., et al. "Cancer Statistics, 2007." *CA: A Cancer Journal for Clinicians* 57, no. 1 (January/February, 2007): 43-66.

Welch, H. G., L. M. Schwartz, and S. Woloshin. "Are Increasing Five-Year Survival Rates Evidence of Success Against Cancer?" *Journal of the American Medical Association* 283, no. 22 (June 14, 2000): 2975-2978.

▶ Other Resources

Centers for Disease Control and Prevention
Health Disparities in Cancer
http://www.cdc.gov/Features/
CancerHealthDisparities/

MayoClinic.com
Cancer Survival Rate: A Tool to Understand Your Prognosis
http://www.mayoclinic.com/health/cancer/CA00049

National Cancer Institute
Overview of Population-Based Cancer Survival Statistics
http://srab.cancer.gov/survival

See also African Americans and cancer; Breast cancer in children and adolescents; Breast cancer in men; Breast cancer in pregnant women; Breast cancers; Bronchial adenomas; Chemotherapy; Chewing tobacco; Childhood cancers; Elderly and cancer; Epidemiology of cancer; Imaging tests; Lung cancers; Melanomas; National Cancer Institute (NCI); Prevention; Prostate cancer; Psycho-oncology; Statistics of cancer; Survivorship issues; Tobacco-related cancers; Young adult cancers.

▶ Survivorship issues

Category: Social and personal issues

Definition: A survivor is anyone who remains alive and continues to function after being treated for cancer. Survivors face many issues—financial, physical, and emotional—as they return to everyday living.

Cancer survival: The survival rate for various types of cancer is the number of people who are alive for a given period of time after diagnosis (usually defined as five years). As of 2009, more than 10 million people in the United States had survived cancer. The overall death rate from cancer began to decline in 1992 and continues to decline. Reasons for the decline include the availability of more effective treatments and more people being diagnosed at earlier, treatable stages of cancer. Also, more people are reducing their cancer risk by stopping smoking, using sun protection, and undergoing screening tests. The number of people being diagnosed with some cancers (lung, bladder, and prostate), however, is increasing.

Issues facing cancer survivors: With increasing survival rates, those involved in cancer care are realizing the importance of addressing the unique needs of cancer survivors. For many patients, enduring and surviving cancer and its treatment become the sole focus of life. Once treatment is over, patients often are faced with worries about the future and decisions about how to transition to life as a survivor. Survivors may face financial issues, difficulties obtaining or returning to employment, or discrimination in obtaining health and life insurance or in finding employment. The experience of surviving cancer also may create emotional reactions, such as depression, guilt, or anxiety, that can evolve into significant emotional difficulties without appropriate help.

Resuming daily life: Cancer affects very basic aspects of patients' lives, such as their daily routines. Those undergoing treatment are faced with a daily, often painful battle simply to survive the illness. Their entire lives and those of their families are consumed by treatments, doctor visits, and hospitalizations. Suddenly, they no longer lead a "normal" life, and daily activities such as going to work or school, buying groceries, or simply visiting with friends become things of the past. Life no longer seems to stretch out in a straight line before them; it no longer is as predictable as it once was.

After treatment, this time line changes, often just as suddenly. Patients may be left wondering what to do. Their daily lives may begin to resume their precancer patterns. Survivors may expect to resume life exactly as it was before cancer but may be impeded by fatigue or other physical changes. It also is possible that survivors will expect the world (jobs, school, and relationships) to be the same as it was before cancer, and they may be disappointed to learn that some things have changed while they were absorbed in cancer treatment.

This change in a person's perception of time can create feelings of anxiety, frustration, anger, sadness, and fear. Feelings of vulnerability, uncertainty, and fear about the future may cause the survivor to feel lost, abandoned by others, and depressed.

Physical changes: After cancer treatment, some patients must face permanent physical changes, such as loss of a limb or a breast. Others may gain significant weight because of medications. Some people must cope with damage to other parts of the body as a result of their treatment. Radiation treatment, for example, not only destroys cancer cells but also can damage organs such as the thyroid gland or the liver. Certain types of chemotherapy may cause toxic effects, such as eye damage or bone degeneration. Women may experience early menopause or infertility resulting from treatment. Survivors simply may look fatigued, with sallow skin and dark circles under the eyes. Some changes, such as hair and nail loss, may be temporary. Experiencing such physical changes may affect survivors psychologically and emotionally. Seeing their changed appearance in the mirror may affect the self-image, self-confidence, and self-identity of survivors.

Disruptions in relationships with others: After surviving cancer, people may expect more from their relationships with spouses or children. They may approach relationships with more intensity if they feel that their lives may be shortened. Likewise, fears that they may not survive for long can cause the survivor to break off relationships with others, to push others away through anger or other behaviors, and to withdraw from social activities. To address these issues, some treatment centers offer coordinated recovery programs for survivors that include continued medical care and help with exercise, nutrition, counseling, and advocacy services.

Amy J. Neil, M.S., M.A.P.

▶ For Further Information

Feuerstein, Michael, and Patricia Findley. *The Cancer Survivor's Guide: The Essential Handbook to Life After Cancer.* New York: Marlowe, 2006.

Hunter, Brenda. *Staying Alive: Life-Changing Strategies for Surviving Cancer.* Colorado Springs, Colo.: WaterBrook Press, 2004.

Levine, Margie. *Surviving Cancer: One Woman's Story*

and Her Inspiring Program for Anyone Facing a Cancer Diagnosis. New York: Broadway Books, 2001.

Nessim, Susan. *Can Survive: Reclaiming Your Life After Cancer.* Boston: Houghton Mifflin, 2000.

▶ Other Resources

American Cancer Society
Cancer Survivors Network
http://www.acscsn.org

Candlelighters Childhood Cancer Foundation
http://www.candlelighters.org

Lance Armstrong Foundation
http://www.livestrong.org

National Coalition for Cancer Survivorship
http://www.canceradvocacy.org

See also Advance directives; Anxiety; Depression; Do-not-resuscitate (DNR) order; End-of-life care; Financial issues; Insurance; Living will; Living with cancer; Psychosocial aspects of cancer; Psycho-oncology; Psychosocial aspects of cancers; Relationships; Self-image and body image; Survival rates; Transitional care.

▶ Symptoms and cancer

Category: Diseases, symptoms, and conditions

Definition: Symptoms are the outward signs—such as swellings, lumps, pain, shortness of breath, rashes, and any number of other unusual conditions—that a person may experience as a result of an underlying disease or other pathology. With regard to cancer, symptoms may be warning signs for undiagnosed, site-specific cancers. Their early or timely recognition is key to treatment and relief of symptoms. As a result of rapid scientific advances, it has become increasingly important that symptoms be managed comprehensively as a vital component of the cancer treatment plan. The notion that quality of life and its maintenance through aggressive symptom management efforts are as important, as maintenance and length of survival is of considerable interest as science and technology can keep individuals alive for lengthening periods albeit often with marginal quality of life. It is also important to differentiate discrete symptoms through refined and evolving assessment strategies, so that treatments aimed at promoting quality of life may be symptom specific.

Symptoms as warning signs: For symptoms to function as warning signs of undiagnosed, site-specific cancers, well-documented, established symptoms and symptom clusters or profiles must be well publicized, using a range of methods that are understandable and palatable to an increasingly diverse American population. Public information should make it easy for people to receive timely medical attention, consisting of a diagnostic workup, definitive medical or surgical recommendations, and timely intervention. Public education regarding signs and symptoms of cancer is vital to promote early diagnosis, not only to promote cure and survival but also to minimize disability and health care costs. Several reliable Internet sites deliver information regarding early symptoms and warning signs for a range of cancer diagnoses. The fact that this information can be accessed in a private, confidential manner may facilitate action among individuals who would otherwise be hesitant to seek medical advice in a timely manner. Nevertheless, attention needs to be paid to recognizing and addressing common psychological issues such as depression, fear, and anxiety that prevent some people from seeking medical attention even when they are aware of symptoms.

Cancer symptoms: The following symptoms may be early warning signs for site-specific cancers and, if experienced, are reason to seek medical attention for a definitive diagnosis:

- Bladder cancer: Blood in the urine, pain or burning upon urination, frequent urination, or cloudy urine
- Bone cancer: Pain in the bone or swelling around the affected site, fractures in bones, weakness, fatigue, weight loss, repeated infections, nausea, vomiting, constipation, problems with urination, weakness or numbness in the legs, bumps and bruises that persist
- Brain cancer: Dizziness; drowsiness; abnormal eye movements or changes in vision; weakness or loss of feeling in arms or legs or difficulties in walking; fits or convulsions; changes in personality, memory, or speech; headaches that tend to be worse in the morning and ease during the day, which may be accompanied by nausea or vomiting
- Breast cancer: A lump or thickening of the breast, discharge from the nipple, change in the skin of the breast, a feeling of heat, enlarged lymph nodes under the arm
- Colorectal cancer: Rectal bleeding (red blood in stools or black stools), abdominal cramps, constipation alternating with diarrhea, weight loss, loss of appetite, weakness, pallid complexion
- Kidney cancer: Blood in urine; dull ache or pain in the back or side; lump in kidney area, sometimes accompanied by high blood pressure or abnormality in red blood cell count

- Leukemia: Weakness; paleness; fever and flulike symptoms; bruising and prolonged bleeding; enlarged lymph nodes, spleen, or liver; pain in bones and joints; frequent infections; weight loss; night sweats
- Lung cancer: Wheezing; persistent cough for months; blood-streaked sputum; persistent ache in chest; congestion in lungs; enlarged lymph nodes in the neck
- Melanoma: Change in mole or other bump on the skin, including bleeding or change in size, shape, color, or texture
- Non-Hodgkin lymphoma: Painless swelling in the lymph nodes in the neck, underarm, or groin; persistent fever; feeling of fatigue; unexplained weight loss; itchy skin and rashes; small lumps in skin; bone pain; swelling in the abdomen; liver or spleen enlargement
- Oral cancer: A lump in the mouth; ulceration of the lip, tongue or inside of the mouth that does not heal within a couple of weeks; dentures that no longer fit well; oral pain or bleeding; foul breath; loose teeth; changes in speech
- Ovarian cancer: Abdominal swelling; in rare cases, abnormal vaginal bleeding; digestive discomfort
- Pancreatic cancer: Upper abdominal pain, unexplained weight loss, pain near the center of the back, intolerance of fatty foods, yellowing of the skin, abdominal masses, enlargement of liver and spleen
- Prostate cancer: Urination difficulties due to blockage of the urethra; bladder retains urine, creating frequent feelings of urgency to urinate, especially at night; bladder not emptying completely; burning or painful urination; bloody urine; tenderness over the bladder; dull ache in the pelvis or back
- Stomach cancer: Indigestion or heartburn, discomfort or pain in the abdomen, nausea and vomiting, diarrhea or constipation, bloating after meals, appetite loss, weakness or fatigue, vomiting blood, or blood in the stool
- Uterine cancer: Abnormal vaginal bleeding, a watery bloody discharge in postmenopausal women, painful urination, pain during intercourse, pain in pelvic area

Symptoms after cancer diagnosis: Identification and treatment of distressing symptoms that occur as a result of cancer or its treatment are paramount so that quality of life and comfort are optimized for the cancer patient. As people live longer following cancer diagnosis, symptom management is an increasingly important aspect of treatment. However, many factors interfere with prompt recognition and treatment of these symptoms.

The period between diagnosis and the start of treatment is marked by medical evaluation, the development of new relationships with unfamiliar medical personnel, and the need to integrate a barrage of information that, at best, is frightening and confusing. Patients and families experience heightened responsibility, concern, and isolation during this period. They are particularly anxious and fearful when receiving initial information regarding diagnosis and treatment. Consequently, care should be taken by professionals to repeat information over several sessions and to inquire about patients' and families' understanding of facts and options. Early assessment by clinicians can help identify individuals at risk for medical or psychological adjustment problems and particularly those who are in the greatest need of ongoing psychosocial support and symptom management. Patients who have ongoing involvement with medical personnel and repeatedly receive accurate and consistent information about what to expect will have less uncertainty and be less likely to develop maladaptive coping strategies based on erroneous beliefs.

Although many studies document the devastating emotional impact of a cancer diagnosis, many individuals cope effectively, experience minimal distress, and have a high quality of life throughout most aspects of the cancer experience. Effective coping strategies, such as taking action and finding favorable aspects of the situation, have been associated with positive treatment experiences. Contrary to the beliefs of many clinicians, denial has been found to assist patients to cope effectively, unless sustained and used to the point that it interferes with obtaining recommended treatment.

Health care providers play a vital role in monitoring physical comfort and psychosocial adjustment and managing problems as they arise. As cancer progresses, patients often report an upsetting scenario that includes frequent pain, disability, increased dependence on others, and diminished functional ability, which often results in psychological symptoms. Investigators studying quality of life in cancer patients have demonstrated a clear relationship between the presence of discomfort and a patient's perception of quality of life. As uncomfortable symptoms increase, perceived quality of life diminishes. Therefore, an important goal in the psychosocial treatment of patients with advanced cancer focuses on symptom control.

Patients who are diagnosed with late-stage disease or have aggressive illnesses with no hope for cure are often the most vulnerable to psychological distress, particularly anxiety, depression, and family problems, and physical discomfort, including pain, fatigue, shortness of breath, and confusion. When physicians cannot offer patients hope for cure, helping them maintain comfort and control promotes adaptation and improved quality of life. One of the highest levels of psychological distress, with an increase in depression, anxiety, and thoughts of suicide, occurs in patients who have a recurrence of their cancer, which is often associated with a negative outcome or advanced disease.

The patient's culture has a significant influence on perception of distressing symptoms such as pain. Some researchers have found that the best predictors of pain intensity are ethnic affiliation and locus of control style. For example, an individual's stoic attitude, which serves to minimize or negate discomfort, may be related to a cultural value learned and reinforced through years of family experiences. Similarly, an individual's highly emotional response to routine events may become exaggerated during the terminal phase of illness and not necessarily signal maladjustment but rather a cultural norm.

Knowledge of an individual's response to illness and symptom expression is enhanced through awareness of the person's family traditions and culture. Understanding a patient's cultural, religious, ethnic, and socioeconomic underpinnings is key to understanding that person's beliefs, attitudes, practices, and behaviors related to illness and death. Cultural patterns play a significant role in determining how patients cope with terminal stages of cancer when symptoms such as delirium, depression, thoughts of suicide, and severe anxiety are common. When severe, these symptoms require aggressive treatment using up-to-date pharmacological and psychotherapeutic treatment strategies.

In spite of the seemingly overwhelming nature of physical discomfort and psychosocial stress associated with cancer, most patients can be relatively symptom free and cope effectively throughout the experience. Differentiating psychiatric complications from adaptive coping and differentiating normal from pathological emotional distress can be challenging. For example, anxiety and depression are normal responses to traumatic events such as a cancer diagnosis or progression of a life-threatening illness and are typical and expected at transitions throughout the cancer experience. Clinicians can distinguish between patients who need aggressive psychiatric intervention and those needing routine support and information by looking at factors such as whether the patient has a prior psychiatric history including hospitalization and has used or is using psychopharmacologic treatments, and the intensity and duration of symptoms and how much they diminish functioning. These factors can also help clinicians determine whether the patient has a lasting psychiatric disorder or transient psychological symptoms that will dissipate without specific treatment.

Psychological symptoms may also emerge when physical discomfort escalates or is not well controlled and diminish following treatment of physical discomfort. Health professionals and family and friends can monitor the patient's symptoms to determine what is normal for the patient and what indicates the need for intervention. They can also observe whether the patient's usual patterns of coping remain effective. In general, when psychological stress worsens over time and does not respond favorably to the usual supports, aggressive psychiatric assessment and management should be instituted.

Jeannie V. Pasacreta, Ph.D., A.P.R.N.

▶ For Further Information

Groenwald, Susan L., et al. *Cancer Symptom Mangement.* Boston: Jones and Bartlett, 1996.

Kelvin, Joanne Frankel, and Leslie B. Tyson. *One Hundred Questions and Answers About Cancer Symptoms and Cancer Side Effects.* Sudbury, Mass.: Jones and Bartlett, 2005.

Lyman, Gary H., and Jeffrey Crawford, eds. *Cancer Supportive Care: Advances in Therapeutic Strategies.* New York: Informa Healthcare USA, 2008.

New England Medical Center EPC. *Management of Cancer Symptoms: Pain, Depression, and Fatigue.* Rockville, Md.: U.S. Department of Health and Human Services, Public Health Service, Agency for Healthcare Research and Quality, 2002.

▶ Other Resources

American Cancer Society
http://www.cancer.org

Cancer.Net
http://www.cancer.net/portal/site/patient

CureSearch
http://www.curesearch.org

Lance Armstrong Foundation
http://www.livestrong.org

National Cancer Institute
http://www.cancer.gov

Oncology Tools
http://www.fda.gov/cder/cancer

See also Bone pain; Coughing; Depression; Diarrhea; Fatigue; Fever; Infection and sepsis; Itching; Lumps; Moles; Nausea and vomiting; Palpation; Personality and cancer; Psychosocial aspects of cancer; Screening for cancer; Weight loss.

▶ Syndrome of inappropriate antidiuretic hormone production (SIADH)

Category: Diseases, symptoms, and conditions
Also known as: Hyponatremia

Related conditions: Dehydration, water intoxication

Definition: Syndrome of inappropriate antidiuretic hormone (SIADH) was first described by Frederic C. Bartter and William B. Schwartz in 1957 when their patient, diagnosed with oat cell carcinoma, was experiencing symptoms related to a low sodium level. Sodium is an electrolyte that is important for the function of many cells within the body. SIADH occurs when there is an excessive release of antidiuretic hormones (ADH, or vasopressin), which causes an increase in fluid retention by the kidneys.

Risk factors: Patients who have small-cell lung cancer are at high risk for developing SIADH. Other cancers that may place the patient at high risk for developing this syndrome are pancreatic cancer, colon adenocarcinoma, olfactory neuroblastoma, lymphoma, and leukemia. Chemotherapy drugs, pain medications, tricyclic antidepressants, general anesthesia, and other drugs used to treat cancer side effects can also cause SIADH.

Etiology and the disease process: Antidiuretic hormone (ADH) is normally produced in the hypothalamus and stored in the posterior pituitary, which are both located in the brain. ADH is released by the pituitary gland but also can be released from a few cancer tumors. It works with the kidneys to regulate the amount of fluid that either remains in the body or is released in the urine. An increase in ADH can cause the kidney to retain fluid, which in turn causes fluid volume overload and dilutes the sodium as well as other electrolytes in the body.

Incidence: SIADH is a rare condition that is the most common cause of hyponatremia. Approximately 1 in 100,000 people are diagnosed with SIADH every year.

Symptoms: Symptoms are related more to the sudden changes in the sodium level than to the sodium level itself. Early signs and symptoms of SIADH include weakness and lethargy, confusion, irritability, altered mental status, nausea, vomiting, increased thirst, abdominal cramping, decreased urine output, and weight gain. Unresponsiveness, muscle cramping, and seizures are symptoms of progressively low sodium levels. Normal blood sodium levels are 135 to 145 milliequivalents of solute per liter of solvent

Common Causes of SIADH

Cancers
- small-cell lung cancer
- bladder cancer
- prostate cancer
- ovarian cancer
- lymphoma
- Hodgkin disease
- oral cancers
- pancreatic cancer
- exocrine cancer
- stomach cancer
- laryngeal cancer
- nasopharyngeal cancer
- thymoma
- brain cancer
- central nervous system cancers
- breast cancer
- melanoma

Chemotherapy drugs
- cisplatin
- cyclophosphamide
- vincristine

Drugs to Treat Side Effects of Cancer
- levamisole
- morphine
- amitriptyline
- carbamazepine

(mEq/l). Symptoms usually start occurring when the sodium level in the blood decreases to 120 to 125 mEq/l.

Screening and diagnosis: Initial blood tests should be taken to evaluate sodium levels. The blood test of a patient with SIADH will commonly reveal low serum (blood) sodium levels. Urine levels will show an increase in sodium levels and an increase in osmolarity. Patients will typically show no edema or volume depletion (dehydration). The patient will have normal renal, adrenal, and cardiac function. The decrease in sodium levels can be a slow gradual process or may have rapid onset.

Additional blood tests include a complete blood count, electrolytes, urea, creatinine, glucose, and serum (blood) osmolarity. Urine can also be tested for electrolytes.

Tests that may also be considered are thyroid-stimulating hormone (TSH) levels, cortisol level, and liver function tests (LFTs). A chest X ray and a computed tomography (CT) scan of the head may also be completed to assist with diagnosis.

Treatment and therapy: SIADH will need to be corrected slowly. Sodium levels that rise too quickly can cause central pontine myelinolysis (CPM), a type of nerve damage caused by the destruction of the layer covering the nerve cells in the brain stem. Symptoms of CPM are mental status changes, weak muscles, and cranial nerve abnormalities. There is no known cure.

Patients with SIADH will be assessed by medical personnel to evaluate for any signs of swelling, increase in thirst, intake and output, urine concentration, daily weights, and what they are currently consuming.

Asymptomatic cases are treated by treating the underlying cause. Symptomatic patients will be initially treated by being placed on fluid restrictions that allow for one half to one liter of fluid every twenty-four hours. Patients may also be placed on a high-protein, high-salt diet. Loop diuretics, such as furosemide (Lasix), may be given to help the body excrete more urine while retaining the sodium. Demeclocycline, a form of tetracycline antibiotic, may also be used to increase urine output. Demeclocycline is a pill that stops the kidneys from responding to the increased ADH, allowing the body to excrete large amounts of urine. For more severe cases, hypertonic saline (3 percent saline) is given intravenously to increase sodium levels within the serum. Furosemide can also be given with the hypertonic saline to help balance the fluid levels.

Prognosis, prevention, and outcomes: Outcomes for SIADH are related to the underlying disease. Prompt treatment of the underlying condition may improve the outcomes for the patient. The more rapid the increase of the sodium levels, the higher the risk of mortality. Patients may have to limit fluid intake for an extended period to ensure that the SIADH does not return if the underlying condition does not improve.

Katrina Green, R.N., B.S.N., O.C.N.

▶ For Further Information

Itano, J. K., and K. N. Toaka. *Core Curriculum for Oncology Nursing.* 4th ed. Philadelphia: Elsevier/Saunders, 2005.

Johnson, B. L., and J. Gross. *Handbook of Oncology Nursing.* 3d ed. Sudbury, Mass.: Jones and Bartlett, 1998.

Lenhard, R. E., R. T. Osteen, and T. Gansler. *The American Cancer Society's Clinical Oncology.* Atlanta: American Cancer Society, 2001.

Otto, S. E. *Oncology Nursing.* 4th ed. St. Louis: Elsevier, 2001.

Yarbro, C. H., M. H. Frogge, and M. Goodman. *Cancer Nursing: Principles and Practice.* 6th ed. Sudbury, Mass.: Jones and Bartlett, 2005.

_____. *Cancer Symptom Management.* 3d ed. Sudbury, Mass.: Jones and Bartlett, 2005.

▶ Other Resources

American Cancer Society
http://www.cancer.org

National Cancer Institute
  http://www.cancer.gov

See also Chemotherapy; Colorectal cancer; Craniotomy; Leukemias; Lung cancers; Lymphomas; Pain management medications; Pancreatic cancers; Paraneoplastic syndromes.

▶ Synovial sarcomas

Category: Diseases, symptoms, and conditions

Related conditions: Soft-tissue sarcomas

Definition: Soft-tissue sarcomas are cancers that begin in fat, cartilage, blood vessels, and muscles. A synovial sarcoma is a distinct type of soft-tissue tumor that arises from tissues that are associated with a joint. Almost all synovial sarcomas are found within 2 inches (5 centimeters, or cm) of a joint. The tumor can be composed of all epithelial cells, all spindle cells, or a mix of the two cell types. These cells form distinct pink, fleshy masses.

Risk factors: Synovial sarcomas appear to develop because of a genetic mutation. About 90 percent of these tumors show a specific genetic defect that is different from that found in all other sarcomas. This defect involves a switch in a small amount of material on chromosome 18 and the X chromosome. As a result, an incorrect protein is formed.

Etiology and the disease process: Exactly why the genetic mutation occurs or how the resulting protein causes cells to become cancerous is not known. About half of synovial sarcomas develop in the legs. The knee joint is the most common tumor location, followed by the ankle and the foot. Primary synovial sarcomas can also develop in arm, wrist, and hand joints and less frequently in the joints of the trunk, head, and neck. Only rarely are primary tumors found in the lungs or abdomen. Synovial sarcomas tend to grow slowly. Often these tumors exist for a long time as hard nodules and then begin to grow suddenly. Sometimes calcium deposits develop in the tumors. Tumors with calcium tend to grow more slowly than those without calcium. Tumors may invade nearby tissues, and about half metastasize to distant sites.

Incidence: Synovial sarcomas account for 8 to 10 percent of all soft-tissue sarcomas and are the fourth most common type of soft-tissue sarcoma. In absolute terms, however, they are quite rare, with only about 800 new cases of synovial sarcoma diagnosed each year in the United States.

Synovial sarcomas are about 1.5 times more common in men than women. They can develop in people of any age, but the median age of diagnosis is about thirty years, with fewer than 30 percent of new cases reported in people younger than twenty.

Symptoms: Most often, the first symptom a person with a synovial sarcoma notices is a swelling that may or may not be painful. Since synovial sarcomas grow slowly, the person may have a hard mass for quite a while, especially if it is not painful, before consulting a doctor. Other symptoms are specific to the location of the tumor. For example, a tumor near a joint may cause pain similar to bursitis or arthritis, or a tumor pressing on a nerve may cause the person to feel numbness and tingling in the surrounding area.

Screening and diagnosis: There are no screening tests specific to synovial sarcoma; however, people who have unexplained swellings or lumps anywhere in the body should consult a physician immediately. Often diagnosis is delayed because these swellings seem nonthreatening and are not painful, so that by the time they are diagnosed, they have already spread to the lymph nodes or beyond.

Exploration of the tumor begins with a magnetic resonance imaging (MRI) scan. However, a definitive diagnosis can be made only by a biopsy (tissue sample) of the tumor. Depending on the location of the tumor, the biopsy process may be complex (for example, a tumor of the hand). The biopsied tissue is examined under the microscope, where a distinctive pattern of cells identifies it as a synovial sarcoma. The tissue also may be tested for the specific chromosomal abnormalities associated with this cancer.

Staging is done using MRI and computed tomography (CT) scans to determine if the sarcoma has metastasized to distant sites.

Treatment and therapy: The treatment of choice is always surgery regardless of the stage of the tumor. These tumors tend to spread along the tissues surrounding joints, and it may be necessary to amputate the entire limb to remove all traces of the sarcoma cells. Surgery is supplemented by radiation therapy before and after tumor removal. The use of chemotherapy in addition to surgery and radiation therapy is controversial, with some studies reporting improved survival rates and others reporting no differences in survival when compared with radiation therapy alone. Clinical trials of biological therapies that use man-made antibodies to target sarcoma cells are under way.

Prognosis, prevention, and outcomes: There is no known way to prevent synovial sarcoma. Outcomes are better with early diagnosis, when tumors are less than 2 inches (5 cm) in diameter, when tumors contain calcium deposits, and when they are located farthest away from the trunk. Recurrence is common, usually within two years of surgery. Amputation of a limb is often necessary. The five-year survival rate is about 50 percent.

Martiscia Davidson, A.M.

▶ **For Further Information**

Pappo, Alberto S., ed. *Pediatric Bone and Soft-Tissue Sarcomas.* New York: Springer, 2005.

Thompson, Lester D. R., and Gretchen S. Folk. "Synovial Sarcoma (Disease Overview)." *Ear, Nose, and Throat Journal* 85 (2006): 418-419.

Verweij, J., and Herbert M. Pinedo. *Targeting Treatment of Soft-Tissue Sarcomas.* Boston: Kluwer Academic, 2004.

▶ **Other Resources**

National Cancer Institute
Synovial Sarcoma: Questions and Answers
http://www.cancer.gov/templates/doc.aspx?viewid=5B6A9BCC-80A4-4FBF-B7C2-7E07D5BD4798

Sarcoma Foundation of America
http://www.curesarcoma.org

See also Amputation; Fibrosarcomas, soft-tissue; Limb salvage; Sarcomas, soft-tissue.

▶ Taste alteration

Category: Diseases, symptoms, and conditions
Also known as: Taste change, taste dysfunction, dysgeusia, hypogeusia, ageusia

Related conditions: Anorexia (loss of appetite), xerostomia (dry mouth), thrush (a fungal disease of the mouth), zinc deficiency, increased levels of calcium

Definition: As the phrase suggests, taste alteration is a change in the way people perceive tastes, or flavors. People can recognize four main tastes: sweet, sour, salty, and bitter. Any one or all four taste sensations can be affected. Taste alteration is a symptom or side effect, not a disease. Infection in the mouth, cancer, and certain cancer treatments can change a person's sense of taste. Taste alteration may emerge as one of three medically recognized abnormalities: dysgeusia (changes in how foods normally taste), hypogeusia (a decreased ability to taste foods), or ageusia (the complete loss of the ability to taste foods). In addition, many cancer patients complain of a medicine-like or metallic taste in the mouth that affects their sense of taste.

Risk factors: Risk factors include having cancer of the mouth, tongue, lips, or throat; receiving radiation treatments to the head or neck; receiving chemotherapy involving certain cancer-fighting drugs; and undergoing surgery to the head or neck.

Etiology and the disease process: Although the exact causes of taste alteration in cancer patients are not known, doctors suspect three principal sources: the disease itself, radiation treatments, and certain cancer-fighting drugs.

Many cancerous tumors, found anywhere in the body, release substances that change the taste of foods or even take away people's desire to eat.

Radiation treatments, especially to the head or neck, can damage taste buds, which changes the way food tastes to a patient. For instance, sour or bitter foods may taste especially strong, or sweet foods may not taste as sweet as they once did. Radiation can also damage the salivary glands, causing them to produce less saliva, which results in a dry mouth. Saliva contributes to the sense of taste by mixing with food particles and carrying them to the tongue. This process stimulates the taste receptors on the tongue, allowing people to experience and distinguish among the four tastes. Taste alteration from radiation may not show up until several weeks after treatment begins.

Chemotherapy seems to change the sense of taste in some patients. Researchers believe that some cancer-fighting drugs affect certain taste cells on the tongue and cause an imbalance of taste, changing the way things normally taste. These changes may result from damage to the cells in the mouth from chemotherapy or by the spread of the drug to the tissues of the mouth.

Taste alteration in itself is normally not a serious problem. Nevertheless, it can lead to problems when patients change their eating habits. Each patient's sense of taste changes differently. Some patients with taste alteration may avoid certain nutritious foods because their taste has changed; others may lose their appetite altogether. Taste alteration is one of the leading causes of malnutrition in cancer patients.

Incidence: Although taste alteration appears to be common among cancer patients receiving radiation treatment or chemotherapy, few studies have confirmed the degree of prevalence. Research may be lacking because the condition usually does not last long and often takes place in the early stages of cancer. When this condition arises in patients in the later stages of cancer, treatment and research focus more on other aspects of care, such as pain relief.

Symptoms: Taste alteration itself is a symptom or a side effect. It can, however, lead to complications in a cancer patient's nutritional status, which causes such symptoms as mouth sores, anorexia, nausea and vomiting, diarrhea, constipation, lack of energy, and weight gain or loss.

Screening and diagnosis: Nutritional screening and assessments are done for nearly all cancer patients before starting radiation therapy or chemotherapy. Screenings identify patients who may be undernourished. Assessments establish the nutritional status of patients and determine which patients need nutritional therapy. Patients who are well nourished are better able to tolerate aggressive cancer treatments.

Chemotherapy Drugs That Can Cause Taste Alteration

- carboplatin
- cisplatin
- cyclophosphamide
- dacarbazine
- dactinomycin
- doxorubicin
- fluorouracil
- levamisole
- mechlorethamine
- methotrexate
- nitrogen mustard
- paclitraxel
- vincristine

Source: Cleveland Clinic Cancer Center

Treatment and therapy: There is no treatment for taste alteration. Results of some studies suggest that increased zinc may be of some benefit. Care management focuses on nutrition therapy to help cancer patients avoid malnutrition, tolerate treatment, maintain their energy and strength, fight infection, heal and recover, and improve their quality of life. In addition, dietitians suggest the following for patients who may have lost their desire to eat:

- Eat with plastic utensils.
- Use sweet marinades or strong sauces with foods.
- Eat chilled rather than hot foods.
- Use extra seasonings, spices, and herbs.
- Drink citrus juices, especially lemon, to stimulate saliva.
- Keep the mouth clean with frequent tooth brushing and rinsing.

Prognosis, prevention, and outcomes: Fortunately, for many cancer patients, taste alteration lasts only a short time and is hardly ever permanent. Normal taste returns within a few weeks up to a few months after treatment ends. In terminal patients, however, taste alteration can cause or exacerbate existing anorexia and cachexia.

Wendell Anderson, B.A.

▶ For Further Information

Bloch, A. *Nutrition Management of the Cancer Patient.* Sudbury, Mass.: Jones and Bartlett, 1990.

Keane, M., and D. Chace. *What to Eat If You Have Cancer: A Guide to Adding Nutritional Therapy to Your Treatment Plan.* New York: McGraw-Hill, 1996.

Whittington, E. "Food for Thought: A Waste of Taste." *CURE* (Fall, 2006).

▶ Other Resources

American Cancer Society
Changes in Taste and Smell
    http://www.cancer.org/docroot/MBC/content/
    MBC_6_2X_When_Things_Arent_Tasting_Right
    .asp?sitearea=MBC

National Cancer Institute
Overview of Nutrition in Cancer Care
    http://www.cancer.gov/cancertopics/pdq/
    supportivecare/nutrition/patient

See also Anorexia; Appetite loss; Cachexia; Calcium; Chemotherapy; Dry mouth; Gastrointestinal complications of cancer treatment; Nausea and vomiting; Nutrition and cancer treatment; Salivary gland cancer.

▶ Teratocarcinomas

Category: Diseases, symptoms, and conditions
Also known as: Teratomas

Related conditions: Germ-cell tumors, nonseminomatous germ-cell tumors (NSGCTs), choriocarcinomas, yolk sac tumors, seminomas, embryonal cell carcinomas, dermoid cysts

Definition: Teratocarcinomas are malignant testicular cancers whose cells are derived from primordial germ cells (spermatozoa precursor cells). The term "teratoma" is sometimes used to refer to a benign form seen in prepubescent boys and may also refer to a benign cancer in the ovary (dermoid cyst), in which cells are derived from all three primitive embryonic tissue layers. Teratocarcinomas contain embryonic stem cells in addition to these cells.

Risk factors: One of the risk factors for the development of a teratocarcinoma is undescended testes (cryptorchidism) during infancy. Anomalies in testicular development such as that found in Klinefelter syndrome may increase the risk of malignancy. Family history, age of descent or correction, location, single or bilateral undescended testes, premature birth, and previous history of testicular cancer have also been implicated.

Etiology and the disease process: The exact mechanisms by which teratocarcinomas develop remain unknown. Studies suggest that primordial spermatozoa cells (gonocytes) in the seminiferous tubules of the testes retain their embryonic characteristics of being able to differentiate into different mature tissues as well as divide uncontrollably when testicular development is interrupted.

Incidence: A history of cryptorchidism increases the risk of testicular malignancy by a factor of 1.6 to 17 times irrespective of prior removal, where carcinoma can still develop in the remaining testis. The incidence of teratocarcinoma in particular is estimated at 7 percent of testicular cancers in male adults and 40 percent in prepubescent boys, although these figures may be grossly underestimated.

Symptoms: Symptoms may include an often painless, palpable mass within the scrotal area. The mass may also be firm and, at times, fixed. Discovery of the mass may be incidental, with no other signs of disease present.

Screening and diagnosis: Diagnosis is primarily clinical. If twisting of the testicle or its blood supply is suspected (causing discoloration and pain), Doppler ultrasound is done to assess blood flow as well as visualize the mass.

Abdominal computed tomography (CT) or magnetic resonance imaging (MRI) is carried out to look for spread outside the scrotum.

Treatment and therapy: Surgical resection of the entire tumor; chemotherapy with cisplatin, bleomycin, and vinblastine; and irradiation are the treatments of choice.

Prognosis, prevention, and outcomes: Prognosis is generally excellent with optimal treatment, approaching 90 percent. However, infertility may occur and should be understood by the patient as a possible side effect of therapy.

Aldo C. Dumlao, M.D.

See also Benign tumors; Carcinomas; Childhood cancers; Choriocarcinomas; Computed tomography (CT) scan; Cryptorchidism; Embryonal cell cancer; Family history and risk assessment; Germ-cell tumors; Infertility and cancer; Magnetic resonance imaging (MRI); Teratomas; Testicular cancer; Yolk sac carcinomas.

▶ Teratomas

Category: Diseases, symptoms, and conditions
Also known as: Germ-cell tumors

Related conditions: Teratocarcinomas, seminomas

Definition: Teratomas are tumors containing cells derived from more than one of the three embryonic germ layers.

Risk factors: Risk factors are unclear. In young men, teratomas in the chest may be associated with other cancers, including acute myelogenous leukemia and small-cell undifferentiated carcinoma. Metastasis risk increases with a tumor stage greater than II and vascular invasion.

Etiology and the disease process: Teratomas can contain structures such as teeth, hair, and bone. They arise from abnormal development of pluripotent cells (cells that have not assumed their final form and function) or germ cells (cells that produce the sperm or eggs) and contain cells from more than one of the three embryonic germ layers. The early embryo has three germ layers: the endoderm (which produces the lining of the digestive tube and its associated organs); the ectoderm (which produces the cells of the epidermis and nervous system); and the mesoderm (which produces the heart, kidney, ovaries, testes, and the connective tissues, including bone, muscles, and blood).

Incidence: Sacroccocygeal teratoma (found at the base of the spine in fetuses) affects 1 in 40,000 births, with 80 percent occurring in girls. In adults, teratomas occur in the neck, brain, ovaries, testes, mediastinum (chest), and retroperitoneum (back of the abdominal cavity). Teratomas of the chest are most commonly diagnosed in young men in their twenties.

Symptoms: Symptoms of teratoma vary with the location of the tumor. Teratomas of the brain in children can produce vision problems, developmental delays, headaches, nausea, and vomiting. Teratomas of the chest may be associated with difficulty breathing, chest pain, cough, and fatigue upon exercise. Ovarian teratomas are associated with abdominal pain.

Screening and diagnosis: Sacroccocygeal teratomas are diagnosed by fetal ultrasound. Other teratomas are diagnosed by physical exam and imaging such as a computed tomography (CT) scan. Teratomas are staged as 0, mature; I, immature; II, immature, possibly malignant; and III, malignant, or teratoma with malignant transformation. Solid teratomas are composed mostly of tissue, and cystic teratomas have pockets of fluid. Mixed teratomas are composed of cysts and tissue. Nonmalignant teratomas can still be highly aggressive and grow quickly.

Treatment and therapy: Sacrococcygeal teratoma is treated surgically. Stage I teratoma is usually treated with a combination of surgery and radiation therapy. Teratoma

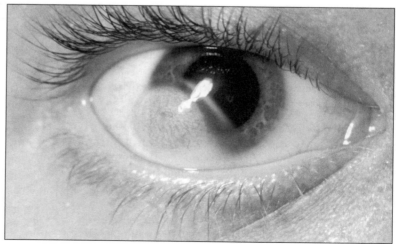

A dermoid cyst (a cystic teratoma that contains developmentally mature skin) in an eye. (Biophoto Associates/Photo Researchers, Inc.)

with malignant transformation is treated surgically, followed by radiation, chemotherapy, or both.

Prognosis, prevention, and outcomes: With sacrococcocygeal teratoma, prognosis is determined by the size and histology of the tumor. These tumors can result in fatalities from secondary effects. Some 20 to 30 percent of adult metastatic teratomas are cured with chemotherapy.

Michele Arduengo, Ph.D., ELS

See also Carcinomas; Childhood cancers; Choriocarcinomas; Cryptorchidism; Embryonal cell cancer; Family history and risk assessment; Germ-cell tumors; Klinefelter syndrome and cancer; Mediastinal tumors; Teratocarcinomas; Testicular cancer; Yolk sac carcinomas.

▶ Testicular cancer

Category: Diseases, symptoms, and conditions
Also known as: Germ-cell tumors, testicular tumors

Related conditions: Testicular tumors, cryptorchidism, germ-cell tumors, decreased fertility

Definition: Testicular cancer is the development of tumors in the testicles, or male sex glands.

Risk factors: The primary risk factor associated with testicular cancer is a history of an undescended testicle (cryptorchidism). Some 5 to 10 percent of patients with this abnormality, which is resolved with surgery, may develop testicular cancer. Research has shown that men who have any type of abnormal development of the testicles are at an increased risk of developing testicular cancer. Additionally, a hypothesized link between some pollutants and testicular cancer has been noted, because of an increase in the diagnoses linked with industrial growth and waste. Although research has not confirmed a link between a hormone taken by mothers during pregnancy, there is an abnormally high rate of testicular cancer in men exposed to diethylstilbestrol (DES) during fetal development.

Etiology and the disease process: In men under the age of sixty, 95 percent of testicular tumors originate in the germ cells, or embryonic cells that develop into sperm cells. These tumors can be divided into seminomas or nonseminomas. Seminomas are responsible for 40 percent of all testicular cancer and are slow to grow and usually remain in the testicle. These types of tumors are very responsive to both radiation therapy and chemotherapy. Nonseminomas are cancers that occur in combination with other types of cancers and arise from more mature germ cells. These can-

cers are more aggressive in growth and respond well to chemotherapy. Rarely tumors leading to testicular cancer include Leydig and Sertoli cell tumors, leiomyosarcoma, rhabdomyosarcoma, and mesothelioma.

Incidence: Approximately 1 in 100,000 men develop testicular cancer each year, and it is the most common malignancy in men between the ages of fifteen and thirty-five. Whites are more likely to be diagnosed than are Hispanics, and the incidence in African Americans has doubled since the 1980's. Male infants and men over sixty have also been diagnosed with the disease.

Symptoms: Symptoms of testicular cancer most often include a lump in one testis or a hardening of the testis and pain or tenderness in the testicles. Some 50 percent of men diagnosed with testicular cancer complain of swelling in the testicles or enlarged testicles. Other symptoms include an increase in fluid in the scrotum, loss of sexual activity, a feeling of heaviness in the scrotum, a dull ache in the groin or lower abdomen, shrinking of the testicle, and enlargement or tenderness of the breasts.

Screening and diagnosis: The most effective screening mechanism for testicular cancer is the testicular self-exam. It involves a manual exam of the testicles to feel for any suspicious lumps and can be performed monthly at home.

If testicular cancer is suspected, the physician conducts a medical history and physical exam. In addition to carefully examining the scrotum, the physician will order an ultrasound, chest X ray, and blood and urine tests.

Age at Diagnosis for Testicular Cancer, 2001-2005

Age Group	Percentage Diagnosed
Under 20	5.8
20-34	46.3
35-44	29.2
45-54	13.3
55-64	3.3
65-74	1.2
75-84	0.6
85 and older	0.2

Source: Data from National Cancer Institute, Surveillance Epidemiology and End Results, Cancer Stat Fact Sheets, 2008
Note: The median age of diagnosis from 2001 to 2005 was thirty-four, with an age-adjusted incidence rate of 5.4 per 100,000 men per year.

A procedure called a serum marker test may be performed to measure the amounts of certain substances released into the blood by organs, tissues, or tumor cells in the blood. Certain substances, called tumor markers, are linked to specific types of cancer when found in increased levels in the blood. Three tumor markers are used in staging testicular cancer: alpha-fetoprotein (AFP), beta-human chorionic gonadotropin (β-HCG), and lactate dehydrogenase (LDH) if ultrasound reveals a solid mass in the testicle.

It is important to note that nearly one-third of all patients diagnosed with testicular cancer are misdiagnosed the first time because testicular cancer is so rare. If there is a lump or mass on the testicle, it is very important to rule out testicular cancer early on. This involves obtaining a second opinion if the patient is not offered an ultrasound at the first discovery of a lump in the testicle.

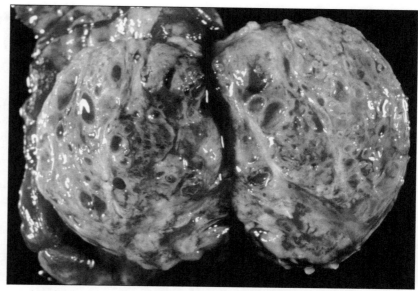

A malignant tumor in a sliced open testicle. (CNRI/Photo Researchers, Inc.)

A procedure called a lymphangiography may also be used to X-ray the lymph system. In this procedure, a dye is injected into the lymph vessels in the feet to observe any possible blockages. This test helps determine whether cancer has spread to the lymph nodes.

The only way to confirm diagnosis of testicular cancer is by removal of the testis (orchiectomy). Biopsy of the tumor is not an option because of the risk of malignancy of any remaining cancerous cells in the testis.

After removal of the suspicious testicle, the tumor is staged by a pathologist. The size of the tumor is irrelevant to the stage of the cancer.

- Stage I: Cancer is only in the testis.
- Stage II: Cancer is in the testis and lymph nodes.
- Stage III: Cancer in the testis has spread to remote sites in the body (for example, the lungs, brain, liver, or bones).

Treatment and therapy: Almost all treatment involves surgically removing the testicle (orchiectomy). This is necessary because of the risk of any remaining cancer cells becoming malignant and spreading to other parts of the body. The risk of surgery is very low, and most men can maintain a normal reproductive life with one testicle. Sometimes surgery will include removing the lymph nodes in the abdomen if the cancer has spread.

Radiation therapy uses high-energy rays to kill localized cancer cells. Seminomas are highly sensitive to radiation, and most men will receive this therapy for their lymph nodes following surgery. Radiation is ineffective with nonseminomas.

Chemotherapy is a treatment whereby drugs are inserted into the bloodstream (either via a vein or taken orally) to treat the entire body. This treatment is used if the physician suspects cancer cells have spread, or if the cells are suspected to remain after surgery or radiation therapy.

Tumor-marker levels are measured again, after radical inguinal orchiectomy and biopsy, to determine the stage of the cancer. This helps to show if all the cancer has been removed or if more treatment is needed. Tumor-marker levels are also measured during follow-up as a way of checking if the cancer has come back.

Prognosis, prevention, and outcomes: Although testicular cancer is the most common malignancy in men between the ages of fifteen and thirty-five, it is the cancer with the highest cure rate. It is almost always curable if discovered early on. It responds well to treatment even when it has spread to other parts of the body.

The most effective method of prevention is the testicular self-exam, which can be performed monthly by men in their own homes. This simple, risk-free exam involves manually examining each testicle for any suspicious lumps, swelling, or hardness.

Men diagnosed with Stage I seminoma have a survival rate of 99 percent. The survival rate of men diagnosed with Stage I nonseminoma is about 98 percent. Cure rates for

Stage II tumors range above 90 percent, while cure rates for Stage III tumors can fall between 50 and 80 percent.

Generally after removal of one testis, a man can lead a life of normal fertility because the remaining testis increases production of testosterone and sperm cells. In the case of men who have decreased fertility before surgery, it may be prudent to consider sperm banking (freezing sperm for later use) if he wants to have children.

Fewer than 5 percent of those diagnosed will have a recurrence in the other testicle. If this occurs, the patient will need to take hormone supplements such as testosterone (produced in the testes) and will be infertile but otherwise will lead a normal life.

Robert J. Amato, D.O.

▶ For Further Information

Johanson, Paula. *Frequently Asked Questions About Testicular Cancer.* New York: Rosen, 2008.

Kurth, K. H., G. H. J. Mickisch, and Fritz H. Schroder, eds. *Renal, Bladder, Prostate, and Testicular Cancer: An Update.* New York: Parthenon, 2001.

Parker, James N., and Philip M. Parker, eds. *The Official Patient's Sourcebook on Testicular Cancer: A Revised and Updated Directory for the Internet Age.* San Diego, Calif.: Icon Health, 2002.

▶ Other Resources

American Cancer Society
Do I Have Testicular Cancer?
http://www.cancer.org/docroot/PED/content/
PED_2_3X_Do_I_Have_Testicular_Cancer.asp

National Cancer Institute
Testicular Cancer
http://www.cancer.gov/cancertopics/types/
testicular/

The Testicular Cancer Resource Center
http://tcrc.acor.org/

See also Cryptorchidism; Desmoplastic small round cell tumor (DSRCT); Diethylstilbestrol (DES); Embryonal cell cancer; Germ-cell tumors; Infertility and cancer; Orchiectomy; Organochlorines (OCs); Paraneoplastic syndromes; Penile cancer; Peutz-Jeghers syndrome (PJS); Renal pelvis tumors; Sertoli cell tumors; Spermatocytomas; Teratocarcinomas; Teratomas; Testicular self-examination (TSE); Urologic oncology; Vasectomy and cancer; Wilms' tumor aniridia-genitourinary anomalies-mental retardation (WAGR) syndrome and cancer; Yolk sac carcinomas; Young adult cancers.

▶ Testicular self-examination (TSE)

Category: Procedures

Definition: Testicular self-examination (TSE) is a procedure done by the patient as a screening tool for early diagnosis of any testicular disorders. The exam is performed by manually examining the scrotum and testes.

Cancers diagnosed: Testicular cancer

Why performed: A self-exam of the testicles is an effective way of becoming familiar with this area of the body and thus enabling the early detection of abnormalities that can lead to testicular cancer. It can be the first line of defense against cancer because testicular cancer comes with virtually no obvious symptoms or pain. Testicular cancer primarily develops in younger men, and it is the most common form of cancer developed by men between the ages of twenty and thirty-five. Therefore, monthly performance of the testicular self-exam is recommended for men over age fourteen.

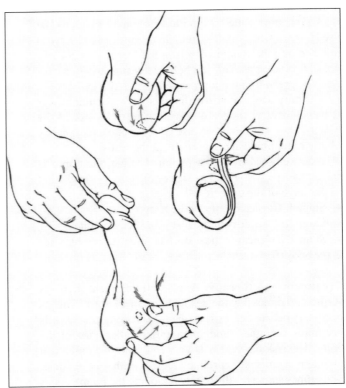

Rolling and palpating the testis in a self-examination. (LifeART© 2008 Wolters Kluwer Health, Inc.-Lippincott Williams & Wilkins. All rights reserved.)

Patient preparation: Because heat relaxes the scrotum, a TSE is best performed after a warm bath or shower.

Steps of the procedure: The first step in TSE is to stand in front of a mirror and observe any possible swelling on the scrotal skin. Next, the patient should elevate one leg for better access and examine each testicle with both hands. With the index and middle fingers under the testicle and the thumbs placed on top, the testicle should be rolled gently between the thumbs and fingers. This process should not be painful, but if pain or tenderness is experienced, the patient should notify a physician. The testicles should feel firm and round, but not hard, and it is normal for one testicle to be slightly larger than the other. It is important to feel for any lumps on the testicle, which can range in size from a pea to a golf ball and are frequently very hard. If any lumps are detected, then it is critical for the patient to see a physician as soon as possible to determine if the lumps are benign (noncancerous) or malignant (cancerous).

The next step in the TSE is to locate the epididymis, a soft, tubelike structure behind the testicle that collects and carries sperm. It is important to become familiar with this structure to avoid mistaking it for a lump or mass.

After the procedure: No aftercare is required.

Risks: There are no risks with this procedure if the patient performs the exam without inflicting pain.

Results: If any abnormalities (swelling, change in color, lumps, hardness, pain) are detected during the testicular self-exam, a physician (urologist) should be consulted. Generally any suspicions can be confirmed or ruled out by the physician with an exam and/or ultrasound.

Robert J. Amato, D.O.

▶ For Further Information

Johanson, Paula. *Frequently Asked Questions About Testicular Cancer*. New York: Rosen, 2007.

Kurth, Karl H., Gerald H. J. Mickisch, and Fritz H. Schröder. *Renal, Bladder, Prostate, and Testicular Cancer: An Update*. New York: Parthenon, 2001.

Parker, James N., and Philip M. Parker, eds. *The Official Patient's Sourcebook on Testicular Cancer: A Revised and Updated Directory for the Internet Age*. San Diego, Calif.: Icon Health, 2002.

See also Embryonal cell cancer; Lumps; Risks for cancer; Symptoms and cancer; Testicular cancer; Ultrasound tests.

▶ Thermal imaging

Category: Procedures
Also known as: Digital infrared thermal imaging (DITI)

Definition: Thermal imaging is a procedure to measure the skin surface temperature by detecting infrared radiation emitted from the circulation. Since tumors have higher metabolic rates than normal tissues, they tend to recruit and/or create more surrounding blood vessels than normal tissues. This process provides nutrients and oxygen for tumor cell survival and increases surface temperature.

Cancers diagnosed: Primarily breast cancer

Why performed: Thermal imaging is an extremely sensitive test performed to detect and monitor cancers. It is an alternative to other screening options that carry the risk of radiation exposure. Additionally, multiple images over time may aid in analyzing responses to treatment.

Patient preparation: Because thermal imaging measures temperature changes, patients should maintain normal circulation and body temperature prior to the imaging, including the avoidance of excessive sun exposure one week prior to testing. Also, patients should avoid hot water exposure and the use of topical analgesics two hours prior to testing, as well as nicotine, caffeine, alcohol, strenuous physical exercise, and hot or cold beverages four hours prior to testing. Medications affecting the sympathetic nervous system may need to be withheld twelve to twenty-four hours prior to the evaluation as well.

Steps of the procedure: Patients will wear a hospital gown and lay on an examination table in a temperature-controlled room (68 degrees Fahrenheit) for approximately ten minutes to equilibrate the patient to the room temperature. Both sides of the body will be scanned with a thermal camera, also called an imaging radiometer, and the scans will be used as a thermal reference because of the body's natural thermal symmetry.

After the procedure: After thermal images are taken, no more action is required by the patient. The emitted infrared radiation will be detected and converted into a monochrome or multicolored image, known as a thermogram, and displayed on a monitor screen.

Risks: The risks of this procedure are negligible, since it is noninvasive and does not use tracer dyes, radiation, or chemicals.

Results: The thermal images are analyzed with the assistance of software programs, where shades or colors represent thermal patterns. The test result would be normal if the sides of the body are mirror images, indicating a symmetrical thermal pattern. Areas of increased heat, however, would indicate a potentially cancerous mass as a result of increased local blood vessels emitting more infrared radiation. Because thermal imagers cannot pinpoint specific tumor sites, an abnormal result would likely be followed up with other imaging or clinical laboratory tests.

Elizabeth A. Manning, Ph.D.

See also Breast cancer in children and adolescents; Breast cancer in men; Breast cancer in pregnant women; Breast cancers; Imaging tests; Risks for cancer.

▶ Thiotepa

Category: Carcinogens and suspected carcinogens
RoC status: Known human carcinogen since 1998
Also known as: TESPA, triethylenethiophosphoramide, TSPA, thio-TEPA

Related cancers: Leukemia

Definition: Thiotepa is a colorless or white crystalline solid that is odorless.

Exposure routes: Some cancer patients are exposed to thiotepa when it is used as a chemotherapy treatment. It is typically administered intravenously. It may be injected into muscle tissue, directly into a tumor, or through a catheter into a body cavity. Potential exposure by direct contact can occur to workers who are involved in the formulation, packaging, preparation, and administration of thiotepa for use in chemotherapy treatments.

Where found: Thiotepa is found at sites where it is manufactured, packaged, and supplied. It can be found at medical facilities where it is prepared and administered during cancer treatments. During the 1970's it was found in some polymeric flame retardants for cotton and in some insecticides.

At risk: Patients who are treated with thiotepa for various cancers, including bladder cancer, ovarian cancer, breast cancer, bronchial cancer, mesotheliomas, and lymphomas, are at high risk. Workers at locations where thiotepa is manufactured, packaged, and supplied for chemotherapy treatments are at risk for contamination. Health care professionals who prepare and administer thiotepa for cancer therapy risk contamination.

Etiology and symptoms of associated cancers: Thiotepa is an alkylating agent that slows or stops the growth of cancer cells in the human body. It can induce deoxyribonucleic acid (DNA) damage, changes in chromosome structure or number, addition or deletion of chromosomes, and cell transformation. It can also control the accumulation of fluids in body cavities that results from various cancers. Side effects of thiotepa chemotherapy include low white and red blood cell counts, decrease in platelets, hair loss, mouth sores, loss of appetite, tightness of the throat, nausea and vomiting, hives, rash, bladder irritation, and painful urination.

History: Thiotepa was first used in cancer therapy treatment of lymphomas and malignant tumors in 1953. Between 1970 and 1978, a link was established between the secondary development of leukemia and exposure to thiotepa. In the *Second Report on Carcinogens* (RoC; 1981), it was listed as a highly probable human carcinogen. By the 1990's, it was produced only in Japan. In the *Eighth Report on Carcinogens* (1998), thiotepa was listed as a known human carcinogen. To a large extent, it has been replaced by nitrogen mustard gas derivatives for chemotherapy treatments. It is still used in combination with other chemotherapy drugs for lymphomas and for bladder, ovarian, breast, lung, and brain cancers.

Alvin K. Benson, Ph.D.

See also Alkylating agents in chemotherapy; Antineoplastics in chemotherapy; Chemotherapy; Leukemias; Occupational exposures and cancer.

▶ Thoracentesis

Category: Procedures
Also known as: Thoracocentesis, pleural tap

Definition: Thoracentesis is the removal of pleural fluid from the layers of the pleura, the membranes lining the lungs and chest cavity. The pleural fluid is removed through a needle inserted through the chest wall, between the ribs, and is analyzed in a laboratory to determine the underlying cause of the fluid accumulation.

Cancers diagnosed or treated: Lung cancer, breast cancer, lymphoma, leukemia

Why performed: A thoracentesis is performed as a diagnostic procedure to determine the cause of a pleural effusion, the abnormal collection of excess fluid between the layers of the pleura. Normally, only a small amount of fluid is present in the pleural cavity to lubricate the pleural surfaces. This procedure is also performed as a therapeutic procedure to remove excess fluid and help reduce pressure on the lungs when an effusion is large and causing symptoms, such as shortness of breath or other breathing problems. A thoracentesis may be used as a palliative treatment to relieve symptoms of advanced cancers.

Patient preparation: Tests performed before the procedure include a chest X ray to confirm the presence of the pleural effusion and identify its location, ultrasound of the chest, and blood tests, such as a complete blood count, to exclude any blood-clotting abnormalities. One week before the procedure, patients must stop taking aspirin and products containing aspirin, ibuprofen, and anticoagulants, as directed by the physician. Other anticoagulant medications may be prescribed if necessary before the procedure. There are no specific eating or drinking guidelines in preparation for a thoracentesis.

Steps of the procedure: The patient usually sits upright on the edge of a chair or bed with the head and arms resting on a table. Sedating medications are not usually given for this procedure. The skin around the procedure site between the ribs and back of the chest is cleansed, and sterile drapes are placed around the area. A local anesthetic is injected into the skin to numb the area. The thoracentesis needle is inserted into the pleural space. Ultrasound guidance may be used to direct the biopsy needle into the effusion. Fluid is withdrawn through a syringe attached to the biopsy needle and collected for analysis in the laboratory.

Sclerosing agents such as talc, doxycycline, bleomycin, and quinacrine may be inserted through a chest tube during thoracentesis to prevent recurring, symptomatic malignant effusions.

The patient may experience mild pain or discomfort at the puncture site. The patient should not cough or breathe deeply during the procedure and must remain as still as possible to prevent injury to the lung. If the patient develops a cough or chest pain during the procedure, then the procedure should be stopped immediately.

After the procedure: Pressure is applied at the site where the needle was inserted. A dressing or adhesive bandage is placed over the site to help prevent infection. Supplemental oxygen may be given to the patient. The patient's breathing will be monitored after the procedure. A chest X ray is performed to ensure that the lung was not injured during the procedure. The patient should immediately report chest pain, shortness of breath, or difficulty breathing to the nurse. After the patient goes home within a few hours of the procedure, he or she should seek emergency treatment if these symptoms occur. A follow-up chest X ray may be scheduled within two to four weeks.

Risks: The risks of a thoracentesis are decreased when the procedure is performed with ultrasound guidance. In most cases, there are few complications. The risks, however, include reaccumulation of fluid in the pleural space or fluid in the lungs (pulmonary edema), bleeding, infection, respiratory distress, or collapse of the lung (pneumothorax). Pneumothorax occurs when air has built up in the pleural space because of a leak in the lung. Pneumothorax often does not require treatment, but in some cases it may require placement of a chest tube thoracostomy, a procedure to drain air from the space around the lungs to allow the lung to reexpand. Rarely, damage to the spleen or liver may occur as a result of a puncture from the thoracentesis needle.

Results: The fluid sample that was removed during the procedure is first examined for color and consistency by the physician and is then analyzed in a laboratory. The fluid may be exudative (protein-rich) or transudative (watery, protein-poor). Pleural fluid analysis is useful in determining the cause of the effusion such as infection, pneumonia, blood in the pleural space (hemothorax), cancer, heart failure, cirrhosis, or kidney disease. It may also help identify other conditions such as pancreatitis, pulmonary embolism, or thyroid disease. The goals of therapeutic thoracentesis include draining excess fluid, treating infection, fully reexpanding the lung, and relieving symptoms such as shortness of breath, chest pain, or dry cough. If a large amount of fluid was removed, then the patient will experience a relief of symptoms soon after the procedure.

A repeat thoracentesis procedure may be needed if the effusion reaccumulates, which often occurs when the underlying cause is a malignancy.

Angela M. Costello, B.S.

▶ **For Further Information**

Colice, Gene L., et al. "Medical and Surgical Treatment of Parapneumonic Effusions: An Evidence-Based Guideline." *Chest* 118 (2000): 1158-1171.

Ferrer, Jaume. "Predictors of Pleural Malignancy in Patients with Pleural Effusion Undergoing Thoracoscopy." *Chest* 127 (2005): 1017-1022.

▶ **Other Resources**

American College of Chest Physicians
http://www.chestnet.org

American Thoracic Society
http://www.thoracic.org

Society of Thoracic Surgeons
http://www.sts.org/sections/patientinformation

See also Bronchoalveolar lung cancer; Lung cancers; Mesothelioma; Needle biopsies; Pleural biopsy; Pleural effusion; Pleurodesis; Radiofrequency ablation; Thoracentesis; Thoracoscopy; Ultrasound tests.

▶ Thoracoscopy

Category: Procedures
Also known as: Pleuroscopy, minimally invasive or video-assisted thoracic surgery

Definition: Thoracoscopy is an endoscopic procedure used to view inside the chest cavity with a thoracoscope (small videoscope). The thoracoscope transmits images of the surgical area onto a computer screen to guide surgeons during the procedure. Compared to open-chest surgery that requires one 6- to 8-inch incision, thoracoscopy uses several small, 1-inch incisions to access the chest, thereby minimizing trauma, decreasing postoperative pain, and promoting a shorter hospital stay and a quicker recovery.

Cancers diagnosed or treated: Pleural effusion, malignant mesothelioma, lung cancer, thymomas, and mediastinal and pericardial tumors

Why performed: Thoracoscopy may be used as a diagnostic procedure to determine the cause of a pleural effusion, perform a lung biopsy, or evaluate tumors. Thoracoscopy may be used to perform therapeutic procedures including thoracoscopic pneumonectomy, lobectomy, or wedge resection for lung cancer treatment; thoracentesis to drain excess pleural fluid; and removal of tumors in the esophagus, mediastinum, pericardium, or thymus.

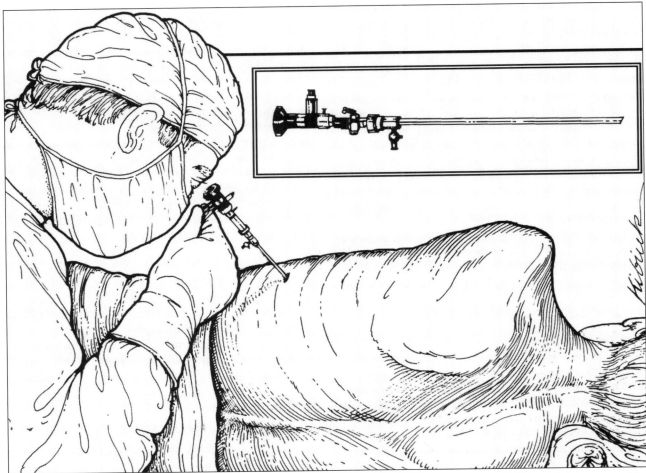

A doctor performs a thoracoscopy. (LifeART© 2008 Wolters Kluwer Health, Inc.-Lippincott Williams & Wilkins. All rights reserved.)

Patient preparation: Preprocedure tests may include a chest X ray and ultrasound, pulmonary function test, computed tomography (CT) scan, electrocardiogram (EKG), and blood tests. In general, patients must not eat or drink for eight hours before the procedure. Depending on the type of procedure to be performed, additional tests or patient preparations may be required.

Steps of the procedure: General anesthesia is used in most cases. The thoracoscope and surgical instruments are inserted through three or four small chest incisions between the ribs. The thoracoscope is manipulated to view the area, and the surgical instruments may be used to remove tissue.

After the procedure: A chest tube drains fluid and removes air that may have accumulated during the procedure. Cardiac function and blood oxygen levels are monitored, and daily chest X rays evaluate lung reexpansion and chest tube placement. The hospital recovery is about three to four days. The chest tube is removed. and the patient receives a follow-up schedule and homegoing instructions. The patient can generally return to normal activities three to four weeks after discharge.

Risks: The risks of thoracoscopy include accumulation of fluid in the pleural space, fluid in the lungs (pulmonary edema), bleeding, infection, respiratory distress, or collapse of the lung (pneumothorax). The risk of death is rare and occurs in about 0.24 percent of patients.

Results: Pleural fluid removed during the procedure is analyzed in the laboratory, and the biopsy tissue is examined for malignancy. The type and extent of disease will help guide the patient's treatment.

Angela M. Costello, B.S.

See also Bronchoalveolar lung cancer; Endoscopy; Gastrointestinal oncology; Hematologic oncology; Lung cancers; Medical oncology; Mesothelioma; Pediatric oncology and hematology; Pleural effusion; Pleurodesis; Surgical biopsies; Thoracentesis; Thymomas.

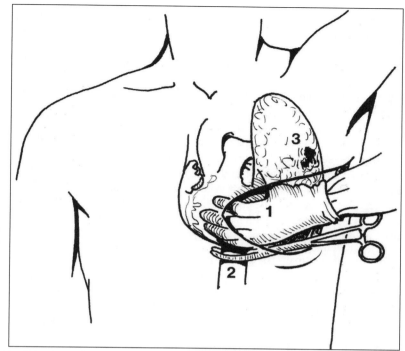

Incisions in a left anterolateral thoracotomy. (LifeART© 2008 Wolters Kluwer Health, Inc.-Lippincott Williams &Wilkins. All rights reserved.)

▶ Thoracotomy

Category: Procedures
Also known as: Lung surgery

Definition: A thoracotomy is the surgical opening of the chest wall so that the lungs, esophagus, or heart may be accessed. It can be performed on the right or left side or the midline of the chest.

Cancers diagnosed or treated: Lung cancer, esophageal cancer, cancer of the heart

Why performed: A thoracotomy is performed to biopsy and/or remove a tumor, to close a bleb (blister) in the external wall of the lung, or to drain an abscess.

Patient preparation: Several days before the thoracotomy, the patient will require blood work and an electrocardiogram (EKG). The patient will have to fast after midnight the day of the procedure.

Steps of the procedure: Before the thoracotomy, the patient will have an intravenous (IV) line inserted and be hooked up to a heart monitor. After the patient is sedated, an endotracheal tube is placed through the patient's nose or mouth into the trachea and attached to a ventilator, which breathes for the patient.

A midline thoracotomy is performed for surgery on the heart or esophagus. The patient lies on the back, and the surgeon splits the sternum to gain access to the chest. A right or left thoracotomy is used for surgery on the lungs. The patient lies on the opposite side with the arm over the head, and the surgeon makes an incision over the fifth intercostal (between the ribs) space.

After the surgery and before the chest wall is closed, one or two chest tubes are placed through the chest wall into the pleural space. They are necessary to reestablish the negative pressure in the chest. The chest tubes are attached to a drainage unit, which has a water seal to keep air from entering the pleural space.

After the procedure: The patient is sent to an intensive care unit (ICU) for close monitoring of vital signs, breathing, heart rhythm, and chest drainage. The patient will remain in the hospital for five or ten days. Usually the chest tubes can be removed after three to five days.

Risks: The risks of a thoracotomy are pneumothorax (collapse of the lung), air leaks, infection, bleeding, local nerve damage, and respiratory failure. After a thoracotomy, the patient may have severe pain with breathing.

Results: The lungs should be fully inflated. The tumor should be removed and the local lymph nodes evaluated.
Christine M. Carroll, R.N., B.S.N., M.B.A.

See also Bilobectomy; Biopsy; Bronchial adenomas; Bronchoalveolar lung cancer; Esophageal cancer; Esophagectomy; Lung cancers; Pleural effusion; Pleurodesis; Pneumonectomy; Surgical biopsies.

▶ Throat cancer

Category: Diseases, symptoms, and conditions
Also known as: Oropharyngeal cancer, laryngeal cancer, pharyngeal cancer, nasopharyngeal cancer

Related conditions: Thyroid cancer, vocal cord cancer, cancer of the glottis, adenoid cystic carcinoma, mucoepidermoid carcinoma, polymorphous low-grade adenocarcinoma

Definition: Throat cancer is a malignant tumor in the pharynx (part of the alimentary canal from behind the nose to the top of the esophagus) or in the larynx (voice box). The pharynx is divided into the nasopharynx (upper part behind the nose), oropharynx (middle part including the

soft palate, base of tongue, and tonsils), and hypopharynx (lower part).

Risk factors: Studies have found that as many as 90 percent of people with head and neck cancers, particularly of the oropharynx, hypopharynx, and larynx, have a history of smoking cigarettes or chewing tobacco, and as many as 80 percent have a history of drinking alcohol. Risk increases with the frequency, duration, and number of "pack-years" of cigarette smoking, independent of alcohol consumption. (One pack-year is defined as equivalent to smoking one pack, or twenty cigarettes, per day for one year.) One study indicated that smoking or chewing tobacco in conjunction with excess drinking of alcohol increases the risk beyond that for those who use either tobacco or alcohol alone. In a study among those who never smoked, only those with excessive amounts of alcohol consumption (three or more drinks per day) were at increased risk of head and neck cancers.

Other factors vary by tumor site and include Chinese ancestry, consumption of preserved and salted foods, wood dust exposure, and infection with the Epstein-Barr virus for nasopharyngeal cancer; poor oral hygiene, a diet low in fruits and vegetables, chewing betel quid, and infection with the human papillomavirus (HPV) for oropharyngeal cancer; Plummer-Vinson syndrome, a disorder characterized by severe anemia and trouble swallowing, for hypopharyngeal cancer; and asbestos exposure for laryngeal cancer. East Asians who drink alcohol and possess a genetic mutation that prevents effective elimination of acetaldehyde, a carcinogen created by metabolism of alcohol, are at greater risk for oropharyngeal cancer.

Etiology and the disease process: Most throat cancers begin in squamous cells lining mucosal surfaces in the throat. Squamous cell cancers grow aggressively. They begin as carcinomas in situ, abnormal cells lining the cells in the epithelieum, before they progress to invasive squamous cell cancers. Salivary gland tumors can develop in the mucosal lining of the oropharynx and oral cavity.

What makes squamous cells become cancerous is unknown, but it is believed that tobacco and alcohol use damage the deoxyribonucleic acid (DNA) in the cells of the mouth and throat, causing changes that lead to cancer.

Incidence: According to the National Cancer Institute, in 2008, there will be an estimated 12,250 new cases of laryngeal cancer and 12,410 new cases of pharyngeal cancer. Some 3,670 people will die of laryngeal cancer, and 2,200 will die of pharyngeal cancer. Cancers of the throat occur more often in men than in women, with men making up 78 percent of those with hypopharyngeal cancer and 69 percent of those with nasopharyngeal cancer. The incidence of head and neck cancers has declined since the 1980's, attributable in part to a drop in the number of people smoking cigarettes. However, the incidence of throat cancers has remained steady and some studies indicate an increase of throat cancer among young adults.

Symptoms: Symptoms of throat cancer may be mild or absent but may include a lump or sore that does not heal or becomes larger, sore throat, trouble swallowing, and a change in voice such as hoarseness. Patients with cancer of the oropharynx or hypopharynx may experience ear pain, and those with cancer of the nasopharynx may have ear pain and difficulty hearing, headaches, and difficulty breathing or talking. Symptoms of cancer of the larynx may include sore throat, hoarseness, ear pain, or a lump in the neck.

Screening and diagnosis: There are no screening tests for throat cancer. If throat cancer is suspected, the physician will take a complete medical history for risk factors and perform a physical exam. During the physical exam, the physician will palpate for lumps in the throat to rule out other conditions related to the symptoms, look for signs of metastasis, and determine the patient's overall health. Then, the physician will most likely perform an endoscopy to view areas that are not visible during a physical exam and to look for lesions. (A laryngoscope examines the larynx; a nasopharyngoscope examines the nasal cavity and nasopharynx.) During this procedure, the physician will excise tissue for examination. Depending on the location of the tumor, the biopsy can be one of three types: an exfoliative biopsy, incisional biopsy, or fine needle aspiration biopsy (commonly done to stage oropharyngeal cancer). The physician may recommend a panendoscopy, a diagnostic procedure done under general anesthesia during surgery to thoroughly examine the nose, throat, voice box, esophagus, and bronchi to look for areas of lesions and obtain a biopsy.

If cancer is present, it will be staged, from Stage 0, localized cancer, to Stage IV, metastasized cancer. Staging depends not only on the pathology results but on clinical data such as results of the endoscopy, findings on physical examination, and results of any imaging studies. Imaging studies may include an X ray to determine if there is cancer in the lungs; computed tomography (CT) scans for a cross-sectional picture of the size, location, shape, and position of the tumor; magnetic resonance imaging (MRI); positron emission tomography (PET) to see if the cancer has spread to nearby lymph nodes; and a barium swallow, a series of X rays to determine if the cancer has spread to the esophagus in the digestive tract and to see if the cancer affects swallowing.

Treatment and therapy: If cancer is present, the physician will discuss treatment options, taking into consideration the patient's overall health, prognosis, staging, psychosocial supports, treatment side effects, and the impact of the cancer and treatment on functions such as swallowing, talking, and chewing. The patient's medical team may consist of otorhinolaryngologists, oral surgeons, pathologists, plastic surgeons, prostodontists, and radiation and medical oncologists. Other allied health professionals—such as dieticians, speech pathologists, physical therapists, and social workers—may be involved as needed.

Surgery and radiation therapies are commonly used for treating throat cancers, particularly when the tumor is small and can be destroyed before spreading to other areas of the body. Radiation therapy may follow surgery if not all the cancer has been removed, or radiation may be used before surgery to preserve the voice. Individuals receiving radiation therapy may experience side effects including nausea, irritation and sores in the mouth, decreased appetite, earaches, and stiffness in the jaw.

If a larger tumor is involved or if the cancer has spread, a combination of radiation and chemotherapy is often successful and can preserve the voice box. Rarely will a laryngectomy be recommended and only in cases in which the larynx and primary tumor must be removed. Palliative care is needed for individuals whose primary throat cancer has spread to other organs or distant parts of the body and cannot be treated.

Relative Survival Rates for Throat Cancer by Site, 1988-2001

Site	Survival Rates (%)					
	1-Year	2-Year	3-Year	5-Year	8-Year	10-Year
Nasopharynx	84.1	73.2	65.3	56.6	48.3	44.7
Oropharynx and tonsils	79.8	65.9	58.8	49.8	43.5	39.3
Hypopharynx	67.4	47.9	38.3	29.5	22.0	18.2
Larynx	87.9	78.4	72.7	65.2	57.6	53.1

Source: Data from L. A. G. Ries et al., eds., *Cancer Survival Among Adults: U.S. SEER Program, 1988-2001—Patient and Tumor Characteristics*, NIH Pub. No. 07-6215 (Bethesda, Md.: National Cancer Institute, 2007)

Prognosis, prevention, and outcomes: The overall five-year survival rate for laryngeal cancer is 65.2 percent; for nasopharyngeal, 56.6 percent; for cancer of the oropharynx and tonsils, 49.8; and for hypopharyngeal cancer, 29.5 percent. If detected early, five-year survival rates climb to 82.5 percent for cancer of the larynx, 78.4 for cancer of the nasopharynx, 56.0 percent for cancer of the oropharynx and tonsils, and 48.7 percent for cancer of the hypopharynx. However, these rates drop when these cancers are detected after metastasis: the larynx to 19.1 percent, the nasopharynx to 46.7 percent, the oropharynx and tonsils to 43.4 percent, and the hypopharynx to 23.2 percent. If the tumor has spread to lymph nodes, it often cannot be controlled with surgery, radiation, or combined treatments. Even when the primary tumor is controlled, distal spread often cannot be avoided.

Rehabilitation is often a critical component in caring for patients treated for throat cancers. Many patients need therapy for assistance in speaking and swallowing following treatment. Patients may need dietary counseling as well. Those who receive a laryngectomy will have a stoma, a surgical opening in the throat, and will need to learn how to care for it and how to speak again if the stoma is permanent.

Follow-up care for those treated for throat cancer is essential to ensure that the cancer does not recur. Individuals with a prior diagnosis of throat cancer are at the highest risk of recurrence of the cancer within two to three years of initial diagnosis. During follow-up visits, the physician will perform a physical exam and sometimes order X rays, blood tests, and imaging studies. Regular dental exams may be necessary as well. If patients received radiation therapy, the physician may monitor functioning of the thyroid and pituitary glands. The treating physician will also urge patients to stop smoking and drinking alcohol, as doing so has been shown to compromise treatment and increase the risk that a second cancer will develop. Second primary tumors, particularly in the aerodigestive tract, have been reported in as many as 25 percent of patients whose initial throat lesions are controlled. It has been reported that daily administration of moderate doses of isotretonin for one year following initial treatment significantly reduces the incidence of second tumors of the oropharynx and larynx. However, survival advantages to this treatment have not yet been demonstrated.

Susan H. Peterman, M.P.H.

▶ For Further Information

Gordon, Serena. "Oral Sex Implicated in Some Throat and Neck Cancer." *Washington Post*, August 27, 2007.

Hashibe, Mia, et al. "Alcohol Drinking in Never Users of Tobacco, Cigarette Smoking in Never Drinkers, and the Risk of Head and Neck Cancers: Pooled Analysis in the International Head and Neck Cancer Epidemiology Consortium." *Journal of the National Cancer Institute* 99 (2007): 777-789.

Lydiatt, William M., and Perry J. Johnson. *Cancers of the Mouth and Throat: A Patient's Guide to Treatment.* Omaha: Addicus Books, 2001.

Spitz, M. R. "Epidemiology and Risk Factors for Head and Neck Cancer." *Seminars in Oncology* 31, no. 6 (2004): 726-733.

▶ Other Resources

MayoClinic.com
Oral and Throat Cancer
   http://www.mayoclinic.com/health/oral-and-throat-cancer/DS00349/DSECTION=1

National Cancer Institute
Throat (Laryngeal and Pharyngeal) Cancer
   http://www.cancer.gov/cancertopics/types/throat/

See also Chewing tobacco; Cigarettes and cigars; Esophageal speech; Head and neck cancers; Hypopharyngeal cancer; Laryngeal cancer; Oral and oropharyngeal cancers; Tobacco-related cancers.

▶ Thrombocytopenia

Category: Diseases, symptoms, and conditions
Also known as: Bleeding disorders

Related conditions: Anemia, neutropenia, pancytopenia

Definition: Thrombocytopenia is any disorder in which the number of platelets (thrombocytes, or blood cells that facilitate clotting) is below average.

Risk factors: Patients who are receiving large doses of chemotherapy, sometimes referred to as dose-dense therapy, or radiation therapy are at risk of developing thrombocytopenia, as are patients with leukemias, myeloma, and lymphomas. As aspirin is a drug known to act against platelets, patients who take aspirin often may be at risk. Serious infections and sepsis also can cause thrombocytopenia.

Etiology and the disease process: Platelets, small cells without a nucleus, are formed from hematopoietic stem cells that develop into megakaryocytes. Megakaryocyte formation is stimulated by the endogenous hormone thrombopoietin. Other hematopoietic growth factors, including interleukin-11 and interleukin-6, are involved in the production of megakaryocytes. Platelets are formed when the megakaryocyte shatters into small pieces. It takes approximately five days for a new platelet to differentiate and mature from a hematopoietic stem cell, which means that a patient receiving chemotherapy or radiation therapy can have a low number of platelets for days; platelets have a life span of only ten days.

The role of platelets is to allow blood to clot normally. Clotting occurs when a platelet encounters and adheres to a rough or jagged edge of damaged tissue. Other platelets adhere to this platelet in the process of platelet aggregation and formation of a plug. Finally, fibrin is released, forming a mesh that traps other platelets and completes the clot.

Chemotherapy and radiation therapy target the rapidly dividing cancer cells as well as other rapidly dividing cells, including hematopoietic stem cells, and reduce the numbers of platelets available for clotting and maintenance of normal blood consistency. Patients with thrombocytopenia can have severe bleeding because of routine blood draws, stiff toothbrushes, vigorous nose blowing, shaving, and ingestion of sharp foods, such as popcorn and peanuts. Under healthy circumstances, tiny ruptures in blood vessels are immediately repaired; when thrombocytopenia is present, this bleeding can go unchecked.

Incidence: At least 25 percent of patients who are receiving chemotherapy or radiation therapy develop thrombocytopenia. Thrombocytopenia makes a patient more susceptible to internal bleeding and stroke and may lead to anemia.

Symptoms: Symptoms of thrombocytopenia include unexplained bruises, nosebleeds, bleeding gums, prolonged bleeding from minor cuts and blood draws, pink or reddish urine, and black or bloody stools.

Screening and diagnosis: Thrombocytopenia is usually confirmed by a blood test. Normal platelet count is 200×10^9/liter to 400×10^9/liter. Sometimes, a bone marrow biopsy is needed to determine the cause of the thrombocytopenia. At 50×10^9/liter, a patient is at great risk of bleeding, and at 20×10^9/liter, at severe risk for bleeding; at this level, thrombocytopenia is a life-threatening condition.

Besides measuring the number of platelets in circulation, platelet function tests also may be done. In the past, the primary test for platelet dysfunction was bleeding time, but this test has fallen out of favor as it is not very sensitive or precise. Normal bleeding time, which requires small, thin cuts on a patient's forearm to assess, is generally 3 to 9.5 minutes but can be affected by aspirin and by

the skill of the laboratory technician. Other tests that may be done on a blood sample include prothrombin time, a measure of how long it takes blood to clot, which normally is 10 to 13 seconds. A partial prothrombin time test is usually done in conjunction with the prothrombin time to measure the function of several clotting factors. Other tests include platelet aggregation studies that measure the response of blood or platelet-rich blood to specific agents known to induce aggregation (clumping) of platelets.

Treatment and therapy: Transfusions of platelets can be used to treat life-threatening thrombocytopenia. Most oncologists, however, prefer not to use transfusions excessively because of the small but inherent risks of infections and immune system complications. Transfusions often involve platelets from a number of volunteer donors. Patients who receive platelets pooled from a number of donors run the risk of developing antibodies to the various proteins on the platelet membranes. If antibodies develop, the patient may no longer respond to transfusions. The risk of immune system reactions can be reduced if a patient who requires platelet transfusions can arrange to receive platelets from one specific donor, preferably a sibling. If antibodies do develop from transfusions of pooled platelets, it may be critical for a patient to receive platelets only from a sibling. A recombinant version of the naturally occurring protein that is responsible for the growth and development of platelets has received marketing approval from the Food and Drug Administration. This product, a recombinant human interleukin-11 (oprelvekin, or Neumega), is administered as a subcutaneous injection and stimulates the bone marrow to produce more platelets.

Prognosis, prevention, and outcomes: Recombinant growth factors and platelet transfusions are standard care for the treatment of severe thrombocytopenia at many cancer centers. Transfusion in particular can rapidly, that is, within hours in some cases, increase platelet counts. Left untreated, the patient is at risk for serious and possibly life-threatening internal bleeding and stroke. Because chemotherapy and radiation therapy carry a risk of thrombocytopenia, the only way to prevent thrombocytopenia is to delay or reduce the amount of chemotherapy or radiation therapy, which is not advised as it lessens the success of the treatments.

MaryAnn Foote, M.S., Ph.D.

▶ **For Further Information**
Kuter, D. J., P. Hunt, W. Sheridan, and D. Zucker-Franklin, eds. "Thrombopoiesis and Thrombopoietins." In *Molecular, Cellular, Preclinical, and Clinical Biology.* Totowa, N.J.: Humana Press, 1997.

McCrae, Keith R., ed. *Thrombocytopenia*. New York: Taylor & Francis, 2006.

▶ **Other Resources**

MayoClinic.com
Thrombocytopenia (Low Platelet Count)
    http://www.mayoclinic.com/health/
    thrombocytopenia/DS00691

MedlinePlus
Thrombocytopenia
    http://www.nlm.nih.gov/medlineplus/ency/article/
    000586.htm

See also Anemia; Angiogenesis inhibitors; Aplastic anemia; Azathioprine; Chemotherapy; Computed tomography (CT)-guided biopsy; Hypercoagulation disorders; Infection and sepsis; Interleukins; Leukemias; Lymphomas; Matrix metalloproteinase inhibitors; Myelosuppression; Neutropenia; Proteasome inhibitors; Topoisomerase inhibitors.

▶ **Thymomas**

Category: Diseases, symptoms, and conditions
Also known as: Epithelial tumors of the thymus, thymic tumors

Related conditions: Thymic cancer, carcinoid tumors, germ-cell tumors, lymphomas

Definition: Thymomas are abnormal tissue masses on the outside of the thymus, a small organ in the upper chest.

Risk factors: Myasthenia gravis is the primary risk factor, occurring in about half of patients with thymomas. Red cell aplasia and hypogammaglobulinemia are tumor-related conditions that may occur with thymomas. Autoimmune diseases increase the risk.

Etiology and the disease process: The World Health Organization's letter grade system identifies thymomas based on their microscopic appearance:
- Type A: Spindle-shaped endothelial cells, few lymphoctyes
- Type AB: Features of type A plus lymphocytes
- Types B1 and B2: Numerous lymphocytes, thymus cells normal (B1) or abnormal (B2)
- Type B3: Few lymphocytes, normal thymus epithelial cells

- Type C (thymic carcinomas): Mature lymphocytes mixed with plasma cells, invasion of surrounding tissues

Incidence: Thymomas and thymic cancers are rare. The American Cancer Society reports about 500 to 700 new cases of malignant thymomas diagnosed annually. The incidence of nonmalignant thymomas is unknown. Thymomas usually affect people aged fory to sixty years.

Symptoms: Symptoms are often related to other coexisting conditions. Thymomas may cause shortness of breath, coughing, and angina when there is added pressure on the nearby airways or blood vessels. About 40 percent of patients do not experience symptoms, but the thymoma is found during examination for another medical condition.

Screening and diagnosis: A needle biopsy may be performed, but thymomas are usually diagnosed, staged, and treated during surgery.
- Stage I: Noninvasive, within thymus boundary
- Stage II: Spread beyond the thymus, affecting fatty tissue or mediastinum
- Stage III: Extending to the pleura, pericardium, lungs, nerves, or superior vena cava
- Stage IVA: Spread throughout the pleura and pericardium
- Stage IVB: Spread to distant organs

Treatment and therapy: Surgical removal of the thymus (thymectomy) and some of the surrounding tissue is recommended. Removal of nearby structures affected by the malignancy may be necessary for Stage III or IV thymomas. Chemotherapy, radiation therapy, or both may decrease the size of the tumor before surgery and may be given after surgery.

Prognosis, prevention, and outcomes: The prognosis depends on the stage of the disease, with the highest survival rates for patients with Stage I and II thymomas that undergo thymectomy. About 25 percent of patients with thymic carcinomas are cured, with a five-year survival rate of 35 percent. There is no known prevention for thymomas.

Angela M. Costello, B.S.

See also Carcinoid tumors and carcinoid syndrome; Carcinomas; Germ-cell tumors; Hemolytic anemia; Lambert-Eaton myasthenic syndrome (LEMS); Lymphomas; Mediastinal tumors; Mediastinoscopy; Myasthenia gravis; Superior vena cava syndrome; Surgical biopsies; Thoracoscopy; Thymus cancer.

▶ Thymus cancer

Category: Diseases, symptoms, and conditions
Also known as: Thymic cancer, thymoma, thymic carcinoma, thymic carcinoids

Related conditions: Myasthenia gravis, red cell aplasia, autoimmune disorders (including lupus and rheumatoid arthritis)

Definition: Thymus cancer is a malignant tumor in the thymus, a small organ in the upper chest where the body makes and matures T lymphocytes (a type of white blood cell involved in immune responses). When thymic cells acquire mutations, normal cells may be replaced by cancerous ones. About 90 percent of thymic cancers are thymomas, with thymic carcinoma and thymic carcinoids being much less common.

Risk factors: Thymic tumors are most prevalent in middle-aged or elderly populations (between fifty and eighty years of age). Men and women have similar incidence rates. There is some evidence that thymomas may be hereditary, although specific gene mutations have not yet been identified.

There are several disorders that predispose one to developing thymic cancer. For instance, myasthenia gravis, characterized by severe muscle weakness, develops in about 30 to 50 percent of people with thymoma, and 15 percent of patients with myasthenia gravis have thymomas. Red cell aplasia, characterized by a lack of red blood cell formation, also develops in about 30 to 50 percent of people with thymoma and occurs in 5 percent of thymoma patients. Additionally, people with autoimmune disorders, in which the immune system incorrectly targets the body's own tissues, also have an increased risk of thymic cancers.

Etiology and the disease process: Two major cell types in the thymus include lymphocytes and epithelial cells. When lymphocytes are transformed into cancerous cells, this may lead to Hodgkin disease and non-Hodgkin lymphomas. Thymic cancers arise from either the cortical or medullary epithelial cells.

One of the early events in the development of thymomas is a *TP53* mutation. The protein produced by this gene is involved in regulating the cell cycle, and loss-of-function mutations can allow damaged or abnormal cells to divide and replicate. Another genetic mutation in thymic cancer is the overexpression of the epithelial growth factor receptor (EGFR), which is involved in signal transduction pathways that activate proteins and transcription factors to subsequently turn on genes involved in survival and proliferation.

The World Health Organization's classification system of thymic cancers is based on their microscopic appearance. The types and prevalence follow:

- Type A (about 5 percent): Cells are spindle-shaped or oval epithelial cells, and they do not appear to be malignant.
- Type AB (about 30 percent): Cells look like Type A, except that there are also some lymphocytes mixed in with the tumor.
- Type B1 (about 10 to 20 percent): Cells look like Type A, except that there are many lymphocytes mixed in with the tumor.
- Type B2 (about 20 to 35 percent): Epithelial cells appear abnormal and have large nuclei, and there are several lymphocytes.
- Type B3 (10 to 15 percent): This type has few lymphocytes and mostly consists of thymic epithelial cells that look pretty close to normal.

While Types A-B3 describe thymomas, Type C thymic cancers are known as thymic carcinomas. Thymic carcinomas have abnormal cells and are likely to spread outside of the thymus. They are divided into low-grade and high-grade carcinomas based on how aggressive the tumor is and how likely it is to spread.

Thymic carcinoids are often associated with disorders of the endocrine system. These tumors are aggressive and can spread outside the thymus.

Incidence: The American Cancer Society estimates 500 to 700 new cases of thymic cancers are diagnosed each year in the United States. Thymomas make up 90 percent of all cases, while the remaining 10 percent are thymic carcinomas and carcinoid tumors.

Symptoms: In about 40 percent of cases, there are no symptoms. However, when they occur, signs include long-lasting coughs, chest pain, and trouble breathing. These symptoms are often the result of thymic tumors constricting air passages or blood vessels. Obstructing blood flow may also lead to swelling in the arms or face. Other symptoms include low levels of red blood cells, fatigue and muscle weakness, and an increased risk of infection.

Screening and diagnosis: An X ray of the chest is often the first procedure performed to detect thymic cancer. Follow-up imaging tests include computed tomography (CT), which is a more sensitive X ray that produces cross-sectional images. CT scans provide information regarding the size, shape, and position of a tumor, as well as identify enlarged lymph nodes that may also have cancerous cells. Magnetic resonance imaging (MRI) scans, which use radio waves and magnets instead of X rays, are another

Relative Survival Rates for Thymus Cancer by Gender, 1988-2001

Gender	Survival Rate (%)			
	1-Year	*3-Year*	*5-Year*	*10-Year*
Men	88.9	75.0	68.5	54.4
Women	85.5	73.9	63.4	46.8
Total	87.4	74.5	66.3	51.3

Source: Data from L. A. G. Ries et al., eds., *Cancer Survival Among Adults: U.S. SEER Program, 1988-2001—Patient and Tumor Characteristics*, NIH Pub. No. 07-6215 (Bethesda, Md.: National Cancer Institute, 2007)

sensitive test that provides sectional scans of the body. Finally, positron emission tomography (PET) is a newer form of imaging that scans the entire body. PET generally uses radioactive glucose (a form of sugar) as a tracer. The radioactivity is absorbed by the cancer cells and then detected with a special camera.

The most definitive procedure to diagnose thymic cancer is a biopsy, in which a piece of the tumor tissue from the thymus is removed by either a needle or surgery, and then analyzed under the microscope.

Thymomas are staged using the Masaoka system. Since thymic carcinomas and thymic carcinoid tumors are rare (about 10 percent of thymic cancers), there is not a separate staging system for these cancer types. However, the Masaoka system is sometimes used for thymic carcinomas. The stages of the Masaoka system are as follows:
- Stage I: The cancer remains within the thymus.
- Stage II: The cancer has spread into the outer layer of the lung or into nearby fat tissue.
- Stage III: The cancer has spread to areas within the chest, including the outer layer of the heart, lungs, or blood vessels.
- Stage IVA: The cancer has spread throughout the heart, lungs, or both.
- Stage IVB: The cancer has spread to organs in other parts of the body.

Treatment and therapy: For Stage I thymoma, surgical removal of the thymus is the standard treatment. In other stages, the thymus and any tissues to which the cancer may have spread are removed. Radiation therapy may be performed if patients are unable to undergo surgery, if the tumor has spread to too many tissues, if there is still a residual tumor mass after surgery, or if the tumor is inoperable because it is next to major arteries or veins in the chest. In the later stages, radiation therapy may also be given after surgery to decrease the risk of recurrence or spreading.

Chemotherapy drugs used to treat thymic cancers include doxorubicin, cisplatin, cyclophosphamide, etoposide, and ifosfamide. These drugs may be used either alone or in combination and may be administered before surgery to reduce tumor size or after surgery if tumor cells still remain.

For tumors where surgery cannot be performed, and patients have not responded to radiation, corticosteroids may be used. A newer therapy for advanced thymic cancers is the drug octreotide. Octreoide blocks the ability of cancerous thymic cells to bind the hormone somatostatin, and this leads to cell death or slower rates of proliferation.

After surgery or therapy, patients should have checkups including blood work and chest X rays every six to twelve months to monitor for recurrence.

Prognosis, prevention, and outcomes: Survival rates depend on the stage of the cancer at diagnosis. Results from a study published in 2000 showed that the average five-year survival rates for thymomas are 96 percent for Stage I, 86 percent for Stage II, 70 percent for Stage III, and 50 percent for Stage IV (staging based on the Masaoka system). However, up to 30 percent of survivors can experience a recurrence. For thymic carcinomas, the five-year survival rates are around 35 percent, and they are approximately 60 percent for thymic carcinoids.

There are no specific guidelines for preventing thymic cancers. However, following a healthy diet, which is high in fruits and vegetables and low in fat, has been shown to prevent the development of many cancers.

Elizabeth A. Manning, Ph.D.

▶ **For Further Information**

Bogot, N. R., and L. E. Quint. "Imaging of Thymic Disorders." *Cancer Imaging* 5 (December 15, 2005): 139-149.

Detterbeck, F. C. "Clinical Value of the WHO Classification System of Thymoma." *Annals of Thoracic Surgery* 81, no. 6 (June, 2006): 2328-2334.

Johnson, S. B., T. Y. Eng, G. Giaccone, and C. R. Thomas, Jr. "Thymoma: Update for the New Millennium." *Oncologist* 6, no. 3 (2001): 239-246.

Nishino, M., et al. "The Thymus: A Comprehensive Review." *Radiographics* 26, no. 2 (March/April, 2006): 335-348.

Suster, S. "Diagnosis of Thymoma." *Journal of Clinical Pathology* 59, no. 12 (December, 2006): 1238-1244.

Suster, S., and C. A. Moran. "Thymoma Classification: Current Status and Future Trends." *American Journal of Clinical Pathology* 125, no. 4 (April, 2006): 542-554.

▶ **Other Resources**

American Cancer Society
Detailed Guide: Thymus Cancer
   http://www.cancer.org/docroot/CRI/
   CRI_2_3x.asp?dt=42

Medline Plus
Thymus Cancer
   http://www.nlm.nih.gov/medlineplus/
   thymuscancer.html

See also Carcinoid tumors and carcinoid syndrome; Carcinomas; Computed tomography (CT) scan; Hodgkin disease; Immune response to cancer; Lymphomas; Thymomas.

▶ Thyroid cancer

Category: Diseases, symptoms, and conditions
Also known as: Malignant neoplasm of the thyroid

Related conditions: Autoimmune thyroiditis, sarcoma of the thyroid, Gardner syndrome, Cowden syndrome

Definition: Thyroid cancer is a malignant tumor in the thyroid gland, a butterfly-shaped gland in the neck that makes a hormone essential for normal body function. The thyroid contains cells that grow and divide to form new ones as needed; however, when this process goes awry, tissue masses called nodules develop; these may be benign or malignant (cancerous). There are several types of thyroid cancer: papillary, the most common type (over 70 percent), has a very high cure rate. It usually appears in people thirty to fifty years old and accounts for 85 percent of thyroid cancers resulting from radiation exposure. About 10 to 15 percent of thyroid tumors are follicular carcinoma. This cancer is more aggressive, occurs in a slightly older age group, and rarely occurs after radiation exposure but is more common in an iodine-deficient environment. Hurthle cell carcinoma is a rare variant. Medullary thyroid cancer (about 5 to 8 percent) is not associated with radiation exposure and is inherited. Anaplastic carcinoma is the rarest type (about 0.5 to 1.5 percent) but the most deadly; it may appear many years following radiation exposure. Thyroid lymphomas account for less than 5 percent of thyroid cancers.

Risk factors: Increased risk of papillary carcinoma is associated with external-beam irradiation to the head and neck areas, especially during childhood. Exposure to ingested radioactive isotopes and radioactive fallout also poses a cancer risk. Having a parent with multiple endo-

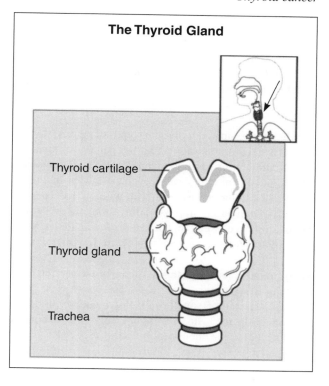

The Thyroid Gland

Thyroid cartilage

Thyroid gland

Trachea

crine neoplasia (MEN) types 2A or 2B or familial medullary cancer increases the chance of having the genetic mutation that causes thyroid cancer by as much as 50 percent. Women are two to three times as likely as men to develop thyroid cancer; women whose last pregnancy occurs at or later than age thirty are also at greater risk. Whites are more susceptible than are blacks, and being Asian or California Asian increases the risk. Other risk factors include dietary iodine deficiency; ingestion of goitrogenic (goiter-causing) or cruciferous vegetables (such as cabbage) and seafood and shellfish, especially when fished from sites near active volcanoes, as in Hawaii and Iceland; and chronic elevation of thyroid-stimulating hormone (TSH).

Etiology and the disease process: In many cases, the etiology, or cause, of thyroid cancer is unknown. Thyroid cancers are either differentiated or undifferentiated. Differentiated cells look and act like normal ones and actually assist in making thyroxine. They reproduce more slowly than undifferentiated ones do. Papillary and follicular carcinoma are two types of differentiated cancer. Around 85 percent of papillary thyroid cancers are caused by radiation exposure. Follicular cancer is more prevalent in countries where people are iodine deficient.

   Undifferentiated cancer is made up of very primitive cells that do nothing but reproduce; this produces the rare anaplastic cancer that is not effectively treatable and therefore has a high mortality rate. Even rarer is medullary thyroid carcinoma (MTC), which is inherited. A specific cell, the C cell, is involved. It makes the hormone calcitonin, which helps regulate calcium in the body, but when it overproduces, medullary carcinoma must be suspected.

Incidence: Compared with other types of cancer, thyroid cancer is uncommon; only about 0.6 percent of men and 1.6 percent of women in the United States are diagnosed with it, and the mortality rate is even lower. The incidence of thyroid carcinoma, especially in women, has been on the rise, due in part to improved diagnosis, but earlier detection, improved treatment, and a decline in the very aggressive anaplastic type have resulted in fewer deaths.

Symptoms: In its early stages, thyroid cancer often does not exhibit symptoms. As the disease progresses, however, the affected person may develop a nodule (lump) in the front of the neck; hoarseness or changes in the normal speaking voice; swollen lymph nodes, especially in the neck; swallowing or breathing difficulty; and pain in the throat or neck.

Screening and diagnosis: More often than not, a nodule felt in the thyroid during a routine physical examination or found incidentally during an imaging test for some other condition signals a tumor's presence. When symptoms suggest thyroid cancer, a number of tests may be performed: An ultrasound scan outlines a growth but does not rule out malignancy. That determination is made with biopsy. Biopsy may be fine needle aspiration (FNA) biopsy, in which a needle is inserted in different parts of a nodule to remove cell samples that are analyzed in a laboratory, or surgical biopsy to remove the nodule and check the tissue for cancer cells.

Blood tests may also be done to detect abnormal levels of thyroid-stimulating hormone in the blood. If a physician suspects medullary cancer, blood tests are run to check for abnormally high levels of calcitonin in the blood or to detect an altered gene (*RET* gene), which aids diagnosis.

Radionuclide scanning involves administering a small

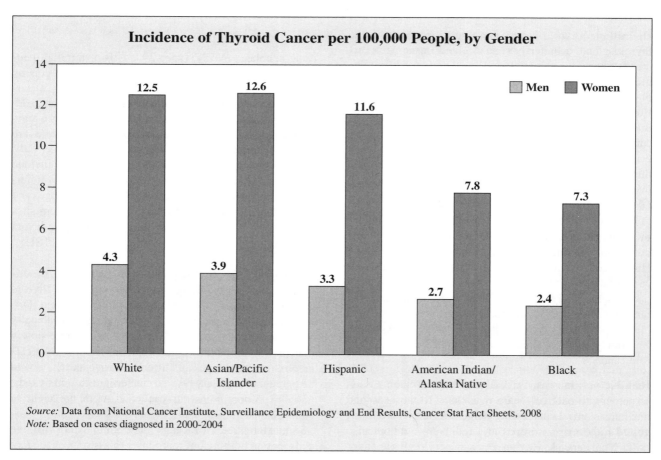

Incidence of Thyroid Cancer per 100,000 People, by Gender

Source: Data from National Cancer Institute, Surveillance Epidemiology and End Results, Cancer Stat Fact Sheets, 2008
Note: Based on cases diagnosed in 2000-2004

amount of radioactive material to make thyroid nodules show up on a picture. When thyroid cancer is diagnosed, tests are done to determine whether the cancer has spread; this process is called staging. Tests such as ultrasonography, computed tomography (CT) scanning, and magnetic resonance imaging (MRI) can help the doctor determine if the cancer has spread to the lymph nodes or to other areas. A special scan may be used to check for the spread of medullary cancer. Staging is essential to choose treatment options and predict odds for cure and long-term survival. A common staging system is that of the American Joint Committee on Cancer (AJCC), called the TNM (tumor/lymph node/metastasis) system. This system looks at the size of the tumor, whether it has spread to the lymph nodes, and whether it has metastasized to distant organs. Stages are described in Roman numerals from I to IV, with values assigned to each one. In the case of papillary or follicular thyroid carcinoma, age is also taken into account. All anaplastic thyroid cancers are considered Stage IV to reflect the poor prognosis of this particular kind of thyroid cancer.

Treatment and therapy: Treatment for thyroid cancer includes surgery, thyroid hormone therapy, radiation, and chemotherapy. Total or near-total surgical removal is the treatment of choice in most cases. Following surgery, thyroid hormone medication is required for life to supply the hormone the thyroid would normally produce. Frequent blood tests are done until the proper dosage can be established. Radioactive iodine may be used for follow-up screening to detect remaining normal or abnormal tissues. Moderate doses can eliminate the normal tissue, and larger doses destroy any cancerous cells. External beam radiation also destroys cancer cells. Chemotherapy may be used when the cancer has metastasized, especially for the medullary type, which does not respond to radioiodine therapy. Other follow-up care includes blood tests for thyroglobulin levels that would indicate recurrence, and imaging such as ultrasonography.

Prognosis, prevention, and outcomes: The type of thyroid cancer affects the prognosis to a large extent. In papillary and follicular cancer, Stages I and II have a 100 percent five-year survival rate. Stage III decreases to 96 percent for papillary and 79 percent for follicular types. Stage IV drops to 45 percent in papillary cancer and 47 percent for follicular. Stage I medullary thyroid cancer has a 100 percent five-year survival rate, then drops to 97 percent and 78 percent, respectively, for Stages II and III; however, the rate falls to only 24 percent for Stage IV. The five-year survival rate for anaplastic thyroid cancer is around 9 percent.

Thyroid cancer prevention measures are limited. However, certain steps can be taken in situations in which there is heightened risk. A genetic test can determine if there is increased risk for medullary thyroid cancer. If the results are positive, thyroid gland removal may prevent development of cancer later in life. Also, government guidelines recommend that people living within ten miles of a nuclear power plant take potassium iodide tablets just before or immediately after exposure to fallout. Anyone who has received radiation to the head and neck during childhood should be examined carefully every year or two. More general measures include diets high in fruit and vegetables and low in animal fats and consumption of unsaturated fats, which contain omega-3 fatty acids. Maintaining a healthy weight may also help.

Victoria Price, Ph.D.

▶ **For Further Information**

Braverman, Lewis E., and Robert D. Utiger, eds. *Werner and Ingbar's The Thyoid: A Fundamental and Clinical Text.* 7th ed. New York: Lippincott-Raven, 1991.

Foley, John R., Julie M. Vose, and James O. Armitage. *Current Therapy in Cancer.* Philadelphia: W. B. Saunders, 1994.

Lenhard, Raymond E., Jr., Robert T. Osteen, and Ted Gansler. *The American Cancer Society's Clinical Oncology.* Atlanta: American Cancer Society, 2001.

Rosenthal, M. Sara. *The Thyroid Sourcebook: Everything You Need to Know.* 3d ed. Los Angeles: Lowell House, 1998.

▶ **Other Resources**

Endocrine Web
Thyroid Cancer
http://www.endocrineweb.com/thyroidca.html

MedlinePlus
Thyroid Cancer
http://www.nlm.nih.gov/medlineplus/thyroidcancer.html

National Cancer Institute
Thyroid Cancer
http://www.cancer.gov/cancertopics/types/Thyroid

See also Childhood cancers; Computed tomography (CT) scan; Cowden syndrome; Cruciferous vegetables; Fibrocystic breast changes; Gardner syndrome; Imaging tests; Multiple endocrine neoplasia type 1 (MEN 1); Multiple endocrine neoplasia type 2 (MEN 2); Radionuclide scan; Surgical biopsies; Ultrasound tests; Young adult cancers; Zollinger-Ellison syndrome.

▶ Thyroid nuclear medicine scan

Category: Procedures

Also known as: Thyroid scintiscan, technetium thyroid scan

Definition: The thyroid nuclear medicine scan is an imaging technique using a gamma camera to help assess the health and anatomy of the thyroid gland following the administration of a radioisotope, a radiation-emitting form of an element. The radioisotopes most commonly used are iodine 123, iodine 131, and technetium pertechnetate. Other isotopes, such as gallium 67 and thallium 201, are also in use for their characteristic correlation in malignancy profiling. Still others are being scrutinized for better visualization of specific thyroid cancers.

When radiation is given off during the procedure, it is recorded by the scanner on radiographic film or on a screen, which allows direct viewing or photographing of the thyroid image. The radioactive substance used often gives name to the procedure, such as a technetium thyroid scan or a radioactive iodine uptake scan (RAIU test). These studies are possible because of the thyroid's special affinity for radioactive substances and its normal uptake of iodine in the production of thyroid hormones.

Cancers diagnosed: Thyroid cancers (papillary, follicular, medullary, or anaplastic)

Why performed: Thyroid scans are helpful in evaluating masses in the neck area, in defining specific types of hyperthyroidism, and in assessing thyroid nodules, metastatic tumors, and thyroid cancer. They are an important tool in determining the position, size, and structure of the thyroid gland and, together with other tests, help assess thyroid function. Scans are especially helpful in evaluating patients with suspected thyroid nodules. Thyroid nodules are either functioning (hot or warm) or nonfunctioning (cold), and this has important implications in assessing malignancy.

The butterfly-shaped thyroid is an endocrine gland consisting of two lobes located on either side of the trachea connected by bridging tissue called an isthmus. Assessing thyroid health is critical because of its central role to basic human physiology. The iodine-laden hormone produced in the thyroid gland regulates oxygen consumption, body temperature, heart function, skeletal growth, skin function, and carbohydrate, lipid, and fat metabolism.

Patient preparation: The scintiscan may be performed either in an outpatient X-ray center or a hospital radiol-ogy department. The patient is instructed to discontinue iodine-containing medications such as thyroid drugs, corticosteroids, phenothiazines, salicylates, anticoagulants, and antihistamines for several weeks to twenty-four hours prior to the scan, depending on the amount of time that the substance takes to clear from the body. If the radioisotope is to be administered orally, then the patient should fast after the midnight preceding the test. Fasting is not required for intravenous (IV) injection.

Steps of the procedure: The patient will receive the radioisotope either intravenously or orally. The patient takes the oral medication (iodine 123 or iodine 131) as either a tasteless liquid or a capsule twenty-four hours prior to imaging or receives an IV injection (pertechnetate) twenty to thirty minutes before imaging. During the scan, the patient will be lying down with the face up. The camera is then positioned over the thyroid area in the neck, and the radioactive response is displayed on a monitor and recorded on X-ray film. The procedure is usually complete in less than thirty minutes.

When evaluating thyroid function, the radioisotope iodine 123 or iodine 131 is measured at six hours and again at twenty-four hours after dosing.

After the procedure: This is a noninvasive procedure, and there are no special precautions or instructions. Regular eating can continue two hours after imaging.

Risks: The radioactive dose is very small and is generally considered harmless, but pregnant or lactating women, as well as patients allergic to iodine, shellfish, or the tracers used in the imaging, should not undergo the procedure.

Results: Many types of thyroid pathology may be revealed through imaging, and fortunately most are not cancerous. One of the ways in which the scintiscan makes this distinction is through the assessment of thyroid nodules. A thyroid nodule is a nonspecific term for a swelling in the thyroid gland. It might be no more than an accumulation of thyroid cells or a cyst. Even though they are common, they might grow large enough to interfere with swallowing or breathing, or they can produce so much hormone that hyperthyroidism results. They can also become cancerous about 5 percent of the time.

On scintiscan, the nodules are seen as hot, warm, or cold. An area of increased radionuclide uptake may be called a hot nodule, signifying that a benign growth has become overactive. An area of decreased radionuclide uptake, representing low thyroid activity, is a cold nodule. A variety of conditions, including cysts, nonfunctioning benign growths, localized inflammation, or cancer, may produce a cold spot. Hot or warm nodules are rarely malignant, while almost all cancerous nodules are cold. A cold nodule is not exclusive to malignancy, however, as most benign nodules, cysts, and localized areas of inflammation are cold as well.

Neoplasms are graded according to cell abnormality and for their potential for invasiveness and growth as a guide to treatment options and prognosis. The minimally invasive, encapsulated, and well-circumscribed growth is a grade I neoplasm. As the neoplasm becomes more aggressive and infiltrates the surrounding gland and the cells become more irregular and mitotic, the neoplasm is considered grade II. Grade III describes even more extensive growth, with possible invasiveness beyond the gland and increased cellular irregularity and mitosis. Further classification is done by anatomic staging, which defines the extent of the disease process.

The results of a thyroid nuclear medicine scan serve as a guide and are almost always used in conjunction with other tests to establish a diagnosis.

Richard S. Spira, D.V.M.

▶ For Further Information

Beers, Mark H., et al., eds. *The Merck Manual of Medical Information, Second Home Edition.* Whitehouse Station, N.J.: Merck Research Laboratories, 2003.

Feld, Stanley. *AACE Clinical Practice Guidelines for the Diagnosis and Management of Thyroid Nodules.* New York: American Association of Clinical Endocrinologists, 1996.

▶ Other Resources

American Thyroid Association
http://www.thyroid.org

MedlinePlus
http://www.nlm.nih.gov

Thyroid Foundation of America
http://www.allthyroid.org

See also Cobalt 60 radiation; Cold nodule; Corticosteroids; Endocrine cancers; Imaging tests; Nuclear medicine scan; Pathology; Pregnancy and cancer; Radionuclide scan; Risks for cancer; Staging of cancer; Thyroid cancer; X-ray tests.

▶ TNM staging

Category: Procedures
Also known as: Tumor/nodes/metastases staging

Definition: TNM (an abbreviation for tumor, node, and metastasis) staging is a system used to describe the extent and severity of solid malignant tumors and how much they have spread.

Cancers diagnosed or treated: Solid tumors such as breast, colorectal, kidney, larynx, lung, and prostate cancers and melanoma

Why performed: Staging of cancer is important because the stage at diagnosis is the most powerful predictor of survival. Doctors use staging information to help plan a patient's treatment, to estimate a patient's prognosis, to select changes in treatment, and to identify appropriate clinical trials for patients.

TNM staging provides a common language with which oncologists and all other members of the health care team can communicate when discussing cancer patients, as well as evaluate and compare the results of clinical trials. Staging data, when collected over time, can be valuable to epidemiologists for analysis of similar types of cancer or for use in special studies.

Patient preparation: Tissue samples are taken from a variety of tumors; patient preparation depends on the type of tumor and its location. Often, samples are taken as part of the surgical process to remove the tumor.

Steps of the procedure: Staging is based on an understanding of the way in which cancer develops. A tumor is formed at the primary site as cancer cells grow and divide in an uncontrolled fashion. As a tumor grows, its cells can invade neighboring tissues or leave the tumor to migrate through the bloodstream or lymph system to new sites in the body, a process called metastasis.

Staging systems for cancer have evolved over time and continue to be upgraded as cancer becomes better understood. The American Joint Committee on Cancer, established in 1988 to address the inadequacies of the traditional method of staging cancer using I-IV, created the TNM system for staging solid tumors throughout the body. Most types of solid tumors have TNM designations, although some do not (for example, cancers of the brain and spinal cord). As of 2008, the TNM system was in its sixth edition. In the TNM system, each factor is evaluated separately and given a number. For instance, a T1N1M0 cancer means that the patient has a T1 tumor, N1 lymph node involvement, and no metastases.

The precise definitions of T, N, and M are specific to each type of cancer, but general definitions of each element are tumor, node, and metastasis. Tumor (T) describes the extent of the primary tumor and carries a number of 0 to 4, with 0 being a tumor that is entirely contained at the local site and 4 being a large primary tumor that has probably invaded other organs. Node (N) describes regional lymph node metastasis and can also be ranked from 0 to 4, with 0 being no lymph node involvement and 4 being extensive involvement. Metastasis (M) describes the presence or absence of distant metastases; it is 1 if distant metastases are present and 0 if not. For example, breast cancer T3N2M1 describes a large tumor that has spread outside the breast to nearby lymph nodes and to other parts of the body, whereas prostate cancer T2N0M0 describes a tumor located only in the prostate that has not spread to the lymph nodes or any other part of the body.

The category X is used in each element where no assessment of that characteristic was made. For example, NX indicates that the status of lymph nodes was not assessed. It is important not to confuse this category with N0, which indicates that no lymph node involvement was found by the diagnostic tools used.

The types of tests that are used for staging depend on the type of cancer but can include physical examination; imaging studies such as X rays, computed tomography (CT) scans, magnetic resonance imaging (MRI), or positron emission tomography (PET) scans; laboratory values such as tests for liver function or tumor markers; pathology reports; and surgical reports. The TNM system has evolved as advances have been made in diagnosis and treatment of different types of cancer. For instance, endoscopic ultrasound imaging of esophageal and rectal tumors has improved the accuracy of the clinical T, N, and M classifications. Advances in treatment have necessitated more detail in some T4 categories.

Clinical TNM staging and pathological TNM staging are distinct evaluations. Clinical staging is based on all available information obtained before pathology results are available. It may include information obtained by physical examination, radiologic examination, and endoscopy, for example. Pathologic staging includes information gained by microscopic examination of the primary tumor and regional lymph nodes. These two categories of staging are denoted by a small *c* or *p* before the stage, such as cT2N2M0 or pT3N4M1. It is also possible to stage a case at recurrence after a disease-free interval, at which time an *r* precedes the TNM designation.

After the procedure: Aftercare depends on the type of biopsy taken and whether the patient was placed under anesthesia. For most types of biopsy for which a patient is not already hospitalized, patients will arrange transportation to and from the health care facility and will have a family member or friend's supervision afterward. Often, a postsurgical hospital stay is required.

Risks: The risks to patients are related to the type of sample taken and the disease involved.

Results: Staging is an important aspect of understanding a patient's cancer. It guides treatment decisions and provides insight into the patient's prognosis.

Jill Ferguson, Ph.D.

▶ **For Further Information**

Bernick, P. E., and W. D. Wong. "Staging: What Makes Sense? Can the Pathologist Help?" *Surgical Oncology Clinics of North America* 9 (2000): 703-720.

Kehoe, J., and V. P. Khatri. "Staging and Prognosis of Colon Cancer." *Surgical Oncology Clinics of North America* 15 (2006): 129-146.

Sobin, L. H. "TNM: Evolution and Relation to Other Prognostic Factors." *Seminars in Surgical Oncology* 21 (2003): 3-7.

▶ **Other Resources**

American Joint Committee for Cancer
General Guidelines for TNM Staging
http://training.seer.cancer.gov/module_staging_cancer/unit03_sec03_part04_ajcc_guidelines.html

National Cancer Institute
Staging: Questions and Answers
http://www.cancer.gov/cancertopics/factsheet/Detection/staging

See also Biopsy; Blood cancers; Breast cancers; Epidermoid cancers of mucous membranes; Head and neck cancers; Imaging tests; Kidney cancer; Lung cancers; Melanomas; Metastasis; Risks for cancer; Staging of cancer; Surgical oncology; Thyroid cancer; Tumor markers; Ultrasound tests.

▶ # Tobacco-related cancers

Category: Diseases, symptoms, and conditions

Definition: Tobacco-related cancers are malignant tumors that are caused wholly or in part by the direct use of or indirect exposure to tobacco and tobacco-based products.

Related cancers: There are many types of cancer related to tobacco. The most well-known condition associated with tobacco is lung cancer. In the United States, lung cancer is the leading cause of cancer death, with 87 percent of these deaths related to tobacco. Other types of cancer related to tobacco include cancers of the bladder, breast, esophagus, kidney, larynx, liver, mouth, nasal cavity, pancreas, pharynx, stomach, and uterus. Tobacco also has been related to endometrial, cervical, and colon cancers, as well as myeloid leukemia.

Tobacco-related products and their risks: Tobacco products include cigarettes, cigars, smokeless tobacco (such as snuff or chew), and pipe tobacco. Interestingly, nicotine is not considered carcinogenic, though it may play a role in cancer. It is the other chemicals in these products as well as what happens to them when vaporized through the process of smoking that are troublesome. For instance, the smoke may contain substances such as ammonia, carbon monoxide, cyanide, and even formaldehyde. Obviously, the way the products are used relates somewhat to the types of cancers produced. For instance, lung cancer is more associated with smoking, while use of smokeless tobacco products is typically linked to cancers of the mouth and throat.

Incidence and statistics: Approximately 30 percent of all cancer deaths are said to be caused by tobacco use. Worldwide, more than three million people die each year from tobacco use. However, it is not just smokers who die, but also nonsmokers exposed to secondhand smoke. Estimates suggest that approximately 3,000 nonsmokers die of lung cancer each year because of secondhand smoke, and 35,000 people who are not current smokers will die each year of heart disease attributed to secondhand smoke exposure. For example, female nonsmokers exposed to secondhand smoke for as little as three hours per day on a regular basis have a threefold increase in risk for cervical cancer over female nonsmokers who are not exposed to secondhand smoke. Secondhand smoke also causes an increase in pet mortality due to cancer. Each year tobacco-related health problems cost Medicare and Medicaid $22.9 billion. In addition, over a lifetime, current and former smokers generate more than $500 billion in health care costs.

Nancy A. Piotrowski, Ph.D.

See also Acute myelocytic leukemia (AML); Air pollution; Bladder cancer; Blood cancers; Breast cancers; Cancer biology; Chewing tobacco; Cigarettes and cigars; Esophageal cancer; Head and neck cancers; Laryngeal cancer; Lung cancers; Malignant tumors; Metastatic squamous neck cancer with occult primary; Oral and oropharyngeal cancers; Pancreatic cancers; Personality and cancer; Prevention; Salivary gland cancer; Smoking cessation; Throat cancer; Uterine cancer.

▶ Topoisomerase inhibitors

Category: Chemotherapy and other drugs
ATC code: 101XX, 101CB

Definition: Topoisomerase inhibitors are a group of anticancer chemotherapeutic drugs. Topoisomerases are important in changing the topology of deoxyribonucleic acid (DNA), allowing for efficient DNA replication and subsequent cell proliferation. Inhibitors of topoisomerases primarily kill tumors by interfering with DNA replication, which results in both a decrease in tumor cell division and an increase in tumor cell death. Because tumors comprise rapidly dividing cells, cancer cells are particularly susceptible to the inhibitory actions of topoisomerase inhibitors. These drugs are often administered in combination with other chemotherapy agents but may also be given as a single-agent therapy.

Cancers treated: Advanced colorectal cancer, testicular tumors, small-cell lung cancer, and acute lymphocytic leukemia; many other cancers that are refractory to first-line therapies

Subclasses of this group: Epipodophyllotoxins, camptothecin and related analogs

Delivery routes: Topoisomerase inhibitors are generally administered orally or intravenously (IV). The two main oral formulations used are either a solution or a soft gelatin capsule. Many of the topoisomerase inhibitors are not water-soluble and therefore to be administered by IV must be dissolved in a special solution of chemicals, including alcohol, polyethylene glycol, and polysorbate 80. This solution is responsible for the hypersensitivity reactions induced in some patients (less than 5 percent) following infusion, such as vasomotor changes in the gastrointestinal and pulmonary systems. Slowing the rate of infusion, as well as administration of steroids or antihistamines, can diminish these hypersensitivity reactions.

How these drugs work: As a cell prepares to undergo division, the DNA must be replicated in order to provide a copy of DNA for each of the resulting cells. Double-stranded DNA is normally tightly coiled in the nucleus of nondividing cells. The supercoiled topology of the DNA strands makes it difficult for the replication protein complexes that are necessary to copy the DNA to properly localize on the DNA strand. Therefore, to properly duplicate the DNA, it must first be "unwound," relaxing the structural topology and allowing access for the replication protein complexes. Topoisomerases are proteins located in

Common Topoisomerase Inhibitors

Drug	Brands	Subclass	Delivery Mode	Cancers Treated
Etoposide, etoposide phosphate	Etopophos, VePeside (VP-16)	Epipodophyllotoxin	IV, oral	Refractory testicular tumors, small-cell lung cancer
Irinotecan hydrochloride	Camptosar (CPT-11)	Camptothecin	IV	Metastatic colon cancer, metastatic rectal cancer
Teniposide	Vumon	Epipodophyllotoxin	IV	Childhood acute lymphocytic leukemia, glioma brain tumors
Topotecan	Hycamtin	Camptothecin	IV	Refractory ovarian cancer, small-cell lung cancer, advanced cervical cancer

the cell nucleus that can act to unwind the DNA. These proteins are enzymes, meaning that they have an intrinsic catalytic activity that allows them to perform a certain function in the cell. Topoisomerases relax the supercoiled DNA by making transient breaks within the DNA strand, allowing it to unwind. Once the topoisomerase cleaves the DNA and relieves the DNA topology, the enzyme then reseals the breakage.

Two types of topoisomerases have been identified, mainly differentiated by how they cleave double-stranded DNA. Type I topoisomerases alter DNA supercoiling by cleaving only one DNA strand. Type II enzymes are capable of cleaving both DNA strands. The current model of both types I and II topoisomerase activity predicts that the enzyme breaks the DNA phosphate backbone, and in an intermediate reaction step, a covalent linkage is formed between the DNA and the enzyme. For type I topoisomerases, the nicked DNA strand is then free to rotate around the unnicked strand, relieving the DNA supercoil. Type II topoisomerases relax the DNA by cleaving the entire DNA strand, inducing the passage of one DNA double-strand through a loop in another DNA double-strand. Without the action of topoisomerases, normal cell division would not be possible. However, these enzymes also play a major role in the growth of cancer cells.

Many natural compounds act to poison topoisomerases. Inhibitors to both types of topoisomerases have shown clinical activity against tumors. The primary mechanism of action of topoisomerase inhibitors is thought to be stabilization of the enzyme while it is bound to the cleaved DNA. By stabilizing this complex, the topoisomerase enzyme is unable to religate the DNA back together, resulting in cleaved DNA strands. Prolonged DNA cleavage induces apoptosis, or cell death. These drugs therefore are thought to kill cells either by increasing the rate of

DNA breakage or by decreasing the rate of DNA religation. Although some of these drugs may also intercolate between DNA bases, DNA binding has been shown not to be a critical component of topoisomerase activity inhibition, as neither camptothecin nor etoposide binds DNA.

Two main groups of topoisomerase inhibitors are currently in clinical use, epipodophyllotoxins and camptothecin analogs. Epipodophyllotoxins, which target topoisomerase II, were synthesized in an effort to chemically improve the efficacy of the antimicrotubule drug podophyllotoxin, isolated from the mandrake plant. The epipodophyllotoxins include etoposide and teniposide. Camptothecin, an inhibitor of topoisomerase I, was discovered in an extract from the Chinese tree *Camptotheca acuminate*. The extreme side effects induced by camptothecin induced the creation of two main derivatives that cause fewer side effects, topotecan and irinotecan.

Resistance to topoisomerase inhibitors can occur through many mechanisms, including changes in the accumulation of these drugs, changes in the topoisomerase enzyme, and changes in the cellular response to the damage induced by these drugs. Because many topoisomerase inhibitors are naturally occurring substances, they are particularly susceptible to natural cellular efflux mechanisms. Cellular efflux results in a "pumping out" of the drugs, causing less total concentration of drug to be available inside the cell. By means of in vitro laboratory techniques, several cancer cell lines have been shown to display resistance to topoisomerase inhibitors. Laboratory studies have found that one mechanism of this resistance is the development of point mutations within the topoisomerase enzyme, genetic alterations that may change the target binding site where these drugs bind to the enzyme, inhibiting the ability of the drug to bind. Another way in which cells evade the effects of topoisomerase inhibitors is by increasing the expression of DNA repair enzymes, which can repair the cleavage induced by the topoisomerases.

Side effects: Topoisomerase inhibitors are generally well tolerated in most patients. The main toxicity resulting from topoisomerase inhibitors is bone marrow suppression, also known as myelosuppression. This is primarily manifested as leukopenia, or a decrease in the number of circulating white blood cells, and thrombocytopenia, a decrease in the number of blood platelets. The decrease in white blood cells increases the risk of patients developing infections, while the decrease in blood platelets may increase the risk of bleeding. Typically, the onset of myelosuppression occurs within five to seven days after the initiation of therapy, peaks within the next week, and is returned to normal approximately twenty-one to twenty-eight days after the original administration. Because of the potential seriousness of myelosuppression, patients receiving topoisomerase inhibitor therapy are required to be closely monitored by a clinician. Patients can effectively manage myelosuppression by avoiding interaction with infected people and by minimizing the risk of cuts and bruises.

Other side effects that result from drug administration mainly involve the gastrointestinal system, including diarrhea, nausea, and vomiting. Many patients often experience hair loss. These side effects can be controlled by reducing the dosage of therapy administered and by administering drugs to control the side effects, such as antinausea agents. Most of these side effects are reversible after drug therapy is stopped.

Despite the powerful effects that these drugs have in inducing tumor cell death, the use of topoisomerase inhibitors has also been linked with the development of secondary cancers in rare cases. For example, use of epipodophyllotoxins such as etoposide has been associated with an increased risk of developing secondary leukemia, at an incidence ranging from 0.7 to 3.2 percent. The reason for this increase is currently unknown.

Lisa M. Cockrell, B.S.

▶ For Further Information

Adams, Val R., and Thomas G. Burke, eds. *Camptothecins in Cancer Therapy*. Totowa, N.J.: Humana Press, 2005.

Andoh, Toshiwo, ed. *DNA Topoisomerases in Cancer Therapy: Present and Future*. New York: Kluwer Academic/Plenum, 2003.

Kantarjian, Hagop M., et al. *The M. D. Anderson Manual of Medical Oncology*. New York: McGraw-Hill, 2006.

Kufe, Donald W., et al., eds. *Holland Frei Cancer Medicine 7*. 7th ed. Hamilton, Ont.: BC Decker, 2006.

Pratt, William B., et al. *The Anticancer Drugs*. 2d ed. New York: Oxford University Press, 1994.

Skeel, Roland T. *Handbook of Cancer Chemotherapy*. 7th ed. Philadelphia: Lippincott Williams & Wilkins, 2007.

▶ Other Resources

American Cancer Society
http://www.cancer.org

National Cancer Institute
Drug Information Summaries
http://www.cancer.gov/cancertopics/druginfo/alphalist

See also Acute lymphocytic leukemia (ALL); Antineoplastics in chemotherapy; Chemotherapy; Drug resistance and multidrug resistance (MDR); Infusion therapies; Leukemias; Lung cancers; Myelosuppression; Plant alkaloids and terpenoids in chemotherapy; Rectal cancer; Testicular cancer.

▶ TP53 protein

Category: Cancer biology
Also known as: Tumor protein 53, p53, cellular tumor antigen p53, tumor suppressor p53, phosphoprotein p53 (pp53), antigen NY-CO-13, guardian of the genome

Definition: The TP53 protein is the product of the *TP53* tumor-suppressor gene. As the molecular weight appears to be 53,000 when electrophoresed in a sodium dodecyl sulfate (SDS) polyacrylamide gel, it is referred to as TP53. The TP53 protein functions as a transcription factor that controls the activity of other genes. The *TP53* gene is often referred to as the "guardian of the genome" because if the cell detects damage to its deoxyribonucleic acid (DNA), TP53 protein prevents the replication of the damaged DNA, stimulates DNA repair, or stimulates cell death (apoptosis) so that damaged DNA is not passed to daughter cells. It also seems to be important in the process of suntanning.

Biological function: The *TP53* tumor-suppressor gene is located on chromosome 17 at 17p13.1 and is essential for cell function. The TP53 protein's anticancer activity is exhibited by one of several mechanisms, many of which have not been clearly elucidated: activating mechanisms that repair DNA, arresting the cell cycle and preventing it from entering the DNA synthesis phase and passing damaged DNA on to daughter cells until damaged DNA can be repaired, and initiating apoptosis to prevent damaged DNA from being replicated and distributed to its daughter cells.

One well-characterized pathway involves the *CDKN1A* (*p21*) gene, so called because its product is a protein of 21,000 daltons. Normally, TP53 is sequestered in the nucleus by the protein HDM2. When bound to HDM2, TP53 is inactive and targeted for breakdown, keeping its cellular concentration low. If the cell detects damage to its DNA, oxidative stress, or membrane damage, TP53 becomes phosphorylated on its N-terminus by enzymes called kinases. These kinases include DNA-PK, CHK1, CHK2, ATM, ATR, CAK, and members of the MAPK (mitogen-activated protein kinase) family. When phosphorylated, TP53 dissociates from HDM2, becomes more stable, increases in concentration, changes its conformation, and becomes an active transcription factor that stimulates transcription of several genes including the *CDKN1A* gene. The CDKN1A protein binds to and inactivates polypeptides that are required for the cell to enter the DNA synthesis phase of the cell cycle. Thus, the cell is prevented from replicating damaged DNA that could cause cancer and passing it on to its daughter cells.

The TP53 protein can also activate genes that stimulate apoptosis of cells with damaged DNA, activate genes necessary for the repair of damaged DNA, and stimulate genes involved with the tanning reaction to protect cells from damaging ultraviolet (UV) light. By these and other mechanisms TP53 prevents cell growth and even causes cell death to suppress the formation of cancer.

Structure of the protein: Active TP53 protein is a tetramer consisting of four identical polypeptides of 393 amino acids each. Many of the amino acid residues can be assigned to distinct functional domains. The 39 amino acid residues at the N-terminus are involved with HDM2 binding and activation of transcription of the *CDKN1A* gene. Residues 80 to 94 are responsible for TP53's apoptosis activity, while amino acid residues 101 to 306 are responsible for TP53's DNA-binding activity, an activity essential to its role as a transcription activator. The ability of TP53 monomers to polymerize into tetramers depends on amino acid residues 307 to 355. The C-terminus amino acids (356 to 393) are responsible for TP53's localization in the nucleus and nonspecific binding to damaged DNA.

Cancer involvement: Mutations, usually simple amino acid replacement (missense) mutations, and deletions in the *TP53* gene that alter the function of its product can severely limit its tumor-suppressor activity. People who inherit one defective *TP53* gene are highly predisposed to developing Li-Fraumeni syndrome, which is characterized by cancer in a variety of tissues. More than 50 per-

cent of all human cancers involve the *TP53* gene, including 60 percent of head and neck cancers, 50 percent of ovarian and lung cancers, 45 percent of colon cancers, 35 percent of stomach cancers, and 30 percent of bladder cancers.

Of the mutations in *TP53* that result in cancer, 90 percent affect the DNA-binding domain (amino acids 101 to 306). These mutations result in the inability of TP53 to bind to the *CDKN1A* gene and stimulate its expression.

Mutations in the *TP53* gene affecting amino acid residues 307 to 355 are in the domain that allows TP53 to form tetramers with other TP53 molecules, a function necessary for its activity. TP53 molecules with one of these mutations form dimers with normal TP53 molecules, preventing their activity. Thus, these mutations are referred to as dominant loss-of-function mutations.

Charles L. Vigue, Ph.D.

▶ **For Further Information**

Hainaut, Pierre, and Klas G. Wiman. *Twenty-five Years of p53 Research.* New York: Springer, 1999.

Mukhopadhyay, Tapas, Steven A. Maxwell, and Jack A. Roth. *p53 Suppressor Gene.* New York: Springer, 1995.

Zambetti, Gerald, ed. *Protein Reviews: The p53 Tumor Suppressor Pathway and Cancer.* New York: Springer, 2005.

▶ **Other Resources**

Cornell University
Tumor Suppressor Genes: Guardians of Our Cells
http://envirocancer.cornell.edu/FactSheet/Genetics/fs6.TSgenes.cfm

HUGO Gene Nomenclature Committee
Symbol Report: TP53
http://www.genenames.org/data/hgnc_data.php?hgnc_id=11998

International Agency for Research on Cancer
IARC TP53 Mutation Database
http://www-p53.iarc.fr

p53 Knowledgebase
http://p53.bii.a-star.edu.sg/index.php

The p53 Web Site
http://p53.free.fr

See also Adenoid cystic carcinoma (ACC); Ataxia telangiectasia (AT); Bowen disease; *BRAF* gene; Breast cancer in pregnant women; Cancer biology; Cytogenetics; Dilation and curettage (D&C); Drug resistance and multidrug resistance (MDR); Endocrine cancers; Endometrial cancer;

Fallopian tube cancer; Family history and risk assessment; Fibrosarcomas, soft-tissue; Free radicals; Gene therapy; Genetics of cancer; Giant cell tumors (GCTs); Gynecologic cancers; Li-Fraumeni syndrome (LFS); Liver cancers; Mutagenesis and cancer; *MYC* oncogene; Nasal cavity and paranasal sinus cancers; Neuroectodermal tumors; Oncogenes; Sarcomas, soft-tissue; Simian virus 40; Spermatocytomas; Thymus cancer; Tumor-suppressor genes; Virus-related cancers; Vulvar cancer.

▶ Tracheostomy

Category: Procedures
Also known as: Tracheotomy, trach tube

Definition: Tracheostomy is a surgical procedure performed to aid breathing. An incision is made in the neck, just below the larynx (voice box), to directly access the trachea (windpipe). A tracheostomy tube is inserted through the opening, called a stoma, to keep the airway open. The tracheostomy tube may be connected to oxygen or mechanical ventilation.

Cancers treated: Neck, laryngeal, thyroid, and some congenital cancers

Why performed: A tracheostomy is performed for patients who have an upper airway obstruction, difficulty breathing, or excess secretions in the airway. It is also performed for patients recovering after tracheal or laryngeal surgery and for patients who are having difficulty being weaned from mechanical ventilation.

Patient preparation: With a planned tracheostomy, patients must stop taking aspirin and products containing aspirin, ibuprofen, and anticoagulants, as directed by the physician, one week before the procedure. Patients must not eat or drink for eight hours beforehand.

Steps of the procedure: The procedure is usually performed by a surgeon in an operating room while the patient is under general anesthesia. In emergent cases, the procedure may be performed at the patient's bedside in an emergency room or an intensive care unit (ICU). If the procedure is emergent, then the patient lies on the back with a rolled-up towel between the shoulders. A local anesthetic is injected and the procedure is performed.

In nonemergent cases, an intravenous (IV) line is inserted into the patient's arm to deliver medications. A small clip placed on the patient's finger is attached to an oximeter monitor to check the patient's blood oxygen level during the procedure. Electrodes, placed on the patient's chest, are attached via wires to an electrocardiograph (EKG) machine to monitor the patient's heart rhythm. The patient receives general anesthesia through the IV. The neck is cleaned, and sterile drapes are placed around the surgical area. Incisions are made in the neck and through the second and third tracheal rings to create an opening in the trachea. The tracheostomy tube is inserted into the opening. Tape or stitches hold the tube in place.

A newer technique, called tube-free tracheostomy, may be performed when a long-term tracheostomy is anticipated. A permanent opening in the trachea is created with skin and muscle flaps. After a one-month recovery period, the patient is usually able to talk efficiently by contracting the neck muscles, without the use of valves or devices.

After the procedure: The patient will not be able to talk or eat by mouth immediately after the procedure and while remaining on mechanical ventilation. Most patients will need several days to adjust to breathing through the trach tube. Nutrition is given directly into the stomach through a

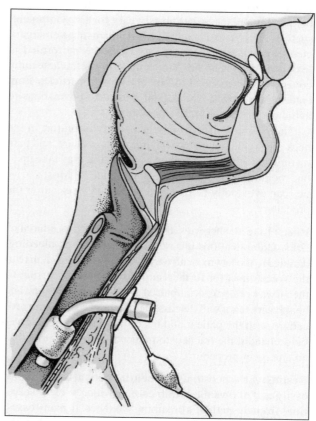

A tracheostomy tube placed in the trachea. (LifeART© 2008 Wolters Kluwer Health, Inc.-Lippincott Williams & Wilkins. All rights reserved.)

percutaneous endoscopic gastrostomy tube until the tracheostomy tube is removed. The patient will communicate with others by writing and nonverbal communication in response to questions. With training and an adaptive valve on the tracheostomy, patients are able to resume speaking as they adjust to the tracheostomy. A speech therapist can help the patient learn to speak with the tube in place.

Antibiotics may be given to reduce the risk of infection. A nurse or respiratory therapist will remove secretions from the trach tube using a suction device to clear the breathing passages.

A tracheostomy is not necessarily permanent. The patient's condition and the purpose of the tracheostomy will determine when and if the tube can be removed. If the tube is eventually removed, then the area heals quickly, leaving a small scar.

The patient and caregiver will learn how to care for the tracheostomy before leaving the hospital. The patient is usually able to go home in three to five days after the procedure, depending on his or her medical condition and rate of recovery. Some patients go home with mechanical ventilation, depending on their condition. A nurse will teach the patient and caregiver how to care for the equipment; suction, clean, and change the tube; and manage emergencies. Routine tracheostomy care must be performed at least once daily at home. A loose covering or tracheostomy cover is recommended to prevent foreign particles from entering the stoma. The patient must take precautions to avoid getting water in the opening.

The patient will feel some pain and discomfort in the neck area for about one week after the procedure, and pain medication will be prescribed as needed. It may take up to one month for the patient to heal completely. Most activities can eventually be resumed within six weeks after the procedure.

Risks: Like all surgeries, the tracheostomy procedure has risks. Complications are rare but may include bleeding, damage to the larynx or airway with a permanent change to the voice, need for further surgery, infection, scarring of the airway or neck, or impaired swallowing function. The health care team will discuss the potential risks of the procedure with the patient and his or her family or caregiver beforehand if the tracheostomy is not being performed as an emergent procedure.

Results: A tracheostomy can help the patient breathe more easily and allows the health care provider to clear secretions from the patient's breathing passages. In many cases, the tracheostomy is temporary and is removed when the patient is able to breathe without the help of a ventilator.

Angela M. Costello, B.S.

► **For Further Information**
Cooper, Sue, ed. *Tracheostomy Care.* Hoboken, N.J.: John Wiley & Sons, 2006.
Lewarski, Joseph. "Management of the Tracheostomy Patient in the Home." *RT for Decision Makers in Respiratory Care*, August, 2006. Available online at http://www.rtmagazine.com.
Pierson, D. J., S. K. Epstein, C. G. Durbin, Jr., et al. "Twentieth Annual New Horizons Symposium: Tracheostomy from A to Z." *Respiratory Care* 50 (2005): 473-549.

See also Infection and sepsis; Laryngeal cancer; Laryngeal nerve palsy; Laryngectomy.

► Transfusion therapy

Category: Procedures
Also known as: Blood transfusion, red cell transfusion, platelet transfusion, plasma transfusion, cryoprecipitate transfusion, granulocyte transfusion

Definition: Transfusion therapy is the infusion of blood components.

Cancers treated: All

Why performed: Cancer patients may need transfusion of blood components because of the disease itself or as a result of cancer treatments. Some cancers, such as those of the digestive system, may cause loss of blood through internal bleeding. Patients with cancers affecting the production or storage of blood cells may need transfusion if blood counts become too low. Treatments such as chemotherapy and radiation may destroy enough cells that patients need transfusion. Patients having surgery for cancer may need blood to replace blood loss during the procedure.

Patient preparation: The physician admits the patient to an inpatient or outpatient facility. The physician discusses benefits and risks of transfusion with the patient or legal guardian and asks him or her to sign an informed consent for transfusion. Patients experiencing previous allergic reactions to blood components are given a pretransfusion medication such as diphendydramine (Benedryl).

Steps of the procedure: A phlebotomist collects a sample of blood. In some facilities, a special transfusion armband is placed on the patient's arm at the time that the blood sample is collected. Other facilities use the standard hospital patient armband for identification. The sample is sent to transfusion services.

Transfusion services staff test the sample to determine the patient's blood type. An antibody screening is also done to detect any unusual antibodies, proteins that may cause adverse reactions if the corresponding antigen is present on the donor cells. These antibodies may be naturally occurring, formed from exposure to a blood cell antigen during previous blood transfusions, or, in females, during childbirth. If unusual antibodies are present, then donor units that lack the corresponding antigen are used for transfusion. Transfusion services staff select appropriate components from storage. If the component is red cells, then a crossmatch is performed to ensure compatibility between the patient's serum and the donor red cells. Platelets, fresh frozen plasma, or cryoprecipitate do not need to be crossmatched. The selected components are tagged with the patient's name and identification number, the component unit number, blood type of the patient and the donor, results of antibody screening, and any special needs.

Special needs that the physician may order are leukoreduction and/or irradiation of cellular components (red cells and platelets). Leukoreduction is the removal of white cells, which decreases exposure to leukocyte antigens and cytomegalovirus (CMV). Irradiation is done to prevent graft-versus-host disease.

A nurse inserts an intravenous (IV) line into the patient's arm. Two nurses verify identification of the patient and that information on the component tag matches the patient and donor information. Before starting the transfusion, the nurse checks and records the patient's temperature, pulse, and blood pressure. During the first fifteen minutes of the transfusion, the nurse stays at the bedside and observes the patient for any signs of adverse reaction. At the end of fifteen minutes, the nurse again checks and records pulse, temperature, and blood pressure. Transfusion of blood components takes as little as fifteen minutes to as long as four hours, depending on the component and the rate of transfusion that the physician orders. At the end of the transfusion, the nurse again checks and records the pulse, temperature, and blood pressure, comparing them with the beginning rates. Changes that are greater than established standards at any time or adverse patient symptoms may result in stopping the transfusion. The physician reviews the information and may order a reaction workup.

In the event of a reaction workup, any remaining component and the transfusion tubing are sent to transfusion services. A phlebotomist collects a new sample of blood and sends it to transfusion services. Nursing staff and transfusion services staff review all patient identification, paperwork, and donor information. Repeat testing is performed on pretransfusion and posttransfusion blood samples and the donor sample. Additional tests such as a cul-

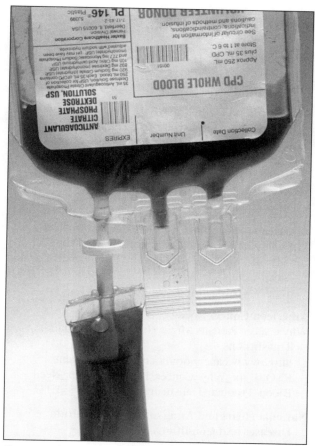

Cancer patients may require blood transfusions because of either the disease itself or cancer treatments. (PhotoDisc)

ture for bacteria or other blood and chemistry tests may be done. A pathologist reviews the results of the transfusion reaction workup and determines the cause. The patient will not be transfused with additional components until the completion of the workup.

After the procedure: The IV line is removed. The nurse advises the patient about signs and symptoms to watch for and report. Blood samples may be collected to test for hemoglobin, platelet count, or clotting factors. If transfusion is done on an outpatient basis, then the patient may be discharged shortly after completion of the transfusion.

Risks: The risks of transfusion are allergic reactions, transmission of viruses or infectious diseases, fever iron overload, lung injury, acute hemolytic reaction, delayed hemolytic reaction, and graft-versus-host disease.

Results: Red cells are given to replace blood loss or correct anemia. Platelet transfusions are given to replace platelets to prevent bleeding. Plasma and cryoprecipitate are given to correct coagulation factors. Rarely, granulocytes are given to increase the white blood cell count.

Wanda E. Clark, M.T. (ASCP)

▶ **For Further Information**

Abeloff, Martin D., et al. *Clinical Oncology.* 3d ed. Philadelphia: Churchill Livingstone Elsevier, 2004.

Klein, Harvey G., and David J. Anstee. *Mollison's Blood Transfusion in Clinical Medicine.* 11th ed. Malden, Mass.: Blackwell, 2005.

▶ **Other Resources**

American Association of Blood Banks, America's Blood Centers, and the American Red Cross
Circular of Information for the Use of Human Blood and Blood Components
http://www.fda.gov/cber/gdlns/crclr.pdf

American Cancer Society
Why Cancer Patients Might Need Blood Product Transfusions
http://www.cancer.org/docroot/ETO/content/ETO_1_4x_Why_Cancer_Patients_Might_Need_Blood_Product_Transfusions.asp?sitearea=ETO

National Heart and Lung and Blood Institute Diseases and Conditions Index
What Is a Blood Transfusion?
http://www.nhlbi.nih.gov/health/dci/Diseases/bt/bt_whatis.html

See also Anemia; Aplastic anemia; Autologous blood transfusion; Biological therapy; Blood cancers; Bone marrow aspiration and biopsy; Fanconi anemia; Hematemesis; Hematologic oncology; Hemochromatosis; Hemolytic anemia; Hepatitis B virus (HBV); Hepatitis C virus (HCV); Infusion therapies; Pathology; Risks for cancer.

▶ Transitional care

Category: Social and personal issues

Definition: Transitional care consists of the needs, services, and resources to consider when helping a person with cancer adjust, as the disease shifts from one phase to another.

The importance of transitions: The course of treatment for cancer can be long and difficult, with many changes in disease state and in treatments. As these changes occur, the needs of the patient and the patient's family or caregivers also change. For example, the patient may move from hospital care to home care, or from home care to hospice care. In other situations, the patient may shift frequently between home care and hospital care, or may require care at a rehabilitation facility or a nursing home. Whatever the case may be, it is important that the patient's (and family's) needs remain the primary consideration and that each transition occurs as smoothly as possible to ensure continuity of care.

What to consider in planning: Ideally, a nurse will develop a comprehensive care plan addressing every aspect of the patient's life that will be affected by the forthcoming transition. This plan should include a detailed assessment of the following:
• The patient's current physical status
• Specific needs of the patient and family if the patient is cared for at home
• The patient's and family's emotional and psychological adjustment
• Requirements for extra support at home
• Transferring records and other information with the patient if health care providers change
• Financial issues, such as insurance coverage, the patient's ability to work, and how the costs of care will be covered
• Spiritual needs of the patient and family
• Legal issues, such as advance directives, a living will, health care proxy, durable power of attorney, and do-not-resuscitate (DNR) orders

The patient (or the patient's caregivers) should receive all legal documents, which should accompany the patient through different stages of care. This helps ensure that the patient's wishes are respected during all stages of care.

Who does the planning: Many people may be involved in planning for transitional care, depending on the needs of the patient and family. Those involved might include the patient and patient's family or caregivers, the patient's doctors and primary nurse, a social worker, psychologist or other mental health professional, advocacy or support personnel from community agencies or cancer support organizations, pastoral counselor or other spiritual adviser, physical therapist, and occupational therapist.

Services available: A variety of services are available, depending on the needs of the patient and family and on available local resources. For example, patients may require specific services, such as visiting nurses, housekeeping or cleaning services, medical equipment and supply services, a home infusion agency, financial or legal consultation, transportation services for medical appointments, counseling, spiritual care, employment services that can help with employment transitions or skills retraining, special services to enable the patient to return to school, and other community services that can assist with various needs, such as home meal delivery and errands.

Other patients may be transferred to a hospice, to a nursing home, or to a rehabilitation center. Many of these facilities provide a social worker, nurse, or other personnel to help the patient and family adjust to the new surroundings, to access needed services, and to ensure that the patient's medical care (including medication) is coordinated among previous and current care providers.

Transition to the patient's or caregiver's home: In this case, health care staff are advised to assess the following aspects of home care:
- Issues of safety and access (stairs, bathing facilities, and the like) that may require modification (ramps, handle bars, lifts)
- If special equipment (hospital beds, medical devices) will be required in the home
- If the home can physically accommodate such equipment
- If the patient or caregiver is able to operate the equipment
- If the patient or caregiver will require physical help (such as with the patient's hygiene or personal care)
- If the patient or caregiver understands and can safely give medications
- If the patient or caregiver can handle the emotional stress of home care
- If the patient or caregiver understands pain control and how to manage symptoms of pain.

The person performing this assessment (for example, an occupational therapist, social worker, or home health nurse) can then work with the patient and appropriate staff to ensure the patient's needs are met.

Amy J. Neil, M.S., M.A.P.

▶ For Further Information

Bellenir, Karen, ed. *Cancer Survivor Sourcebook*. Detroit: Omnigraphics, 2007.

Brennan, James. *Cancer in Context: A Practical Guide to Supportive Care*. New York: Oxford University Press, 2004.

Houts, Peter, ed. *Home Care Guide for Cancer*. Philadelphia: American College of Physicians, 1996.

Stern, Theodore, and Mikkael Sekeres. *Facing Cancer: A Complete Guide for People with Cancer, Their Families, and Caregivers*. New York: McGraw-Hill, 2004.

▶ Other Resources

Hospice Foundation of America
http://www.hospicefoundation.org

International Association for Hospice and Palliative Care
http://www.hospicecare.com

National Cancer Institute
Transitional Care Planning
http://www.cancer.gov/cancertopics/pdq/supportivecare/transitionalcare/patient

National Care Planning Council
http://www.longtermcarelink.net

National Family Caregivers Association
http://www.nfcacares.org

National Patient Advocate Foundation
http://www.npaf.org

Patient Advocate Foundation
http://www.patientadvocate.org

See also Advance directives; Caregivers and caregiving; Do-not-resuscitate (DNR) order; Financial issues; Home health services; Hospice care; Infusion therapies; Insurance; Living will; Occupational therapy; Oncology social worker; Psychosocial aspects of cancer; Rehabilitation.

▶ Transitional cell carcinomas

Category: Diseases, symptoms, and conditions
Also known as: Transitional cell cancer, bladder cancer, renal pelvic tumors, TCCs

Related conditions: Bladder cancer, kidney cancer, renal cell carcinoma

Definition: Transitional cell carcinoma is a cancer that forms in transitional cells in the lining of the bladder, kidney, or ureter (tube connecting the kidney to the bladder).

Risk factors: Common risk factors for this disease include smoking, misusing certain pain medicines for an extended period of time, and exposure to some chemicals and dyes used in the textile, leather, plastic, and rubber industries.

Etiology and the disease process: The lining of the bladder, ureter, and kidney contain transitional cells, which can change shape and stretch without breaking apart as needed in organs that expand in the urinary tract. Transitional cell carcinoma begins in these cells and can move

Stage at Diagnosis and Five-Year Relative Survival Rates for Bladder Cancer, 1996-2004

Stage	Cases Diagnosed (%)	Survival Rate (%)
Localized[a]	75	92.1
Regional[b]	19	44.6
Distant[c]	4	6.4
Unstaged	3	59.3

Source: Data from National Cancer Institute, Surveillance Epidemiology and End Results, Cancer Stat Fact Sheets, 2008

[a]Cancer still confined to primary site
[b]Cancer has spread to regional lymph nodes or directly beyond the primary site
[c]Cancer has metastasized

from the lining of the organs to invade the internal areas of the organ, as well as other nearby organs.

Transitional cell carcinoma that begins as a superficial tumor may grow through the lining and into the muscular wall of the bladder, kidney, or ureter. This invasive cancer may extend into a nearby organ such as the uterus, vagina, or prostate gland or to nearby lymph nodes, in which case cancer cells may have spread to other lymph nodes or other sites, such as the lungs, liver, or bones.

Incidence: The incidence of transitional cell carcinoma is equivalent to that of bladder and kidney cancer, though almost 90 percent of bladder and ureter cancers are caused by transitional cell carcinoma. According to the National Cancer Institute, bladder cancer is the fourth most common type of cancer in men and the eighth most common in women. Whites get bladder cancer twice as often as blacks and Hispanics. People with family members who have bladder cancer are more likely to get the disease, as well as people who have previously had bladder cancer.

Symptoms: The most common symptom is blood in the urine (hematuria). Some patients experience pain or burning during urination or a change in urinary habits, such as painful urination or a frequent urge to urinate. Other symptoms include back pain, lethargy, and weight loss.

Screening and diagnosis: Diagnosis of transitional cell carcinoma is confirmed with a physical exam, urinalysis, and urine cytology tests. The urinalysis determines if abnormalities such as blood, protein, sugar, and solids exist

in the urine. Urine cytology is a microscopic examination of urine to detect any abnormal cells that have sloughed off the walls of the bladder or kidney and been released in the urine. If necessary, cytoscopy is performed; a very narrow tube with a light and camera is inserted through the urethra to examine the inside of the bladder and ureter. Further imaging studies can help determine if the cancer has spread to other layers of the organs, as well as outside the urinary tract. If bladder or kidney cancer is suspected, a physician may order a computed tomography (CT) scan, pyelography, or biopsy. The CT scan is helpful for a three-dimensional view of the urinary tract to determine if any masses or tumors exist in the bladder or if the cancer has spread to other organs. Pyelography involves injecting a special dye into the vein or urethra and examining a series of timed-interval X rays of the urinary system to determine if abnormalities exist. The biopsy is typically performed during cytoscopy, and abnormal cells can be detected with a microscope.

Treatment and therapy: Treatment for transitional cell carcinoma depends on the stage and location of the cancer. Typically surgery to remove the entire kidney, the ureter, and the bladder cuff (connecting the ureter to the bladder) will be performed. When the cancer is superficial and in the lower third of the ureter, another procedure called a segmental resection of the ureter is performed. In this surgery, part of the ureter is removed and the ends of the ureter are reattached.

Radiation therapy uses high-energy rays to kill localized cancer cells to shrink the tumor before surgery or if surgery is not an option. Chemotherapy uses one drug or a combination of drugs to kill cancer cells. Superficial bladder cancer can be treated with local chemotherapy by inserting a catheter through the urethra and leaving it in the bladder for several hours, once per week for several weeks. If the cancer has deeply invaded the bladder or spread to lymph nodes or other organs, chemotherapy may be used to treat the entire body.

Prognosis, prevention, and outcomes: The outcome of transitional cell carcinoma varies depending on the exact location of the cancerous cells and whether the cancer has metastasized. Cancer localized to the kidney or ureter can be cured with surgery. Cancer that has metastasized to other organs is usually not curable, though there are exceptions. Preventive measures include not smoking, wearing protective equipment if exposed to toxic chemicals, and following the physician's advice concerning the use of all pain medications, including over-the-counter pain medications. Treatment given after the primary treatment to increase the chances of a cure is called adjuvant therapy and may include chemotherapy, radiation therapy, hormone therapy, or biological therapy.

Robert J. Amato, D.O.

▶ For Further Information

Ellsworth, Pamela. *One Hundred Questions and Answers About Bladder Cancer.* Sudbury, Mass.: Jones and Bartlett, 2005.

Raghavan, Derek. *Bladder Cancer: A Cleveland Clinic Guide—Information for Patients and Caregivers.* Cleveland: Cleveland Clinic Press, 2008.

Schrier, Robert W., ed. *Diseases of the Kidney and Urinary Tract.* 8th ed. Philadelphia: Wolters Kluwer Health/ Lippincott Williams & Wilkins, 2007.

▶ Other Resources

American Cancer Society
Detailed Guide: Bladder Cancer
http://www.cancer.org/docroot/CRI/
CRI_2_3x.asp?dt=44

American Urological Association
UrologyHealth.org
http://www.urologyhealth.org

National Cancer Institute
Bladder Cancer
http://www.cancer.gov/cancertopics/types/bladder

See also Bladder cancer; *HRAS* gene testing; Kidney cancer; Phenacetin; Urethral cancer; Urinary system cancers.

▶ Transrectal ultrasound

Category: Procedures
Also known as: Prostate sonography

Definition: Transrectal ultrasound is a procedure that uses ultrasonic waves to evaluate the prostate gland, primarily by acting as a guide for prostate biopsies.

Cancers diagnosed: Prostate cancer

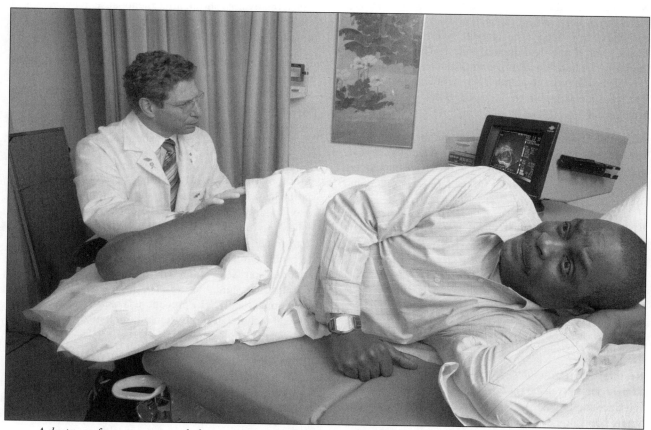

A doctor performs a transrectal ultrasound of a patient's prostate gland. (©Yoav Levy/Phototake—All rights reserved)

Why performed: Since the sensitivity of transrectal ultrasound is only 60 to 70 percent for the detection of prostate cancer, it is not a screening test. Therefore, the primary role of transrectal ultrasound is to guide prostate biopsies. The sonographic appearance of prostate cancer is variable, with approximately 70 percent of cancer appearing hypoechoic (lower in density) compared to the peripheral zone. The remainder of prostate cancer can appear hyperechoic (higher in density) or a mixture of both and can be either nodular or infiltrative. Cystic cancer is rare. Although classically cancer of the prostate presents as a hypoechoic nodule in the peripheral zone, only 20 to 30 percent of such nodules actually represent cancer. Benign conditions that can be visualized on transrectal ultrasound include prostatitis, atrophy, fibrosis, infarct, and benign prostatic hyperplasia (BPH).

Patient preparation: The scan is usually performed as an outpatient procedure, and patients are not asked to perform any special preparation.

Steps of the procedure: The patient is placed on his side on a table, and the technologist or the radiologist applies a water-based conducting gel to the probe in order to study the organ or body part of interest, in this case the prostate gland. The transducer is designed to be inserted inside the rectum, and it may feel uncomfortable. The sonographer then rubs the handheld probe or transducer across the surface of the the prostate gland. There will be some discomfort from pressure, but the ultrasound waves themselves are painless.

After the procedure: The scan is generated by the computer attached to the ultrasound probe and read by the radiologist the same day. The patient will need to contact his doctor or health care provider for the radiology report and for any follow-up therapy,

Risks: The study is painless and relatively harmless, as no radiation is involved. Use of the transrectal probe is a decision made by the health care provider, not the sonographer or radiologist. The patient should consult his health care provider if he has any questions or concerns regarding use of the transrectal probe and talk to his health professional about any concerns regarding the need for the ultrasound, its risks, how it will be done, and what the results indicate.

Results: The results are dependent on the type of scan performed and the reason for the study. If evidence of cancer is found, additional tests will be ordered to confirm the diagnosis and suggest a course of treatment.

Debra B. Kessler, M.D., Ph.D.

See also Benign prostatic hyperplasia (BPH); Endorectal ultrasound; Prostate cancer; Prostate-specific antigen (PSA) test; Prostatitis; Screening for cancer; Ultrasound tests.

▶ Transvaginal ultrasound

Category: Procedures
Also known as: Transvaginal sonogram

Definition: Transvaginal ultrasound is a diagnostic procedure that uses an internal probe or transducer to enter the vagina.

Cancers diagnosed: Uterine, ovarian, and endometrial cancers; noncancerous fibroids

Why performed: Transvaginal ultrasound is a diagnostic procedure used to evaluate women with dysfunctional uterine bleeding to detect pelvic masses, ectopic pregnancy, and pelvic inflammatory disease. In postmenopausal women, the thickness of the endometrium is evaluated to check for overgrowth (hyperplasia) or cancer. Since the ovaries shrink after menopause, a gynecologist cannot feel them during a routine pelvic examination. The ovaries can be examined by transvaginal ultrasound.

Patient preparation: Little preparation is needed for the transvaginal ultrasound. The patient undresses from the waist down and lies face-up on the examination table. Either the patient will place her feet in stirrups or a bolster is placed under the hips to tilt the pelvis upward for insertion of the probe as well as the examination. The bladder is empty.

Steps of the procedure: Often the woman inserts the probe herself (similar to inserting a tampon). Warm gel is used to lubricate the probe. There may be slight pressure when the transducer is inserted. A transducer is used to transmit high-frequency sound waves, which bounce back to produce images that can be seen on a video monitor or recorded on X-ray film. There is no radiation exposure during transvaginal ultrasound, and the results are available immediately. The procedure is performed by a radiological technician or physician radiologist and read by a physician radiologist.

After the procedure: The patient can resume normal activities immediately. There may be a small amount of leakage from the gel used, which can be absorbed by using a sanitary pad.

Risks: No risks are associated with this procedure.

Results: The results of a transvaginal ultrasound may be normal or abnormal. Normal results mean that no abnormal areas are found in the uterus. It is normal in shape and size with no abnormal thickness, masses, or growths. Abnormal results include growths (masses or cysts) and unanticipated thickness. Because there is a risk of false positive results, abnormal findings should be evaluated and confirmed by magnetic resonance imaging (MRI) or biopsy.

Marcia J. Weiss, J.D.

See also Endometrial cancer; Gynecologic cancers; Hereditary leiomyomatosis and renal cell cancer (HLRCC); Imaging tests; Pelvic examination; Ultrasound tests; Uterine cancer.

▶ Trichilemmal carcinomas

Category: Diseases, symptoms, and conditions

Related conditions: Trichilemmomas, Cowden syndrome

Definition: Trichilemmal carcinomas are rare and slow-growing malignant tumors that start in the outer sheath of a hair root; they most often occur on skin that has had a lot of exposure to the sun, such as the face or arms.

Risk factors: There are no known risk factors, although exposure to the sun may be a reason for development of trichilemmal carcinoma.

Etiology and the disease process: The cause of trichilemmal carcinoma is not known. The carcinoma is slow-growing and does not cause pain.

Incidence: Trichilemmal carcinoma usually occurs in individuals over the age of fifty, with equal incidence in men and women.

Symptoms: A trichilemmal carcinoma appears as a small (approximately ¼-inch to ¾-inch in diameter) tan, flesh-colored, or purplish spot on the face, scalp, trunk, or extremities; usually it is a single spot. The tumor may look like a wart and may have a hair in it. Less likely, the trichilemmal carcinoma may be on a part of the body that is not exposed to the sun, and it may appear as multiple spots. There are no other symptoms of a trichilemmal carcinoma.

Screening and diagnosis: Any spot on the skin that fits the description of a trichilemmal carcinoma should be looked at by a dermatologist. Trichilemmal carcinoma is diagnosed by biopsy and histological examination (when the tissue is viewed under a microscope by a pathologist). Trichilemmal carcinoma is probably the malignant form of a noncancerous tumor called a trichilemmoma. A trichilemmal carcinoma is not the same as a malignant proliferating trichilemmal tumor (usually seen on the scalp or the back of the neck).

Treatment and therapy: The trichilemmal carcinoma spot is usually easily removed by a surgeon during an outpatient surgical procedure; the procedure is considered low risk, and additional therapy is not necessary. It is possible that the spot may recur in the same location, and surgical removal should be repeated. Spread (metastasis) of a trichilemmal carcinoma is very unlikely.

Prognosis, prevention, and outcomes: The prognosis for individuals who have had a trichilemmal carcinoma removed is very good. There are no recommended preventive strategies for trichilemmal carcinoma since the underlying cause is not known.

Vicki Miskovsky, B.S., R.D.

See also Carcinomas; Cowden syndrome; Family history and risk assessment; Metastasis; Sunscreens.

▶ Tuberous sclerosis

Category: Diseases, symptoms, and conditions
Also known as: Tuberous sclerosis complex (TSC), Bourneville disease, epiloia

Related conditions: Benign tumors

Definition: Tuberous sclerosis is a genetic disease characterized by the growth of benign tumors in the brain and other organs.

Risk factors: Tuberous sclerosis develops because of a genetic mutation, but only 35 percent of tuberous sclerosis cases are known to be inherited; the other 65 percent are the result of spontaneous genetic mutations. The cause of these spontaneous mutations is unknown.

Etiology and the disease process: Two genes have been shown to be important in the development of tuberous sclerosis: the hamartin gene (*TSC1*) and the tuberin gene (*TSC2*). Both of these genes are tumor suppressors, and mutations that suppress their function have been linked with uncontrolled cell growth. Because these genes are thought to act in concert together, inactivation of only one gene is sufficient to produce symptoms of tuberous sclerosis.

Incidence: Tuberous sclerosis is a relatively rare disease, affecting all ethnicities and both genders equally. Currently, nearly 1 million people worldwide are estimated to be afflicted with the disease; approximately 50,000 of these cases are in the United States.

Symptoms: The growth of benign, tumor-like nodules is a common feature of tuberous sclerosis. These growths, also termed hamartomas, have the potential to form in almost every organ, resulting in distinct consequences. For example, brain growths can lead to seizures and mental retardation, while hamartomas that form in and around the heart, called cardiac rhabdomyomas, can lead to valve dysfunction and arrhythmia. Kidney growths, or renal angiomyolipomas, may eventually grow so large that the normal kidney function is compromised. Many children with tuberous sclerosis exhibit small, reddish facial growths, called angiofibromas.

Screening and diagnosis: There is no particular hallmark sign used to diagnosis tuberous sclerosis. Instead, the recognition of a combination of major and minor symptomatic features is used to establish a clinical diagnosis.

Treatment and therapy: Currently no cure exists for tuberous sclerosis. Surgery has become an important approach to remove harmful nodule growths and preserve the function of the affected organ. Drugs to alleviate the symptoms may also be used, including antiepileptic drugs to control seizures.

Prognosis, prevention, and outcomes: The prognosis for individuals with tuberous sclerosis depends on the severity of symptoms. Many patients with mild tuberous sclerosis lead productive lives with a normal life span. However, if these patients are not treated appropriately, complications arising from hamartoma growth in vital organs can result in premature death.

Lisa M. Cockrell, B.S.

See also Benign tumors; Brain and central nervous system cancers; Fibrosarcomas, soft-tissue; Sarcomas, soft-tissue.

▶ Tubular carcinomas

Category: Diseases, symptoms, and conditions
Also known as: Pure or mixed tubular carcinomas, tubulolobular carcinomas

Related conditions: Infiltrating ductal carcinomas

Definition: Tubular carcinomas are a type of invasive ductal carcinoma, a well-differentiated form of breast cancer, characterized by invasion of the stroma by small epithelial tubules.

Risk factors: The risk factors for the development of tubular carcinoma may be the presence of a radial scar, lobular proliferative lesions, and ductal carcinoma.

Etiology and the disease process: Tubular breast carcinoma is estrogen dependent and human epidermal growth factor receptor 2/neu (HER2/neu) negative. The tumor varies in size and cell division time. Tubular carcinomas are a genetically distinct group of breast cancers. In particular, pure tubular carcinomas are a separate morphologic entity and have more than 70 percent tubularity. Carcinomas with less than 70 percent tubularity are often ductal and aggressive, and are referred to as mixed tubular carcinomas. Another type of tubular carcinoma is tubulolobular carcinoma, which consists of tubular and infiltrating lobular elements. Tubular carcinoma is usually a unicentric lesion, but in about 20 percent of the cases, it exhibits multifocality. Multifocality is found in more than 30 percent of mixed tubular or tubulolobular carcinomas. Contralateral development of cancers, such as infiltrating ductal tumors, has been reported in 10 percent of patients with tubular carcinoma.

Incidence: Although invasive cancers containing tubular elements are common, tubular carcinoma is rare and accounts for less than 2 percent of all breast cancers. It occurs most frequently in women between the ages of forty and sixty.

Symptoms: Tubular carcinoma often manifests as a palpable mass. Infiltrating ductal carcinoma is characterized by a hard lump with irregular borders, and the skin over the area or the nipple may retract.

Screening and diagnosis: Tubular carcinoma is usually detected by mammography, appearing as a small mass and spicules or microcalcifications when the mass is less than 1 centimeter (cm) in diameter. The spicules are often due to malignant cells and fibrous stroma. Under a microscope, the cancer cells in tubular carcinoma resemble tiny tubes that are well differentiated.

Treatment and therapy: Treatment for tubular carcinoma resembles that for estrogen-responsive breast cancer, and it may include mastectomy.

Prognosis, prevention, and outcomes: Pure tubular carcinoma typically does not metastasize, and patients with this disease have an excellent survival rate. However, the differentiation between the types of tubular carcinomas is important for more precise prognosis. With the increase of nontubular elements in a tumor, the likelihood of metastatic spread and multifocality also increase.

Anita Nagypál, Ph.D.

See also Breast cancer in children and adolescents; Breast cancer in men; Breast cancer in pregnant women; Breast cancers; Calcifications of the breast; Ductal carcinoma in situ (DCIS); Invasive ductal carcinomas; Invasive lobular carcinomas.

▶ Tumor flare

Category: Diseases, symptoms, and conditions
Also known as: Hormone flare, hormonal flare

Related conditions: All cancers

Definition: Tumor flare is a sudden and temporary worsening of symptoms or markers, which can include an increase in the size a tumor, heightened pain, and abnormal blood chemistry values. Tumor flare can occur in all types of cancer and often follows administration of a cancer therapy. This can be considered a positive sign that the cancer is responding to the treatment; however, tumor flare can be life-threatening.

Risk factors: Risk factors for tumor flare depend on the type of tumor and the stage of the cancer.

Etiology and the disease process: The cause of tumor flare varies depending on the type of cancer and the tumor. Tumor flare typically involves intense exacerbation of symptoms followed by diminished symptoms.

Incidence: Tumor flare is a common adverse reaction to chemotherapy in patients with cancer.

Symptoms: Symptoms of tumor flare can include but are not limited to an increase in the size of the tumor, bone and tumor pain, paralysis (depending on the location of the tumor), and wide variations in blood laboratory values that can lead to life-threatening conditions.

Screening and diagnosis: Tumor flare typically is not difficult to diagnose, as many of the symptoms are detectable by the patients. Further evaluation, however, can also include blood tests and biopsy.

Treatment and therapy: Treatment for tumor flare includes supportive therapy for the symptoms, such as pain medications and treatments that counteract the potential variation in blood chemistry values. Hormonal therapy can also be used to reduce the symptoms of tumor flare.

Prognosis, prevention, and outcomes: Prognosis for tumor flare depends on the type of cancer exacerbated by the flare. As a flare can be life-threatening but is not in every case, it is not possible to predict a prognosis. Tumor flare can be prevented by administration of antiandrogen therapy in some cases.

Anna Perez, M.Sc.

See also Androgen drugs; Antiandrogens; Chemotherapy; Hormonal therapies; Malignant tumors; Metastasis.

▶ Tumor lysis syndrome

Category: Diseases, symptoms, and conditions

Related conditions: Acute renal failure, cardiac arrhythmia, metabolic acidosis

Definition: Tumor lysis syndrome is a potentially life-threatening metabolic emergency caused when tumor cells are destroyed and broken down faster than the body can get rid of them. This causes an increase in various electrolyte levels in the blood. The rapid increase of uric acid and phosphate may also cause acute renal failure. These cells are destroyed by chemotherapy, radiation, or the disease process itself. Tumor lysis syndrome can occur up to seven days after the initiation of treatment. The increase in destroyed cells can occur rapidly and cause patient death.

Risk factors: People at risk are those who are diagnosed with a rapidly growing cancer that responds well to chemotherapy. Common cancers that place patients at risk for tumor lysis syndrome are leukemia, non-Hodgkin lymphoma, breast cancer, testicular or germ-cell cancer, soft-tissue sarcoma, small-cell lung cancer, and medulloblastomas. The more involved or aggressive the disease is, the more the risk for developing tumor lysis syndrome.

People who have preexisting kidney failure and are diagnosed with a cancer that involves rapidly growing cells are also at increased risk for developing tumor lysis syndrome.

Etiology and the disease process: Chemotherapy causes the patient's cancer cells to lyse, or break down, releasing the contents of the cancer cell into the bloodstream. This causes an increase in the serum potassium, phosphate, and uric acid levels and a decrease in the calcium levels. The levels change at such a rapid rate that the body is unable to maintain a balance and lethal symptoms arise.

Incidence: The exact incidence of tumor lysis syndrome is not known. Patients who are diagnosed with leukemia in blast crisis have a higher incidence of tumor lysis syndrome.

Symptoms: Symptoms include the following changes in blood values:

- Hyperkalemia: Increased levels of potassium in the blood. Normal potassium levels are about 3.5 to 5.0 millimoles/deciliter (mmol/dl). In tumor lysis, the potassium will increase to greater than 7 mmol/dl. Symptoms commonly associated with an increase in potassium levels are muscle weakness, muscle cramps, and paralysis. High potassium levels also contribute to cardiac problems including a racing heart rate, decrease in heart rate, and sudden death. Additional symptoms associated with high potassium levels include nausea, vomiting, diarrhea, and loss of appetite.
- Hyperphosphatemia: Increased levels of phosphorus in the blood. Cancer cells contain about four times more phosphorus than normal cells. When the cancer cells are killed, the phosphorus is released into the blood. This increased level of phosphate can cause the kidneys to misfunction and can cause acute renal failure. The increase in the phosphorus combines with the increased calcium levels and affects the kidney and muscle tissue. This causes a rapid decrease in calcium levels, which can then cause the patient to experience severe muscle cramping and twitching, and problems with the heart.
- Hypocalcemia: Decreased levels of calcium in the blood. When phosphate increases, the calcium decreases. Symptoms of hypocalcemia can include seizures, Parkinson-like movements, swelling of the optic disk, agitation or anxiety, painful muscle spasms, and muscle weakness.
- Hyperuricemia: Increased levels of uric acid in the blood. This can cause acute renal failure. Symptoms may include nausea, vomiting, diarrhea, and loss of appetite.

Screening and diagnosis: Patients who are at high risk of developing tumor lysis syndrome should have baseline labs drawn before therapy begins. Many times patients may not exhibit any signs and symptoms but will begin to have altered lab values. It is important that the patient who is at risk have frequent blood tests taken to monitor for changes. Blood tests should be drawn at least every two to six hours to monitor the calcium, potassium, phosphate, magnesium, and uric acid levels.

Treatment and therapy: The best treatment is prevention. Treatment is targeted to the altered laboratory value as well as symptoms as they arise. Intravenous (IV) fluids should be initiated in patients before therapy begins and continue to be infused throughout therapy. If high flow rate is used for IV fluids, then a diuretic, such as furosemide (Lasix), may be added to assist with urine excretion.

Patients are also given allopurinol, an antigout medication, to stop the formation of uric acid. Urine alkalization may be done by adding sodium bicarbonate to the IV fluids. More severe cases of tumor lysis syndrome may require kidney dialysis to help support the patient through the crisis. The dialysis helps remove the excess potassium and phosphorus when the patient's kidneys are unable to do so.

Patients who have increased potassium levels are treated with sodium polystyrene (Kayexalate). Sodium polystyrene draws the potassium into the bowel to be excreted. Diuretics can also be used to help eliminate the potassium in the urine. In severe cases of elevated potassium, patients are treated with insulin and dextrose, which causes the cells to take in more potassium, decreasing the potassium levels in the blood.

Increased phosphorus is treated with oral doses of aluminum hydroxide. Aluminum hydroxide will draw the phosphorus into the bowel to be excreted. Diuretics can also be given to increase the amount of phosphorus excreted in the urine. Decreasing the phosphorus level causes the calcium level to increase.

Low calcium levels are not typically treated unless the patient becomes symptomatic and then the patient receives calcium gluconate.

Prognosis, prevention, and outcomes: Tumor lysis may be prevented by administering intravenous fluids and allopurinol. Tumor lysis syndrome can occur rapidly, within hours, and have a poor prognosis. As lab values can start changing before the patient experiences side effects, patients who are at risk for tumor lysis syndrome should be hospitalized with preventive therapy initiated, allowing for aggressive treatment to start before the patient's condition worsens.

Katrina Green, R.N., B.S.N., O.C.N.

▶ **For Further Information**

Itano, J. K., and K. N. Toaka. *Core Curriculum for Oncology Nursing.* 4th ed. Philadelphia: Elsevier/Saunders, 2005.

Johnson, B. L., and J. Gross. *Handbook of Oncology Nursing.* 3d ed. Sudbury, Mass.: Jones and Bartlett, 1998.

Lenhard, R. E., R. T. Osteen, and T. Gansler. *The American Cancer Society's Clinical Oncology.* Atlanta: American Cancer Society, 2001.

Otto, S. E. *Oncology Nursing.* 4th ed. St. Louis: Elsevier, 2001.

Yarbro, C. H., M. H. Frogge, and M. Goodman. *Cancer Nursing: Principles and Practice.* 6th ed. Sudbury, Mass.: Jones and Bartlett, 2005.

Yarbro, C. H., M. H. Frogge, and M. Goodman. *Cancer Symptom Management.* 3d ed. Sudbury, Mass.: Jones and Bartlett, 2005.

▶ **Other Resources**

American Cancer Society
http://www.cancer.org

National Institutes of Health
http://www.nlm.nih.gov

See also Calcium; Chemotherapy; Cobalt 60 radiation; Diarrhea; Gastrointestinal complications of cancer treatment; Medical oncology; Nausea and vomiting; Oncology.

▶ Tumor markers

Category: Procedures
Also known as: Biomarkers, cancer markers, tumor-associated antigens, tumor-specific antigens

Definition: Tumor markers are molecules whose presence or abnormal concentration in body fluids or tissue samples is associated with malignancy. They are most often individual, well-characterized proteins or nucleic acids. Increasingly, multiple tumor markers are interpreted in combination.

Cancers identified: Many, notably prostate, ovarian, and gastrointestinal cancers

How tumor markers are used: Tumor markers have been sought for every type of cancer, and tumor-marker determinations can be used in several contexts. In risk assessment, mutations in the *BRCA1* and *BRCA2* genes confer an increased risk of breast and ovarian cancer, and mutations in the *APC* gene are associated with increased colorectal cancer risk. Knowledge of increased risk can motivate more frequent screening procedures or more aggressive treatment decisions if cancer is eventually diagnosed.

In early detection efforts, three serum tumor markers are widely used:
- Cancer antigen 125 (CA 125) for ovarian cancer
- Carcinoembryonic antigen (CEA) for gastrointestinal cancer
- Prostate-specific antigen (PSA) for prostate cancer

Because of the need for very high specificity, only one tumor marker (PSA) is recommended for screening of asymptomatic individuals; most early detection efforts focus on clinical and radiological findings. In diagnostic con-

firmation procedures, markers such as alpha-methylacyl-CoA racemase (AMACR) can be interrogated on biopsy specimens; the presence of AMACR in prostate tissue helps rule out benign mimickers of prostate cancer. In molecular classification efforts, tumor markers can resolve different types of cancer that might otherwise be misdiagnosed. Four malignancies appearing histologically as small round blue cell tumors—neuroblastoma, non-Hodgkin lymphoma, rhabdomyosarcoma, and Ewing sarcoma—fall into this category; tumor markers are needed to distinguish among them.

Therapy selection can also be guided by tumor markers, such as the ABCB1 (more commonly known as MDR1) protein and the estrogen and progesterone receptors (ER/PR). Low levels of MDR1 correlate with better response to treatment in ovary and lung cancer patients, whereas presence of the ER/PR tumor marker in advanced breast cancer patients correlates with a high response rate to endocrine ablation. Breast cancer patients whose tumors overexpress the HER2/neu (also known as ERBB2, c-erb-B2) protein are another important subgroup identified by tumor-marker analysis, since these patients are uniquely appropriate for therapy with anti-HER2-based therapies such as trastuzumab. Tumor-marker concentrations often correlate with tumor burden or activity, providing information on the effectiveness of treatment. Rapid normalization of serum CA 125 levels following ovarian cancer treatment, for example, has favorable prognostic significance.

The next important application of tumor markers is in long-term follow-up of patients with previously diagnosed and treated cancer, because early detection of recurrent or metastatic disease can hasten intervention and improve outcome. The tumor markers CA 15-3 (breast), CEA (colorectal), CA 125 (ovary), and PSA (prostate) are used in this context.

Finally, scientists performing cancer research are seeking improved diagnostic assays and clues to novel therapies; tumor markers are an integral part of these efforts. Overexpression of fatty acid synthase, for example, was noted in several types of tumors; subsequent efforts to inhibit the enzyme demonstrated this to be a promising therapeutic modality.

Significant barriers exist to more extensive use of tumor markers in oncology. Primarily, the clinical value of the marker must be proven; that is, the result should trigger or remand a treatment decision that benefits patients, this benefit must be demonstrated in a large and rigorous trial, and the benefits must outweigh the costs of implementation and follow-up. After this is accomplished, oncologists must be convinced of the need to change their established practices by incorporating the marker.

Data analysis: After the appropriate material is obtained from the patient, several options exist for tumor-marker determination and data analysis. The method for tumor-marker quantification depends both on the marker and on the specimen; the method of analysis depends largely on the form and amount of data present.

Serum protein markers are typically measured with specific antibody-based assays. A popular immunoassay format is the enzyme-linked immunosorbent assay (ELISA), which provides a numerical readout of the marker's concentration. Protein markers can also be determined in tissue biopsy slices or individual cells by immunohistochemistry (IHC) or immunocytochemistry (ICC). In contrast to the ELISA, samples analyzed by IHC or ICC must be assessed visually for an estimate of tumor-marker abundance. However, IHC and ICC allow precise localization of the tumor marker within the cell. IHC and ICC are appropriate for tumor markers that are not shed into the extracellular space. Enzymes such as lactate dehydrogenase are sometimes employed as tumor markers; their concentration is inferred from their catalytic activity. Highly complex protein mixtures present in body fluids such as serum or urine can be analyzed by protein chips coupled with surface-enhanced laser desorption ionization/time-of-flight mass spectrometry (SELDI/TOF-MS). In this case, the relative abundance of hundreds to thousands of proteins in a sample is determined in a single run.

Tumor markers that are products expressed by genes (messenger ribonucleic acid, or mRNA, molecules) can be measured by the reverse transcriptase polymerase chain reaction (RT-PCR) or on a larger scale by oligonucleotide microarrays. In reverse transcriptase polymerase chain reaction, the mRNA sample is first reverse-transcribed into deoxyribonucleic acid (DNA), then amplified by standard polymerase chain reaction. Relative quantification is achieved by monitoring the abundance of the polymerase chain reaction products spectrophotometrically during the thermal cycling process. Messenger RNA-based tumor-marker assays can estimate the risk of breast cancer recurrence in women who are diagnosed with Stage I or II hormone-responsive cancer that has not spread to the surrounding lymph nodes. In this setting, the abundance of multiple different transcripts in breast tumor tissue is determined by reverse transcriptase polymerase chain reaction.

Tumor markers that exist as mutated or disrupted genes can be analyzed by several methods. Chromosomes can be inspected microscopically to confirm changes in genomic DNA. For example, abnormal amplification of *MYCB* (also known as *N-myc*) in neuroblastoma can be visualized as a homogenous staining region on chromosome 2p.

Other tumor risk markers, such as mutated *APC*, can be detected through DNA sequencing or single-strand conformational polymorphism.

Tumor markers that exist as small organic compounds such as 5-hydroxyindoleacetic acid (carcinoid tumors) are measured with chemical techniques such as high-performance liquid chromatography.

Results: Numerical results (concentrations) for single tumor markers can be interpreted only with knowledge of the marker's normal concentration range and its sensitivity, specificity, and positive and negative predictive value for the tumor type in question. Also essential are knowledge of the tumor's prevalence and the patient's clinical history. Serial tumor-marker determinations offer additional information by demonstrating the rate of the tumor marker's increase or decrease. In the case of PSA, a short time to doubling may prompt more concern than higher levels that remain steady. No single tumor marker reaches the ideal standards of 100 percent sensitivity and specificity. Many proposed tumor markers are ultimately rejected by practitioners because of unacceptably low sensitivity or specificity.

Results from multiplexed assays consist of patterns of individual data points that can yield more biologically relevant and clinically useful information than single markers. Analysis requires sophisticated and sometimes proprietary pattern-matching algorithms. Protein chips coupled with SELDI/TOF-MS, for example, have identified tumor-marker patterns that correctly classified individuals with and without early-stage ovarian cancer with high sensitivity and specificity. Gene expression chips (oligonucleotide microarrays) have also shown remarkable accuracy in identifying the primary sites of poorly differentiated metastatic lesions. Test results are highly reproducible and provide information to aid the physician and patient in making treatment decisions.

John B. Welsh, M.D., Ph.D.

▶ **For Further Information**

Bigbee W., and R. B. Herberman. "Tumor Markers and Immunodiagnosis." In *Cancer Medicine*, edited by James F. Holland and Emil Frei. 6th ed. Hamilton, Ont.: BC Decker, 2003.

Diamandis, E. P., et al., eds. *Tumor Markers: Physiology, Pathobiology, Technology, and Clinical Applications*. Washington, D.C.: AACC Press, 2002.

Hartwell, L., et al. "Cancer Biomarkers: A Systems Approach." *Nature Biotechnology* 24 (2006): 905-908.

Nakamura, R. M., et al., eds. *Cancer Diagnostics: Current and Future Trends*. Totowa, N.J.: Humana Press, 2004.

Perkins, G. L., et al. "Serum Tumor Markers." *American Family Physician* 68 (2003): 1075-1082.

Petricoin, E. F., et al. "Use of Proteomic Patterns in Serum to Identify Ovarian Cancer." *Lancet* 359 (2002): 572-577.

Taube, S. E., et al. "Cancer Diagnostics: Decision Criteria for Marker Utilization in the Clinic." *American Journal of Pharmacogenomics* 5 (2005): 357-364.

▶ **Other Resources**

Lab Tests Online
Tumor Markers
   http://www.labtestsonline.org/understanding/
   analytes/tumor_markers/glance.html

National Cancer Institute
Tumor Markers: Questions and Answers
   http://www.cancer.gov/cancertopics/factsheet/
   Detection/tumor-markers

See also Alpha-fetoprotein (AFP) levels; Bone cancers; CA 15-3 test; CA 19-9 test; CA 27-29 test; CA 125 test; Carcinoembryonic antigen antibody (CEA) test; Carcinomas; Embryonic cell cancer; Endocrine cancers; Germ-cell tumors; Gynecologic oncology; Lactate dehydrogenase (LDH) test; Liver cancers; Malignant tumors; Neuroendocrine tumors; Placental alkaline phosphatase (PALP); Proteomics and cancer research; Testicular cancer; TNM staging.

▶ Tumor necrosis factor (TNF)

Category: Chemotherapy and other drugs; cancer biology

Also known as: Tumor necrosis factor-alpha (TNF-α), tumor necrosis factor-beta (TNF-β, or lymphotoxin); the colloidal gold-bound form of TNF is also called Aurimmune

Definition: TNF is a protein belonging to the class of cytokines (immunoregulatory proteins) that is made by the body's white blood cells in response to an infection, or antigen. It can also be synthesized in the laboratory. Because it causes necrosis (cell death), it is being investigated as a possible immunotherapeutic drug to induce death of some types of tumor cells.

Cancers treated: Breast, ovarian, colon, kidney, and liver cancers, as well as melanomas; tests carried out with a variety of other tumors

Delivery routes: Tumor necrosis factor is generally delivered as an injection in a vein or muscle. Injection may also be under the skin. A colloidal form of TNF bound to small particles of gold has also been tested for improved specificity for cancer tissue, reducing the ability of the drug to bind normal tissue and possibly permitting systemic delivery.

How this drug works: The term TNF actually refers to a family of trimeric proteins produced by certain types of white blood cells that can attack blood vessels in tumors, thereby destroying certain types of cancer cells. The most common forms are TNF-α and TNF-β. TNF-α is the form used for cancer therapy. Its existence was discovered fortuitously in the early twentieth century when physicians observed that certain types of tumors would spontaneously regress in the presence of bacterial infections. It was subsequently discovered that TNF production is a part of the immune response and is induced in the presence of bacterial endotoxin (lipopolysaccharide).

The response to TNF is dose-dependent and can result either in inflammation, augmenting the immune response, or in binding to a cell surface, inducing the destruction of that cell. The induction of apoptosis, or "cell suicide," appears to be the primary mechanism by which TNF may cause tumor regression. Depending upon the state of the particular cell, either tumor cells or the cells of the blood vessels that feed those tumors may express receptors on their respective surfaces for the drug. Binding of TNF sets in motion a series of intracellular signals that results in the death of the cell.

Testing has also been carried out using a human recombinant form of TNF (rTNF), as well as treatments utilizing a combination of chemotherapies in conjunction with TNF.

Side effects: Like other forms of chemotherapy, TNF has the potential to interact with other medications. Since TNF may interact with other cells of the immune system, vaccinations should be avoided during the course of treatment. Specific side effects of TNF may include a mild fever, chills or sweating, fatigue, and vomiting. Since most cells in the body have surface receptors to which TNF may bind, the drug is potentially toxic if given systemically.

Richard Adler, Ph.D.

See also Biological therapy; Cancer biology; Chemotherapy; Crohn disease; Cytokines; Gene therapy; Histiocytosis X; Hyperthermic perfusion; Immune response to cancer; Immunotherapy; Liver cancers.

▶ Tumor-suppressor genes

Category: Cancer biology

Definition: Tumor-suppressor genes are genes found in normal cells that function to control cell division, repair damage to deoxyribonucleic acid (DNA), and tell cells when to die. Mutated tumor-suppressor genes can cause a loss of growth control and can lead to cancer.

What they do: Tumor-suppressor genes regulate cell division and growth through many biochemical mechanisms. The quality the mechanisms have in common is that the loss of each increases the likelihood that a cell will undergo transformation from a normal cell to a cancerous one. Tumor-suppressor genes code for proteins that inhibit the division of cells if proper conditions for growth are not met. Conditions that could inhibit division include DNA damage, a lack of growth factors, or a malfunction of the cell's division machinery. Scientists have identified about thirty tumor-suppressor genes.

Types of tumor-suppressor genes: There are several types of tumor-suppressor genes. Some control cell division and growth. The retinoblastoma (*RB1*) gene is an example of this type. A second type is involved in repairing errors in DNA. The process of DNA replication leads to occasional mistakes, and cells have a set of proteins that function to repair these mistakes. A third type is responsible for inducing a cell to undergo programmed cell death, or apoptosis, if its DNA is damaged beyond repair or if the cell division process malfunctions. In this way the cell's well-being is monitored, protecting the organism from the effects of runaway replication of wayward cells by activating the apoptotic pathway in such cells. The *TP53* (also known as *p53*) gene is an example of this type of tumor-suppressor gene.

Because the presence of tumor-suppressor genes contributes to normal cell division and function, both copies of a tumor-suppressor gene must be inactivated to result in a maximum increased risk of cancer development. An increased risk of developing a specific type of cancer in some families is often the result of the presence of one defective copy of a tumor-suppressor gene. Although there is a low likelihood that the good copy of the tumor-suppressor gene will be mutated in any given cell, there is a much higher likelihood that the necessary second mutation will occur somewhere in the vast number of cells in a human body. Many of the identified tumor-suppressor genes have been shown to be implicated in familial cancers. Inheritance of a defective copy of one of these genes carries a greatly increased risk of developing one or more specific types of cancer, often types that are otherwise rare. In some cases, mutant copies of these genes are linked to susceptibility to multiple cancer types, as is the case with the retinoblastoma (*RB1*) gene. The two most important tumor-suppressor genes code for the TP53 protein and the retinoblastoma protein (RB1 or pRB).

***TP53* gene:** The *TP53* gene has been found to be involved in numerous cellular processes and is considered to be one of the most important cancer-related genes. The TP53 protein belongs to a class of proteins containing covalently bound phosphate groups, called phosphoproteins. It is located in the nucleus of the cell and interacts directly with the cell's DNA to function as a transcription factor by binding to a specific DNA sequence in the control regions of the genes it controls. The number of bound phosphate groups modulates the activity of TP53. Normal TP53 function results in a global transcriptional response that can negatively regulate cell division, or induce apoptosis. TP53 function is activated in response to various kinds of cell stress that increase the cell's need for DNA repair and surveillance of the cell's physiological status, including irradiation, lack of oxygen, oncogene activation, and DNA damage.

The *TP53* gene is the single most frequently inactivated gene in human cancers. More than 90 percent of small-cell lung cancers and more than 50 percent of breast and colon cancers have been shown to be associated with mutant forms of *TP53*.

Retinoblastoma (*RB1*) gene: The *RB1* gene encodes another phosphoprotein located in the nucleus of the cell. The RB1 protein acts as a negative regulator of cell division by binding to other transcription factors to alter their function. The action of these other transcription factors in turn regulates the level of expression of a number of other genes. The number of phosphate groups bound to the RB1 protein controls its ability to bind to other transcription factors and varies in a regular controlled manner during a normal cell cycle. The RB1 protein is responsible for a major "checkpoint," or regulatory step, in the cell cycle, in which cells must make a decision whether to undergo another round of cell division. Normal RB1 protein function results in a coordinated progression of the cell through the division process. Loss of the RB1 protein leads to unregulated and increased cell division, characteristic of cancer cells. The *RB1* gene is mutated in many types of cancer, including retinoblastoma (a cancer of the eye from which the gene got its name), as well as bone, lung, breast, and bladder cancers.

Jill Ferguson, Ph.D.

► For Further Information

Hanahan, D., and R. A. Weinberg. "The Hallmarks of Cancer." *Cell* 100 (2000): 57-70.

Sherr, C. J. "Principles of Tumor Suppression." *Cell* 116 (2004): 235-246.

Strano, S., et al. "Mutant *p53*: An Oncogenic Transcription Factor." *Oncogene* 26 (2007): 2212-2219.

Weinberg, R. A. *The Biology of Cancer.* New York: Garland Science, 2007.

► Other Resources

American Cancer Society
Oncogenes and Tumor Suppressor Genes
Http://www.cancer.org/docroot/ETO/content/ETO
_1_4x_oncogenes_and_tumor_suppressor_genes.asp

Emory University
CancerQuest: Important Tumor Suppressors
http://www.cancerquest.org/index.cfm?page=52

Tumor Suppressor Genes
http://users.rcn.com/jkimball.ma.ultranet/
BiologyPages/T/TumorSuppressorGenes.html

See also APC gene testing; *BRCA1* and *BRCA2* genes; Cancer biology; Cowden syndrome; Endocrine cancers; Gene therapy; Genetic testing; Genetics of cancer; Mutagenesis and cancer; Oncogenes; Oncogenic viruses; *RB1* gene; *RhoGD12* gene; TP53 protein.

► Turcot syndrome

Category: Diseases, symptoms, and conditions
Also known as: Brain tumor-polyposis syndrome, glioma-polyposis syndrome

Related conditions: Malignant tumors of the central nervous system (CNS), familial polyposis of the colon, familial adenomatous polyposis (FAP), Gardner syndrome, hereditary nonpolyposis colorectal cancer (HNPCC)

Definition: Turcot syndrome is a rare genetic disorder clinically characterized by the concurrence of a primary brain tumor and multiple colorectal adenomas. This syndrome is characterized by adenomatous polyps (benign growths) in the mucous lining of the gastrointestinal tract and tumors of the central nervous system, including medulloblastoma and malignant glioma. It was first reported by Canadian surgeon Jacques Turcot in 1959.

Risk factors: Turcot syndrome has been linked to various mutations in a number of genes. Turcot syndrome seems to be inherited in an autosomal recessive manner. Mutation or mismatch of the adenomatous polyposis coli (*APC*) gene in chromosome 5q is most likely involved in the disease. Mismatch repair genes, such as *MLH1* or *PMS2*, were found in some families. The types of brain tumor differ, depending on the type of mutation; *APC* mutations are more commonly associated with medulloblastoma, while mismatch repair genes are associated with glioblastoma. The gene map locus is 7p22, 5q21-q22, or 3p21.3.

Etiology and the disease process: It has been debated whether Turcot syndrome is a variant of familial adenomatous polyposis or a separate disorder. The cause of Turcot syndrome is not known, but it has been characterized genetically.

In this syndrome, there may be three types of polyposis coli in combination with central nervous system tumors. Type 1 is characterized by multiple colonic polyps numbering between twenty and one hundred; some of these may exceed 3 centimeters (cm) in diameter. These polyps frequently undergo malignant transformation in the second and third decades of life. In several of the type 1 cases, a familial cluster has been described. In type 2, the number of colonic polyps is usually less than ten, and the mode of inheritance is uncertain. In type 3, there are numerous small colonic polyps present, and the mode of inheritance may be autosomal dominant with respect to colonic lesions.

Turcot syndrome may be divided into two distinct entities. The first entity includes patients who have gliomas and colorectal adenomas without polyposis. This type is associated with hereditary nonpolyposis colorectal cancer (HNPCC), which is characterized by germ-line mutations in the mismatch repair genes *MLH1* and *PMS2*. The second entity includes patients who develop a central nervous sytem tumor (familiar adenomatous polyposis cases). These patients carry germ-line mutations in the *APC* gene, indicating a predisposition to brain tumors.

Incidence: The normal onset of Turcot syndrome occurs between the ages of fifty and eighty. Turcot syndrome is strongly associated with an underlying genetic cause. The most common brain tumors associated with Turcot syndrome are medulloblastoma (79 percent) and glioblastoma multiforme. The glioblastomas and colorectal tumors often have replication errors characteristic of hereditary nonpolyposis colorectal cancer.

Symptoms: The symptoms of Turcot syndrome are associated with polyp formation, and they include diarrhea, bleeding from the rectum, fatigue, abdominal pain, and weight loss. Because of the development of brain tumors, patients with this disease may also experience neurological symptoms, depending on the type, size, and location of the tumors. Patients with Turcot syndrome commonly complain of skin abnormalities, including café-au-lait spots, multiple lipomas (fatty tumors), and multiple scalp basal cell carcinomas (skin cancers of the scalp). Turcot syndrome polyps are somewhat fewer in number than in familial adenomatous polyposis, but they tend to be larger in size (greater than 3 cm in diameter). Many patients with Turcot syndrome have *APC* gene mutations, pigmented ocular fundus lesions, epidermal inclusion cysts, or osteosclerotic jaw lesions consistent with Gardner syndrome.

Screening and diagnosis: Patients with Turcot syndrome often have multiple adenomatous colon polyps or colorectal cancer along with glioblastoma or medulloblastoma. Generally, blood tests can confirm mutation in the *APC* gene or in the *MLH1* gene. Testing for mutations in *PMS2* is still in development. If a specific gene mutation is found, family members are also tested for Turcot syndrome.

Treatment and therapy: Typically tumors, such as adenomatous sigmoid polyps, are removed. Brain tumors, depending on their location, are more difficult to remove surgically. Colectomy and gastrectomy are also common treatments for patients with Turcot syndrome.

Prognosis, prevention, and outcomes: In most cases, a complete resection of the brain tumors is difficult and the colonic polyps are malignant at the time of diagnosis, resulting in poor prognosis. Better prognosis can be expected with early diagnosis.

Anita Nagypál, Ph.D.

▶ **For Further Information**

De Vos, M., et al. "Novel *PMS2* Pseudogenes Can Conceal Recessive Mutations Causing a Distinctive Childhood Cancer Syndrome." *American Journal of Human Genetics* 74 (2004): 954-964.

Dupuis, M. J. M., and C. Verellen-Dumoulin. "Gastrointestinal Polyposis and Nonpolyposis Syndromes." *New England Journal of Medicine* 332 (1995): 1518.

Hamilton, S. R., et al. "The Molecular Basis of Turcot's Syndrome." *New England Journal of Medicine* 332 (1995): 839-847.

Lionel, J., N. Bathurst, D. Mohan, and D. Beckly. "Turcot's Syndrome." *Diseases of the Colon and Rectum* 31 (1998): 11.

Van Meir, E. G. "Turcot's Syndrome: Phenotype of Brain Tumors, Survival, and Mode of Inheritance." *International Journal of Cancer* 75 (1998): 162-164.

▶ **Other Resources**

American Cancer Society
http://www.cancer.org

American Society of Clinical Oncology
http://opl.asco.org

National Cancer Institute
http://www.cancer.gov

National Organization for Rare Disorders
Turcot Syndrome
http://www.rarediseases.org/search/
rdbdetail_abstract.html?disname=
Turcot%20Syndrome

See also Adenomatous polyps; Astrocytomas; Brain and central nervous system cancers; Colon polyps; Colorectal cancer; Gardner syndrome; Gliomas; Hereditary mixed polyposis syndrome; Hereditary polyposis syndromes; Neuroectodermal tumors; Rectal cancer.

▶ **Tyrosine kinase inhibitors**

Category: Chemotherapy and other drugs
ATC code: 101XE

Definition: Tyrosine kinase inhibitors are a class of antitumor drugs that act by specifically targeting tyrosine kinase enzymes. Tyrosine kinase inhibitors are particularly effective in slowing tumor growth and killing tumor cells because of the importance of these enzymes in determining cellular fate, including survival and proliferation.

Cancers treated: Chronic myeloid leukemia, gastrointestinal stromal tumors, non-small-cell lung cancer, pancreatic cancer, renal cell carcinoma, breast cancer, colorectal cancer

Subclasses of this group: Small molecule inhibitors, biologic antibody inhibitors

Delivery routes: The small molecule tyrosine kinase inhibitors are orally active and administered in a tablet form. Biologic antibody tyrosine kinase inhibitors are administered by a slow intravenous (IV) infusion, usually over the course of a few hours.

How these drugs work: Through basic scientific research, several proteins critical for cellular growth, survival, and proliferation have been identified. One of the largest classes of these proteins is known as tyrosine kin-

Common Tyrosine Kinase Inhibitors

Drug	Brands	Subclass	Delivery Mode	Cancers Treated
Cetuximab	Erbitux	Biologic antibody therapy	IV	Metastatic colorectal cancer, head and neck cancer
Dasatinib	Sprycel	Small molecule inhibitor	Oral	Chronic myeloid leukemia, Philadelphia chromosome-positive acute lymphoblastic leukemia
Erlotinib	Tarceva	Small molecule inhibitor	Oral	Advanced non-small-cell lung cancer, advanced pancreatic cancer
Gefitinib	Iressa	Small molecule inhibitor	Oral	Advanced or metastatic non-small-cell lung cancer
Imatinib	Gleevec	Small molecule inhibitor	Oral	Philadelphia chromosome-positive chronic myeloid leukemia, gastrointestinal stromal tumor
Lapatinib	Tykerb	Small molecule inhibitor	Oral	Advanced or metastatic HER2-positive breast cancer
Sorafenib	Nexavar	Small molecule inhibitor	Oral	Advanced renal cell carcinoma
Sunitinib	Sutent	Small molecule inhibitor	Oral	Advanced renal cell carcinoma, gastrointestinal stromal tumor
Trastuzumab	Herceptin	Biologic antibody therapy	IV	HER2-positive breast cancer

ases. Kinases are enzymes, proteins that can perform a specific activity or function. Kinases act by transferring a phosphate group onto a substrate protein, a process called phosphorylation. In particular, tyrosine kinases add a phosphate group onto specific tyrosine amino acid residues in the substrate protein. Phosphorylation can perform many different functions, including activating the substrate protein through an "on-off" mechanism, inducing protein-protein interaction, and changing protein localization. The functional changes induced in the substrate protein are used in many different signaling pathways, including those important to relay growth and proliferation signals in cells.

Cells can react to many external stimuli, including circulating growth factors and hormones, through binding of these ligands to cell surface receptors. Many of these receptors are actually tyrosine kinases themselves, or signal directly to downstream tyrosine kinases after being activated. Therefore, the activity of tyrosine kinases is a critical part of the signaling required to transmit information from the outside of the cell to the cellular interior, affecting the fate of the cell. Tumor cells often hijack the normal essential function of tyrosine kinases, mutating these proteins so that they remain in a constitutive "on" state. Because the kinase activity is then unable to be halted, the signaling pathways are continuously activated, and uncontrolled cell growth and proliferation ensue.

Because of their importance in determining cellular fate, especially whether a cell will live or die, tyrosine kinases are a very attractive target for anticancer chemother-apy. There are two major categories of tyrosine kinase inhibitors, small molecule inhibitors and targeted biological therapy. The major mechanism of action of small molecule inhibitors is to inhibit the binding of adenosine triphosphate (ATP) to the kinase. Because tyrosine kinases use ATP as a source of phosphate groups to perform phosphorylation, the enzyme cannot phosphorylate substrate proteins, thereby reducing the activation of the downstream signaling pathways. The second major class of tyrosine kinase inhibitors is targeted therapy, using antibodies that are generated against the tyrosine kinase receptors that reside on the cellular surface. These antibodies mainly work by blocking the ligand-binding sites on these receptors, inhibiting the binding and thus the activation of these receptors. One of the main benefits of using tyrosine kinase inhibitors as an anticancer chemotherapy is that they can selectively target tumor cells compared to normal cells because tumor cells often develop a dependence on overactivated and overexpressed tyrosine kinases.

Side effects: The most common side effects of the oral small molecule inhibitors are nausea and vomiting, fatigue, muscle pain, fluid retention (swelling), and rash. In most cases, these symptoms can be effectively managed with medication, so that treatment can continue. The side effects caused by biologic antibody therapies are mainly induced by the actual administration of the drug. Many patients (approximately 40 percent) experience flulike symptoms, including fever, chills, muscle aches, and nausea. These side effects are generally lessened with the administration of drugs such as acetaminophen.

Lisa M. Cockrell, B.S.

▶ For Further Information

Fabbro, Doriano, and Frank McCormick, eds. *Protein Tyrosine Kinases: From Inhibitors to Useful Drugs.* Totowa, N.J.: Humana Press, 2006.

Kantarjian, Hagop M., et al. *The M. D. Anderson Manual of Medical Oncology.* New York: McGraw-Hill, 2006.

Kufe, Donald W., et al., eds. *Holland Frei Cancer Medicine 7.* 7th ed. Hamilton, Ont.: BC Decker, 2006.

Pratt, William B., et al. *The Anticancer Drugs.* 2d ed. New York: Oxford University Press, 1994.

Skeel, Roland T. *Handbook of Cancer Chemotherapy.* 7th ed. Philadelphia: Lippincott Williams & Wilkins, 2007.

▶ Other Resources

American Cancer Society
http://www.cancer.org

National Cancer Institute
Drug Information Summaries
http://www.cancer.gov/cancertopics/druginfo/alphalist

See also Biological therapy; Breast cancers; Bronchial adenomas; Carcinomas; Chemotherapy; Chronic myeloid leukemia (CML); Gastrointestinal complications of cancer treatment; Gastrointestinal stromal tumors (GISTs); Infusion therapies; Leukemias; Lung cancers; Medical oncology; Nausea and vomiting; Oncology; Pancreatic cancers; Rectal cancer.

▶ Ultrasound tests

Category: Procedures
Also known as: Sonogram, echogram

Definition: An ultrasound test is a type of radiologic study that utilizes sound waves to detect an abnormality in an organ of the body under evaluation using a principle similar to sonar used in ship navigation. Ultrasound waves are mechanical pressure waves that occur at a higher frequency compared to audible sound waves, hence the name ultrasound. These high-frequency sound waves reflect off body surfaces and structures. Different tissues in the body have different acoustic velocities or speeds of sound propagating through them. The time that it takes for a pulsed sound wave to travel from a transducer to a reflector and back again can be measured and then, along with the known acoustic velocity of a tissue, can be used to calculate their separation and thus the depth from the skin surface of the organ or organ part under study. Bone, for example, has a higher acoustic velocity than soft tissue. One would expect higher-amplitude echoes from soft tissue-bone interfaces and lower-amplitude reflection or echoes from soft tissue-soft tissue interfaces because of the almost matched acoustic velocities among the latter.

The ultrasound transducer converts the amplitude of the mechanical energy received from the organ under study into an electrical signal and vice versa. The emitting and receiving element of an ultrasound transducer is a piezoelectric crystal. The electrical signals from the transducer are fed into a computer, and an image is produced that can be stored on compact disc (CD), printed on film, or viewed on a computer monitor by the sonographer and the radiologist, who is ultimately responsible for the quality and interpretation of the study.

Cancers diagnosed: Breast, thyroid, testicular, uterine, ovarian, prostate, renal (kidney), bladder, gallbladder, liver, spleen, and pancreatic cancers; cancers associated with pregnancy, such as gestational trophoblastic disease; unsuspected adenopathy often detected as an incidental finding during ultrasound examination, especially during examination of the thyroid, breast, and abdomen

Why performed: Ultrasound is used to diagnose primary cancers, both be-nign and malignant, as well as secondary cancers (also known as metastases). It is also used to diagnose ailments depending on the patient's symptoms, including but not limited to the following: right-upper-quadrant abdominal pain caused by acute and chronic cholecystitis (both calculus and acalculus) and postoperative leaks following cholecystectomy (gallbladder and right-upper-quadrant ultrasound); goiter, Hashimoto's thyroiditis, and ectopic parathyroid (thyroid ultrasound); mastitis and Paget disease of the breast (breast ultrasound); pain in the right lower quadrant of the abdomen caused by appendicitis (ultrasound of the appendix); scrotal pain caused by testicular torsion, testicular trauma, orchitis, epididymitis, and hydrocele, as well as undescended testes (testicular ultrasound); pain in the back caused by kidney stones, kidney obstruction, or infection (renal ultrasound); pain and swelling in the legs caused by deep venous thrombosis (DVT study); pain in the epigastric area caused by pancreatitis (abdominal ultrasound); pain in the left upper abdomen caused by splenic infarct or splenic trauma (abdominal ultrasound); pain in the right upper quadrant caused by liver trauma, liver infection, or liver cysts and evaluation for the presence of ascites (abdominal ultrasound); valvular heart disease (cardiac ultrasound or echocardiography); atherosclerosis of the lower-extremity arteries, abdominal aortic aneurysm, and carotid artery atherosclerosis (vascular or arterial Doppler ultrasound); and polycystic ovarian syndrome or pelvic pain and/or bleeding caused by ovarian torsion, uterine polyps, uterine fibroids, and retained products of conception (pelvic and transvaginal ultrasound).

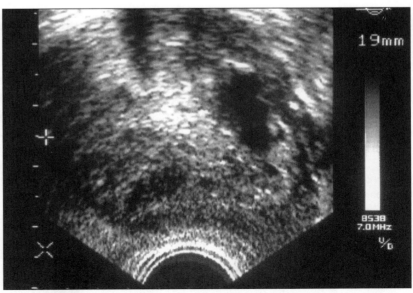

A sonogram showing prostate cancer. (James Cavallini/Photo Researchers, Inc.)

In addition, pregnancy in all three trimesters is evaluated by ultrasound. Ultrasound is also useful in guiding amniocentesis for evaluation of possible fetal anomalies such as Down syndrome (trisomy 21) involving sampling of fluid surrounding the fetus; sampling and removal of fluid from various body cavities in the adult, such as the lung (pleural effusion tap) and abdominal cavity (ascites); and guiding biopsy of various organs in the adult, such as liver, breast, thyroid, and kidney.

Patient preparation: Patients are asked to fast at least four to eight hours prior to gallbladder ultrasound, as food causes the gallbladder to contract and minimizes the area visible for the ultrasound evaluation. Patients are asked to drink at least four glasses of water at least one half hour prior to pelvic ultrasound in order to distend the bladder, which acts as an acoustic window for the study (sound travels well through water). This enables the sonographer, usually a technologist, to evaluate the baby and the womb during pregnancy and to evaluate the state of the uterus, cervix, and ovaries in both the pregnant and the non-pregnant state.

Steps of the procedure: The patient is placed on the back on a table, and the technologist and/or the radiologist applies a clear, water-based conducting gel to the skin over the organ or body part of interest. The gel helps in the transmission of sound waves and may feel wet and cold. The sonographer then rubs a handheld probe or transducer across the surface of the organ of interest. There will be some discomfort from pressure on a full bladder, but the ultrasound waves themselves are painless. Some transducers are designed to be inserted inside a body cavity, such as a transvaginal probe or transrectal probe, which may feel uncomfortable.

After the procedure: The scan is generated by the computer attached to the ultrasound probe and read by the radiologist the same day. The patient will need to contact his or her doctor or health care provider for the radiology report and for follow-up therapy.

Risks: The study is painless and relatively harmless, as no radiation is involved; transvaginal ultrasound is generally done early in a pregnancy to determine fetal age or to detect a suspected ectopic pregnancy. Use of the transvaginal probe late in pregnancy is a decision made by the health care provider, not the sonographer or radiologist.

Results: The results are dependent on the type of scan performed and the reason for the study. Some ultrasound tests are screening tests and may be normal, while others are ordered by a health care provider when an abnormality is suspected.

Debra B. Kessler, M.D., Ph.D.

▶ **For Further Information**
Bushong, Stewart C. *Diagnostic Ultrasound.* New York: McGraw-Hill, 1999.
Curry, Thomas S., III, James E. Dowdey, and Robert C. Murry, Jr. *Christensen's Physics of Diagnostic Radiology.* 4th ed. Philadelphia: Lea & Febiger, 1990.
Rumak, Carole M., S. R. Wilson, and J. W. Charboneau. *Diagnostic Ultrasound.* St. Louis: Mosby-Year Book, 1991.

See also Breast ultrasound; Endorectal ultrasound; Pregnancy and cancer; Screening for cancer; Transrectal ultrasound; Transvaginal ultrasound.

▶ Ultraviolet radiation and related exposures

Category: Carcinogens and suspected carcinogens
RoC status: Solar radiation and exposure to sunlamps or sun beds, known carcinogens since 2000; broad-spectrum ultraviolet radiation (UVR), known carcinogen since 2002; ultraviolet A, B, and C (UVA, UVB, and UVC), reasonably anticipated carcinogens since 2002
Also known as: UV, ultraviolet light, black light, UVR, UVA, UVB, UVC

Related cancers: Melanoma and nonmelanocytic skin cancers

Definition: Ultraviolet light is electromagnetic radiation that lies between X rays and visible light in the spectrum, with wavelengths between 100 and 400 nanometers (nm). UV is divided into long-wave UVA (315-400 nn), UVB (280-315 nm), and short-wave UVC (100-280 nm).

Exposure route: Through skin

Where found: Sunlight, tanning beds

At risk: Individuals chronically exposed to sunlight or occupationally exposed to ultraviolet (UV) light sources, especially those with fair skin

Etiology and symptoms of associated cancers: The damage caused by exposure to UV radiation depends on the intensity and wavelengths of the radiation, the duration of exposure, and many other highly individual factors.

Cancers caused by UV radiation are based on damage to cellular deoxyribonucleic acid (DNA) and suppression of the immune system. Since UV radiation is absorbed efficiently by the skin, this is the primary carcinogenic target, and UV radiation-caused skin cancers occur mostly on sun-exposed areas. The interaction of UV radiation with DNA results in abnormal dimerization of adjacent pyrimidine bases, damage to individual bases, strand breakage, and cross-linkages between DNA and adjacent proteins. Such DNA damage contributes to cancer formation through the release of cytokines, induction of latent viruses, or mutations that cause functional changes in encoded protein molecules. Skin cancers are typically noted and diagnosed by inspection before producing systemic illness.

History: Hippocrates, a physician in ancient Greece, recognized that depression was more common in the winter months and recommended sunbathing to treat both medical and psychological maladies. Ultraviolet light as a component of sunlight and its interactions with matter were first demonstrated in the early 1800's. Ultraviolet radiation's ability to injure the eyes was noted in 1843 in welders, and papers from 1889 confirmed that ultraviolet rays cause skin burns. An epidemiologic study published in 1907 first associated sun exposure and skin cancer. A causal relationship was demonstrated in a 1928 publication that described induction of skin cancer in mice by exposure to UV radiation. The peak carcinogenic response of UVB at 310 nm was identified in 1975. Reduction of UVB in favor of UVA rays is a current strategy to reduce the carcinogenicity of tanning beds. Liberal use of sunscreens is a current recommendation to reduce the incidence of melanoma.

John B. Welsh, M.D., Ph.D.

See also Basal cell carcinomas; Carcinogens, known; Electromagnetic radiation; Melanomas; Merkel cell carcinomas (MCC); Moles; Occupational exposures and cancer; Premalignancies; Skin cancers; Squamous cell carcinomas; Sunlamps; Sunscreens.

▶ Umbilical cord blood transplantation

Category: Procedures
Also known as: Cord blood transplantation

Definition: Umbilical cord blood transplantation is the administration of healthy stem cells obtained from umbilical cord blood into an individual after his own bone mar-

row has been eradicated by chemotherapy with or without radiation. These healthy stem cells move into the bone and reconstitute the bone marrow, producing new, healthy blood cells.

Cancers treated: Leukemia, lymphoma, myeloma, and neuroblastoma; other disorders treated include immunodeficiency, hemaglobinopathies, and metabolic disorders

Why performed: In patients with various cancers and diseases, a cure can be achieved when the patient's affected bone marrow is obliterated and replaced with healthy stem cells. Umbilical cord blood is discarded after birth. Donated umbilical cord blood is an accepted source of hematopoietic stem cells for marrow reconstitution. Two transplant-dependent variables affect long-term recipient survival: donor-recipient human leukocyte antigen (HLA) match grade and the dose of stem cells. HLA is a genetic fingerprint on white blood cells and platelets, composed of proteins that play a critical role in activating the body's immune system to respond to foreign agents. There are six HLA factors. The more of these factors that match between the donor and the recipient, the more likely the transplant is to be successful and complications to be prevented.

Patient preparation: A repeat HLA tissue typing is done to confirm donor-recipient match. Then the recipient's bone marrow is destroyed by chemotherapy with and without radiation. This process kills diseased bone marrow. The patient must be protected to prevent infection, since his or her own immune system has been obliterated.

Steps of the procedure: An intravenous (IV) device is placed in the recipient's vein, and a solution containing the donor stem cells is infused.

After the procedure: The patient will be monitored for engraftment, the process in which stem cells enter the bone marrow and begin to produce blood cells. The patient will remain in an environment free from infectious agents until the new stem cells engraft and produce disease-fighting white blood cells. The patient will be monitored for relapse (return) of the original disease.

Risks: The risks of this procedure are infection, graft failure (the absence of or inadequate production of blood cells), and graft-versus-host disease (GVHD), in which the donor stem cells attack the recipient's body. GVHD can be either acute or chronic.

Results: Umbilical cord blood stem cells produce less GVHD than other forms of stem cell transplants. Umbilical cord blood transplant is limited in adults because of the relatively limited number of stem cells that can be harvested from one placenta and umbilical cord.

Wanda Todd Bradshaw, R.N.C., M.S.N.

See also Acute lymphocytic leukemia (ALL); Bone marrow aspiration and biopsy; Bone marrow transplantation (BMT); Chemotherapy; Chronic lymphocytic leukemia (CLL); Chronic myeloid leukemia (CML); Graft-versus-host disease (GVHD); Leukemias; Lymphomas; Myeloma; Stem cell transplantation.

▶ Upper gastrointestinal (GI) endoscopy

Category: Procedures
Also known as: Esophagogastroduodenoscopy (EGD)

Definition: An upper gastrointestinal (GI) endoscopy is a diagnostic procedure in which a thin tube with a light and camera is inserted into the throat to evaluate the inside of the esophagus, stomach, and first part of the small intestine (duodenum).

Cancers treated: Esophageal cancer, gastric (stomach) cancer, duodenal cancer

Why performed: An upper endoscopy helps identify the cause of unexplained abdominal or chest pain, nausea and vomiting, heartburn, bleeding, and swallowing disorders. It can evaluate tumors, ulcers, and areas of inflammation.

Patient preparation: Patients who have heart valve disease, rheumatic heart disease, and some other cardiovascular conditions may need to take an antibiotic before the procedure to reduce the risk of infection. Patients must not eat solid foods for eight hours before the procedure, but clear liquids may be allowed until a few hours before the procedure, depending on the specific guidelines of the testing center. Before the procedure, an assessment of the patient's health history is conducted, and the potential risks of the procedure will be discussed.

Steps of the procedure: The patient will change into a hospital gown. An intravenous (IV) line is inserted into a vein in the patient's arm to deliver medications. A blood pressure cuff is placed on the patient's arm to monitor blood pressure, a small clip placed on the patient's finger is attached to an oximeter monitor to check the patient's blood oxygen level, and the patient's pulse is monitored during the procedure.

The patient lies on the left side during the procedure. A sedative is given (conscious or moderate sedation), so the patient is awake but relaxed and able to respond to the physician's instructions during the procedure. A pain-relieving medication is infused in the IV, and a local anesthetic is applied via a spray at the back of the patient's throat to numb it and reduce the natural gag reflex. A mouthpiece is placed in the patient's mouth through which the endoscope is passed. The physician may ask the patient to swallow several times to help pass the endoscope down the throat to the stomach. An endoscope is a long, thin, lighted flexible instrument with a camera on the end that transmits images of the esophagus, stomach, and duodenum onto a video monitor to guide the physician during the procedure. The procedure lasts from twenty to thirty minutes.

If an abnormality such as a polyp or lesion is found during the procedure, then instruments can be inserted through the endoscope to remove it. Tissue samples (biopsy) can be removed through the endoscope. If bleeding is found during the procedure, then a sclerosing agent can

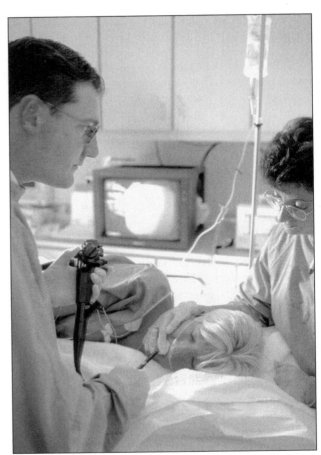

A physician performs an upper gastrointestinal endoscopy. (Will & Deni McIntyre/Photo Researchers, Inc.)

be injected or another instrument can be inserted through the endoscope to stop the bleeding.

After the procedure: The patient is observed in a recovery room for one to two hours as he or she recovers from the effects of the sedation. The patient will receive homegoing instructions from the nurse, including diet restrictions and medication and activity guidelines. The patient should not drive or operate machinery for eight hours after the procedure and should avoid vigorous physical activity after the procedure, as directed by the physician. The patient may have temporary throat soreness for a few days after the procedure, which can be relieved with throat lozenges. If a polyp or tissue sample was removed, then the patient may need to avoid aspirin and products containing aspirin, ibuprofen, and anticoagulants for one week. The physician will provide specific guidelines. Within seventy-two hours after the procedure, the patient should call the physician if he or she experiences severe abdominal pain, black or bloody stools, a continuous cough, fever, chills, chest pain, nausea, or vomiting.

Risks: Complications associated with an upper endoscopy procedure are rare but may include bleeding and puncture of the stomach lining. The risk of complications associated with the sedation given during the procedure is also rare, occurring in less than 1 in every 10,000 people, according to the American College of Gastroenterology. In general, most patients experience only a mild sore throat after the procedure.

Results: If the results of the test indicate that prompt treatment is needed, then the physician will discuss the treatment options with the patient and his or her family and the necessary arrangements will be made. The abnormal tissue or biopsy sample is sent for analysis in the laboratory to determine if there is a malignancy. If bleeding in the stomach lining or duodenum is found, then a peptic or duodenal ulcer may be diagnosed and a proton pump inhibitor or H$_2$ antagonist medication may be prescribed. Barrett esophagus (a condition that increases the risk of esophageal cancer) is revealed by upper endoscopy in up to 5 percent of high-risk patients with gastroesophageal reflux disease (GERD), according to the American College of Gastroenterology.

When the laboratory results are available within two to three days, the physician will notify the patient with the results. If another physician referred the patient for the procedure, then he or she will also receive a copy of the results.

Angela M. Costello, B.S.

▶ **For Further Information**
Cohen, J., et al. "Quality Indicators for Esophagogastroduodenoscopy." *American Journal of Gastroenterology* 101 (2006): 886-891.
Faigel, D. O., et al. "Quality Indicators for Gastrointestinal Endoscopic Procedures: An Introduction." *American Journal of Gastroenterology* 101 (2006): 866-872.

▶ **Other Resources**

American College of Gastroenterology
http://www.acg.gi.org

American Gastroenterological Association
http://gastro.org

American Society for Gastrointestinal Endoscopy
http://www.askasge.org

International Foundation for Functional Gastrointestinal Disorders
http://www.iffgd.org

National Digestive Diseases Clearinghouse, National Institute of Diabetes and Digestive and Kidney Diseases
http://digestive.niddk.nih.gov/index.htm

See also Barrett esophagus; Duodenal carcinomas; Endoscopy; Esophageal cancer; Gastrointestinal complications of cancer treatment; Gastrointestinal oncology; *Helicobacter pylori*; Infection and sepsis; Nausea and vomiting; Small intestine cancer.

▶ Upper gastrointestinal (GI) series

Category: Procedures
Also known as: Barium swallow, upper GI and small bowel series

Definition: An upper gastrointestinal (GI) series is a radiographic examination of the upper digestive tract, including the esophagus, stomach, and small intestine. Moving X-ray images of the digestive tract are produced with a fluoroscopy machine.

Cancers diagnosed: Esophageal, gastric, duodenal, and laryngeal cancers

Why performed: An upper GI series helps identify structural or functional abnormalities of the upper digestive tract, including a tumor in these organs, hiatal hernia, nar-

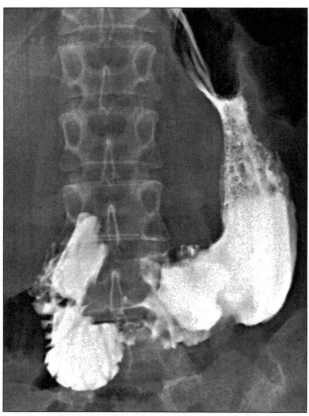

An upper GI series reveals a large cancerous ulceration on the anterior stomach wall. (©ISM/Phototake—All rights reserved)

rowing of the esophagus, esophageal muscle disorders, esophageal varices (enlarged veins), gastroesophageal reflux disease (GERD), achalasia, ulcers, strictures, polyps, diverticula, some causes of intestinal inflammation, and certain swallowing disorders. It also may be performed to determine the cause of frequent heartburn or unexplained abdominal pain.

Patient preparation: Specific dietary restrictions may be given to be followed for a few days before the procedure. A laxative may need to be taken the day before the procedure to clear the digestive tract. Patients must not eat or drink anything or smoke after midnight the night before the procedure. In most cases, the patient can continue taking regularly scheduled medications, but they must be taken with small sips of water. Patients with diabetes should ask how to adjust their meal plans, insulin, or other diabetes medications in preparation for the test. Patients should tell the physician if they are allergic or sensitive to contrast dyes, certain medications, iodine, shellfish, or latex. Female patients should tell the physician if they are pregnant or think

they might be pregnant; this test is not advised for pregnant women, so another test may be recommended.

Steps of the procedure: The patient will change into a hospital gown. The X-ray technician will first take a regular X ray of the stomach and abdomen. A medication may be injected into a vein in the patient's arm to temporarily slow bowel movement. The patient is asked to drink 16 to 20 ounces of a barium solution that coats the lining of the esophagus, stomach, and duodenum to allow these organs to be seen on the X rays. Using a fluoroscope, a radiologist passes a continuous X-ray beam through the part of the digestive system being examined, and detailed pictures of the organ and its motion are transmitted on a monitor as the barium moves through the digestive system. The patient will be asked to hold his or her breath as each picture is taken so that the movement of breathing does not interfere with the images. The patient may be lying on a table or standing during the test and will be asked to turn in different positions as the barium moves through the digestive system. In some cases, the table may move to tilt the patient in different positions. The patient may be asked to swallow a "fizzy" tablet that produces air bubbles in the stomach. After the fluoroscopy part of the test, another regular X ray is taken of the stomach and abdomen. The procedure lasts about one to two hours, including the barium preparation time.

After the procedure: The patient will receive homegoing instructions from the nurse, including diet restrictions and medication and activity guidelines. The patient can go home right after the procedure and resume regular activities and diet, unless otherwise instructed by the physician. The patient should increase the intake of fluids and high-fiber foods to help flush the barium. The patient will pass what remains of the barium during the next few days after the procedure, and the stool may be light-colored or white. If constipation occurs after the procedure, then the patient should ask his or her doctor about taking a laxative. The patient should call the physician if he or she experiences abdominal pain within twenty-four hours after the procedure or constipation for more than two days after the procedure.

Risks: There are no significant risks of the upper GI series. There is a low exposure of radiation during the test, but the amount of radiation is minimal and not likely to cause any health problems. The patient may find the taste of the barium solution unpleasant and may experience constipation after the procedure.

Results: Normal values indicate that there are no structural abnormalities found on the upper GI examination.

The physician will notify the patient within two to three days about the test results after the radiologist has reviewed the fluoroscopy films. If a structural or functional problem was identified during the procedure, then the physician will discuss the appropriate treatment options with the patient. If another physician referred the patient for the procedure, then he or she will receive a copy of the test results.

Angela M. Costello, B.S.

▶ For Further Information

Allen, J. I., et al. "Best Practices: Community-Based Gastroenterology Practices." *Clinical Gastroenterology and Hepatology* 4 (2006): 292-295.

McPhee, Stephen J., Maxine A. Papadakis, and Lawrence M. Tierney, eds. *Current Medical Diagnosis and Treatment, 2008.* New York: McGraw-Hill Medical, 2007.

▶ Other Resources

American College of Gastroenterology
http://www.acg.gi.org

American Gastroenterological Association
http://gastro.org

American Society for Gastrointestinal Endoscopy
http://www.askasge.org

International Foundation for Functional Gastrointestinal Disorders
http://www.iffgd.org

National Digestive Diseases Clearinghouse, National Institute of Diabetes and Digestive and Kidney Diseases
http://digestive.niddk.nih.gov/index.htm

See also Barium swallow; Cobalt 60 radiation; Colon polyps; Duodenal carcinomas; Endoscopy; Fiber; Gastrointestinal oncology; Imaging tests; Laryngeal cancer; Laryngeal nerve palsy; Laxatives; Polyps; Pregnancy and cancer; Risks for cancer; Small intestine cancer; X-ray tests.

▶ Urethral cancer

Category: Diseases, symptoms, and conditions
Also known as: Urethral neoplasm, urethral carcinoma

Related conditions: Squamous cell carcinoma of the urethra, transitional cell carcinoma of the urethra, adenocarcinoma of the urethra

Definition: Urethral cancer is a cancer of the urethra, the tube that carries urine from the bladder to outside the body. In women, the tube is about 3 centimeters (cm) in length, whereas in men it is about 20 cm in length.

Risk factors: Patients with the disease may have a history of bladder cancer, frequent urinary tract infection, chronic irritation of the urethra, or chronic inflammation of the urethra caused by a sexually transmitted infection. Additional risk factors include a history of cigarette smoking and age older than sixty years. Approximately 37 to 44 percent of individuals with urethral cancer have had a sexually transmitted infection, and some researchers believe the human papillomavirus is associated with urethral cancer.

Etiology and the disease process: The urethral mucosal tissue consists of transitional epithelial cells near the bladder and squamous epithelial cells near the urethral opening. These cell types thus classify urethral cancer either as squamous cell carcinoma (the most common type of this cancer), transitional cell carcinoma (the second most common), or adenocarcinoma (in which transitional cells undergo metaplasia).

Incidence: Urethral cancer is exceedingly rare; only about 700 cases are diagnosed in the world each year. In the United States, it is diagnosed more often in whites than in blacks and more often in women than in men. It has been reported in Americans between the ages of thirteen and ninety. Most patients are in their sixties when they are diagnosed.

Symptoms: Because chronic irritation, inflammation, and infection tend to interfere with the natural reproductive mechanisms of the urethral mucosal cells, these processes usually precede urethral cancer. Patients with urethral cancer may be entirely asymptomatic for up to three years.

Symptoms may include voiding problems such as frequency, diminished stream and straining to void, increased nighttime urination, itching, painful urination, bladder opening obstruction, overflow incontinence, blood in the urine or semen, and malodorous or watery discharge as well as perineal, pelvic, or penile pain.

Screening and diagnosis: Urethral cancer is difficult to diagnose, in part because it is so rare and patients generally do not seek early treatment. Like most cancers, however, early detection leads to a greater chance of cure. Once urethral cancer develops, it often invades nearby structures (such as the bladder), and thus becomes difficult to treat with traditional surgical and radiation techniques. Ure-

Relative Survival Rates for Urethral Cancer (Papillary Transitional Cell), 1988-2001

Years	Survival Rate (%)
1	83.5
3	63.4
5	55.9
10	49.6

Source: Data from L. A. G. Ries et al., eds., *Cancer Survival Among Adults: U.S. SEER Program, 1988-2001—Patient and Tumor Characteristics*, NIH Pub. No. 07-6215 (Bethesda, Md.: National Cancer Institute, 2007)

thral cancer might be suspected if a urethral fistula (an unusual drainage of urine) or an abscess occurs or tissue necrosis is present. Most patients are in an advanced stage of the disease when it is diagnosed. Screening may consist of a chest X ray; a computed tomography (CT) scan of the pelvis and abdomen; magnetic resonance imaging (MRI) of the urethra, nearby lymph nodes, and other soft tissue; blood chemistry studies; and a complete blood count.

Urethral cancer is staged on the basis of what part of the urethra is affected and how widespread the cancer is. Anterior urethral cancer means the cancer affects parts of the urethra closest to the outside of the body, whereas posterior urethral cancer occurs in deeper parts of the body, near the bladder. In men, this often means the prostate is affected as well. Most clinicians categorize urethral cancer using the following criteria:

• Stage 0: The urethral lining contains abnormal cells that may become cancerous and spread to nearby normal tissue.

• Stage A: Cancer is present and has spread into the tissue adjacent to the lining of the urethra.

• Stage B: Cancer is present in the muscle surrounding the urethra. In men, nearby tissues in the penis may be affected.

• Stage C: Cancer has spread beyond the tissue surrounding the urethra. In women, cancer may be present in the vagina, the vaginal labia, and nearby muscle; in men, cancer may be present in the penis or in nearby muscle.

• Stage D1: Cancer has spread to the nearby lymph nodes in the pelvis and groin.

• Stage D2: Cancer has spread to distant lymph nodes and other organs in the body.

Treatment and therapy: Treatment options depend on a patient's general health, the stage and location of the cancer, when the diagnosis is made, and whether the cancer has recurred. The most common treatment is surgery; several different types of surgery may be pursued depending on the stage and severity of cancer. Some patients may receive radiation therapy or chemotherapy to kill any remaining cancer cells.

Prognosis, prevention, and outcomes: Prognosis depends on a patient's general health, the stage and size of the cancer, where in the urethra the cancer first developed, when the diagnosis was made, and whether the cancer has recurred.

In most patients, the cancer is locally advanced when a diagnosis is made, and the prognosis is generally poor. Invasive urethral cancer treated with surgery, radiation, and chemotherapy combined occurs in about 50 percent of patients. The five-year survival rate for patients with noninvasive urethral cancer receiving surgical or radiation therapy is 60 percent.

Terry A. Anderson, B.S.

▶ For Further Information

Parisi, S., et al. "Role of External Radiation Therapy in Urinary Cancers." *Annals of Oncology* 18 (2007): vi157-vi161.

Swartz, M. A., et al. "Incidence of Primary Urethral Carcinoma in the United States." *Urology* 68, no. 6 (2006): 1164.

▶ Other Resources

American Urological Association
http://www.urologyhealth.org

National Cancer Institute
Urethral Cancer
  http://www.cancer.gov/cancertopics/types/urethral

See also Anal cancer; Benign prostatic hyperplasia (BPH); Bladder cancer; Cigarettes and cigars; Cystoscopy; Dilation and curettage (D&C); Enterostomal therapy; Exenteration; Gynecologic cancers; Gynecologic oncology; Human papillomavirus (HPV); Hysteroscopy; Kidney cancer; Laparoscopy and laparoscopic surgery; Penile cancer; Prostate cancer; Renal pelvis tumors; Urinalysis; Urinary system cancers; Urography; Urologic oncology; Vulvar cancer.

▶ Urinalysis

Category: Procedures

Also known as: UA, routine urinalysis, complete urinalysis

Definition: A routine complete urinalysis is the physical, chemical, and microscopic examination of the urine and a comprehensive overview of kidney function.

Cancers diagnosed: While urinalysis is the most cost effective and least invasive evaluation of kidney and urinary tract function, it is not a screening method for the detection of cancer. Suspicious cells may be seen, however, upon microscopic review of the urine sediment and forwarded for cytological examination and further pathology review to rule out cancer of the bladder or kidney.

Why performed: Urinalysis is the single most important evaluation of kidney function. It may detect urinary tract infections, systemic diseases such as diabetes mellitus, glomerulonephritis, and malignancy.

Patient preparation: First morning voided urine of a minimum of 10 milliliters is the preferred specimen for a urinalysis. A random urine sample taken at any time during the day is acceptable. The patient collects the urine sample at midstream while urinating.

The source of the urine sample may also be through the catherization of the bladder through the urethra or, rarely, through a suprapubic transabdominal needle aspirate of the bladder.

If the physician suspects a urinary tract infection, then the urine must be a clean-catch sample in which contaminating bacteria are absent. For more detailed studies, a twenty-four-hour urine specimen may be required. A sample contaminated by vaginal discharge or hemorrhage will be rejected for analysis.

Steps of the procedure: After the patient voids the urine sample into a cup or other container, it is labeled and sent to the clinical laboratory. A sample might have to be collected again if the transport to the clinical laboratory has been delayed, the quantity is insufficient, or there is bacterial overgrowth.

The clinical laboratory completes three evaluations of the urine. The physical characterization of the urine includes a description of the color (pale yellow, yellow, red orange, or brown), appearance or transparency (clear to cloudy to opaque), odor if abnormal, and specific gravity. The chemical evaluation includes the pH, protein, glucose, occult blood, ketones, leukocyte esterase, nitrite, bilirubin, and urobilinogen. These chemistry detection systems are each impregnated on a series of reagent pads on a dipstick that are activated when dipped into the urine and can be read manually or with an instrument. The microscopic examination of the urine sediment looks for bacteria, cells, and other formed elements such as casts, squamous epithelial cells, and crystals.

After the procedure: The urine sample is analyzed as soon as possible after voiding, ideally in less than two hours after collection. The results are sent to the physician who ordered the test.

Risks: There are no risks to collecting a routine urine sample other than inconvenience.

Results: Fresh normal urine is sterile, pale to dark yellow or amber in color, clear, and faintly aromatic, with a specific gravity between 1.003 and 1.035 grams per milliliter and a pH of 4.5 to 8.0. The dipstick chemistries are negative, and the microscopic observation is absent of cells or other elements. The normal twenty-four-hour urine volume is 750 to 2,000 milliliters.

Urine from a healthy individual is yellow to amber in color. A pale urine may suggest diabetes insipidus. A

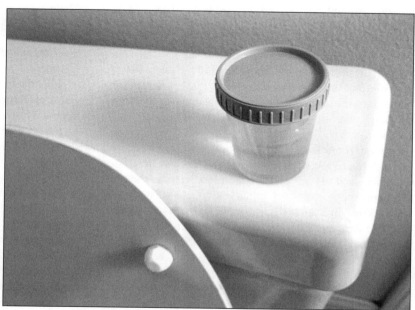

Urinalysis is invaluable for evaluating kidney function. (PhotoDisc)

milky urine may be caused by fat globules or by white cells in a urinary tract infection. A red urine may be the result of red blood cells, medications, or certain foods. A greenish urine suggests the presence of bile associated with jaundice. A brown/black urine suggests hemorrhage or poisoning.

Normal urine is clear, through which newsprint can be read. Cloudy to turbid urine may be the result of precipitation of mucin or calcium phosphates, neither of which merits pathological significance. Milky urine may suggest the pathological presence of fat globules. Turbid urine can point to a urinary tract infection.

Normally urine presents a faintly acrid odor. A pleasantly sweet-smelling urine may suggest ketone production associated with diabetes mellitus. Strong acrid odors may be the result of medications or ingestion of certain foods, such as an acrid odor associated with asparagus.

The urinary specific gravity is a reliable indicator of a person's hydration status.

The body maintains a narrow acid-to-base ratio (pH) in order to sustain life. The kidney monitors metabolic activity, and excess acid or base ions are excreted in the urine to maintain that balance.

In healthy persons, protein is not present in urine in detectable amounts. Proteinuria is the excretion of more that 150 milligrams per day or 10 to 20 milligrams per deciliter of protein in the urine and is a classic symptom of renal disease. The proteinuria may be transient or persistent. If the proteinuria is persistent, then additional studies will determine if the cause is glomerular, tubular, or the result of overflow in which low-molecular-weight proteins overwhelm the ability of the system to reabsorb filtered proteins.

In healthy persons, glucose is filtered by the glomerulus and reabsorbed in the proximal tubule. Glucose appears in the urine when the amount of glucose overwhelms the ability of the tubule to reabsorb it. Further evaluation determines the source of the glycosuria: diabetes mellitus, Cushing syndrome, liver and pancreatic diseases, or Fanconi syndrome.

A positive test for occult blood indicates the presence of hemoglobin or myoglobin. A finding of blood in the urine chemistry and the presence of red blood cells in the microscopic examination of urinary sediment (hematuria) requires the clinician to determine the source of the bleeding. The hematuria may be caused by an infection; glomerular, tubular, renovascular, or metabolic disorders; tumors; or calculi (stones). The hematuria may be induced by exercise, such as long-distance running.

Ketones are the end products of the body's fat metabolism and are not usually detected in the urine. The clinician determines the cause of the presence of ketones (ketonuria): carbohydrate-free dieting, uncontrolled diabetes, or starvation.

Normally, fresh voided urine is sterile. In the case of urinary tract infections and subsequent pyuria, the white blood cells produce leukocyte esterase, which is detected on the dipstick reagent strip.

A healthy person does not have nitrites in the urine. In the case of a urinary tract infection, gram-negative and some gram-positive microorganisms reduce the nitrates in the urine to nitrites, which can be detected.

Normally, unconjugated bilirubin is water insoluble and cannot pass through the glomerulus. Conjugated bilirubin is water soluble, however, and appears in the urine, suggesting liver disease or biliary obstruction.

The urine is also tested for urobilinogen, a colorless derivative of bilirubin formed by the action of intestinal bacteria.

Urinalysis also checks for microscopic formed elements. Except for an occasional epithelial, white, or red cell, the microscopic examination of normal healthy urine sediment is without comment. Any of the following may or may not suggest pathology and require clinical interpretation in context of patient history: white blood cells (leukocytes), red blood cells (erythrocytes), casts, crystals, and bacteria.

Casts are cylindrical bodies with a protein matrix, formed in the lumen of the renal tubules. They may demonstrate a homogenous or cellular matix and include any of the following types: hyaline, waxy, erythrocyte, leukocyte, epithelia, bacteria, granular, fatty, or broad. Crystals result from the precipitation of urinary solute out of the urine. They are not normally present in fresh voided urine, and many are not clinically significant. Examples include calcium oxalate, uric acid, triple phosphate (struvite), and cystine.

Five bacterial organisms per high-power field from a clean-catch urine sample is the classic diagnostic criteria for bacteriuria and a diagnosis of a urinary tract infection. Typically five organisms per high-power field represents 100,000 colony-forming units when the urine is cultured.

Jane Adrian, M.P.H., Ed.M., M.T. (ASCP)

▶ **For Further Information**

Brunzel, Nancy A. *Fundamentals of Urine and Body Fluid Analysis*. 2d ed. Philadelphia: W. B. Saunders, 2004.

Ringsrud, Karen Munson, and Jean Jorgenson Linne. *Urinalysis and Body Fluids: A Colortext and Atlas*. Philadelphia: Elsevier, 1994.

Simerville, Jeff A., William C. Maxted, and John J. Pahira. "Urinalysis: A Comprehensive Review." *American Family Physician*, March 15, 2005, 1153.

Strasinger, Susan King, and Marjorie Schaub Di Lorenzo. *Urinalysis and Body Fluids*. 5th ed. Philadelphia: F. A. Davis, 2008.

▶ Other Resources

American Urological Association
http://www.auanet.org

Lab Tests Online
http://www.labtestsonline.org

Onco Link
http://www.oncolink.com

See also Calcium; Cushing syndrome and cancer; Exercise and cancer; Fanconi anemia; Hematuria; Pathology; Risks for cancer; Tubular carcinomas; Urethral cancer.

▶ Urinary system cancers

Category: Diseases, symptoms, and conditions
Also known as: Bladder cancer, kidney and renal pelvic cancer, renal cell carcinoma, cancer of the urothelium, transitional cell cancer of the renal pelvis and ureter, urethral cancer, urethral neoplasms, squamous cell carcinoma of the urethra

Related conditions: Birt-Hogg-Dubé syndrome, von Hippel-Lindau disease, hereditary leiomyomatosis

Definition: Urinary system cancers are malignancies occurring anywhere in the organs that make up the urinary tract, including the kidney, ureter, bladder, and urethra. The kidney removes wastes and water from the blood, creating urine, which collects in the renal pelvis in the kidney. A tube called a ureter carries the urine to the bladder, which stores urine. Typically the bladder is flat when empty and balloons when full with urine, triggering the urge to urinate. The urethra, another tube, carries urine from the bladder to the outside of the body. Nine out of ten kidney cancers are renal cell carcinomas. Cancers that form in the renal pelvis and ureters develop from transitional cells. Some 98 percent of bladder tumors occur in the transitional cells that line the bladder. Urethral cancers are most commonly squamous cell cancers, followed by transitional cell cancers.

Risk factors: Risk factors vary by type of urinary tract cancer. Risk factors for kidney cancer include cigarette smoking (40 percent greater risk), obesity, high blood pressure, long-term dialysis, and occupational exposure to

carcinogens such as asbestos, benzene, cadmium, herbicides, and organic solvents. Several hereditary disorders also increase the risk of kidney cancer: von Hippel-Lindau (VHL) disease (about 25 percent of those afflicted develop the clear cell type of renal carcinoma), hereditary papillary renal cell carcinoma, Birt-Hogg-Dubé syndrome, hereditary leiomyomatosis, and hereditary renal oncocytoma. People with any of these hereditary conditions or a prior renal cell carcinoma should be evaluated frequently. Renal cancer affects more men than women, in part because men are more likely to smoke cigarettes and to be exposed to occupational carcinogens.

Cigarette smokers have two to three times the risk of developing bladder cancer than do nonsmokers. Smokers account for 50 percent of bladder cancer cases. Other risk factors implicated in the development of bladder cancer are occupational exposure to benzene or benzidene (20 to 25 percent of cases), a high-fat diet, excessive use of drugs containing the pain reliever phenacetin, and infection from *Schistosoma haematobium*, a type of fluke endemic in Europe, North America, and regions of Northern Africa. There has also been an association found between chlorinated drinking water and incidence of bladder cancer.

A history of bladder cancer and being the age of sixty or older are the major risk factors for urethral cancer. Some studies have implicated chronic urinary tract infections and irritation as causing urethral cancer cells to grow. A history of sexually transmitted infections, particularly the human papillomavirus (HPV), has also been associated with increased risk of urethral cancer.

Etiology and the disease process: Exactly what causes urinary tract cancers is not known, although many cases are found in active or past cigarette smokers. Renal cell carcinomas are primarily of the clear cell type (80 percent), followed by papillary renal carcinoma (10 to 15 percent). The clear cell type has cells that look very pale under a microscope; the papillary type is characterized by finger-like projections.

The bladder wall is lined with transitional cells and squamous cells. More than 90 percent of bladder cancers begin in transitional cells and 8 percent in squamous cells. Cancer occurring only in cells that line the bladder is referred to as superficial bladder cancer (carcinoma in situ). Cancers that begin in the transitional cells may spread through the bladder's lining and into the muscular wall of the bladder. In women, this type of bladder cancer may invade adjacent organs such as the vagina or uterus. In men, it may invade the prostate gland. In either gender, it may spread to the wall of the abdomen. When the cancer spreads outside the bladder, nearby lymph nodes are often involved. Distant disease may develop when a primary bladder cancer spreads to another part of the body.

Most urethral cancers invade locally, but they tend to be aggressive, metastasizing to nearby tissue. Often they are locally advanced by the time a diagnosis is made. However, the majority of urethral cancers do not spread distally. Cancer of the urethra manifests differently in men and women, differing in the type of cancer cells involved (squamous cell, transitional cell, or adenocarcinoma).

Incidence: The median age of diagnosis for cancer of the kidney and renal pelvis is sixty-five years. Renal cell carcinoma accounts for approximately 70 percent of kidney cancers and renal pelvis cancers for about 15 percent. The incidence rate for kidney cancer adjusted for age is 12.8 per 100,000 men and women per year. The incidence rate is approximately twofold in men versus women across ethnic groups, with the highest incidence in black men, a rate of 20.4 cases per 100,000 population.

Bladder cancer is the most common type of malignancy affecting the urinary system. About 50,000 cases of bladder cancer are diagnosed each year, making it the fourth most common cancer in men and the eighth most common cancer in women. The incidence is higher in men than women, with 40.5 cases per 100,000 population for white men. Bladder cancer occurs twice as often in whites as in blacks and Hispanics. The age-adjusted incidence for both men and women for bladder cancer is 21.1 cases per 100,000 people per year. Two-thirds of cases of bladder cancer occur in individuals over the age of sixty-five.

Urethral cancer usually develops in the squamous cells that line the urethra. Most urethral cancer in women occurs in the labia, vagina, or bladder neck, while in men it occurs in the vascular spaces of the corpora and periurethal tissue, deep tissue in the perineum, urogenital diaphragm, prostate, or penial and scrotal skin. Urethral cancer is a very rare condition occurring in less than 1 percent of all cancer cases. It is the only genitourinary system cancer that has greater incidence in women than in men. Although most urethral cancers are squamous cell cancers (78 percent of cases in men), the second most common type for both genders is transitional cell cancer. Adenocarcinoma occurs in the glands near the urethra in both men and women.

Symptoms: People with urinary tract cancer often experience hematuria, or blood in the urine, which in most cases is visible to the naked eye or upon inspection under a microscope. A thorough diagnostic evaluation following a finding of hematuria is essential to eliminate other conditions such as kidney stones or a urinary tract infection.

Patients with renal cell carcinoma may complain of hematuria, pain in the side, an abdominal lump, anemia, loss of appetite, and unexplained weight loss. Symptoms of transitional cell cancer of the renal pelvis and ureters include hematuria, back pain, fatigue, unexplained weight loss, frequent urination, or pain on urination. Common symptoms of bladder cancer include hematuria, lower back pain, frequent urination, and pain during urination. Patients with urethral cancer may have no symptoms early on or may experience hematuria, trouble with urinary flow (such as interrupted flow), a discharge, a lump or thickness

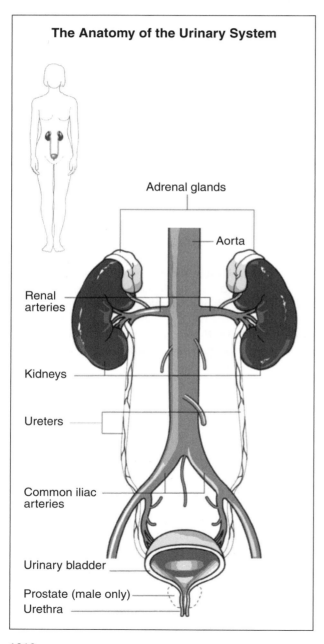

The Anatomy of the Urinary System

Adrenal glands

Aorta

Renal arteries

Kidneys

Ureters

Common iliac arteries

Urinary bladder

Prostate (male only)

Urethra

Lifetime Risk of Developing Common Urinary System Cancers, Based on Rates from 2003-2005

Cancer Type	Lifetime Risk: %	Lifetime Risk: No.	Probability of Developing Cancer
Urinary bladder cancer	2.38% of people born today will be diagnosed with bladder cancer in their lifetime	1 in 42 people will be diagnosed with bladder cancer in his or her lifetime	1.22% of men and 0.35% of women will develop bladder cancer between their 50th and 70th birthdays
Kidney and renal pelvis cancer	1.38% of people born today will be diagnosed with kidney or renal pelvis cancer in their lifetime	1 in 72 people will be diagnosed with kidney or renal pelvis cancer in his or her lifetime	0.85% of men and 0.43% of women will develop kidney or renal pelvis cancer between their 50th and 70th birthdays

Source: Data from National Cancer Institute, Surveillance Epidemiology and End Results, Cancer Stat Fact Sheets, 2008

in the penis or perineum, and enlarged lymph nodes in the groin area.

Screening and diagnosis: There are no standard screening tests for cancers of the urinary tract. Often kidney cancer is detected during a physical examination conducted for another purpose. When a person complains of symptoms consistent with a urinary system cancer, the physician will perform a complete physical exam, feeling the abdomen for any masses or abnormalities, and take a medical history, asking about risk factors such as cigarette smoking and occupational exposure to environmental carcinogens.

If the patient complains of hematuria, blood and urine tests will be ordered. A urine cytology test reveals markers in the urine associated with cancer cells or cancer cells coming from the lining of the bladder. A cystoscopy, in which a cystoscope (lighted tube) is inserted into the bladder through the urethra, checks for abnormal areas that can then be biopsied. (If the scope is extended into the ureter and renal pelvis, the test is called a ureteroscopy.) Another tool is an intravenous pyelogram (IVP), in which a contrast dye is injected into a vein and a series of X rays is taken to look for blockages in the kidney, ureter, and bladder. If cancer is detected, imaging studies such as computed tomography (CT) scans, magnetic resonance imaging (MRI), or ultrasound may be used to assess tumor growth and spread and to stage the cancer.

Urinary system cancers follow various staging systems. Most systems divide cancers into stages according to the size of the tumor and its extent of spread (localized, regional, or distant areas of the body). Many systems also grade the tumor, depending on how aggressively the cancer is growing.

Treatment and therapy: Surgery, radiation therapy, chemotherapy, and biological therapy are typical treatment options for urinary system cancers.

In renal cell carcinoma, surgery is the common option. A partial nephrectomy removes the tumor in the kidney and some tissue with it; a simple nephrectomy removes only the kidney; and a radical nephrectomy removes the kidney, surrounding tissue, adrenal gland, and lymph nodes. A radical nephrectomy may be more likely to cure the cancer in individuals with Stage II or Stage III tumors. Patients sometimes receive radiation therapy or chemotherapy after surgery to remove any remaining cancerous cells. Minimally invasive surgeries such as laparoscopy can be used for partial or radical nephrectomies. These techniques are gaining acceptance, since the use of laparoscopy reduces blood loss during surgery, requires less use of narcotics for pain, and shortens hospital stays and recovery time.

Surgery is not undertaken for Stage IV renal cell cancers since the cancer cannot be cured. In these cases, a technique called arterial embolization is used. Gelatin sponges are used to block the flow of blood to the kidney and kill the cancerous cells. Newer targeted chemotherapies such as sorafenib, sunitinib, and temsirolimus seem to be helpful. Patients at this stage in otherwise good health may be able to tolerate the side effects associated with interleukin 2 (IL-2) or cytokine therapy. The patient's physician may recommend that the kidney be removed before starting this therapy to enhance the response to treatment.

For transitional cell cancer of the renal pelvis and ureter, standard surgical options include removing part of the ureter (in superficial cases) or a nephroureterectomy, which removes the kidney, ureter, and the tissue that connects the ureter to the bladder.

For bladder cancer, standard treatment includes surgery, radiation therapy, chemotherapy, and biological therapy. Surgical options include transurethral resection (TUR) with fulguration, in which high-energy electricity is used to burn away cancerous areas during a cytoscopy; a segmental cystectomy, in which part of the bladder is removed; and a radical cystectomy, in which the bladder, lymph nodes, and nearby organs (prostate and seminal vesicles in men; uterus, ovaries, and part of the vagina in women) are removed. If the bladder is removed, the surgeon creates another outlet in which urine is stored and leaves the body, referred to as a urinary diversion. Chemotherapy or radiation therapy may be performed following surgery to eliminate any remaining cancer cells or retard their growth.

In cases of bladder cancer, radiation therapy is used externally and internally through radioactive seeds placed in the body near the cancer. Chemotherapy is delivered orally or by injection, placed directly in an affected area or delivered through a tube inserted into the bladder. Biological therapy may be used to bolster an affected individual's immune system to fight the cancer.

The standard treatments for urethral cancer are surgery, radiation therapy, and watchful waiting. Surgery may remove the cancer by excision, burning with high-energy electricity (electroresection with fulguration), or laser surgery. Depending on the cancer's spread, other surgeries performed include lymph node dissection (removal of lymph nodes in groin and pelvis), cystourethrectomy (removal of bladder and urethra), cystoprostatectomy (removal of bladder and prostate), anterior exenteration (removal of urethra, bladder, and vagina), partial penectomy (removal of part of penis near urethra), and radical penectomy (removal of entire penis).

External and internal radiation therapy are also used for urethral cancer. Some patients are simply monitored for signs that the cancer has developed to the point where further treatment is necessary.

Patients should consult with their physician regarding treatment options, including those in clinical trials. Decisions should be based on the stage and grade of cancer, the patient's age and overall health, and the expected quality of life following treatment.

Prognosis, prevention, and outcomes: Outcomes experienced by those with urinary system cancers depend on many factors, including the stage of their cancers, whether they are superficial or invasive, the degree of metastasis, and patients' overall health and age. It is estimated that one-third of renal cell cancers and more than half of renal pelvic and ureter cancers could be eliminated if people stopped smoking cigarettes.

The overall five-year relative survival rate for those with renal cell cancer is about 50 percent, and for those with renal pelvic or ureter cancers, it is about 65 percent. The overall five-year relative survival rate for bladder cancer is 79.8 percent. The five-year relative survival rate rises to 92 percent if bladder cancer is diagnosed while still localized, falling to 45 percent when diagnosed when regional and 6 percent when the cancer has spread to distant areas. Urethral cancer, if noninvasive and treated surgically or with radiation, has five-year survival rates of about 60 percent.

Susan H. Peterman, M.P.H.

▶ **For Further Information**

Campbell, Steven C., et al. *One Hundred Questions and Answers About Kidney Cancer*. Sudbury, Mass.: Jones and Bartlett, 2009.

Eble, John N., Guido Sauter, Jonathan Epstein, and Isabell Sesterhenn, eds. *Pathology and Genetics of Tumours of the Urinary System and Male Genital Organs*. Vol. 7 in *World Health Organization Classification of Tumours*. Lyon, England: International Agency for Research on Cancer Press, 2003.

Ellsworth, Pamela, and Brett Carswell. *One Hundred Questions and Answers About Bladder Cancer*. Sudbury, Mass.: Jones and Bartlett, 2006.

Schrier, Robert W., ed. *Diseases of the Kidney and Urinary Tract*. 8th ed. Philadelphia: Wolters Kluwer Health/Lippincott Williams & Wilkins, 2007.

Tekes, Aylin, et al. "Dynamic MRI of Bladder Cancer: Evaluation of Staging Accuracy." *American Journal of Roentgenology* 184, no. 1 (January, 2005): 121-127.

▶ **Other Resources**

American Cancer Society
http://www.cancer.org

American Urological Association
http://www.aunet.org

National Cancer Institute
http://www.cancer.gov

Urologychannel: Your Urology Community
http://www.urologychannel.com

See also Bladder cancer; Coke oven emissions; Cystography; Epidermoid cancers of mucous membranes; Exenteration; Kidney cancer; Nephrostomy; Renal pelvis tumors; Transitional cell carcinomas; Urethral cancer; Urography; Urologic oncology; X-ray tests.

▶ Urography

Category: Procedures

Also known as: Intravenous pyelography (IVP), oral urography, retrograde urography, magnetic resonance urography, computed tomography urography

Definition: Urography allows an assessment of the health and functioning of the urinary system by injecting a contrast material (dye) into the bloodstream. When this contrast material reaches the urinary tract, its soft-tissue structures become visible on imaging scans, so that abnormalities can be detected.

Cancers diagnosed: Cancers of the kidney (renal cell carcinoma), ureters, and bladder

Why performed: The urinary system is composed of the kidneys, ureters, bladder, and urethra. The kidneys are two bean-shaped organs located in the lower back below the rib cage. Their function is to filter blood, remove waste products, and help maintain the proper balance of fluid in the body. The ureters carry excess water and waste materials from the kidney to the bladder, where these waste materials are stored. The urethra removes this urine from the body. Urography allows these structures to be examined for cancer and other abnormalities in a noninvasive way.

Most often, urography is done for reasons unrelated to cancer. Kidney stones, for example, can cause obstruction in the urinary system accompanied by extreme pain. In this case, urography is done on an emergency basis to locate the obstruction. Cancer tumors can also cause obstruction or blood in the urine. Urography to detect cancer is done on a nonemergency basis in a radiology center or other outpatient setting.

Urography can be done in several different ways using various imaging techniques. Sometimes it is necessary to use more than one method in order to acquire precise information about the location of tumors. In intravenous pyelography (IVP), a dye containing iodine is injected into a vein in the hand or arm. When the dye reaches the urinary tract, the tissues become visible on conventional X rays. The only difference between oral urography and IVP is that the individual drinks the dye instead of having it injected. Retrograde pyelography is similar to an IVP, only the dye is placed directly in the urinary tract by way of a catheter (thin tube)

inserted into the urethra. In computed tomography (CT) urography, contrast material is injected into the bloodstream, but instead of using conventional X rays to visualize the kidneys, ureters, and bladder, a CT scanner takes multiple cross-sectional images of the body and uses a computer to compile a three-dimensional image. In magnetic resonance imaging (MRI) urography, contrast material is injected, and then the individual is placed in a special tube while a three-dimensional picture is obtained through MRI. This type of urography is used most often to locate bladder cancer that has spread into the pelvic region.

Patient preparation: For nonemergency urography, the physician will review the patient's medications to make sure that they do not interact with the contrast material. Patients should tell their physicians if they are allergic to seafood or iodine, as this increases the likelihood that they may have an allergic reaction to the contrast dye. Women who are or think they might be pregnant should not have urographic tests that expose them to X rays.

The night before the test, the patient takes a laxative to empty the bowel and should not eat or drink on the day of the test. During the test, the patient will wear a hospital gown.

Steps of the procedure: The contrast material is injected into a vein (most commonly), injected into the urethra, or given by mouth. The patient may briefly feel a warm, tingling sensation. In rare cases, the patient can develop breathing problems or experiences swelling in the throat

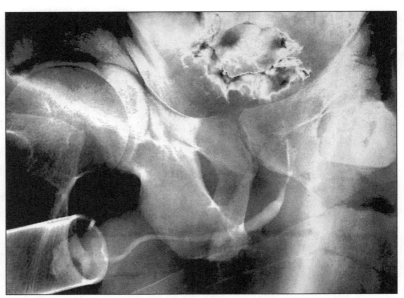

An intravenous urogram showing a polyploid cancer of the bladder. (©ISM/ Phototake—All rights reserved)

or elsewhere. This is a sign of an allergic reaction, and the physician should be notified immediately.

The patient is placed on the X-ray table, and a series of X rays are taken at timed intervals, usually at zero, five, ten, twenty, and sometimes forty minutes. While each X ray is being taken, the patient must remain still. Between X rays, the patient may move. For the final X ray, the patient is asked to urinate, and an X ray is taken of the bladder. CT and MRI urography are very similar. MRI urography takes about one hour and requires the patient to remain still during that time.

After the procedure: After the procedure, the patient may eat, drink, and resume normal activities. The patient may have a mild headache or slight nausea from the contrast material. Urine will appear normal; the contrast material does not change its color.

Risks: This is a minimally invasive procedure with few risks. Rarely does a patient have a serious allergic reaction to the contrast material. Although X rays are very safe, pregnant women should not have them because of potential damage to the developing fetus. These women can have MRI or CT urography, neither of which uses X rays.

Results: In a healthy kidney, the dye will show up on the X rays soon after it is injected. In people with kidney damage, the dye takes longer to appear in the X rays.

Martiscia Davidson, A.M.

▶ For Further Information

Anderson, E. M., et al. "Multidetector Computed Tomography Urography (MDCTU) for Diagnosing Urothelial Malignancy." *Clinical Radiology* 62, no. 4 (April, 2007): 324-332.

Guermazi, A., ed. *Imaging of Kidney Cancer.* New York: Springer, 2006.

Strum, Stephen, and Donna L. Pogliano. *A Primer on Prostate Cancer: The Empowered Patient's Guide.* Hollywood, Fla.: Life Extension Media, 2002.

▶ Other Resources

eMedicinehealth.com
Intravenous Pyelogram
    http://www.emedicinehealth.com/
    intravenous_pyelogram/article_em.htm

See also Bladder cancer; Gastrointestinal complications of cancer treatment; Hematuria; Imaging tests; Kidney cancer; Nephrostomy; Prostate cancer; Urethral cancer; Urinary system cancers; X-ray tests.

▶ Urologic oncology

Category: Medical specialties
Also known as: Genitourinary oncology

Definition: Urology is the study of the male and female urinary systems and the male reproductive system. Oncology is the study of the development, diagnosis, treatment, and prevention of cancer. Urologic oncology is the diagnosis, treatment, and prevention of cancers involving the urinary and male reproductive system.

Cancers treated: Urologic oncologists treat bladder, kidney, penile, and testicular cancer in men and bladder and kidney cancer in women.

Training and certification: Urologic oncologists are doctors who are board certified in urology. In the hierarchy of medicine, urology is classified as a surgical subspecialty. This means the doctor has specialized training in surgery. Doctors who are fellows of the American College of Surgeons (FACS) have achieved more advanced qualifications in surgery.

To become board certified in urology in the United States, the doctor must have graduated from an approved medical school and have completed an accredited urology residency program that involved at least five years of training. In the course of the residency training program, there must be one year of training in general surgery, three years in clinical urology, and at least six months in general surgery, urology, or another specialty relevant to urology. The doctor must be a senior or chief resident in urology during the last year of the program.

Within five years of completing the education program, the doctor must complete a qualifying examination followed by a certifying examination to become board certified. The qualifying examination consists of a one-day written exam to assess the doctor's knowledge of the entire field of urology and related subjects. The certification examination is designed to assess clinical competence. During the two-day certification process, the doctor is evaluated to ensure the existence of an approved practice log and a favorable professional reputation among peers. Additionally, the urologist is tested on knowledge in the areas of immunology, molecular biology, hypertension, transplantation, sexual dysfunction, urologic imaging, pathology, and problems with urination, such as benign prostatic hyperplasia (BPH) and incontinence. There are also questions that pertain to infections, inflammatory diseases, fertility problems, obstructive diseases, cancer, anatomy, fluid imbalances, and pediatric urology. The practicing urologist needs to have obtained a high level of expertise in all these areas to become board certified. Doctors who were certified after January 1, 1985, must undergo a recertification process every ten years.

There is no recognized board-certified subspecialty of urologic oncology. Doctors who choose to practice medicine in urologic oncology can receive additional training in this area of expertise through fellowship programs, attending conferences and other training programs, and membership in organizations such as the Society of Urologic Oncology.

Services and procedures performed: Urologic oncologists are surgeons who specialize in the management and treatment of cancer. This includes evaluation, diagnosis, and treatment of cancer or suspected cancer in the prostate, bladder, kidney, and testicles. Additionally, conditions such as urinary retention and blood in the urine are treated.

Typically, the doctor asks a series of questions on the first visit to assess the problem. After the patient's initial examination, a series of tests may be recommended to determine the type and extent of disease. Some of these diagnostic tests may include a blood test, urine test, cystoscopy (insertion of a small scope to view the inside of the bladder and ureter), digital rectal exam, biopsy, cystourethrogram (an X ray taken of the bladder and urethra while urinating), ultrasound, or other imaging studies.

Depending on the test results, the doctor devises a treatment plan, which may be aggressive to rid the body of disease or simply palliative to alleviate symptoms associated with the cancer. When the cancer is localized, meaning limited to an organ or specific area, aggressive treatment is often undertaken to get rid of disease. When the cancer has spread to other areas of the body, called metastasis, treatment often involves minimizing symptoms and discomfort instead of trying to cure the body of disease.

Some of the procedures performed by urologic oncologists include laparotomy (incision in the abdominal wall to view inside the abdomen), transurethral resection (to diagnose and remove cancer of the bladder or prostate), cystectomy (partial or complete removal of the bladder), and prostatectomy (partial or complete removal of the prostate gland). In addition to surgery, treatment may include the use of hormone therapy, radiation, chemotherapy, or combinations of these therapies. When other treatment options are considered, a urologic oncologist may include other members on the team who specialize in these different types of cancer treatments.

Related specialties and subspecialties: Many urologic oncologists work with specialists in oncology fields such as radiation, chemotherapy, and immunotherapy. Pathologists are also intimately involved in the diagnostic process.

A pathologist is a doctor who specializes in identifying diseases by examining tissues and cells under a microscope to determine if cancer cells are present and, if they are, how aggressive the disease may be. The pathologist's report is critical in setting the stage for treatment of the disease.

A radiation oncologist uses radiotherapy, which is high-energy waves or particles, to destroy or damage cancer cells. It can be done using electron beam therapy, X-ray therapy radiation treatment, or cobalt therapy. This type of treatment is primarily used to treat localized cancer, though in some instances it is used for total body irradiation in preparation for a bone marrow transplant.

A medical oncologist specializes in using chemotherapy, hormone therapy, and biological therapy for the treatment of cancer. Chemotherapy is often used when the cancer has metastasized or spread throughout the body. This can be delivered intravenously, by injection, or with a pill. Hormone therapy, commonly used in the treatment of prostate cancer, involves administering hormones to suppress the production of testosterone in the body. This helps stop the production of cancer cells. Immunotherapy, sometimes called biological therapy or biotherapy, uses treatments to stimulate the body's immune system to fight disease. This can be done by administering a drug or by stimulating the body's own immune system to work harder to fight disease. This type of treatment is often used in conjunction with other therapies to enhance the effect.

When cancer is not contained within the urinary or male reproductive systems, assistance may be required from doctors who specialize in treating other areas of the body, such as gynecologists. It is not uncommon to have a treatment team consisting of specialists in urologic oncology, pathology, radiation therapy, chemotherapy, immunotherapy, and other areas who all work together to fight the disease.

Vonne Sieve, M.A.

▶ **For Further Information**

Ellsworth, Pamela, and Anthony Caldamone. *The Little Black Book of Urology.* Sudbury, Mass.: Jones and Bartlett, 2007.

Society of Urologic Oncology. "Advances in the Treatment of Genitourinary Cancer: Highlights from the Third Annual Meeting of the Society of Urologic Oncology, December 13-14, 2002, Washington, D.C." *Reviews in Urology* 5, no. 4 (Fall, 2003): 232-234.

_____. "Report from the Society of Urologic Oncology: Highlights from the Fourth Annual Meeting of the Society of Urologic Oncology, December 5-6, 2003, Bethesda, Md." *Reviews in Urology* 6, no. 4 (Fall, 2004): 193-199.

▶ **Organizations and Professional Societies**

American Association of Clinical Urologists
  http://www.aacuweb.org
  Two Woodfield Lake
  1100 E. Woodfield Road, Suite 520
  Schaumburg, IL 60173

American Association of Genitourinary Surgeons
  http://www.aagus.org
  University of Michigan
  Department of Urology
  3875 Taubman Center SPC 5330
  1500 East Medical Center Drive
  Ann Arbor, MI 48109-5330

American Board of Urology
  http://www.abu.org
  2216 Ivy Road, Suite 210
  Charlottesville, VA 22903

American Urological Association
  http://www.auanet.org
  1000 Corporate Boulevard
  Linthicum, MD 21090

National Cancer Institute, Center for Cancer Research: Urologic Oncology Branch
  http://ccr.cancer.gov/labs/lab.asp?labid=92
  10 Center Drive, MSC 1501 10/2B47
  Bethesda, MD 20892

Society of University Urologists
  http://www.suunet.org
  1100 E. Woodfield Road, Suite 520
  Schaumburg, IL 60173

Society of Urologic Oncology
  http://www.societyofurologiconcology.org
  1100 E. Woodfield Road, Suite 520
  Schaumburg, IL 60173

▶ **Other Resources**

American Urology Association
  http://www.urologyhealth.org

Journal of Urology
  http://www.jurology.com

See also Benign prostatic hyperplasia (BPH); Chemotherapy; Digital rectal exam (DRE); Fertility drugs and cancer; Fertility issues; Imaging tests; Kidney cancer; Nephrostomy; Prostate cancer; Testicular cancer; Urethral cancer; Urinary system cancers; Urography; Urostomy; X-ray tests.

▶ # Urostomy

Category: Procedures
Also known as: Urinary diversion

Definition: A urostomy is a surgical opening (stoma) through the abdominal wall that allows urine to drain from the diseased bladder into an artificial pouch, to be emptied intermittently, when long-term drainage from the bladder is not possible. A urostomy can be conventional or standard, with an ileal conduit, or feature a continent urinary reservoir.

Cancers treated: Bladder cancer

Why performed: When a bladder is diseased, the body must have a way to excrete urine, liquid human waste. A surgeon creates a urostomy to drain urine from the kidney.

Patient preparation: The surgeon discusses the risks and benefits of the urostomy with the patient and examines the patient's abdomen to locate the best place for the stoma. Some patients try flat pouches at the predetermined place to see if the location allows maximum comfort and minimal interference in activities of daily living. Patients should tell the surgeon if their work or hobbies need special consideration.

Steps of the procedure: The steps of the procedure depend on the type of surgery performed. In a conventional urostomy, a small pouch or urine reservoir is created surgically from a small bowel segment. A passage is created from the kidney and ureters to the ileal segment that bypasses the bladder (which may or may not be removed). The far end of the ileal segment is brought through the abdominal wall to make a stoma.

After the procedure: Education regarding how to care for a pouch after surgery is provided by an ostomy specialist. After surgery, the stoma may swell but will decrease in size over six to eight weeks. Most health care facilities have ostomy visitors who have experienced a urostomy and understand concerns about body image. They can answer questions that the patient may have after surgery. Support groups are also useful.

Risks: Typical risks include urinary crystals, infection, and skin irritation. A pouch that fits well along with adequate fluid intake and appropriate skin care with a protectant barrier can minimize problems. The patient should notify the health care provider if bleeding occurs from the stoma, if ulcers form on the skin around the stoma, or if fever or a strong odor in the urine (a sign of a kidney infection) occurs.

Results: The urostomy can improve quality of life for the bladder cancer patient, who can return to most normal activities. Managing the urostomy will become routine with practice.

Marylane Wade Koch, M.S.N., R.N.

See also Bladder cancer; Enterostomal therapy; Exenteration; Nephrostomy; Self-image and body image.

▶ Uterine cancer

Category: Diseases, symptoms, and conditions
Also known as: Endometrial carcinoma, cancer of the uterus, adenocarcinoma of the uterus, carcinosarcoma of the uterus, clear cell endometrial carcinoma, papillary serous carcinoma of the uterus, adenosquamous carcinoma of the uterus, endolymphatic stromal myosis, heterologous uterine sarcoma, homologous uterine sarcoma, leiomyosarcoma of the uterus, malignant mixed Mullerian tumor of the uterus, serous endometrial carcinoma, endometrial stromal sarcoma, rhabdosarcoma of the uterus, osteosarcoma of the uterus, chondrosarcoma of the uterus

Related conditions: Cancer of the cervix, cancer of the Fallopian tube, bladder cancer, rectal cancer, vaginal cancer, cancer of the ovary

Definition: The uterus has a body (also called the corpus), which is located within the lower portion of the abdominal cavity between the bladder and the rectum, and a vaginal portion, referred to as the cervix. Although the uterus and cervix are continuous, they are considered as separate structures with respect to cancer. Further, the uterus has a covering (the serosa), a layer of muscle (the myometrium), and a layer of cells (the endometrium) lining the uterine cavity (the uterine cavity is the site for fetal growth during pregnancy). Cancer of the uterus most often involves the endometrium, with the myometrium the less fequent site of cancer. The Fallopian tubes are connected to the top of the uterus on either side but are not considered part of the uterus. Cancer of the uterus is thus defined as cancer of the body of the uterus (the endometrium or myometrium), as opposed to cancer arising from the cervix or metastatic from an adjacent structure (such as the vagina, Fallopian tube, ovary, bladder, or rectum).

Risk factors: There are factors that increase a woman's risk of developing cancer of the uterus and those that decrease it. Factors that increase the risk are the use of estrogen-containing medications without the addition of progesterone (called the unopposed estrogen effect; progesterone neutralizes the stimulatory effect of estrogen on the endometrium of the uterus), late menopause (after reaching the age of fifty-two), obesity, not having given birth to a child (also known as nulliparity), diabetes, estrogen-secreting ovarian tumors, polycystic ovarian syndrome, high blood pressure, increased dietary fat intake, radiation therapy to the pelvis for other reasons, and the use for more than two years of the medication tamoxifen in the treatment of breast cancer.

The factors known to decrease a woman's risk of cancer of the uterus include interrupted ovulation (during and shortly after pregnancy or while using oral contraceptives, which prevent ovulation), use of progesterone, menopause before the age of forty-nine, normal weight, and having given birth to more than one child (also known as multiparity). In fact, use of oral contraceptives has been shown to reduce a woman's risk of cancer of the uterus by approximately 50 percent, the benefit emerging after one year of use and lasting for up to fifteen years after discontinued use.

Etiology and the disease process: Cancer of the uterus most often occurs in women in the menopause or those approaching the menopause (that is, perimenopause), with a peak occurrence between the ages of fifty and sixty-five. In women who have long-term unopposed estrogen stimulation, the endometrium undergoes hyperplastic changes that are benign but precede the development of cancer. In most cases, hyperplastic changes can be reversed with the discontinuation of estrogen or the addition of progester-

---

Age at Diagnosis of Uterine Cancer, 2001-2005

Age Group	Cases Diagnosed (%)
Under 20	0.0
20-34	1.5
35-44	6.4
45-54	18.9
55-64	28.8
65-74	22.8
75-84	16.5
85 and older	5.1

Source: Data from National Cancer Institute, Surveillance Epidemiology and End Results, Cancer Stat Fact Sheets, 2008

Note: The median age of diagnosis from 2001 to 2005 was sixty-two, with an age-adjusted incidence rate of 23.4 per 100,000 women per year.

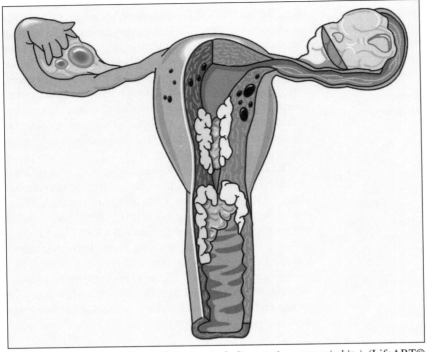

A number of possible uterine pathologies, including uterine cancer (white). (LifeART© 2008 Wolters Kluwer Health, Inc.-Lippincott Williams &Wilkins. All rights reserved.)

one. The risk of hyperplasia progressing to cancer is age dependent: 11 percent for women less than the age of thirty-five, 12 percent for women between the ages of thirty-six and fifty-four, and 28 percent for women over the age of fifty-five.

Incidence: Cancer of the uterus is the most frequent cancer involving the female reproductive tract in the United States and the fourth most frequent cancer affecting women, behind breast, lung, and colorectal cancer. There are approximately 41,000 new cases of uterine cancer each year with about 7,300 deaths. An individual woman's lifetime risk of cancer of the uterus is about 1 in 50 (compared with 1 in 8 for breast cancer).

Symptoms: Abnormal bleeding through the vagina is the most common symptom associated with cancer of the uterus, occurring in about 90 percent of cases. Such bleeding may arise from the vagina, bladder, or rectum and must be thoroughly evaluated. Fortunately, abnormal bleeding is a sign of uterine cancer in only 10 to 20 percent of all cases. For premenopausal women, the bleeding may take the form of breakthrough, prolonged, or heavy bleeding, all of which generally reflect an underlying hormonal imbalance and can be treated as such. For postmenopausal women, any bleeding should be considered abnormal and should be evaluated by a gynecologist.

Screening and diagnosis: Unlike cancer of the cervix or breast cancer, which have well-accepted and effective screening tests (Pap smears and mammography, respectively), no such screening test exists for cancer of the uterus. Nevertheless, two screening tests are available for anyone at high risk: endometrial sampling and measurement of the endometrial thickness (or lining).

Endometrial sampling is an office-based procedure in which a small, flexible, plastic catheter is inserted into the uterus, and the cells lining the uterus (endometrial cells) are aspirated (sucked) into the catheter. Endometrial sampling is a relatively painless procedure, although some women experience mild uterine cramping. The aspirated cells are sent to a laboratory for microscopic evaluation, similar to a Pap smear. Endometrial sampling can also serve as the diagnostic test for endometrial cancer. In some cases, if the diagnosis of uterine cancer is in question based on endometrial sampling, a dilation and curettage (D&C) can be performed as an outpatient procedure in which more extensive sampling of the uterine cavity can be undertaken without causing discomfort to the patient. In rare cases, the diagnosis of uterine cancer is made at the time of a hysterectomy being performed for other indications.

Measurement of the endometrial thickness is also an office-based procedure but in some cases is done by a radiologist. An ultrasound probe is inserted through the vagina (transvaginal ultrasound) to messure the thickness of the lining of the uterus. The procedure is painless and takes only a few minutes to perform. Measurement of the endometrial thickness is most appropriate for menopausal women. An endometrial thickness less than 4 millimeters (mm) is rarely associated with a uterine malignancy in a woman not taking hormones, or less than 8 mm in a woman on hormones.

Staging of uterine cancer is according to the International Federation of Gynecology and Obstetrics (FIGO) as follows:

- Stage I: Cancer limited to the endometrium or myometrium

- Stage II: Cancer extending from the body of the uterus to the cervix
- Stage III: Cancer protruding through the serosa or metastases to the vagina, pelvis, or lymph nodes adjacent to the aorta
- Stage IV: Metastases to the bladder, bowel, or organs outside the pelvis in the abdomen

Treatment and therapy: Surgery, typically a hysterectomy with removal of the Fallopian tubes and ovaries and sampling of the local lymph nodes, is the mainstay of treatment. Radiation therapy is reserved for patients who are poor surgical candidates (such as patients with severe heart or respiratory diseases) or have unresectable disease. Chemotherapy is usually of limited value, being used primarily for women with metastatic disease. The blood test for cancer antigen 125 (CA 125) is not diagnostic of cancer of the uterus but can be used to monitor a patient for recurrence.

Prognosis, prevention, and outcomes: Prognostic factors for uterine cancer include age at the time of diagnosis, race (whites have a better prognosis than blacks), tumor stage, tumor grade, type of tumor (adenocarcinoma, clear cell adenocarcinoma, papillary serous adenocarcinoma, sarcoma, and so on), size of the uterus at the time of diagnosis, depth of invasion of the tumor into the layer of uterine muscle, presence of tumor in the blood vessels supplying the uterus, and spread of the tumor outside the uterus to other organs or lymph nodes. It is important to remember that cancer of the uterus is diagnosed more often than other cancers of the female reproductive tract and that fewer women die of cancer of the uterus than cancers of the cervix and ovary combined. The overall five-year survival rates for cancer of the uterus by stage at diagnosis are 87 percent for Stage I, 72 percent for Stage II, 51 percent for Stage III, and 9 percent for Stage IV.

D. Scott Cunningham, M.D., Ph.D.

▶ **For Further Information**

Creasman, W. T., F. Odicino, and P. Maigonnueve. "FIGO Annual Report on the Results of Treatment in Gynecological Cancer: Carcinoma of the Corpus Uteri." *Journal of Epidemiology and Biostatistics* 23 (1998): 35-61.

Parazzini, F., C. La Vecchia, L. Bocciolone, and S. Franceschi. "The Epidemiology of Endometrial Cancer." *Gynecologic Oncology* 41 (1991): 1-16.

▶ **Other Resources**

American Cancer Society
Overview: Endometrial Cancer
http://www.cancer.org/docroot/CRI/
CRI_2_1x.asp?rnav=criov&dt=11

National Cancer Institute
Cancer of the Uterus
http://www.cancer.gov/cancertopics/wyntk/uterus

See also Adenocarcinomas; Adenomatoid tumors; Bladder cancer; Carcinosarcomas; Endometrial cancer; Fallopian tube cancer; Fertility drugs and cancer; Gynecologic cancers; Gynecologic oncology; Hormonal therapies; Hysterectomy; Ovarian cancers; Ovarian cysts; Rectal cancer; Vaginal cancer.

▶ Vaccines, preventive

Category: Chemotherapy and other drugs
ATC code: J07BC01, J07BM01, J07BM02

Definition: Vaccines are biological drugs used to induce immunity against a germ (virus or bacterium) without causing disease. After vaccination, the body's immune system develops antibodies that then kill or neutralize the germ if exposed to it. These antibodies circulate in the bloodstream. The immune response induced by a vaccine may decrease or wane over time, requiring a booster dose—some vaccines require three or more doses to provide full protection against the germ.

Vaccines may contain live germs that have been weakened so that they cannot cause disease; killed or inactivated viruses that cannot cause an infection but can stimulate antibody production; toxoids (harmless bacterial toxins) that do not cause illness but stimulate production of antibody; and parts or components of bacteria or viruses, which cannot cause disease but generate an immune response.

Cancers treated: Liver cancer, cervical cancer

Subclasses of this group: Recombinant DNA hepatitis B vaccine, plasma-derived hepatitis B vaccine, quadrivalent human papillomavirus (HPV) vaccine

Delivery routes: The hepatitis B vaccine is administered by intramuscular injection in the anterolateral thigh of infants twenty-four months of age and younger and in the deltoid muscle (shoulder) of older children, adolescents, and adults. Most people should receive three doses of the vaccine.

The HPV vaccine is also administered by intramuscular injection of 0.5 milliliter in three doses. The second and third doses should be administered two and six months after the first dose.

How these drugs work: Hepatitis B vaccine prevents hepatitis B disease and its serious consequences, such as hepatocellular carcinoma (liver cancer). The recombinant hepatitis B vaccine is made by copying the genetic sequence of a protein contained in the hepatitis B virus into a yeast cell, which is then cultured and purified. The immunization series with hepatitis B vaccines is 95 percent effective at inducing immunity.

Plasma-derived hepatitis B vaccines are made by harvesting particles of the hepatitis B surface antigen (HBsAg) from plasma of people with chronic hepatitis B infection. HBsAg is a component of the hepatitis B virus that appears in the blood before symptoms of the disease. The HBsAg particles are purified and inactivated with heat or chemicals to produce the vaccine.

Available HPV vaccines protect against two types of the virus that cause about 70 percent of cervical cancer cases—types 16 and 18. The vaccine is produced by assembling the L1 protein of HPV types 16 and 18 into virus-like-particles (VLPs). VLPs look like the virus to the immune system but do not contain deoxyribonucleic acid (DNA), so they cannot replicate and cause disease. The HPV vaccine will only protect women who have not previously been infected with HPV. The other two types included in the quadrivalent version of the vaccine—HPV 6 and HPV 11—are intended to protect against genital warts, not cancer.

The quadrivalent HPV vaccine has been tested in thousands of women sixteen to twenty-six years of age. Clinical trials showed the vaccine to be 100 percent effective in preventing cervical precancers caused by types 16 and 18 in women who had not been previously exposed to these HPV types. Also, the vaccine was almost 100 percent effective in preventing vulvar and vaginal precancers and genital warts caused by the HPV types in the vaccine.

People vaccinated against hepatitis B or HPV can still develop liver cancer or cervical cancer. Chronic hepatitis B infection is only one of many risk factors for liver

Licensed Anticancer Vaccines

Drugs	Brands	Subclasses	Delivery Mode	Cancers Treated
Hepatitis B vaccine	Engerix-B, Recombivax HB, Comvax, Twinrix, Pediarix	Recombinant DNA hepatitis B vaccine, plasma-derived hepatitis B vaccine	Injection	Liver cancer
Human papillomavirus (HPV) vaccine	Gardasil, Cervarix	Quadrivalent human papillomavirus (HPV) vaccine	Injection	Cervical cancer, anogenital cancers

cancer, and 30 percent of cervical cancer cases are caused by HPV types not included in the current HPV vaccines.

Side effects: Of those who receive the hepatitis B vaccine, 65 percent do not experience any side effects. Only 3 percent of recipients will develop pain and tenderness where the injection has been given, and between 1 and 6 percent of recipients will have a low-grade fever. Serious allergic reactions occur in less than 1 out of 10,000 vaccines given, or about 0.001 percent. Serious allergic reactions include anaphylaxis, a rapid life-threatening allergic response affecting more than one part of the body—it may also affect the whole body, causing the airway to swell, close off, and prevent the intake of oxygen.

Studies of more than 11,000 women between nine and twenty-six years of age around the world have shown that the quadrivalent HPV vaccine causes no serious side effects, but 84 percent of vaccine recipients experienced pain at the injection site. Other mild-to-moderate side effects were swelling and redness at the injection site.

Diego Pineda, M.S.

▶ **For Further Information**

Offit, Paul A. *Vaccinated: One Man's Quest to Defeat the World's Deadliest Diseases.* New York: Collins, 2007.

Offit, Paul A., and Louis M. Bell. *Vaccines: What You Should Know.* New York: Wiley, 2003.

Plotkin, Stanley A., Walter A. Orenstein, and Paul A. Offit, eds. *Vaccines.* 5th ed. Philadelphia: Saunders/Elsevier, 2008.

▶ **Other Resources**

Liver Cancer Network
   http://www.livercancer.com

National Cancer Institute
Human Papillomaviruses and Cancer: Questions and Answers
   http://www.cancer.gov/cancertopics/factsheet/Risk/HPV

National Network for Immunization Information
   http://www.immunizationinfo.org

See also Biological therapy; Complementary and alternative therapies; Immune response to cancer; Immunotherapy; Infectious cancers; Prevent Cancer Foundation; Prevention; Vaccines, therapeutic; Virus-related cancers.

▶ **Vaccines, therapeutic**

Category: Chemotherapy and other drugs
Also known as: Biological therapy, immunotherapy

Definition: Therapeutic vaccines treat cancer by stimulating the body's natural immune system. Therapeutic vaccines contain the whole cancer cell, parts of cells, or components of the body's immune system.

Cancers treated: The Food and Drug Administration (FDA) does not currently license any therapeutic vaccines. Advanced phase III clinical trials are now in progress to evaluate vaccines against a variety of cancers.

Subclasses of this group: Whole cell vaccines, heat shock proteins, antigen/adjuvant vaccines, dendritic cell vaccines, anti-idiotype vaccines, DNA vaccines

Delivery routes: Cancer vaccines may be delivered by scarification (scratch), subcutaneous or intramuscular injection, or intranasally. The delivery route depends on the type of vaccine and cancer.

How these drugs work: The immune system is very complex and interconnected. It consists of various types of white blood cells (lymphocytes) and cytokines. The immune system is stimulated when it identifies foreign molecules known as antigens. The immune response can be either humoral (body fluids) or cellular. In the cellular process, phagocytes (macrophages and dendritic cells) engulf and digest cells and particles. The resultant fragments are attached to a molecule known as the major histocompatibility complex (MHC) and are presented on the cell surface. They are therefore known as antigen presenting cells (APCs). If helper T cells recognize the fragments as antigens, then they can either activate B cells to produce antibodies or activate cytotoxic T cells to kill the foreign invader or cancer cell directly. Another process involves natural killer (NK) cells. These cells are activated to destroy cancer cells when they recognize abnormalities on the surfaces of cells. Cytokines are soluble proteins secreted by activated immune cells. They facilitate communication and function among immune system components and enhance the immune response.

Therapeutic vaccines are used to treat existing cancers, in contrast to the traditional role of vaccines to prevent infectious diseases. The immune response is very specific, so cancer vaccines have been developed to selectively destroy cancer cells without harming normal cells. Unfortunately, the field has been fraught with disappointments over the last century. A basic problem lies with the fact that cancer cells are derived from normal cells. Success de-

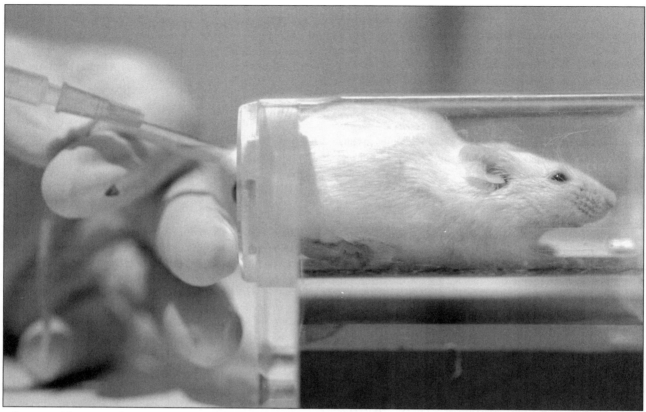

A mouse with cancer is being injected with a therapeutic vaccine developed by the Pasteur Institute. (©Vo Trung Dung/Corbis Sygma)

pends on the immune system recognizing very small molecular differences between normal and cancer cells. Although the immune system does respond naturally to the presence of cancer cells, this response is often weak and the cancer may be tolerated.

Cancer cells develop many methods to evade the immune system. They can hide their identity by repressing display of their antigens. They can alter their metabolism to become resistant to attacks by the immune system. They can secrete cytokines that kill lymphocytes. Cancer cells can actively suppress the activation and function of dendritic cells and T cells.

A variety of therapeutic vaccines have been developed. A key goal of the vaccines is to enhance the immune system's response to cancer antigens. Preparations include whole cell vaccines, heat shock proteins, antigen/adjuvant vaccines, dendritic cell vaccines, anti-idiotype vaccines, and DNA vaccines.

Whole cell vaccines are prepared from the patient's whole cancer cells. Whole cell vaccines do not require the identification of antigens but presumably contain the full array of cancer antigens. Unfortunately, early whole

cell vaccines were not very effective. Researchers discovered that T cells are activated only when a second co-stimulatory molecule is present. Current whole cell vaccines are genetically modified to secrete cytokines or express co-stimulatory molecules.

Heat shock proteins are found in most cells and serve to repair protein structure. They are often found in excess in cancer cells. Vaccines are prepared by purifying heat shock proteins from tumor tissue removed from the patient and linking these to tumor antigen. Administration of the vaccine results in uptake and processing by APCs and a strong T-cell response.

Antigen/adjuvant vaccines are prepared by combining a known cancer antigen with a chemical known as an adjuvant, which enhances the effect of the antigen.

Dendritic cell vaccines have been found very effective. To prepare the vaccines, dendritic cells are removed from the patient, exposed to the patient's own cancer antigens in the laboratory, and grown in culture. When the resultant vaccine is injected into the patient, the T cells in the immune system are stimulated to attack the tumor cells.

Anti-idiotype vaccines have been developed for use

against cancers that poorly present antigens. Antibodies that are produced in response to an antigen have unique antigen regions called idiotypes. The body can produce antibodies to these idiotypes that are called anti-idiotypes. Anti-idiotype vaccines can be prepared in the laboratory, often using synthetic monoclonal antibodies. Since these anti-idiotype vaccines appear to be like the tumor antigen, they stimulate a stronger immune response.

DNA vaccines are based on genes that code for antigen proteins. When these vaccines are administered, they are taken up by APCs. The vaccines are delivered to the APCs by means of vectors, such as modified viruses, bacteria, or synthetic polymers. Within the APCs, antigen protein is produced and presented to the T cells. This method provides a continuous supply of antigen to maintain the immune response.

Side effects: The primary concern with therapeutic vaccines is the development of autoimmune responses, although this seldom occurs. Some patients may experience a skin reaction or mild flulike symptoms.

David A. Olle, M.S.

▶ **For Further Information**

Finn, Olivera J. "Cancer Vaccines: Between the Idea and the Reality." *Nature Reviews Immunology* 3, no. 8 (August, 2003): 630-641.

Greten, Tim F., and Elizabeth M. Jaffe. "Cancer Vaccines." *Journal of Clinical Oncology* 17, no. 3 (March, 1999): 1047-1060.

Orentas, Rimas, James W. Hodge, and Bryon D. Johnson, eds. *Cancer Vaccines and Tumor Immunity.* Hoboken, N.J.: Wiley-Interscience, 2008.

Weinberg, Robert A. *The Biology of Cancer.* New York: Garland Science, Taylor & Francis, 2007.

▶ **Other Resources**

American Cancer Society
Cancer Vaccines
http://www.cancer.org/docroot/ETO/content/ETO_1_4X_Cancer_Vaccines_Active_Specific_Immunotherapies.asp?sitearea=ETO

National Cancer Institute
Cancer Vaccine Fact Sheet
http://www.cancer.gov/cancertopics/factsheet/cancervaccine

See also Bacillus Calmette Guérin (BCG); Biological therapy; Chemoprevention; Complementary and alternative therapies; Cytokines; Duke Comprehensive Cancer Center; Immune response to cancer; Immunotherapy; Vaccines, preventive.

▶ **Vaginal cancer**

Category: Diseases, symptoms, and conditions
Also known as: Squamous cell carcinoma of the vagina, clear cell adenocarcinoma, malignant melanoma of the vagina, leiomyosarcoma of the vagina, endodermal sinus tumor, yolk-sac tumor, sarcoma botryoides, embryonal rhabdomyosarcoma, pseudosarcoma botryoides

Related conditions: Cancers of the vulva, cervix, uterus, ovary, colon and rectum

Definition: The vagina is a muscular, tubelike structure that extends from the vulva, or the visible external genitalia, to the uterus. Cancer of the vagina involves a tumor that arises within the vagina rather than as an extension, metastasis, or recurrence from the cervix or vulva.

Risk factors: Risk factors for vaginal cancer include age, human papillomavirus (HPV) infection, exposure to diethylstilbestrol (DES, banned in the United States in 1971), a history of cervical cancer, vaginal adenosis, uterine prolapse, cigarette smoking, chronic vaginal irritation, low socioeconomic status, hysterectomy at an early age, and vaginal trauma.

Etiology and the disease process: Precancerous changes involving the vagina are much less common than precancerous changes affecting the cervix or vulva. Although not proven, it is thought that the lack of glands in the vagina is the basis for the rarity. Most vaginal cancers are metastatic, originating from cancers of the cervix or vulva with spread to the vagina, although metastases have been reported to occur from the uterus, ovaries, colon, rectum, breast, and even the kidney. Metastasis to the vagina occurs by spread from the lymphatics or blood.

Incidence: There are approximately 2,000 new cases of vaginal cancer in the United States each year. The actual incidence of vaginal cancer is 0.42 case per 100,000 women. Vaginal cancer accounts for 1 to 2 percent of malignancies involving the female reproductive tract.

Symptoms: The most common symptoms associated with cancers of the vagina are abnormal bleeding or an excessive, nonodorous, watery discharge; less frequent symptoms include pelvic pain, an increased frequency of urination or pain with urination, and constipation.

Screening and diagnosis: Screening for vaginal cancer should be performed in the context of a woman's annual physical examination, sometimes called a well-woman examination. During the examination, the gynecologist in-

Age at Diagnosis of Vaginal Cancer, 1988-2001

Age Group	Cases Diagnosed (%)
20-34	1.0
35-44	4.1
45-54	10.4
55-64	15.1
65-74	20.2
75-84	25.1
85 and older	24.2

Source: Data from L. A. G. Ries et al., eds., *Cancer Survival Among Adults: U.S. SEER Program, 1988-2001—Patient and Tumor Characteristics*, NIH Pub. No. 07-6215 (Bethesda, Md.: National Cancer Institute, 2007)

spects the vaginal walls for lesions, areas of discoloration, or abnormal discharge. Proper inspection of the vagina requires rotation of the speculum during the examination so that all areas of the vaginal wall are visualized, with continued inspection during removal of the speculum.

A diagnosis of vaginal cancer is made, based on a tissue biopsy, after an abnormality is seen on physical examination. Because symptoms of vaginal cancer are often absent or nonspecific, its diagnosis is often missed or delayed. Although useful in determining the extent of disease, computed tomography (CT) and magnetic resonance imaging (MRI) are not used to make the initial diagnosis of cancer of the vagina.

The most common types of vaginal cancer include squamous cell carcinoma, adenocarcinoma (including a rare variant, known as clear cell adenocarcinoma), and melanoma. Squamous cell carcinomas are by far the most common, accounting for 90 percent of all cases, and usually occur in women in their fifties. Squamous cell carcinomas usually occur high in the vagina and have the appearance of ulcerating masses that look like large warts or fleshy lesions. Unlike cancer of the cervix, in which infection with HPV has been clearly linked to the development of cancer, HPV is causal in the majority of true cancers of the vagina in adults in only 50 percent of the cases.

Adenocarcinomas of the vagina have peak occurrences in women younger than thirty and then again in women older than seventy. It appears that women with late-onset adenocarcinoma have a genetic predisposition, but the precipitating factor has not been identified. The subtype of adenocarcinoma known as clear cell adenocarcinoma occurs in women with known exposure to DES as a fetus (in

utero exposure) by maternal use to counteract the risk of pregnancy loss. It is known that DES exposure does not affect all such women; in fact, only 1 in 1,000 women exposed to DES in utero will develop clear cell adenocarcinoma. Nevertheless, women so exposed should undergo more frequent screening at the discretion of the physician and patient. It is generally recommended that women with exposure to DES as a fetus should undergo their initial gynecologic examination at the time of menarche (onset of menstrual activity) and have increased lifelong surveillance at the discretion of their physician. Vaginal melanomas are rare and usually affect women older than sixty.

Infants and children are also affected by tumors of the vagina, usually of the three following types: endodermal sinus tumor (yolk sac tumor), sarcoma botryoides (embryonal rhabdomyosarcoma), and pseudosarcoma botryoides.

Endodermal sinus tumors are rare tumors of the ovary that originate in the vagina, usually in infants less than two years old. Girls younger than eight years are those most often diagnosed with the rare sarcoma botryoides. This tumor usually manifests as a mass protruding from the vaginal opening. Pseudosarcoma botryoides is a rare, benign tumor that resembles sarcoma botryoides.

Cancer of the vagina is staged according to the International Federation of Gynecology and Obstetrics (FIGO).
- Stage 0: Carcinoma in situ; the cancer is localized without apparent spread.
- Stage I: Cancer is limited to the vaginal wall.
- Stage II: Cancer has extended to the subvaginal tissues but not to the pelvic wall.
- Stage III: Cancer involves the pelvic wall.
- Stage IV: Cancer has spread beyond the pelvis or has extended to the bladder or rectum.

At the time of diagnosis, between 18 and 23 percent of women are found to have Stage I vaginal cancer, while 46 to 58 percent of women are found to have Stage II.

Treatment and therapy: Although surgery and radiation therapy have been used to treat squamous cell carcinomas of the vagina, radiation therapy is preferred. Initially, external radiation is used to shrink the tumor mass; this is followed by internal radiation therapy to maximize the toxic effect. Surgical treatment of squamous cell carcinoma can range from local procedures (such as destruction of lesions with laser treatment or surgical excision of the lesions) to more radical procedures (such as removal of part or all of the vagina or vaginectomy; hysterectomy; or pelvic exenteration, a hysterectomy with removal of the bladder, bowel, or both).

Because most patients with clear cell adenocarcinoma are young, removal of the uterus (hysterectomy) and partial or complete removal of the vagina (vaginectomy), followed by creation of a new vagina (neovagina) with skin grafts, is the standard treatment.

Vaginal melanomas are best treated with complete excision and dissection of the lymph nodes. Because of the depth of invasion, vaginal melanomas do not respond well to radiation or chemotherapy, and the goal is complete excision with clear surgical margins (in other words, the excised specimen has a central tumor with normal tissue completely surrounding the tumor).

Endodermal sinus tumors are generally treated with surgery and radiation, but most affected children have died. Sarcoma botryoides is a very aggressive tumor and has been treated with radical surgery and multiagent chemotherapy. Pseudosarcoma botryoides can be successfully treated with local excision. Recurrent vaginal cancers are best treated with chemotherapy

Prognosis, prevention, and outcomes: The prognosis for vaginal cancer is directly related to the stage at the time of diagnosis. The overall five-year survival rate for squamous cell carcinoma of the vagina is about 45 percent. By stage, five-year survival rates are 69 percent for Stage I, 45 percent for Stage II, 21.8 percent for Stage III, and 5 percent for Stage IV.

With respect to clear cell adenocarcinoma of the vagina, patients older than nineteen have a better prognosis than patients less than fifteen years of age. Five-year survival rates for clear cell adenocarcinoma have been reported to be 91 percent for Stage I, 82 for Stage II, 37 percent for Stage III, and 0 percent for Stage IV. Vaginal melanomas frequently recur, and the five-year survival rate is about 20 percent.

D. Scott Cunningham, M.D., Ph.D.

▶ **For Further Information**

Creasman, W. T., J. L. Phillips, and H. R. Menck. "The National Cancer Data Base Report on Cancer of the Vagina." *Cancer* 83 (1998): 1033-1040.

Peters, W. A., N. B. Kuman, and G. W. Morley. "Carcinoma of the Vagina: Factors Influencing Treatment Outcome." *Cancer* 55 (1985): 892-897.

▶ **Other Resources**

Detailed Guide: Vaginal Cancer
http://www.cancer.org/docroot/CRI/content/
CRI_2_4_1X_What_is_vaginal_cancer_55.asp

National Cancer Institute
Vaginal Cancer
http://www.cancer.gov/cancertopics/types/vaginal

See also Adenocarcinomas; Brachytherapy; Cervical cancer; Computed tomography (CT) scan; Endoscopy; Gynecologic cancers; Hysterectomy; Ovarian cancers; Ovarian cysts; Ovarian epithelial cancer; Pelvic examination; Pregnancy and cancer; Uterine cancer; Vulvar cancer.

▶ **Vascular access tubes**

Category: Procedures
Also known as: Peripherally inserted central catheters (PICC), subcutaneous ports, Hickman catheters, Groshong catheters, Broviac catheters

Definition: A vascular access tube is a catheter inserted into the veins of the arm, neck, or just beneath the collarbone for long-term intravenous access (greater than seven to ten days). The catheter can also be used to draw blood for lab tests. Patients receiving long-term chemotherapy, pain medications, nutrition, or antibiotics will have vascular access.

Cancers treated: All requiring long-term therapy

Why performed: Many patients have poor veins or are unable to receive treatment without access.

Patient preparation: Vascular access lines can be placed at the bedside, in the operating room (OR), or in vascular radiology. Procedures at the bedside have no preprocedure preparation. Patients going to the OR or vascular radiology are not allowed to eat or drink for at least eight hours before line placement as a result of the anesthesia.

Steps of the procedure: All lines are placed using sterile technique. For peripherally inserted central catheters (PICC), a catheter is inserted through the antecube to be threaded up the arm and to end in the superior vena cava. PICC lines are flushed at least once a day and their dressings are changed once a week.

For ports, a small titanium or plastic reservoir is inserted and stitched into place in the upper chest. The catheter is attached to the reservoir and inserted into the vein and then threaded into the superior vena cava. The reservoir is accessed through the patient's chest wall with special needles. Ports must have a needle inserted and flushed at least once a month to prevent clotting. This line can be placed in the OR or vascular radiology.

Hickman, Broviac, or Groshong catheters are also placed in the upper chest wall. The line is inserted through a small incision and into the vein and follows until the end rests in the superior vena cava. It is held into place by a small cuff located under the skin; typically stitches are not used. The patient or caregiver will be responsible for flushing the access and changing the dressing every seven days.

After the procedure: Line placement is verified by a chest X ray. Once the line has been verified, it can be used to infuse therapy or for lab sampling. The patient or caregiver is responsible for home care, including flushing the access and changing the dressing.

Risks: The risks associated with vascular access lines are pneumothorax (collapsed lung), bleeding, and infection.

Results: The result of this procedure is reliable venous access to receive therapy and for blood draws.

Katrina Green, R.N., B.S.N., O.C.N.

See also Caregivers and caregiving; Chemotherapy; Infection and sepsis; Nutrition and cancer treatment; Pain management medications; Superior vena cava syndrome.

▶ Vasectomy and cancer

Category: Procedures
Also known as: Sterilization, permanent birth control

Related cancers: None

Definition: Vasectomy, a form of permanent birth control for men, is a commonly performed procedure that results in sterilization and is more than 99 percent effective in preventing pregnancy. No link has been established between having this procedure and developing cancer.

Vasectomy facts: More than 13 million vasectomies have been performed in the United States. Of the men who had vasectomies, 91 percent were married or cohabiting, 87 percent were white, and 81 percent were educated beyond high school. Although vasectomy is effective at preventing pregnancy, it does not prevent or protect from sexually transmitted diseases.

History: In 2004, prostate cancer was the most commonly identified new cancer in American men and the second highest cause of cancer mortality in men. Some questions were raised about a possible association between vasectomy and cancer, with the greatest concern being an association with prostate cancer. The cause of prostate cancer is unknown, and therefore there was concern that an association might be found between cancer and vasectomy.

Several studies have been conducted in an effort to determine if there is a causal relationship between the two. The major studies done in 1993 found that it was not pos-

sible to show a correlation. There were too many other factors that introduced bias into the ability to draw the conclusion. Similarly, it has been impossible to identify a correlation between vasectomy and testicular cancer. Testicular cancer is a cancer of young men (ages fifteen to thirty-four), while prostate cancer is seen in older men.

A 2002 study looked at vasectomy and the risk of prostate cancer and concluded that the association was small and could be explained by bias. This means that there were too many factors that interfered with the ability to scientifically make an association. The researchers concluded that studies should continue because of the popularity of vasectomy. Men should discuss any cancer concerns with their physician prior to having a vasectomy, but there is no evidence to show that a man should not have a vasectomy because of concerns about cancer.

Janet R. Green, M.S.P.H.

See also Birth control pills and cancer; Fertility issues; Pregnancy and cancer; Prostate cancer; Relationships; Sterility; Testicular cancer.

▶ Veterinary oncology

Category: Medical specialties
Also known as: Animal cancer management, companion animal cancer management, domestic animal cancer management

Definition: Veterinary oncology is officially defined as the study of tumors in animals, excluding humans. The most common usage of the term currently refers to the study and management of cancer in domestic and, more typically, companion animals. Most veterinary oncologists are trained primarily in the care of cancer in dogs and cats. However, many also become involved in diagnosing and treating or directing the management (in cooperation with the attending small, large, or exotic animal veterinarian) of cancer in other companion species such as birds, rodents, rabbits, horses, pet ruminants, aquatic animals, and exotic animals.

Veterinary oncology is informative for the study and treatment of cancer in people because some animals can serve as models of human neoplasia. These cancers can either occur naturally in these animals or be experimentally induced. One example of naturally occurring cancer in animals possibly informing the treatment of humans involves the use of dogs as models of osteosarcoma in children, since the tumors show very similar behavior in dogs and children (growing most often on the metaphysis and acting aggressively) and are associated with rapid bone growth (which occurs in large-breed dogs), trauma (such as bone fractures), and gender (male canines and humans are both more susceptible), among other correspondences. Another example is the recent development of the canine melanoma vaccine at the University of Wisconsin School of Veterinary Medicine. Animals also serve as models of experimentally induced neoplasia or metastasis, such as nude mice that receive implants of cancerous human cells to test pharmaceutical interventions and study tumor biology.

Subspecialties: Veterinary oncology is divided into two specialties: veterinary medical oncology and veterinary radiation oncology. Medical oncologists are diplomates of the American College of Veterinary Internal Medicine. Radiation oncologists are diplomates of the American College of Veterinary Radiology. An unofficial specialty is surgical oncology. There is no diplomate status in this field, but these veterinarians are trained in special surgical procedures and techniques to remove cancerous tissue from animals (mostly dogs and cats).

Cancers treated: The increase in life expectancy in companion animals due to vaccines, antiparasitic medications, and general improvements in health care has resulted in increased cancer incidence associated with advanced age. Some cancers are more prevalent in certain species and more responsive to treatment than in others.

One of the most common blood cancers in all domestic animals is lymphoma (lymphosarcoma), which is comparable to non-Hodgkin lymphoma in people. In dogs, the incidence rate is about 30 cases per 100,000, and it is the most common blood cancer in this species, with a higher incidence recorded in boxers and golden retrievers, among others. This disease can generally be managed for a few years, if caught early, but not cured. Cats have an even higher prevalence of lymphoma than dogs or people but the use of the feline leukemia virus (FeLV) vaccine in cats beginning in the late 1990's has lowered the incidence of certain forms of lymphoma in cats. However, feline lymphoma is generally less responsive to treatment than the canine variety. Another blood cell cancer, mast cell tumor, is the most common skin malignancy in dogs. Certain breeds, such as boxers, bull dogs, and Boston terriers, have shown increased incidence of this disease, which is amenable to treatment if caught early. An internal form of this disease in dogs and cats is less responsive to treatment.

Other veterinary cancers treated include hemangiosarcoma, which is a very aggressive tumor of mesenchymal origin affecting the blood vessels and seen most commonly in dogs (about 2 percent of all canine cancers), with higher prevalence noted in German shepherds, golden retrievers, and poodles, among others. This condition generally has a very poor prognosis, despite treatment.

Another cancer with a very poor prognosis is vaccine-associated sarcoma in cats. This is an unusually aggressive, but relatively rare, sarcoma that is believed to be promoted by inflammation accompanying the administration of certain vaccines and possibly other injected medications in cats. It has proven to be unresponsive to most treatment modalities, including surgery, and the location of the growth is a key prognostic factor. Vaccination guidelines, stating that certain vaccines (FeLV, rabies) be inoculated subcutaneously on the distal leg instead of in the interscapular region, have decreased the likelihood that an inoperable growth will develop on the trunk. If an aggressive sarcoma develops on the leg, the limb can be amputated, increasing the chance of a cure.

Another aggressive cancer, osteosarcoma, occurs primarily in large-breed dogs and is also most successfully treated with surgery (generally amputation of the affected limb) but difficult to catch before it metastasizes—usually to the lungs.

Mammary cell tumors are the most common neoplasia in female dogs and are third after skin tumors and lymphoma in cats. About 40 to 50 percent of canine mammary tumors are benign, while about 80 to 90 percent of feline mammary tumors are malignant. The best treatment for dogs is actually prevention, since spaying before the first heat virtually eliminates the risk of development of this tumor. Treating cats with progestin drugs increases their risk of developing mammary cancer. Complete surgical resection offers the best chance of a cure in dogs, while in cats the disease has usually metastasized to the lungs by the time of its diagnosis.

Other cancers commonly treated by veterinary oncologists are bladder cancers (transitional cell carcinoma most commonly), prostate cancer (dogs are the only nonhuman species with a significant occurrence of this neoplasia), melanomas, oral and cutaneous squamous cell carcinoma (common in cats), transmissible venereal tumors, and various other sarcomas, carcinomas, and round-cell tumors in cats, dogs, and other species.

Training and certification: For medical oncology, candidates for certification and diplomate status must apply for membership in the American College of Veterinary Internal Medicine (ACVIM). The college requires these candidates to be graduates of an accredited or approved veterinary school, licensed to practice veterinary medicine in a state, province, or other country; to be in satisfactory moral and ethical standing; and to pass both the general medicine and oncology certification examinations.

The general exam for medical oncology consists of two parts: comprehensive, which tests knowledge of general medicine common to all species, and a more specialized section oriented toward the individual's field of interest— that is, small animals (mostly dogs and cats) or large animals (mostly horses and ruminant species). To take the general exam, qualified veterinarians must have completed an approved one-year internship (or equivalent) in either small- or large-animal medicine and surgery and a two-year residency in veterinary oncology under the direct supervision of a diplomate of the ACVIM. To take the certification exam in veterinary medical oncology, veterinarians must additionally submit a letter from the supervisor of their oncology training program, other letters of recommendation, a case log, and publications.

For radiation oncology, a candidate for certification must be a graduate of an accredited or approved veterinary school, maintain proper ethical and moral standing, be licensed to practice veterinary medicine and surgery in one or more states, and have completed a one-year internship in either small- or large-animal medicine and surgery. The candidate must also have successfully completed a pro-gram in veterinary radiation oncology approved by the executive council of the American College of Veterinary Radiology (ACVR). Additionally, the candidate must have completed a two-year residency training program in veterinary oncology, submit references, and pass the written and oral exams in general and radiation oncology. The written exam tests the candidate's knowledge of general veterinary oncology, radiation physics and dose calculations, radiation biology, and clinical aspects of radiation oncology.

Surgical oncologists are diplomates of the American College of Veterinary Surgeons (ACVS). The unofficial designation of "surgical oncologist" follows successful completion of a fellowship in surgical excision of tumors and cancerous tissue from animals.

Services and procedures performed: Veterinary oncologists diagnose, stage, and plan treatment strategies for their animal patients. Most of the time, they are not expecting or planning a cure for the malignant or metastatic conditions. Rather, they are looking to effect a remission or control the tumor's growth to provide a good quality of life

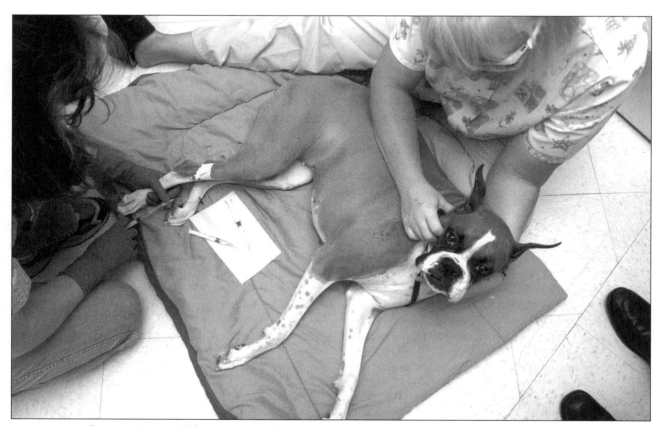

Lacey, a six-year-old boxer, receives chemotherapy to treat her lymphoma. (AP/Wide World Photos)

for the animal. Generally, extremely toxic treatment modalities are avoided in animals because of their shorter life spans, high costs, inconvenience to owners (traveling to distant treatment centers, caring for a sick pet, and so on), and the fact that animals primarily live in the moment (and cannot rationalize discomfort).

For diagnosis and staging, veterinary oncologists examine blood work (complete blood count, blood chemistries); employ various imaging modalities, depending on need, availability, and cost (X rays, magnetic resonance imaging, computed tomography); and analyze the results of biopsies, cytologies, and bone marrow aspirates. For some conditions, such as mast cell tumors, the cancer cells are graded by a histopathologist. Not all tests are conducted in all animals. Staging is an extremely important part of planning the treatment process and forming a prognosis. Once this is completed, the veterinary oncologist will often work with a surgeon if the tumor is resectable. If spread to distant lymph nodes or metastases are found, most medical oncologists will plan adjunctive chemotherapy. Chemotherapy is also prescribed for diffuse cancers, such as lymphoma, that are not amenable to surgical intervention. Growths that cannot be resected or can be only partially resected are often treated with local radiation therapy directed by a radiation oncologist. Some veterinary referral or academic centers offer their own orthovoltage or megavoltage (linear accelerator, cobalt, or cesium) units. However, others outsource these therapies to human cancer treatment clinics that work directly with the veterinary oncologist. Other forms of radiotherapy, such as brachytherapy or systemic radiotherapy (offered for thyroid tumors in cats) are also offered to veterinary patients.

Animal oncology employs just about every chemotherapeutic agent used for human chemotherapy, and specially trained veterinary nurses often administer the drugs under the direct supervision of the oncologist. The veterinary oncologist can also offer therapy for pain and the side effects of treatment, such as nausea and vomiting following chemotherapy, or oral mucositis following radiation therapy. The oncologist follows the animal's progress over the course of treatment and modifies the protocol in the event of complications such as severe bone marrow suppression. The veterinary oncologist should ultimately provide a good idea of the animal's prognosis and help the client make informed decisions about treatment options while considering costs and quality of life for the animal and owner.

Related specialties and subspecialties: Veterinary oncologists and clients work closely with practitioners in the fields of veterinary pathology, veterinary clinical pathology, veterinary dermatology, veterinary emergency and critical care, veterinary small-animal internal medicine, veterinary large-animal internal medicine, and veterinary surgery for the treatment and diagnosis of neoplastic conditions.

Lisa J. Shientag, V.M.D.

▶ **For Further Information**

Birchard, Stephen J., and Robert G. Sherding. *Saunders' Manual of Small Animal Practice.* 3d ed. Philadelphia: Elsevier, 2006.

Downing, Robin. *Pets Living with Cancer: A Pet Owner's Resource.* Lakewood, Colo.: AAHA, 2000.

Eldredge, Debra M., and Margaret H. Bonham. *Cancer and Your Pet: The Complete Guide to the Latest Research, Treatments, and Options.* Sterling, Va.: Capital Books, 2005.

Ettinger, Stephen J., and Edward C. Feldman. "Section X: Cancer." In *Textbook of Veterinary Internal Medicine.* 6th ed. Philadelphia: Elsevier, 2005.

Meuten, Donald J., ed. *Tumors in Domestic Animals.* 4th ed. Malden, Mass.: Blackwell, 2002.

▶ **Organizations and Professional Societies**

American College of Veterinary Internal Medicine
http://www.acvim.org
1997 Wadsworth, Suite A
Lakewood, CO 80214-5293

American College of Veterinary Radiology
http://www.acvr.org
777 East Park Drive
P.O. Box 8820
Harrisburg, PA 17105-8820

American College of Veterinary Surgeons
http://www.acvs.org
19785 Crystal Rock Dr., Suite 305
Germantown, MD 20874

Veterinary Cancer Society
http://www.vetcancersociety.org
P.O. Box 1763
Spring Valley, CA 91979

▶ **Other Resources**

Morris Animal Foundation: Canine Cancer Campaign
http://www.curecaninecancer.org

NetVet Veterinary Resources
http://netvet.wustl.edu/vet.htm

Oncolink Vet
Types of Cancer
   http://www.oncolink.com/types/
   section.cfm?c=22&s=69

ThePetCenter.com
Cancer in Dogs and Cats
   http://www.thepetcenter.com/gen/can.html

Vaccine-Associated Feline Sarcoma Task Force
   http://www.avma.org/vafstf/contact.asp

See also Amputation; Arsenic compounds; Carcinomas; Chemotherapy; Imaging tests; Leukemias; Living with cancer; Medical oncology; Oncology; Pathology; Staging of cancer; Vaccines, preventive.

▶ Vinyl chloride

Category: Carcinogens and suspected carcinogens
RoC status: Known human carcinogen since 1980
Also known as: Chloroethene, chloroethylene, ethylene monochloride

Related cancers: Liver cancer, possibly brain and lung cancers

Definition: Vinyl chloride is a toxic, colorless, combustible gas that has a sweet odor.

Exposure routes: For the general public, exposure to vinyl chloride occurs through inhalation of contaminated air, ingestion of contaminated foods and drinking water, or skin contact with consumer products containing vinyl chloride. Occupational exposure occurs by inhalation or skin contact during the production or use of vinyl chloride.

Where found: More than 95 percent of all vinyl chloride is used to manufacture polyvinyl chloride (PVC) and copolymers. The rest is used in organic synthesis and miscellaneous applications. PVC, a plastic resin, is used in myriad applications, including pipes, automotive parts, furniture, electrical insulation, videodiscs, flooring, windows, toys, wrapping plastic, medical supplies, credit cards, and storage containers.

At risk: People who work where vinyl chloride is produced; where plastics, rubber, resins, PVC, furniture, or automotive parts are manufactured; or around railroad cars that carry vinyl chloride have a high risk for vinyl chloride contamination. People who live near industries that manufacture or use vinyl chloride in their products or who live near hazardous waste sites or landfills also risk exposure to vinyl chloride. Between 1958 and 1974, hair sprays contained vinyl chloride, causing beauty salon workers and hair spray users to be exposed.

Etiology and symptoms of associated cancers: Breathing high levels of vinyl chloride for short periods of time can cause dizziness, sleepiness, and unconsciousness. Extremely high levels over short periods of time can result in death. Breathing vinyl chloride over long periods of time can decrease blood flow to the hands, making hand bones brittle, and can produce permanent liver damage, nerve damage, immune reactions, and liver cancer. Exposure of the skin to vinyl chloride can produce numbness, redness, and blisters. Dioxins produced as by-products of vinyl chloride production and from burning waste PVC can suppress the immune system, cause a variety of cancers, and produce endometriosis.

History: Vinyl chloride has been in existence since at least the early part of the nineteenth century. It was first produced commercially in the 1920's. In the late 1960's vinyl chloride was definitely linked to liver cancer. It has become one of the highest-volume chemicals produced in the United States. Approximately 15 billion pounds of vinyl chloride were manufactured annually in the United States during the mid-1990's.

Alvin K. Benson, Ph.D.

See also Bisphenol A (BPA); Brain and central nervous system cancers; Bronchial adenomas; Carcinogens, known; Carcinogens, reasonably anticipated; Di(2-ethylhexyl) phthalate (DEHP); Dioxins; Endotheliomas; Fibrosarcomas, soft-tissue; Gliomas; Hemangiosarcomas; Liver cancers; Lung cancers; Occupational exposures and cancer; Organochlorines (OCs); Plasticizers; Sarcomas, soft-tissue.

▶ Viral oncology

Category: Medical specialties

Definition: Viral oncology is the study of cancers caused by viruses and other such infectious agents.

Cancers treated: Cancers known to be associated with viral agents, including cervical carcinoma, hepatocarcinoma, nasopharyngeal carcinoma, and several forms of lymphoma

Subspecialities: Retrovirology

Training and certification: Viral oncology represents a discipline within the general area of medical oncology, the study of cancer. Although a small proportion of cancers may be directly caused by infectious agents, particularly viruses, most oncologists associated with medical aspects of the disease are involved with the diagnosis and treatment of cancer rather than the study of the molecular basis of the disease. Certainly this is true for most physicians specializing in branches of oncology. Those physicians who both practice medical oncology and carry out research in the field of viral oncology are generally associated with medical schools that allow for research and study of the disease as well as diagnosis and treatment. These individuals divide their time between seeing patients and directing a laboratory that includes technicians and postdoctoral trainees.

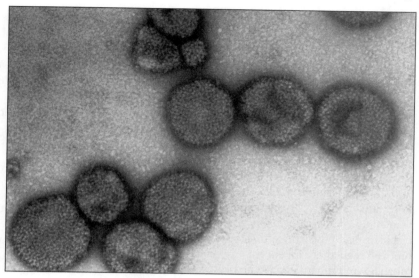

Tumor viruses. (Biophoto Associates/Photo Researchers, Inc.)

Viral oncology primarily involves research into the molecular changes produced by viral infections that transform normal cells into malignant ones. Training may involve either medical school, the outcome of which is a medical degree, or a research, which may result in a doctoral degree. Although postdoctoral training is not required, most people with doctorates in the sciences and an interest in cancer research, viral or otherwise, generally pursue additional training after receiving their degrees.

A number of universities and medical schools, supported by a variety of federal grants and fellowships, provide specialized training in the field of viral oncology. Generally these programs are postdoctoral, requiring either a medical or a doctoral degree. In these two- to three-year programs, the individual studies and carries out research with highly regarded individuals in the field. Training may be in any of a wide range of specialties, including the study of tumor viruses, pathogenesis following infection by these viruses, and the regulation of cell processes affected by such viruses. Those who complete such programs frequently move on to jobs at universities or medical schools, specializing in aspects of medical oncology.

Services and procedures performed: The primary concerns of physicians who deal with cancer are identifying the form, staging, treatment, and prognosis of cancer. Approximately 15 to 20 percent of cancers are associated with infections by viruses and other agents. Viral oncologists study cancers caused by viruses to understand the underlying molecular mechanisms that result in the initial transformation of a cell from a normal, properly regulated entity to one that progressively evolves into a malignant cell. They also develop therapeutic strategies to control the disease or prevent the transformation of normal cells into malignant ones. Viral oncologists may study samples obtained from cancerous tissue to determine the presence of or possible role played by the virus. Generally, however, they are not involved in the actual treatment of the disease.

The work carried out by viral oncologists depends on the interests of the individual. Some viruses leave "footprints" in the cell following infection: the presence of viral genetic material as well as the products—protein or ribonucleic acid (RNA)—encoded by the virus. The researcher may use either biopsy material or other cancerous tissue samples for analysis of viral information or evidence of viral expression. The results of such analysis may provide clues as to the mechanism of malignant transformation. Clues into the cause of the disease may provide ideas for research into treatment.

Treatment of virus-induced cancers may also involve clinical trials, in which pharmaceuticals may be studied to determine their efficacies. Most such studies involve cooperation between hospitals and pharmaceutical companies.

Related specialties and subspecialties: Viral oncologists specialize in the specific forms of cancers that may follow certain viral infections. Human papillomaviruses (HPV), associated in the mind of many with warts, have also been shown to be the etiological agents behind development of cervical carcinomas. The study of these deoxyribonucleic acid (DNA)-containing viruses and the mechanism by which they initiate cancer represent a field of active investigation among some virologists.

Retroviruses are a subclass of viruses that contain a genome consisting of RNA. These are relatively simple viruses that encode a relatively small number of genes, often as few as four to five, one of which is considered an oncogene, a gene that when unregulated may convert a normal cell into a malignant one. These viruses also encode an enzyme called an RNA-directed DNA polymerase, more commonly called a reverse transcriptase, which copies the RNA genome into DNA. The DNA copy then integrates into the host genome. Such viruses are frequently called RNA tumor viruses. Retrovirologists are viral oncologists who study such viruses, their genome makeup, and the mechanisms by which their encoded oncogene may disrupt cell regulation. Like most viral oncologists, retrovirologists are primarily concerned with the mechanism of malignant transformation rather than the treatment of patients.

A subclass of retroviruses includes agents such as hepatitis B virus (HBV), associated with certain forms of viral hepatitis, but which may also serve as the etiological agent for hepatocarcinoma, cancer of the liver. HBV is a DNA virus but one that replicates through an RNA intermediary. HBV also is the subject of extensive study by retrovirologists interested in this unusual form of replication. Some universities and medical schools provide specialized programs in this area. For example, because hepatitis B infection often results in a lifelong chronic infection, viral oncologists may specialize not only in the study of the disease but also in the maintenence of quality care for the patient and education of the patient's family.

Some forms of lymphomas and leukemias also appear to be the result of viral infections, including T-lymphocyte leukemia. Evidence suggests Hodgkin disease may be the result of viral infection. Certain non-Hodgkin lymphomas are known to be associated with infection. For example, both Burkitt lymphoma and nasopharyngeal carcinoma are the result of infection by a type of herpesvirus called the Epstein-Barr virus, which is most commonly associated with infectious mononucleosis. Subspecialties in the field of viral oncology exist for the study of these diseases as well.

Richard Adler, Ph.D.

▶ For Further Information

Boshoff, Chris, and Robin Weiss. *Kaposi Sarcoma Herpesvirus: New Perspectives.* New York: Springer-Verlag, 2006.

Pitot, Henry. *Fundamentals of Oncology.* 4th ed. New York: Marcel Dekker, 2002.

Strauss, James, and Ellen Strauss. *Viruses and Human Disease.* 2d ed. Burlington, Mass.: Elsevier Academic Press, 2008.

Tannock, Ian, et al. *The Basic Science of Oncology.* Columbus, Ohio: McGraw-Hill, 2005.

▶ Organizations and Professional Societies

American Society for Microbiology
http://www.asm.org
1752 N Street, NW
Washington, D.C. 20036

American Society for Virology
http://www.asv.org
University of Toledo College of Medicine
3000 Arlington Avenue, Mail Stop 1021
Toledo, OH 43614

▶ Other Resources

Fred Hutchinson Cancer Research Center
Virology Laboratory Core
http://www.fhcrc.org/science/clinical/id/research/vlc.html

National Cancer Institute
Center of Excellence in HIV/AIDS and Cancer
Virology, CCR
http://ccr.cancer.gov/initiatives/CEHIV

See also Antiviral therapies; Burkitt lymphoma; Carcinomas; Cervical cancer; Epstein-Barr virus; Hepatitis B virus (HBV); Hepatitis C virus (HCV); HIV/AIDS-related cancers; Hodgkin disease; Human papillomavirus (HPV); Infection and sepsis; Kaposi sarcoma; Leukemias; Lymphomas; Non-Hodgkin lymphoma; Oncogenes; Oncogenic viruses; Oncology; Proto-oncogenes and carcinogenesis; Virus-related cancers.

▶ Virus-related cancers

Category: Diseases, symptoms, and conditions

Related conditions: Cervical cancer, hepatocarcinoma, Kaposi sarcoma, T-cell lymphomas, B-cell lymphomas

Definition: Cancer is a malignant disease characterized by uncontrolled growth of anaplastic cells that invade or spread into sites beyond their origin. While most human cancers are the product of genetic mutations, some cancers are the result of infection by viruses.

A Primer on Viruses

A virus consists of nucleic acid, either ribonucleic acid (RNA) or deoxyribonucleic acid (DNA), inside a protein coat, or capsid, which is enclosed in an outer membrane. On its own, a virus cannot replicate itself.

To infect a person, a virus must first find a way into the individual. Usually, this is not through the skin but rather the mouth, lungs, penis, vagina, gastrointestinal tract, or breaks in the skin (wounds, sores). The virus attaches to its host cell and injects genetic material. The cell begins to make viral DNA or RNA and produces viral proteins instead of its usual products. The host cell creates new viruses, which are released, destroying the host cell. The new viruses find other cells and begin the process anew.

Retroviruses, like the human immunodeficiency virus (HIV), have RNA in a protein capsid with a lipid envelope that contains receptor-binding proteins used to attach to the host cell. The retrovirus injects RNA plus the enzyme reverse transcriptase (Rtase) into the cell. This allows the cell to make viral DNA, then a complementary strand of DNA. The double-strand copies of DNA become part of the host cell's chromosome.

Risk factors: Viruses associated with cancer—human immunodeficiency virus (HIV) and hepatitis B and C viruses (HBV, HCV)—are most commonly spread through sexual relations or contamination of intravenous fluids. The pooling of blood fluids for isolation of the clotting factor VIII during the early years of the acquired immunodeficiency syndrome (AIDS) epidemic was the primary factor in the infection of hemophiliacs with HIV. Unprotected sexual relations with infected partners and intravenous drug use, in which infected users shared needles, also transmitted HIV and the hepatitis viruses. The human papillomavirus (HPV), the etiological agent for cervical carcinoma, is commonly transmitted by infected sexual partners.

Etiology and the disease process: Most human cancers are not infectious in that they are not the direct result of microbial infection. However, certain groups of viruses have long been known to be associated with malignancies in animals, and several members of these groups have been shown to cause certain human cancers. Viruses can cause genetic changes in oncogenes—genes that directly regulate cell division such as growth factors and their receptors, signal mechanisms, and tumor suppressors—and disrupt regulation of cell growth. However, people can be infected with these viruses and not develop cancer, so how they become activated is unknown.

More than one hundred types of human papillomaviruses have been identified, of which about half are capable of causing cervical cancer. Some 75 percent of cervical cancer cases are associated with three serotypes of HPV. Three genes encoded by these viruses appear to be linked to the disease, the most important of which is known as *E7*. The *E7* gene product inhibits tumor-suppressor proteins such as the retinoblastoma (Rb) molecule, a protein that regulates the steps necessary for cell replication. Infection of cervical cells by these strains of the virus may eventually result in uncontrolled growth and a malignancy.

Hepatocellular carcinoma (liver cancer) is among the most common cancers worldwide and has been shown to result from infection with the hepatitis B virus (HBV) and less commonly the hepatitis C virus (HCV). Both HBV and HCV are associated with potentially severe forms of liver disease, and a person with a chronic hepatitis infection or a long-term carrier may eventually develop liver cancer. Little is understood as to how infection results in cancer, as no viral protein having oncogenic ability has been described. However, one protein encoded by HBV, the *X* gene product, appears to bind the p53 protein, a tumor-suppressor molecule that regulates activation of genes associated with cell division. The core protein of HCV has also been shown to bind p53, suggesting tumor induction in a similar manner.

Kaposi sarcoma is believed to be caused by human herpesvirus 8 (HHV-8), which produces gene products that induce cell replication. Classic Kaposi sarcoma, a rare form of the disease not associated with HIV infection, appears to involve both viral and genetic factors. The population at risk for this form of Kaposi sarcoma appears to be limited to men from the Mediterranean region, indicating a possible genetic link, but HHV-8 infection may also play a role.

A variety of B-cell and T-cell lymphomas are also associated with viral infections. The human T-cell lymphotropic virus (HTLV) has been shown to be the etiological agent for certain forms of T-cell disease. T-cell lymphomas resulting from HTLV infection are most commonly found in southern Japan, Africa, and portions of the Caribbean. About 5 percent of persons infected by HTLV develop cancer. The mechanism by which cancer is induced is unclear but appears to involve a disruption of the cell's signaling mechanism, which regulates cell replication.

There are numerous non-Hodgkin lymphomas (NHLs), some of which are associated with viral infection. The Epstein-Barr virus (EBV), a member of the herpesvirus family, is the etiological agent behind Burkitt lymphoma, an illness in which malaria is a cofactor, and nasopharyngeal carcinoma, an illness found among those whose ancestry can be traced to southern China. The precise mechanism by which EBV infection results in cancer is unclear but appears to involve a translocation event with the cell chromosome, activating a cellular oncogene.

Incidence: Incidence rates for virus-related cancers vary widely by virus and affected site. Incidence rates for cancers that have viral and nonviral causes are generally not broken down by cause.

Approximately 500,000 cases of cervical cancer are reported annually worldwide. In the United States, cervical cancer accounts for some 5,000 deaths each year. Incidence rates in the United States are about 7 per 100,000 women per year.

Liver cancer is estimated to result in 500,000 deaths worldwide each year. Liver cancers account for one-quarter of all cancers in developing countries. In Africa and Southeast Asia, the incidence rate is 20 per 100,000 people, while in the United States, it is about 5 per 100,000 people. Most of these cases result from infection by HBV, though HCV has been shown to be increasingly associated with cases of liver cancer. A precise number is unavailable, since the extent of HCV in the population is unknown; however, studies from Japan have found HCV in 75 percent of cases of liver cancer. Most cases of liver cancer in the United States are found in immigrant populations from areas in which the disease is endemic.

An increasing number of cases of Kaposi sarcoma began to appear in the late 1980's as a result of the AIDS epidemic. Incidence rates grew to 9.5 per 100,000 men in 1989 and fell to 1.3 in 2005.

In the United States, non-Hodgkin lymphomas (all types) are the fifth most common forms of cancer, with an incidence rate of about 20 per 100,000 people per year.

Symptoms: Symptoms of virus-related cancers vary depending on the site affected. For cervical cancer, the early stages are generally asymptomatic, and as the disease progresses, women experience unusual vaginal bleeding or pain.

For liver cancer, the symptoms include abdominal pain, unexplained weight loss, and a sudden onset of jaundice. A physician performing a physical examination will usually find an enlarged and tender liver and can hear turbulent bloodflow through the liver because it has an extensive vascular system. Blood tests may reveal elevation of certain liver proteins such as alpha-fetoprotein.

The first symptoms of Kaposi sarcoma are generally purplish lesions or nodules on or under the skin or mucous membranes.

Symptoms of lymphomas are general, usually mani-

festing as swollen lymph nodes, fever, or unexplained weight loss.

Screening and diagnosis: A standard screening test exists for cervical cancer, but the other virus-related cancers do not have routine screening procedures.

Early diagnosis of cervical cancer results from the observation of abnormal cervical cells following a Pap test. Although not all abnormal-appearing cells are cancerous, their presence may indicate a precancerous state. A colposcopy, the visual observation of the cervix, may help the physician in deciding whether to perform a biopsy. As with most cancers, the extent of the disease is the basis for staging.

If a patient's symptoms suggest liver cancer, the physician will investigate further, using a variety of imaging scans. Ultrasound is generally the first choice because it is noninvasive and easily performed. This may be followed up with a computed tomography (CT) scan or magnetic resonance imaging (MRI). Ultimately, a biopsy is necessary to confirm the cancer. Staging of liver cancer is based on the size of the tumor and the extent of spread.

Kaposi sarcoma is diagnosed by taking the patient's history and examining the skin for the lesions typical of the disease. Biopsies are performed to confirm the disease, and imaging tests are used to find lesions in the stomach or lungs. Because Kaposi sarcoma is AIDS related, its staging is based on the extent of the tumor, the state of the immune system, and the amount of systemic illness.

Non-Hodgkin lymphoma is commonly diagnosed by biopsy of an enlarged lymph node that does not respond to antibiotic treatment. If cancer is found in the sample, imaging tests such as X ray, CT scans, MRI, and positron emission tomography (PET) scans can help determine how much the cancer has spread. Staging for non-Hodgkin lymphoma uses the Ann Arbor system, which is based on the degree of spread. In addition, two prognostic systems, one for slow-growing and one for fast-growing lymphomas, have been developed. These systems attempt to describe a patient's risk of dying and help physicians select appropriate courses of treatment.

Treatment and therapy: Treatment for virus-related cancers varies depending on the site but generally involves surgery, radiation therapy, chemotherapy, or a combination of therapies.

Treatment of cervical cancer generally starts with surgery to remove as much cancerous tissue as safely possible. Additional treatments depend on the stage of the disease. Radiation therapy may be external or internal using a radioactive implant. Chemotherapy, usually intravenous, is recommended if metastasis has occurred.

A small liver tumor can be removed surgically. Historically, a liver transplant had been recommended for most forms of liver cancer, though later it was determined that such a radical approach might not be necessary in the absence of extensive involvement. Extensive liver cancer may require chemotherapy, though other approaches have also been shown to be useful. Transarterial chemoembolization (TACE), the embolization of tumor blood vessels using a gel or coil; radiofrequency ablation (RFA), the insertion of an electrical probe directly into the tumor, followed by ablation of the tissue; and proton beam therapy have all been shown to be useful in reducing the size of localized tumors.

Treatment of Kaposi sarcoma depends on the extent of the tumor and can involve either surgical removal or radiation therapy and chemotherapy.

Non-Hodgkin lymphoma in HIV-infected patients is complicated by the patients' low blood cell counts, although the use of highly active antiretroviral therapy has made it easier for patients to endure chemotherapy.

Prognosis, prevention, and outcomes: Prognosis and prevention of virus-related cancers varies depending on the specific cancer and virus. Prevention generally involves attempting to avoid the spread of viruses that cause cancers. The screening of donated blood has reduced the risk of viral infection through transfusion. Safe-sex practices (such as condom use) help prevent the spread of sexually transmitted viruses such as HPV, HIV, HBV, and HCV. Efforts have been made to educate intravenous drug users about the dangers of sharing needles and thereby spreading viruses. Vaccines have been developed for HBV and HPV. The HBV vaccine can prevent most infections by this virus. Since 80 percent of cases of liver cancer are associated with this virus, immunization should reduce the incidence rate. In 2006, a vaccine for HPV, Gardasil, was approved by the U.S. Food and Drug Administration. While the long-term results of vaccine use are unknown and questions as to its efficacy still exist, it is hoped that early immunization for HPV may serve to protect women against most forms of the virus.

The prognosis for patients with cervical cancer depends on the stage of the disease and its response to therapy. Early diagnosis can result in the elimination of the disease, while once metastasis has taken place, the outcome becomes increasingly poor.

Liver cancer is curable if caught early and the tumor removed. None of the techniques used to treat advanced cancer is effective long-term, and the prognosis for patients with advanced liver cancer remains poor, with death generally resulting within a year of diagnosis.

The prognosis for those with HIV-related Kaposi sarcoma is improving because of better treatments for AIDS patients. If detected early, the five-year survival rate can reach 90 percent; however, if the disease has reached the lungs, the survival rate drops to 30 percent. Similarly, the outlook for HIV-infected patients with lymphoma depends largely on how well their AIDS is controlled.

Richard Adler, Ph.D.

▶ **For Further Information**

Fields, Bruce, ed. *Fields Virology*. Philadelphia: Lippincott-Raven, 1996.

Grand, J. A., ed. *Viruses, Cell Transformation, and Cancer*. New York: Elsevier, 2001.

Pelengaris, Stella, and Michael Khan, eds. *The Molecular Biology of Cancer*. Malden, Mass.: Blackwell, 2006.

Strauss, James, and Ellen Strauss. *Viruses and Human Disease*. New York: Academic Press, 2002.

Tabor, Edward, ed. *Viruses and Liver Cancer*. New York: Elsevier, 2006.

▶ **Other Resources**

American Cancer Society
http://cancer.org

The Leukemia and Lymphoma Organization
http://www.leukemia-lymphoma.org

National Cancer Institute
http://www.cancer.gov

See also Antiviral therapies; Burkitt lymphoma; Carcinomas; Cervical cancer; Epstein-Barr virus; Hepatitis B virus (HBV); Hepatitis C virus (HCV); HIV/AIDS-related cancers; Human papillomavirus (HPV); Infection and sepsis; Kaposi sarcoma; Leukemias; Liver cancers; Lymphomas; Retinoblastomas; Vaccines, preventive; Viral oncology.

▶ Von Hippel-Lindau (VHL) disease

Category: Diseases, symptoms, and conditions
Also known as: Von Hippel-Lindau syndrome, angiomatosis retinae

Related conditions: Renal cysts; clear cell form of renal cell carcinoma; hemangioblastomas of the brain, spinal cord, and retina; pheochromocytoma; endolymphatic sac tumors

Definition: A hereditary cancer syndrome, von Hippel-Lindau (VHL) disease is associated with renal cell carcinoma (kidney cancer); pheochromocytoma (an adrenal gland tumor that releases stress hormones); catecholamine-secreting paraganglioma (a tumor that releases stress hormones like a pheochromocytoma but is located outside the adrenal gland); hemangioblastomas (blood vessel tumors) of the brain, spinal cord, and retina; neuroendocrine tumors (nerve-cell tumors that may produce hormones) of the pancreas; and endolymphatic sac tumors (inner ear tumors). Approximately 40 percent of individuals with VHL develop renal cell carcinoma, which is the leading cause of VHL-associated death. Several distinct clinical presentations of VHL have been described based on the risk for pheochromocytoma and renal cell carcinoma. The types of tumors and the severity of the disease vary within and between families.

Risk factors: Because von Hippel-Lindau disease is hereditary, the main risk factor is having a family history of this syndrome. Each child of a person with von Hippel-Lindau disease has a 50 percent chance of inheriting the disease.

Etiology and the disease process: The underlying genetic cause of von Hippel-Lindau disease is a mutation, or a genetic change, in the *VHL* gene. Normally, the protein made by the *VHL* gene acts as a tumor suppressor, which means that it helps stop uncontrolled cell growth and proliferation. Mutations in the *VHL* gene either prevent the protein from being made or cause the protein to be made incorrectly, which leads to the multistep process of tumorigenesis (formation or production of tumors).

Usually, each person has two normal copies of the *VHL* gene. A mutation in one copy of the gene is sufficient to cause von Hippel-Lindau disease, which is why this condition is referred to as autosomal dominant (autosomal means the *VHL* gene is located on one of the twenty-two pairs of autosomes, which are the non-sex chromosomes). A person with von Hippel-Lindau disease has a *VHL* gene mutation from the time of conception in the womb; however, symptoms of the disease may not manifest until later in life. Symptoms can occur before the age of five, and nearly all people with a *VHL* gene mutation have symptoms of the disease by the age of sixty-five.

Different types of mutations in the *VHL* gene lead to different clinical presentations. Therefore, a person with von Hippel-Lindau disease may be more likely to have pheochromocytoma, renal cell carcinoma, or both.

Incidence: Approximately 1 in 36,000 people has von Hippel-Lindau disease. Some 80 percent of people with von Hippel-Lindau disease inherit the disease from a parent, but 20 percent of people with the disease have a new gene mutation, meaning the mutation occurs for the first time in that individual.

Symptoms: Symptoms depend on where the tumors are located. Hemangioblastomas of the brain or spinal cord can cause headaches, vomiting, coordination problems, and walking difficulties. Retinal (eye) hemangioblastomas can lead to vision problems. Pheochromocytomas and catecholamine-secreting paragangliomas release catecholamines (stress hormones) that can cause dangerously high blood-pressure levels. Neuroendocrine tumors of the pancreas usually do not produce hormones and may have no associated symptoms. Tumors of the endolymphatic sac can result in deafness, which may occur suddenly and be severe to profound.

Screening and diagnosis: Von Hippel-Lindau disease is clinically diagnosed in a person who has two or more tumors associated with this condition. However, if a person has a family history of the disease, just one of the characteristic findings is needed to make a diagnosis. Tools used to check for disease include computed tomography (CT) or magnetic resonance imaging (MRI) to look for pheochromocytomas, endolymphatic sac tumors, or tumors of the brain and spinal cord. Ultrasound or CT may be used to examine the kidneys and pancreas, and urine testing may be done to check for catecholamines and metanephrines released by pheochromocytomas or paragangliomas. Ophthalmologic examination (an eye exam) is performed to check for retinal hemangioblastomas.

Because von Hippel-Lindau disease is caused by mutations in the *VHL* gene, genetic testing is a valuable tool to confirm a suspected diagnosis or to test a family member who is at risk for the disease but has no symptoms. Genetic testing detects nearly 100 percent of *VHL* gene mutations.

Treatment and therapy: The main focus of treatment for von Hippel-Lindau disease is surgery to remove tumors. Early surgery offers the best outcome for most of the tumors associated with von Hippel-Lindau disease, including renal cell carcinoma. Renal cell carcinoma may also be treated with chemotherapy, radiation therapy, ablation therapy (using probes to destroy the tumor with heat or cold), biological therapy (using the patient's immune system to fight the cancer), and targeted therapy (using drugs that attack cancer cells without damaging normal cells).

Prognosis, prevention, and outcomes: Because von Hippel-Lindau disease is a genetic condition, its manifestations cannot be prevented. However, monitoring of individuals who are at risk for the disease based on their family history or who are known to have a *VHL* gene mutation can detect problems early and lead to more effective treatment and better outcomes. Such monitoring includes yearly ophthalmologic screening, yearly blood pressure checks, yearly urine testing for catecholamines and metanephrines, yearly abdominal ultrasounds, periodic MRI of the brain and spinal cord, and hearing evaluation if symptoms of hearing loss are present. The medical team caring for patients decides the age at which monitoring should start.

Abbie L. Abboud, M.S., C.G.C.

▶ **For Further Information**

Linehan, W. M., B. Zbar, and D. R. Klausner. "Renal Carcinoma." In *The Metabolic and Molecular Bases of Inherited Disease*, edited by Charles R. Scriver, Arthur L. Beaudet, David Valle, and William S. Sly. 8th ed. New York: McGraw-Hill, 2001.

Molino, D., J. Sepe, P. Anastasio, and N. G. De Santo. "The History of Von Hippel-Lindau Disease." *Journal of Nephrology* 10 (2006): S119-S123.

Woodward, E. R., and E. R. Maher. "Von Hippel-Lindau Disease and Endocrine Tumour Susceptibility." *Endocrine Related Cancer* 32 (2006): 415-425.

▶ **Other Resources**

Genetics Home Reference
Von Hippel-Lindau Syndrome
http://ghr.nlm.nih.gov/
condition=vonhippellindausyndrome

Kidney Cancer Association
http://www.kidneycancer.org

VHL Family Alliance
http://www.vhl.org

See also Brain and central nervous system cancers; Hemangioblastomas; Hereditary leiomyomatosis and renal cell cancer (HLRCC); Hereditary non-VHL clear cell renal cell carcinomas; Islet cell tumors; Kidney cancer; Pheochromocytomas; Renal pelvis tumors; Spinal axis tumors; Urinary system cancers.

▶ **Vulvar cancer**

Category: Diseases, symptoms, and conditions
Also known as: Vulvar carcinoma

Related conditions: Human papillomavirus (HPV), vaginal cancer, vaginal intraepithelial neoplasia (VAIN), vulvar intraepithelial neoplasia, malignant melanoma, squamous cell carcinoma, Paget disease, adenocarcinoma, verrucous carcinoma, basal cell carcinoma, Bowen disease

Age at Diagnosis of Vulvar Cancer, 1988-2001

Age Group	Cases Diagnosed (%)
20-29	1.2
30-39	5.2
40-49	11.9
50-59	12.4
60-69	16.5
70-79	26.9
80 and older	25.8

Source: Data from L. A. G. Ries et al., eds., *Cancer Survival Among Adults: U.S. SEER Program, 1988-2001—Patient and Tumor Characteristics*, NIH Pub. No. 07-6215 (Bethesda, Md.: National Cancer Institute, 2007)

Definition: Vulvar cancer is the name for malignant growths that originate from the vulva, the visible part of the female external genitalia. The vulva is the collective term for the labia majora, labia minora, clitoris, and perineum. The parts of the vulva are similar in tissue type, which suggests the cancers that can arise from them. The most common tissue type is squamous cell, which makes up the lining of many organs such as the skin and mucous membranes of the vagina and mouth. This type accounts for about 90 percent of all types of vulvar cancer. Individual cells from this type of carcinoma appear flattened, immature, disordered, multilayered, and with dark-staining nuclei on light microscopy. The second most common type is melanoma, which is derived from the pigment cells of the skin (melanocytes). Other, less common types include Paget disease of the vulva, sometimes associated with adenocarcinoma and verrucous, Bartholin gland and basal cell carcinomas.

Risk factors: The risk factors for acquiring vulvar cancer include older age, smoking, age of first sexual intercourse less than nineteen years, having more than two sexual partners, and low socioeconomic status. Abnormal Pap smears, long-standing vulvar dystrophy associated with diabetes, a compromised immune system, exposure to herpes simplex virus 2 (HSV2) and human papillomavirus (HPV) types 16 or 18 are also risk factors. Vulvar cancer has also been associated with a prior history of cervical or vaginal cancer. Precursor lesions such as lichen sclerosis and vulvar intraepithelial neoplasia grade III may also be risk factors.

Etiology and the disease process: As with most cancers, the development of vulvar cancer is closely linked to damage to deoxyribonucleic acid (DNA) and the mechanisms that regulate cell division, particularly the *TP53* tumor-suppressor gene. Multiple factors accumulate and contribute to the probability of inducing a cell to become cancerous. Toxic substances in cigarette smoke or replicating viral DNA that is spliced with cell DNA can cause damage to replicating or unwound DNA in tissue with high cell turnover and division (such as that in the skin and intestinal tract). Replication errors can also occur in aging cells.

Incidence: Vulvar cancer occurs in about 1 percent of all women. However, the proportion of vulvar cancer occurring in women under the age of fifty has increased by almost a factor of ten over twenty years.

Symptoms: Persistent itching of the vulva in an elderly woman with involvement of the surrounding skin, with or without the presence of a vulvar lesion, may be the first sign of vulvar cancer, as it is associated with increased proliferation of vulvar tissue. The itching may have been previously treated but unsuccessfully. The patient may have a wartlike lesion, lump, or an ulcer that has appeared and has been recalcitrant to treatment. A mass in or near the groin area that persists even after antibiotic treatment can be suggestive of cancer that has spread to the lymph

Treatment for genital warts on the vulva, probably caused by HPV. Some types of this virus are suspected of causing cancer. (LifeART© 2008 Wolters Kluwer Health, Inc.-Lippincott Williams & Wilkins. All rights reserved.)

nodes draining the vulvar area. Many clinical situations can preclude this, including more common etiologies of an infectious origin. Physical examination of the vulva may also be nominal in early-stage vulvar cancer. However, an irregularly shaped, changing and persistent ulcer or solid mass that may or may not be movable in the vulvar area, accompanied by a suggestive clinical history, increases the probability of cancer.

Screening and diagnosis: There is no screening test for vulvar cancer. However, if a lesion on the vulva does not respond to treatments for common etiologies, a wedge biopsy—removal of lesions less than 2 centimeters (cm) at greatest breadth with a margin of normal skin and underlying stroma—should be performed to confirm the diagnosis. Care must be taken to ensure groin lymph nodes are truly absent, as their presence can alter disease management. The margin of normal tissue is necessary to assess the microscopic extent of the cancer and correctly stage the cancer. The diagnosis of vulvar cancer is confirmed when microscopic examination of the cells and tissue architecture shows changes characteristic of cancer cells. In addition, the gross specimen is evaluated in terms of depth of penetration of the lesion into the stroma and its widest visible breadth.

Because of the possibility of microscopic spread to other organs, other diagnostic tests may include a cervical Pap smear, vaginal and cervical colposcopy to look for other lesions, pelvic computed tomography (CT) scan or magnetic resonance imagery (MRI) that includes the groin area to look for enlarged lymph nodes that were missed in the physical examination, a chest X ray, and blood tests before surgery.

The International Federation of Gynecology and Obstetrics (FIGO) uses the following surgical staging system to classify the severity of vulvar cancer by tumor size, lymph node involvement, and the presence or absence of distal metastasis:

• Stage 0: Carcinoma in situ or preinvasive carcinoma

• Stage I: Vulvar cancer is confined to the vulva or vulva and perineum and measures 2 cm or less at greatest breadth.

• Stage II: Vulvar cancer is confined to the vulva or both the vulva and perineum and measures greater than 2 cm at greatest breadth.

- Stage III: Invasive vulvar cancer has encroached into the lower urethra, vagina, or anus or has spread to corresponding right- or left-draining lymph nodes.
- Stage IV: Invasive vulvar cancer has encroached into the bladder mucosa, rectal mucosa, or upper urethral mucosa or is fixed to underlying bone, involves bilateral lymph nodes, or has invaded other, distant organs starting from the pelvic lymph nodes.

Surgical staging is not complete until the furthest extent of spread is evaluated, and it does not change afterward with treatment.

Treatment and therapy: For cancer confined within the epithelium or precancerous lesions such as vulvar intra-epithelial neoplasia located on the lateral aspect of the labia majora outward, local excision of vulvar epithelium with a 0.5 to 1.0 cm margin is warranted. Lesions of the labia minora inward may be amenable to local excision, with laser ablation as an alternative. For Stage IA lesions that are 2.0 cm or less in breadth and less than 1.0 millimeter (mm) in depth, wide local excision is recommended.

There are essentially two procedures used in treatment of vulvar cancer beyond Stage IA: wide surgical excision of the lesion, surrounding vulvae, and perineal area; and dissection and biopsy of inguinal lymph nodes at the femoral region of the thigh. During the 1960's, a conservatory approach to radical vulvectomy that involved preservation of as much normal tissue as possible and separate right and left inguinal incisions to dissect lymph nodes was adapted and became the standard approach. Bulky tumors that encroach into adjacent organs preclude conservation, where diseased areas are excised while preserving functionality where feasible.

Postoperative radiation therapy may be warranted in Stage III and IV vulvar cancer if surgical intervention was insufficient to address spread into the vagina, bladder, urethra, rectum, or microscopic spread of tumor cells to neighboring lymph nodes.

Prognosis, prevention, and outcomes: The overall five-year survival rate of women with vulvar cancer approaches 70 percent. Earlier diagnosis means a higher survival rate: Being in Stage I at diagnosis correlates with a survival rate of 96 percent; Stage II, 85 percent; Stage III, 74 percent; and Stage IV, 31 percent. When lymph node status is considered, positive nodes have a 52.4 percent survival rate regardless of stage. Positive pelvic lymph nodes have an 11 percent survival rate.

Preventive measures include modification of risk factors and early detection of disease. Smoking cessation, practice of safe sexual behaviors, and good hygiene are recommended. Yearly Pap smears, visual inspection of the vulvar area, and biopsy of suspicious lesions are also advised. Vaccination with the HPV vaccine has also been seen to deter the development of precancerous lesions.

Aldo C. Dumlao, M.D.

▶ **For Further Information**

Byers, Tim, Susan J. Curry, Maria Elizabeth Hewitt, and the National Cancer Policy Board. *Fulfilling the Potential of Cancer Prevention and Early Detection.* Washington, D.C.: National Academies Press, 2003.

Ko, A., E. H. Rosenbaum, and M. Dollinger. *Everyone's Guide to Cancer Therapy: How Cancer Is Diagnosed, Treated, and Managed Day to Day.* 5th ed. Kansas City, Mo.: Andrews McMeel, 2007.

Morra, Marion E., and Eve Potts. *Choices.* 4th ed. New York: HarperCollins, 2003.

▶ **Other Resources**

American Cancer Society
Detailed Guide: Vulvar Cancer
http://www.cancer.org/docroot/cri/content/
cri_2_4_3x_how_is_vulvar_cancer_diagnosed.asp

American College of Obstetrics and Gynecologists
http://www.acog.org

National Cancer Institute
Vulvar Cancer
http://www.cancer.gov/cancertopics/types/vulvar

See also Adenocarcinomas; Adenoid cystic carcinoma (ACC); Basal cell carcinomas; Bowen disease; Cervical cancer; Gynecologic cancers; Gynecologic oncology; Herpes simplex virus; Human papillomavirus (HPV); Infectious cancers; Pelvic examination; Sexuality and cancer; Vaccines, preventive; Vaginal cancer.

▶ Waldenström macroglobulinemia (WM)

Category: Diseases, symptoms, and conditions
Also known as: Lymphoplasmacytic lymphoma, Waldenström's macroglobulinemia

Related conditions: Multiple myeloma

Definition: Waldenström macroglobulinemia (WM) is a slow-growing form of non-Hodgkin lymphoma distinguished by a significantly elevated level of immunoglobulin-M (IgM) in the blood, often leading to hyperviscosity (thickening) of the blood. The disease was named for Jan Gosta Waldenström, a Swedish physician who identified "monoclonal gammopathy" in patients experiencing a thickening of their serum (1944). In a 1961 report, he described two patients with bleeding from the gums and nose, high platelet count, low red blood cell count (anemia), high sedimentation rate, and swollen lymph nodes. He ruled out multiple myeloma based on bone marrow biopsy tests and a lack of bone pain. In the serum he found a large amount of a single, unknown globulin (protein) with an extremely high molecular weight (macroglobulin). This macroglobulin is now known as IgM.

Risk factors: Researchers have found few risk factors for WM. At least some cases of WM (up to 20 percent) are familial, being passed from generation to generation. For others the cause is unknown. There is some evidence that infection with the hepatitis C virus may increase the incidence of WM in some individuals, as does prior diagnosis with monoclonal gammopathy of undetermined significance. Being older, white, and a man are known risk factors. None of these risk factors is controllable, so prevention remains elusive.

Etiology and the disease process: B cells are an important part of the immune system of the human body. They are the antibody-secreting cells that are a principal part of the adaptive immune system (which creates immunity for specific invaders, such as bacteria, viruses, and so on). There are five types of antibody (immunoglobulin or Ig) secreted by B cells: IgA, IgD, IgE, IgG, and IgM. Of these, IgM is by far the largest (approximately 900,000 Daltons), hence the name "macroglobulin." Some B cells circulate throughout the blood, while others reside in the lymph nodes of the body. Immature B cells are found in the bone marrow.

The lymph nodes are small, pea-sized collections of immune system cells (B cells, T cells, and macrophages) found in recognizable locations throughout the body. The predominant nodes are in the underarm area, the groin, both sides of the neck, the chest, and the abdomen. Small amounts of lymphoid tissue are also found in the digestive tract and the respiratory system.

For unknown reasons, early B cells, predominantly in the bone marrow, can multiply out of control. As they do this, they can crowd out the normal red blood cell production, leading to a low blood cell count. As they mature and circulate, these B cells secrete much larger amounts of IgM than normal. This leads to hyperviscosity (thickening of the serum) as more and more large protein is secreted and trapped in the bloodstream. Other symptoms, such as swelling of the lymph nodes and other parts of the immune system, are also related to the overpopulation of B cells and the overproduction of this macroglobulin.

The cancerous cells found in individuals with WM are similar to those found in people suffering from multiple myeloma (cancer of plasma cells) and non-Hodgkin lymphomas (cancer of lymphocytes, including B cells). The cancer cells of WM are lymphoplasmacytoid, similar to both plasma cells and lymphocytes. These are the cells that secrete the large amounts of IgM and create the various symptoms of the disease.

Incidence: Approximately 1,500 new cases are confirmed each year in the United States. The incidence is higher in whites than in blacks or Latinos, and higher in men than in women. The chance of developing this disease increases with age (mostly because of its slow nature), with the median age of diagnosis at sixty-three. It is very rare in people under the age of fifty but has been reported as early as age twenty-seven.

Symptoms: Many patients are asymptomatic; in others the symptoms vary widely. The most common symptoms of WM are weakness, swollen lymph nodes, swollen liver or spleen, severe fatigue (often the result of severe anemia), low appetite and weight loss, and bleeding from the gums and nose (often the first signs of increased platelet activity). In addition, many patients experience visual problems (most likely due to bleeding of the small blood vessels inside the eyes) or neurological problems (dizziness, headache, vertigo), probably caused by slowed circulation of blood to the brain.

Pain or numbness in the extremities may also be noted, a sign of early nerve damage. Heart problems often arise as a result of damage caused to the heart muscle by the high levels of IgM and because the heart has to work extra hard to pump the very thick blood through the body. Symptoms can vary widely depending on the severity of the disease and the amount of IgM being secreted. None of these symptoms by themselves are diagnostic of WM, since they are also found in many other cancers and noncancerous diseases.

Screening and diagnosis: There are no tests available that can screen for early WM. When signs and symptoms first appear, diagnosis can generally be made based on blood and urine tests along with a bone marrow biopsy or fine needle aspiration biopsy. Tests of blood viscosity are extremely important, as are measurements of the amount of IgM and other immunoglobulins in the serum.

There is no standard staging system for WM (as there is for most other cancers). The amount of lymphoplasmacytoid cells in the bone marrow, the degree of anemia, the degree of viscosity, and age of the patient are all used to determine prognosis.

Treatment and therapy: Although there is no cure for WM, there are several treatments that can help to control the symptoms. Since this is a slow-growing type of cancer, there is no rush to start treatment immediately upon diagnosis. Treatments are generally aimed at relieving symptoms, which vary tremendously from one individual to an-

other. The decision about which treatment to use generally depends on the results of viscosity tests and bone marrow biopsies.

Patients with high viscosity may undergo plasmapheresis. Blood from the patient is removed through a machine that separates the cellular part of the blood from the plasma (the liquid fraction containing the IgM). The cellular portion is returned to the patient along with a plasma substitute. Since this treatment removes only the IgM currently in the system and does not stop the body from producing more, it is only a temporary solution, but it does relieve symptoms, especially in newly diagnosed individuals.

Most patients also undergo either chemotherapy (anticancer drugs) or biological therapy to destroy the IgM-producing cells and stimulate the immune system into attacking the cancer. The most often used regimen has been chlorambucil and prednisone in combination. Other anticancer drugs being used include cyclophosphamide, doxorubicin, fludarabine, and cladribine. Most treatments are given during outpatient therapy over a period of sev-

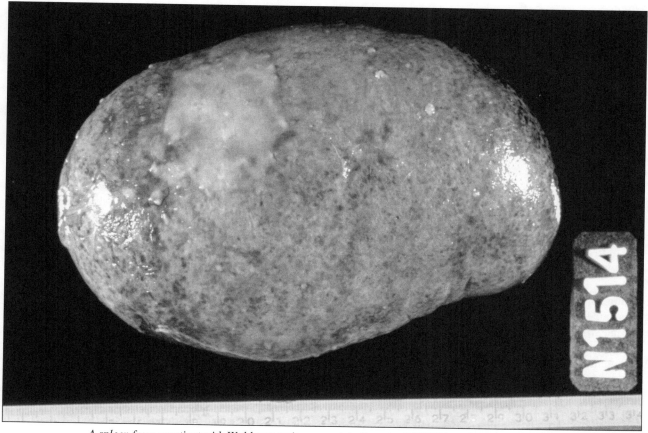

A spleen from a patient with Waldenström's macroglobulinemia. (CNRI/Photo Researchers, Inc.)

eral days. Blood tests of IgM levels, physical examination of lymph nodes, and scans of lymph nodes are often used to determine whether a particular drug is working for the patient. All of these drugs have side effects that may include nausea, vomiting, loss of appetite, hair loss, lowered resistance to infection, and easy bruising. Careful monitoring is important.

Biological therapies may include the use of interferon (a protein produced by lymphocytes to help fight infections) and monoclonal antibodies designed to attack lymphoma cells (rituximab).

A few other treatments have been tried with a variety of successes. These include spleenectomy (removal of an enlarged spleen, where much IgM may be produced), and high-dose chemotherapy followed by stem cell transplantation (cells that will migrate to the bone marrow and replace those blood-forming and immune system cells destroyed by the chemotherapy). Additionally, drugs such as thalidomide and bortezomib, which have been used to treat multiple myeloma (a related type of cancer) have been tried in some patients. Researchers continue to look for new drugs, combinations of drugs, and new biological therapies.

Prognosis, prevention, and outcomes: The prognosis for WM is extremely variable. Many textbooks describe a life span of five to seven years after diagnosis, but since the average age of diagnosis is sixty-three, there is a great likelihood of dying from other causes. According to the International Waldenström's Macroglobulinemia Foundation, patients have been known to live for twenty-five or more years after diagnosis.

Kerry L. Cheesman, Ph.D.

▶ **For Further Information**

Bjorkholm, Magnus. "Lymphoplasmacytic Lymphoma/ Waldenström's Macroglobulinemia." In *The Lymphomas*, edited by George P. Canellos, T. Andrew Lister, and Bryan D. Young. Philadelphia: Elsevier/Saunders, 2006.
Chen, C. I. "Treatment for Waldenström's Macroglobulinemia." *Annals of Oncology* 15 (2004): 550-558.
Johnson, Stephen A. "Waldenström's Macroglobulinemia." *Reviews in Clinical and Experimental Hematology* 6, no. 4 (2002): 421-434.
Rohatiner, Ama Z. S., Nancy L. Harris, Riccardo Dalla-Favera, and T. Andrew Lister. "Lymphoplasmacytic Lymphoma and Waldenström's Macroglobulinemia." In *Non-Hodgkin's Lymphomas*, edited by Peter Mauch et al. Philadelphia: Lippincott Williams & Wilkins, 2004.

▶ **Other Resources**

American Cancer Society
Detailed Guide: Waldenström's Macroglobulinemia
http://www.cancer.org/docroot/CRI/ CRI_2_3x.asp?dt=76

International Waldenström's Macroglobulinemia Foundation
http://www.iwmf.com

See also Immunoelectrophoresis (IEP); Lymphomas; Myeloma; Non-Hodgkin lymphoma.

▶ **Watchful waiting**

Category: Social and personal issues
Also known as: Expectant management, active surveillance

Definition: Watchful waiting is a conservative approach to disease management that delays treatment for slow-growing, indolent cancers and those that are incurable. Watchful waiting is also referred to as expectant management and active surveillance.

Usage: When watchful waiting is used with precancerous lesions, it requires frequent monitoring to ensure early intervention when signs of cancer appear. This management strategy is often an option for a variety of slow-growing cancers including prostate cancer and non-Hodgkin lymphoma. However, research and development of new targeted therapies for cancer treatment may reduce the need for this wait-and-see option in the future.

Treatment criteria: The watchful waiting approach is for individuals who meet disease-specific criteria for delaying treatment. For example, in prostate cancer, the prostate-specific antigen (PSA), Gleason score, and PSA doubling time are used to determine when watchful waiting is appropriate. This approach is considered for low-grade cancers when the patient is asymptomatic and for older men who will more likely die of another cause. Guidelines for this form of treatment involve scheduled monitoring and an established plan that is instituted to document disease growth. Laboratory studies, diagnostic imaging, and other test findings are assessed at predetermined intervals. The most important consideration is that the patient is comfortable with the option to delay treatment and is educated about the signs and symptoms to watch for that may indicate progression.

Advantages: The major advantage is postponement of the toxic effects of therapy and cumulative doses of drugs until it is determined that the cancer is growing. The time gained can be used to evaluate treatments and make a choice before it is necessary to initiate treatment. Those with existing conditions that could make the side effects of cancer treatment worse may prefer this option to preserve quality of life. Watchful waiting does not preclude treating other symptoms, such as pain.

Disadvantages: Delaying treatment is perceived as risky and irresponsible by some individuals. The anxiety and stress this choice would create for them make it unworkable. Also, it is possible that cancer growth could accelerate before it is detected, reducing the window of opportunity for early intervention. For others, however—especially those diagnosed very late in life—watchful waiting may be preferable to aggressive treatments that can compromise quality of life. The patient must be comfortable with the choice to derive the benefit of extending quality of life by avoiding the side effects of treatment.

Linda August Vrooman, R.N., B.S.N., O.C.N.

See also Adjuvant therapy; Elderly and cancer; Gleason grading system; Leiomyomas; Myeloproliferative disorders; Neuroblastomas; Overtreatment; Stress management.

▶ Weight loss

Category: Diseases, symptoms, and conditions
Also known as: Unintentional weight loss, anorexia (loss of appetite), cachexia (extreme weight loss)

Related conditions: Fatigue, malnutrition, illness, infection, poor wound healing, reduced response to physiological and psychological stress, diminished physical and mental performance, inferior response to treatment, and shorter survival time are all complications of less than optimal weight in cancer patients.

Definition: Weight loss is a reduction in body mass marked by a decrease in body fluid, fat, and muscle. Unintentional weight loss is involuntary weight loss.

Risk factors: Medical research has identified more than 360 causes of weight loss, of which cancer is one. Weight loss is one of the most common symptoms of cancer and a common side effect of many cancer treatments. Cancer, then, is a risk factor for weight loss. Weight loss itself is not a risk factor for cancer. In fact, many physicians and nutritionists believe that normal, controlled weight loss to reach optimal weight for health may help in preventing some cancers. However, unintentional rapid weight loss is a sign of a serious health problem and reason to see a doctor.

Etiology and the disease process: As body weight—along with fluids, fat, and muscle—decreases, normal physiological functions in cancer patients degenerate, contributing to a host of medical problems and even death. Being below optimal weight for health impedes treatment efforts.

Metabolic changes brought about by cancer can lead to a condition known as malabsorption. Patients affected by malabsorption may seem to consume enough food, but they do not absorb enough of the nutrients from the food and are unable to produce enough energy to fuel the body. This leads to a loss of fat and muscle, a wasting syndrome known as cachexia, which accounts for the emaciated look of some cancer patients.

Infection, fever, and hot flashes—common symptoms of cancer or side effects of treatment—increase body temperature. To cope with a rise in body temperature, the body needs increased energy, which is furnished by the calories in food. Patients need to increase their intake of calories by 10 to 13 percent for each degree above 98.6 degrees Fahrenheit (37 degrees Celsius).

A cancerous tumor also places demands on the body for added energy, which comes from the intake of extra calories. One theory, not yet proven, suggests that the tumor benefits more than the patient does from the extra calories because the tumor is exceptionally efficient at using calories from food for its own growth. Moreover, a tumor can affect the appetite and the normal digestive process. Studies have shown that tumors produce chemicals that change the way the body makes efficient use of nutrients.

Chemical changes in the body are common with cancer. One theory is that cancer produces chemicals that lead to anorexia, the loss of desire to eat. Anorexia is common among cancer patients, however, and is linked to a number of factors associated with cancer and cancer treatment: changes in smell or taste, dry mouth, mouth sores and infections, difficulty in swallowing, nausea, diarrhea, constipation, and the psychological and emotional impact of cancer, which can lead to anxiety or depression. Anxiety and depression, in turn, can lead to anorexia.

To fully benefit from aggressive cancer treatments such as certain types of chemotherapy and radiation therapy, patients need stores of energy. Weight loss or less than optimal weight can diminish the effectiveness of treatment. To speed up normal tissue repair following aggressive cancer therapies, patients need sufficient calories and adequate amounts of the macronutrients: protein, carbohy-

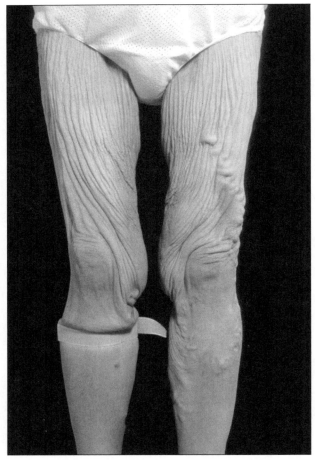

Excessive weight loss in this patient with uterine cancer resulted in loose skin on her thighs. (Custom Medical Stock Photo)

drates, and fat. Poor nutrition weakens the body's capability to tolerate certain treatments. For instance, a decrease in the dose of drugs or radiation to compensate for the patient's low tolerance to a particular treatment could undermine the effectiveness of the treatment.

Incidence: Virtually every cancer patient can expect to suffer weight loss sometime during the course of the disease. Unintentional rapid weight loss is a common symptom of cancer.

Symptoms: Weight loss is a symptom of many possible diseases, including cancer. The primary symptom in relation to cancer is a rapid, *unexplained*, reduction of body mass. The cause of such weight loss will be identified by analysis of other symptons and test results.

Screening and diagnosis: Because weight loss leads to nutrition problems such as malnutrition or anorexia, diag-

nosing weight loss in cancer patients is done through nutrition screening and assessment. Screening identifies patients who may be at risk of complications from weight loss. Assessment establishes the overall nutritional status of a patient and helps doctors and nutritionists determine if the patient needs nutrition therapy. Nutrition screening and assessment are done before cancer treatment begins. Finding and treating nutrition problems in the early stages of the disease can improve the patient's response to treatment and chance of recovery.

Nutrition screening is done by gathering information about the patient such as the following:
- Changes in weight over the past six months
- Changes in the amount and types of food the patient normally eats
- Problems that affect eating such as dry mouth, mouth sores, diarrhea, constipation, and changes in taste and smell
- The patient's ability to reason, walk, and perform normal daily activities
- The patient's perceived quality of life

Nutrition assessment also involves a complete physical exam. The examining physician checks for general health and signs of disease, along with fluid buildup in the body and the loss of fat or muscle. Nutrition assessment and monitoring, done by both doctors and nutritionists, continue throughout treatment of cancer.

Treatment and therapy: Preventing weight loss or encouraging weight gain is a major part of cancer treatment. Before actual treatment of the cancer, doctors treat any complications that may arise from weight loss. Drug therapy and medical nutrition therapy help patients gain or maintain a healthful weight, along with stores of energy, to better battle the cancer.

Drugs are used to relieve both symptoms of weight loss and side effects of treatment. The drugs are meant to achieve the following:
- Prevent nausea, vomiting, or diarrhea
- Promote bowel movements (laxatives)
- Relieve pain
- Prevent infections
- Heal sores in the mouth
- Stimulate saliva
- Encourage the action of pancreatic enzymes, proteins released by the pancreas that help break down food during digestion and create energy for the body
- Battle anxiety or depression

Medical nutrition therapy is a major component of cancer treatment. Depending on the condition of the patient and the stage of the cancer, medical nutrition therapy involves one of three types of nutrition: oral, enteral, and parenteral.

Oral nutrition is nutrition taken by mouth. This includes the normal intake of food, special diets prescribed by nutritionists, and nutritional supplements, including beverages and formulas, to build and maintain healthful nutrition levels.

Enteral nutrition is providing nutrients through a tube placed in the nose, stomach, or small intestine. Tube feeding is for patients who do not meet their nutritional needs from food and beverages and who do not have problems with vomiting or diarrhea. Tube feeding can be used to supply supplements to a patient's diet or as the only source of nutrition.

Parenteral nutrition—also known as hyperalimentation or total parenteral nutrition (TPN)—delivers nutrients intravenously, through a blood vein, bypassing the digestive system. It is for patients who are unable to absorb nutrients through the gastrointestinal tract because of continual vomiting or severe diarrhea and for those undergoing high-dose chemotherapy or radiation and bone marrow transplantation. It is possible for patients to receive all the vitamins, minerals, protein, and calories they need through total parenteral nutrition.

Prognosis, prevention, and outcomes: Studies have shown that maintaining nutritional health improves the chances of survival from cancer. However, maintaining a healthful weight is no guarantee that cancer can be prevented or successfully treated. Too many other factors are involved. Often the cancer eventually overwhelms the entire system. During the later stages of cancer, sometimes the best treatment for patients is to allow them to eat what they want and to preserve the more pleasant and social aspects of eating.

Wendell Anderson, B.A.

▶ **For Further Information**

Fearon, Kenneth C., Anne C. Voss, and Deborah S. Hustead. "Definition of Cancer Cachexia: Effect of Weight Loss, Reduced Food Intake, and Systemic Inflammation on Functional Status and Prognosis." *American Journal of Clinical Nutrition* 83, no. 6 (June, 2006): 1345-1350.

Ko, A., E. H. Rosenbaum, and M. Dollinger. *Everyone's Guide to Cancer Therapy: How Cancer Is Diagnosed, Treated, and Managed Day to Day.* 5th ed. Kansas City, Mo.: Andrews McMeel, 2007.

McIlwain, Harris H. *The Fifty-Plus Wellness Program.* Hoboken, N.J.: John Wiley and Sons, 1991.

▶ **Other Resources**

American Cancer Society
Nutrition for the Person with Cancer
    http://www.cancer.org/docroot/MBC/
    MBC_6.asp?sitearea=ETO

National Cancer Institute
Overview of Nutrition in Cancer Care
    http://www.cancer.gov/cancertopics/pdq/
    supportivecare/nutrition/Patient

See also Anorexia; Appetite loss; Artificial sweeteners; Cachexia; Carcinoma of unknown primary origin (CUP); Chemotherapy; Depression; Diarrhea; Dry mouth; Fatigue; Laxatives; Nausea and vomiting; Nutrition and cancer prevention; Nutrition and cancer treatment; Obesity-associated cancers; Psychosocial aspects of cancer; Side effects; Small intestine cancer; Stress management; Symptoms and cancer.

▶ Wilms' tumor

Category: Diseases, symptoms, and conditions
Also known as: Nephroblastoma, renal (kidney) embryoma

Related conditions: Clear cell carcinoma of the kidney, rhabdoid tumor of the kidney, neuroepithelial tumor of the kidney, cystic partially differentiated nephroblastoma, mesoblastic nephroma, renal carcinoma

Definition: Wilms' tumor is a solid tumor of the kidney that may spread to the lungs, liver, brain, bone, or lymph nodes. The majority of cases of Wilms' tumor occur in children younger than five years old. Wilms' tumors are categorized at the cellular level or histologically as tumors with either favorable histology or anaplastic histology. Wilms' tumors with favorable histology are composed of the three types of cells normally found in the kidney and account for 90 percent of the Wilms' tumor cases. The remaining 10 percent of Wilms' tumor cases have cells that are anaplastic, which are primitive or undifferentiated cells that have large, distorted nuclei. The anaplastic cells can be focal, meaning located in a distinct area, or diffuse throughout the tumor.

Risk factors: Wilms' tumors usually occur in otherwise healthy children, although 10 percent of Wilms' tumor cases occur in children with certain genetic and developmental abnormalities present at birth. These abnormalities are categorized as overgrowth or nonovergrowth syndromes. Overgrowth syndromes include Beckwith-Wiedemann syndrome, hemihypertrophy, Perlman syndrome, Sotos' syndrome, and Simpson-Golabi-Behemel syndrome. Nonovergrowth syndromes include aniridia, trisomy 18, WAGR syndrome, Blooms' syndrome, and Denys-Drash syndrome. Wilms' tumors in both kidneys, called bilateral Wilms' tumor, are more common in children with associated developmental abnormalities. Children with diffuse hyperplastic perilobar nephroblastomatosis, characterized by abnormal tissue growth on the outer part of one or both kidneys, are also at higher risk for Wilms' tumor.

Etiology and the disease process: The exact cause of Wilms' tumor is unknown, although the association of Wilms' tumor with genetic and developmental abnormalities suggests that mutations in one or more genes may play a role. Researchers are studying the association of Wilms' tumor with changes in the deoxyribonucleic acid (DNA) of the Wilms' tumor 1 (*WT1*) gene, several genes that are either tumor-suppressor or tumor-progressive genes, and a chromosomal area identified as Wilms' tumor 2 (*WT2*). Although genetic mutations are most likely involved with the development of Wilms' tumor, only 1 to 2 percent of patients have a family member with Wilms' tumor.

Many Wilms' tumors arise from nephrogenic rests, which are clusters of embryonic kidney precursor cells left over from development. These early building blocks of kidneys usually develop into the cells of a mature kidney, go dormant, or die off. Wilms' tumor arises when the embryonic cells divide and grow out of control. Genetic mutations may cause nephrogenic rests to be abnormally retained.

Incidence: Approximately 500 cases of Wilms' tumor are diagnosed annually. A majority of patients are between the ages of one and five, with the average age of two to three years. Rates of Wilms' tumor decrease as age increases. Adult Wilms' tumor cases (sixteen years or older) are rare and associated with a poor prognosis. Bilateral Wilms' tumors in both kidneys diagnosed at the same time or at different times make up approximately 4 to 5 percent of Wilms' tumor cases. Wilms' tumor accounts for the majority (95 percent) of childhood renal tumors diagnosed each year and for 6 to 7 percent of all childhood cancers.

Symptoms: Wilms' tumors are typically not detected until they become large enough to be felt as a mass in the abdomen; however, most are found before they metastasize. Additional symptoms may include blood in the urine, unexplained fever, high blood pressure, constipation, reduced appetite, abdominal pain, and weight loss.

Screening and diagnosis: Unless a child is at risk for developing Wilms' tumor, routine screenings are not typically done. Screening of a symptomatic child includes a physical exam; assessment of health history; blood tests to examine the number of blood cells, amount of hemoglobin, and the presence of certain substances improperly released by organs and tissues; urine tests to check for blood, bacteria, sugar, or proteins; liver function tests; renal function tests; and imaging tests to visualize the kidneys. The most common imaging test is an ultrasound, but computed tomography (CT), magnetic resonance imaging (MRI), and X rays may also be used.

If a mass in the kidney is detected through imaging, diagnosis is established through surgery, rather than biopsy. Biopsies are avoided because they could rupture the tumor, causing the cancerous cells to spread outside of an otherwise contained area. If possible, the entire affected kidney is removed during surgery in a procedure called a nephrectomy. A pathologist examines the removed tissue to confirm the diagnosis of Wilms' tumor and to assess the histology.

The stage is determined by results of imaging studies, surgery, and the pathology report. Since stages are independent of histology type, they are reported together (for example, Stage I, favorable histology). The stages characterized by the Wilms' Tumor Study Group are most commonly used:

• Stage I: Cancer is found in only one kidney and was completely removed by surgery. The kidney and tumor

---

Prevalence of Wilms' Tumors Among Total Renal Cancers in Children, 1975-1995

Age Group	Number of Cases	Percentage of Total Renal Cancers
Under 5	880	96.2
5-9	260	95.9
10-14	39	66.1
13-19	21	35.0
Under 15	1,149	94.7
Under 20	1,200	92.0

Source: L. A. G. Ries et al., eds., *Cancer Incidence and Survival Among Children and Adolescents: United States SEER Program, 1975-1995*, NIH Pub. No. 99-4649 (Bethesda, Md.: National Cancer Institute, SEER Program, 1999)

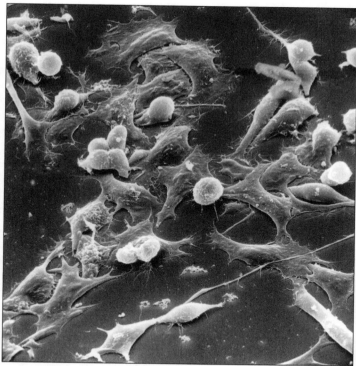

The Wilms' tumor is round when it attaches to a surface and then spreads out. (Science Source)

were intact before removal, and the tumor was not biopsied prior to surgery. There is no evidence that the cancer entered the blood vessels or the regions beyond where it was removed. The majority of patients are diagnosed at Stage I.

• Stage II: The tumor is completely removed; however, before it was removed, the cancer spread to tissues and structures within and near the kidney.

• Stage III: The cancer spread beyond the kidney to nearby lymph nodes and other structures in the abdomen. It could not be completely removed by surgery. The tumor may have broken open before or during surgery, was biopsied before surgery, or was removed in more than one piece.

• Stage IV: Cancer spread to distant structures such as lungs, liver, brain, bone, or distant lymph nodes.

• Stage V: The cancer is in both kidneys at the same time. Each kidney gets a separate stage rating.

Treatment and therapy: Treatment depends on the stage and histology of the Wilms' tumor. In general, tumors with anaplastic histology require more aggressive treatments and tend to be more resistant to chemotherapy than those with favorable histology. Stages I and II involve a ne-

phrectomy and removal of nearby lymph nodes, followed by adjuvant chemotherapy. A dual chemotherapy regimen of vincristine and dactinomycin is typically used.

Stages III and IV require a nephrectomy followed by combination chemotherapy (dactinomycin, vincristine, and doxorubicin, or dactinomycin and vincristine) with radiation. Depending on the size and location of the tumor, chemotherapy may be given before surgery to shrink the tumor.

Stage V involves removal of the tumors in both kidneys while retaining kidney function (a partial nephrectomy). A biopsy in Stage V cases may be done preoperatively to determine the stage of the tumors in each kidney. Chemotherapy and radiation therapies are given based on the stages of the tumors in the kidneys.

Wilms' tumor is so rare that patients should be treated by specialists with experience (pediatric oncologists, pediatric surgeons, and pediatric radiation oncologists) and should be considered for a clinical trial.

Prognosis, prevention, and outcomes: Prognosis is related to the stage of disease at diagnosis, histological features, tumor size, patient age, whether Wilms' tumor is diagnosed for the first time or is recurrent, the presence of abnormal chromosomes or genes, and access to experts with Wilms' tumor experience. Some 90 percent of cases with a favorable histology respond to treatment, and four-year overall survival rates of Stages I through IV with favorable histology range from 98 to 90 percent. Anaplastic histology is associated with a less favorable prognosis, ranging from 82.6 to 44 percent four-year overall survival rates. Anaplastic histology is also associated with a higher rate of relapse.

There are no known preventive measures in children who are otherwise healthy. Children with congenital abnormalities who have been treated for Wilms' tumor, as well as those with other risk factors, should undergo ultrasound screening every three to six months until the age of eight.

Children who have been exposed to high-intensity radiation or chemotherapy treatments are at risk for developing a second malignant neoplasm elsewhere in the body and congestive heart failure later in life. This is referred to the late effects of treatment for childhood cancer. Patients are candidates for a kidney transplant if they have been free of Wilms' tumor for one to two years.

Amanda McQuade, Ph.D.

▶ For Further Information

Janes-Hodder, Honna, and Nancy Keene. *Childhood Cancer: A Parent's Guide to Solid Tumor Cancers*. 2d ed. Sebastopol, Calif.: O'Reilly, 1999.

Steen, R. Grant, and Joseph Mirro, eds. *Childhood Cancer: A Handbook from St. Jude Children's Research Hospital*. New York: Perseus, 2000.

Woznick, Leigh A., and Carol D. Goodheart. *Living with Childhood Cancer: A Practical Guide to Help Families Cope*. Washington, D.C.: APA Life Tools, 2002.

▶ Other Resources

National Cancer Institute
  http://www.cancer.gov

National Wilms' Tumor Study
  http://www.nwtsg.org

Pediatric Oncology Resource Center
  http://www.acor.org/ped-onc

See also Beckwith-Wiedemann syndrome (BWS); Childhood cancers; Computed tomography (CT) scan; Denys-Drash syndrome and cancer; Genetics of cancer; Kidney cancer; Malignant rhabdoid tumor of the kidney; Nephroblastomas; Pediatric oncology and hematology; Proto-oncogenes and carcinogenesis; Wilms' tumor aniridia-genitourinary anomalies-mental retardation (WAGR) syndrome and cancer.

▶ Wilms' tumor aniridia-genitourinary anomalies-mental retardation (WAGR) syndrome and cancer

Category: Diseases, symptoms, and conditions
Also known as: Nephroblastoma

Related condition: Wilms' tumor in the absence of the associated abnormalities of WAGR syndrome

Definition: Wilms' tumor aniridia-genitourinary anomalies-mental retardation (WAGR) syndrome is a combination of abnormalities, which includes Wilms' tumor, aniridia (loss of vision), genitourinary abnormalities, and mental retardation.

Risk factors: The risk factor for WAGR syndrome is the combination of aniridia, genitourinary abnormalities, and mental retardation resulting from a defect or loss of genetic material from chromosome 11.

Etiology and the disease process: The underlying cause of the syndrome is a genetic abnormality characterized by loss of a portion of the short arm of chromosome 11 (11p13 deletion). Genetic information in this region includes the *WT1* gene, a transcription factor that functions in an unknown manner as a Wilms' tumor-suppressor gene. Loss of function contributes to genitourinary malformations.

A second gene, *PAX6*, is considered a master control for the regulation of eye and neural development of the central nervous system. Mutation or deletion of the gene may result in aniridia and mental retardation. The association of this gene with formation of the Wilms' tumor is indirect, the result of a deletion of the region on chromosome 11.

Incidence: The combination of abnormalities inherent in WAGR syndrome is uncommon and the incidence undetermined. However, children with the combination of aniridia, genitourinary abnormalities, and mental retardation have a greater than 30 percent chance of developing Wilms' tumor. The incidence of Wilms' tumor in the general population is 8 per 1 million, slightly higher among African Americans, and represents the most common form of kidney tumors in children. Most cases are not associated with known chromosomal mutations. Cases are most common before the age of five.

Symptoms: The abnormalities of WAGR syndrome are generally observed immediately following birth, though diagnosis of mental retardation may not take place for months to years. Genitourinary abnormalities may include undescended testicles in male infants and abnormal development of the ovaries or uterus in female infants. Undescended testicles also pose a risk for development of testicular cancer.

Children with aniridia may lack an iris, a condition apparent at birth, or have limited development of this region of the eye. The result is significant loss of visual acuity. Lack of an iris may also result in sensitivity to light, a problem that may be handled as the child grows through wearing of sunglasses.

Symptoms of Wilms' tumor include combinations of pain or swelling in the lower back, blood in the urine, and indistinct symptoms such as nausea or vomiting and loss of appetite. Any combination of such symptoms may be followed by more direct examination of the kidneys. Since blood pressure is regulated in part by the kidneys, elevated blood pressure may also result from the presence of the tumor.

Mental retardation, generally referred to as cognitive impairment, may not be apparent, since the mental capacity in many of these children does not deviate from that of the average child. Diagnosis often does not take place until testing following admittance to the educational system and often presents no significant difficulty for the child.

Screening and diagnosis: Children known to have been born with the chromosomal deletion may be routinely screened for development of a tumor. Diagnosis of the syndrome otherwise results from recognition of the combination of abnormalities, particularly genitourinary malformations. Kidney function is assessed through several tests, including measurement of blood urea nitrogen (BUN), measurement of creatinine levels, and X-ray or computed tomography (CT) examination of the kidneys or abdominal region. If a mass is detected in the kidney, biopsy is performed. Staging is determined by the size and possible spread of the tumor:

- Stage I: The tumor is confined to the kidney.
- Stage II: The tumor extends into the capsule of the kidney.
- Stage III: The tumor is confined to the region but has spread beyond the surface of the kidney.
- Stage IV: Metastasis is taking place.
- Stage V: The tumor is present on both kidneys.

Treatment and therapy: Treatment is largely palliative. However, Wilms' tumor can be removed surgically. Regional lymph nodes may be removed for determination of possible metastasis, as well as observation of other organs. If metastasis has occurred, radiation or chemotherapy may be included in the course of treatment.

Prognosis, prevention, and outcomes: Aniridia, genitourinary abnormalities, and mental retardation present lifelong problems for patients but are not life-threatening. Prognosis of Wilms' tumor depends on early diagnosis of the tumor. In general, prognosis is highly favorable, with more than 95 percent of patients with Stage I tumors showing no symptoms after five years. Even patients diagnosed at Stage IV have an 80 percent survival rate after five years.

Once metastasis has occurred, the tumor may be found in most other organs, including bone, lungs, and brain. Such spread is problematic, and chances for recovery are reduced. If both kidneys are involved, reduced kidney function may result following removal of the tumor.

Richard Adler, Ph.D.

Symptoms Sometimes Associated with WAGR Syndrome

- Autism
- Obsessive-compulsive disorder
- Attention deficit disorder
- Anxiety disorders
- Depression
- Polyphagia, hyperphagia (eating excessively)
- Obesity at an early age and high cholesterol levels
- Chronic renal failure after age twelve
- Breathing problems: asthma, sleep apnea, pneumonia
- Frequent childhood infections of the ear, nose, and throat
- Crowded or uneven teeth
- Problems with muscular strength and tone, particularly among infants and small children
- Epilepsy
- Inflammation of the pancreas

Source: National Human Genome Research Institute

▶ **For Further Information**

Pai, G. S., et al. *Handbook of Chromosomal Syndromes.* Hoboken, N.J.: John Wiley & Sons, 2003.

Parker, James N., and Philip M. Parker, eds. *The Official Parent's Sourcebook on Wilms' Tumor: A Revised and Updated Directory for the Internet Age.* San Diego, Calif.: Icon Health, 2002.

Scott, Tamara. *Wilms' Tumor: A Handbook for Families.* Glenview, Ill.: Association of Pediatric Oncology Nurses, 2002.

Wright, Kenneth, et al. *Handbook of Pediatric Eye and Systemic Disease.* New York: Springer Science, 2006.

▶ **Other Resources**

International WAGR Syndrome Association
http://www.wagr.org/

National Organization for Rare Disorders
WAGR Syndrome
http://www.rarediseases.org/search/rdbdetail_abstract
.html?disname=WAGR%20Syndrome

See also Childhood cancers; Denys-Drash syndrome and cancer; Nephroblastomas; Pediatric oncology and hematology; Wilms' tumor.

▶ Wine and cancer

Category: Lifestyle and prevention

Definition: Red wine is a rich source of the natural antioxidants flavonoid and resveratrol. Antioxidants protect cells from the oxidative damage caused by free radicals, which have been implicated in cancer cell development.

How red wine protects: Red wine is a rich source of active phytochemicals (plant chemicals) called polyphenols. Polyphenols are naturally found in the seeds and skins of grapes. Red wine contains more polyphenols than white wine because when white wine is made the skins are removed after the grapes are crushed. The polyphenols found in red wine are the naturally occurring antioxidants known as flavonoid and resveratrol. These antioxidants help clear cancer-causing free radicals from the body. Resveratrol also functions as an anti-inflammatory agent, inhibiting enzymes that promote tumor development and cancer cell proliferation. The flavonoid present in red wine may be especially effective against cancer during the initiation, promotion, and progression phases.

Colorectal cancer and red wine: According to a report published by the American College of Gastroenterology, consuming three or more glasses of red wine per week may reduce a person's risk of developing colorectal cancer. In a New York study that included 1,700 people who underwent routine colorectal cancer screening, 10 percent of those patients who did not drink alcohol had colorectal cancer, while only 3.4 percent of patients who routinely drank red wine had colorectal cancer.

Prostate cancer and red wine: According to a study conducted by investigators at the Fred Hutchinson Cancer Research Center, men who drank four or more glasses of wine per week reduced the risk of prostate cancer by 50 percent. Moreover, there was a 60 percent lower incidence of aggressive types of prostate cancer. Resveratrol, according to the Fred Hutchinson Cancer Research Center, may reduce circulating testosterone levels. This is important because circulating testosterone can promote prostate cancer cell growth.

Leukemia and red wine: Resveratrol has also been effective in causing apoptosis, cancer cell death, in patients with acute promyelocytic leukemia. Resveratrol works by inhibiting deoxyribonucleic acid (DNA) synthesis in the leukemia cells, which causes cell death.

Collette Bishop Hendler, R.N., M.S.

See also Alcohol, alcoholism, and cancer; Antioxidants; Beta-carotene; Bioflavonoids; Biopsy; Breast cancers; Calcifications of the breast; Calcium; Carotenoids; Coenzyme Q10; Complementary and alternative therapies; Curcumin; Dietary supplements; Free radicals; Herbs as antioxidants; Isoflavones; Mammography; Medical marijuana; Microcalcifications; Needle localization; Nutrition and cancer prevention; Prevention; Resveratrol; Ultrasound tests.

▶ Wire localization

Category: Procedures
Also known as: Needle localization

Definition: Wire localization is the insertion of a fine wire under radiologic guidance to mark for biopsy areas of breast density or calcifications that can be seen on mammograms but are not detectable by touch.

Cancers diagnosed: Breast cancers

Why performed: Certain types of images seen on mammograms may indicate precancer or developing cancer. Some of these lesions cannot be seen with the naked eye or felt by touch. Wire localization enables the surgeon to accurately target areas for biopsy. A follow-up radiologic image after the biopsy assures that the suspect tissue was removed.

Conditions of concern that require wire localization include microcalcifications and certain types of breast densities. Microcalcifications are tiny calcium deposits in the breast tissue, which show up on mammograms as white specks. Microcalcifications are generally only of concern when they appear in irregular patterns or are concentrated in one area of the breast. In these patterns or concentrations, they may indicate the rapid cell growth associated with precancer.

Patient preparation: Patients usually get a local anesthetic to numb feeling in the area of the breast where the wire will be inserted.

Steps of the procedure: To locate the area for biopsy, the surgeon uses radiologic images in which the wire site is marked. X ray is the preferred method used for wire localization. Ultrasound can also be used, but conditions requiring wire localization are often not visible by ultrasound. Guided by radiologic images of the breast, a radiologist locates the area in question, first inserts a thin, hollow needle into the area and then, through the needle, a fine wire with a hook. The hook keeps the wire in place in the breast and marks the specific area for biopsy. The wire in the breast provides a guide for where the incision is made. The wire is removed along with the breast tissue.

After the procedure: After the biopsy, the patient remains in the operating room until a repeat radiologic image confirms that the suspect area was removed. If the target area was missed, then another biopsy can be done immediately.

Risks: The risks of wire localization are minimal and include minor pain, possible bruising, and limited radiation exposure.

Results: Wire localization and follow-up radiologic images assure accurate targeting of the area for biopsy.

Charlotte Crowder, M.P.H., ELS

See also Biopsy; Breast cancers; Calcifications of the breast; Calcium; Mammography; Microcalcifications; Needle localization; Ultrasound tests.

▶ Wood dust

Category: Carcinogens and suspected carcinogens
RoC status: Known human carcinogen since 2002
Also known as: Sawdust, wood flour, sander dust

Related cancers: Cancer of the nasal cavities and the sinuses

Definition: Wood dust is composed of fine particles of the hard, fibrous substance that grows beneath the bark of trees in their trunks and branches. Woodworking tools release many lightweight specks of wood into the air. Electric and manual tools create wood dust when they chip, saw, turn, drill, sand, or carve wood. Outdoor compost piles also create visible clouds of wood dust when their layers of wood and leaves are agitated.

Exposure routes: Inhalation

Where found: Sawmills and other wood-processing mills, lumberyards, woodworking shops, furniture and cabinet-making industry, carpentry industry, composting facilities

At risk: Woodworkers in manufacturing industries; wood products press operators; workers who handle wood compost; wood carvers

Etiology and symptoms of associated cancers: The carcinogenic actions of wood dust in the nose and sinuses are not clearly understood. Animal tests show that wood dust damages deoxyribonucleic acid (DNA) and breaks chromosomes. Human studies indicate that exposure to it is associated with nasal adenocarcinoma, sinus squamous cell carcinoma, and cancer of the nasopharynx.

The active biological components of wood dust, cellulose and lignins (substances that make wood rigid), might cause these cancers. Organic chemical components, such as resin acids, terpenes, and tannins, might also be involved. Also, the particulate nature of wood dust most likely adds to its carcinogenicity.

Symptoms of these cancers include spontaneous epistaxis (nosebleed) and chronic obstruction of the nasal or sinus passages.

History: Studies in England in the 1960's showed that rare nasal cancers occurred in woodworkers. During a 1970's National Cancer Institute study, a high percentage of woodworkers died of these cancers.

In 1995 the International Agency for Research on Cancer (IARC) classified wood dust as a Group 1 human carcinogen. In 2002 the National Toxicology Program of the Department of Health and Human Services declared wood dust to be a human carcinogen in the *Tenth Report on Carcinogens* (RoC). In 2005 the National Institutes of Health estimated that the occupations of 2 million people worldwide expose them to the carcinogenic effects of wood dust.

The Occupational Safety and Health Administration (OSHA), the National Institute for Occupational Safety and Health (NIOSH), the IARC, and the American Conference of Governmental Industrial Hygienists (ACGIH) have established exposure limits, and their recommendations include avoidance, use of dust masks, daily removal of wood dust, and ventilation.

Susan E. Ullmann, M.T. (ASCP), M.A.

See also Air pollution; Carcinogens, known; Carcinogens, reasonably anticipated; Carcinomas; Head and neck cancers; Occupational exposures and cancer; Prevention; Throat cancer.

▶ X-ray tests

Category: Procedures

Also known as: Radiology, medical imaging, radiologic procedures, radiographic imaging

Definition: An X-ray test uses a machine to produce radiation that is passed through a particular body part. The size and density of the part show up as light and dark tones in the image on radiographic film, which helps the doctor diagnose the patient. Radiology encompasses many diagnostic types of imaging. Body parts, regions, and systems that can be seen by radiography include the chest, abdomen, skeletal system (skull, pelvis, spine, facial bones, extremities), brain, sinus, circulatory system (veins, arteries), lymphatic system, glands, muscles, urinary system, digestive system, reproductive system, cysts and tumors, and any soft tissues or organ in the body.

Radiologic exams may include routine X rays; computed tomography (CT) scans, previously known as a computed axial tomography (CAT) scans; angiography to study the veins and arteries; intravenous urography (IVU), previously known as intravenous pyelogram (IVP), which uses tomography imaging to view the kidneys, ureters, and bladder; upper gastrointestinal (UGI) series, also known as barium swallow, to show the esophagus, stomach, and small intestines; colon imaging, also known as barium enema or lower GI, to demonstrate the large intestine, colon, rectum, and appendix; dental radiography and panoramic tomography, also known as Panorex imaging, to view the teeth, jaw, and tempromandibular joint; sinus radiography to view the paranasal sinus; bone densitometry scans to evaluate bone porosity; digital subtraction angiography (DSA) to illustrate the blood vessels; ER, also known as emergency room, portables, and trauma, to take radiographic images during emergency situations in surgery and in the emergency room; fluoroscopy, which shows an actively moving video image of the part being evaluated; mammography, which takes medical images of the breasts; single photon emission computerized tomography (SPECT) scans which shows an increase in blood flow; and nuclear medicine and positron emission tomography (PET) which use radioactive tracer materials or radiopharmaceuticals that are injected, inhaled, or swallowed by the patient to create images of the whole body and show areas of increased radioactive uptake according to the organ's functioning ability.

Other imaging technologies that fall outside the scope of X-ray technologies include magnetic resonance imaging (MRI), ultrasound, and endoscopy, which do not use radiation to produce an image. MRI uses a powerful magnet to produce images on film, ultrasound uses sound waves to create its images, and an endoscope is a flexible viewing camera inserted orally or rectally to take internal pictures.

Cancers diagnosed: Medical imaging using X rays is designed to help diagnose cancers, metastases, diseases, fractures, or abnormalities. These diagnostic tests are not to be confused with radiation therapy, which is used to destroy cancers. Most cancers can be seen with the use of radiographic imaging; however, all cancers vary widely in their visibility. Some cancers hide until late in the disease process and then metastasize (grow and spread) quickly.

X-ray tests help diagnose bone cancers, bone marrow cancers, soft-tissue cancers, cancers of vital organs, blood-related cancers, lung cancers, lymph node and lymphoma cancers, spinal cord cancers, abdominal and pelvic cancers, head and neck cancers, liver and gallbladder cancers, reproductive organ cancers, breast cancers, leukemia, esophageal and colon cancers, Hodgkin and non-Hodgkin diseases, advanced skin cancers, brain cancers, and metastases.

Why performed: Diagnostic X rays are used to identify fractures, pneumonias, cancers, sinus infections, bowel obstructions, foreign objects, and anatomical abnormalities, or to confirm that there are no abnormalities. CT, MRI, nuclear medicine scans, and angiography are extremely helpful in locating diseases and cancers that are hard to find. Clinical observation and laboratory tests, combined with X-ray imaging, give the physician a more complete view of the extent of a particular disease. The combination of all tests and exams helps the doctor form a treatment plan for the patient. Any of these imaging devices may also be used to assist with guiding a biopsy, in needle placement, or to verify the location of wires and instruments during surgical procedures.

Patient preparation: Because there is such a wide variety of exams and a vast range of reasons for a radiology exam, it is best for the patient to consult with the medical doctor or discuss the preparation with the technologist three days prior to the exam. Some of the tests are routine, involving no preparation. Others may require eating or drinking restrictions, an increase in the amount of fluids in the bladder, or ingestion of contrast preparations for enhanced viewing in certain areas.

Steps of the procedure: The patient should tell the X-ray technician if there is any chance of pregnancy. If pregnancy is not a factor, then the patient is positioned between the X-ray tube and the radiographic film. Depending on the procedure and part being radiographed, the patient may be sitting, standing, or lying on a table for the exam. A lead shield (radiation protection device) is placed on the area surrounding, but not on, the region to be radiographed. Technique is set according to the size and density of the part. The length of time for procedures varies from five minutes to two hours depending on the test. Often, several images using different angles are needed. Some X-ray exams require the use of a contrast medium (dye). It may be taken orally or injected into the patient prior to or during the imaging process. Contrast materials are used when specific parts need to be enhanced or defined on film.

Contrast materials include barium sulfate (for upper GI and colon studies), iodine-based media (for IVP, CT, and angiography), gadolinium (for MRI), radioactive pharmaceutical materials and radioactive isotopes (for nuclear medicine scans), and xenon gas (for lung scans).

After the procedure: A radiologist will view the X-ray images and document the findings. The report will be given to the patient's doctor. At a follow-up appointment, the results will be discussed. If the imaging used a contrast material, then it is often suggested that the patient drink plenty of fluids to flush the contrast from the body. Over the next several days, the contrast will be eliminated through the body's waste products. Depending on the type of contrast and amount used, an unpleasant taste can linger in the mouth for a few weeks.

Risks: The physician will evaluate the patient's medical situation and determine if the diagnosis and treatment from the radiographic knowledge outweigh the potential risk from the X rays. If the patient is pregnant, then the procedure may be canceled or rescheduled or the patient may be double-shielded to protect the fetus. With the use of high-speed film, fast and accurate imaging equipment, collimation, and lead shielding, radiation is kept to a minimum for the patient. Diagnostic X-ray procedures carry no obvious short-term effects; however, any amount of radiation has the potential to harm cell structure. High doses of

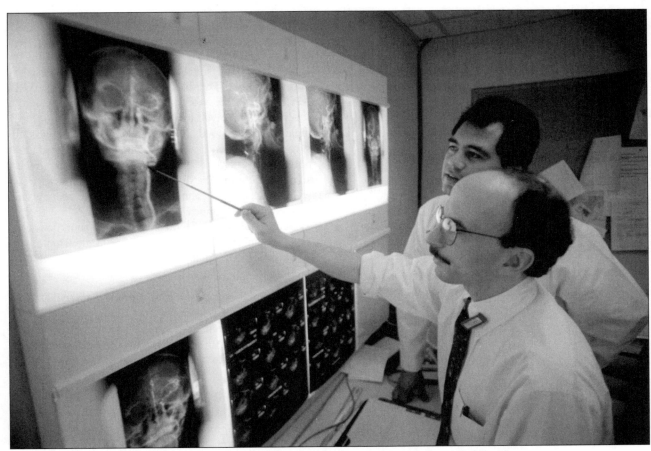

Radiographic images help doctors detect and treat cancers. (Digital Stock)

radiation that produce ill effects are seen in radiotherapy for cancer treatments. Long-term or high-dose effects of radiation can cause fetal or genetic defects, mutations or cancers, nausea, diarrhea, vomiting, or death.

In addition to medical and dental X rays, the general population is exposed to background radiation that increases their total body exposure when they live in a brick house, walk by a brick building, fly in an airplane, smoke or breathe secondhand smoke, live at higher elevation levels, heat their home with natural gas, breathe air pollution, work with natural elements or radiation in their profession, watch television, and work or play on a computer. One can calculate the radiation dose from many potential sources at http://www.epa.gov/radiation/students/calculate.html.

Other risks of X rays include claustrophobia in CT or MRI scanners and allergic reactions to contrast materials. Allergic reactions can include rash, itching, hives, nausea, vomiting, coma, or death.

Results: The radiographic image is developed and viewed by the radiology technician, who gives the film to the physician or radiologist. Depending on the procedure, the patient may receive a preliminary diagnosis or may have to wait until the final report from the radiologist, which may be several days later. The patient's current health status and extent of disease help determine a treatment plan.

Suzette Buhr, R.T.R., C.D.A.

▶ For Further Information

Frank, Eugene D., Bruce W. Long, and Barbara J. Smith. *Merrill's Atlas of Radiographic Positions and Radiologic Procedures.* 11th ed. St. Louis: Mosby/Elsevier, 2007.

Goldmann, David R., and David A. Horowitz, eds. *American College of Physicians Complete Home Medical Guide.* New York: DK, 2003.

Putman, Charles E., and Carl E. Ravin. *Textbook of Diagnostic Imaging.* 2d ed. Philadelphia: W. B. Saunders, 1994.

▶ Other Resources

American Cancer Society
http://www.cancer.org

University of Iowa Hospital and Clinics
Radiation Exposure: The Facts vs. Fiction
http://www.uihealthcare.com/topics/
medicaldepartments/cancercenter/prevention/
preventionradiation.html

See also Barium enema; Barium swallow; Brain and central nervous system cancers; Breast cancers; Computed tomography (CT) scan; Endoscopy; Imaging tests; Lymphomas; Mammography; Radiation therapies; Upper gastrointestinal (GI) series; Urography.

▶ Xeroderma pigmentosa

Category: Diseases, symptoms, and conditions
Also known as: Xeroderma pigmentosum

Related conditions: Skin cancer, eyelid tumors, telangiectasia, photophobia, mental retardation

Definition: Xeroderma pigmentosa is an inherited genetic disease characterized by sensitivity to ultraviolet (UV) light. Patients with this disease have an extremely high risk of developing skin cancer and often die from skin cancer at an early age. Different classes of xeroderma pigmentosa have greater or lesser risks due to the severity of their disease. Dark skin color does not protect xeroderma pigmentosa patients from skin cancer.

Risk factors: The main risk factor for xeroderma pigmentosa is having a family member with the disease.

Etiology and the disease process: Xeroderma pigmentosa is caused by loss of function of genes responsible for repairing deoxyribonucleic acid (DNA) damage caused by ultraviolet light. The disease is classified as XPA, XPB, XPC, XPD, XPE, XPF, or XPG, depending on which of seven genes involved in nucleotide excision repair (DNA repair) are damaged. XP-variant (XPV) is a class for xeroderma pigmentosa patients who have a mutated DNA polymerase eta gene. Xeroderma pigmentosa is a recessive genetic trait. The disease is staged as follows:

• Stage I: After six months of age, freckling, redness, and pigment changes appear on the skin.
• Stage II: Patches of light and dark skin (poikiloderma) develop, and spider veins (telangiectasia) develop.
• Stage III: Malignant skin cancers develop, including eyelid tumors.

Incidence: In populations of European descent, xeroderma pigmentosa occurs in 1 in 250,000 people. In the Japanese population, xeroderma pigmentosa has been estimated at 1 in 40,000 people. Tunisia is noted to have a high proportion of xeroderma pigmentosa cases. Other parts of the world have not been systematically studied.

Symptoms: Common symptoms in xeroderma pigmentosa are freckling, changes in skin pigmentation, and the eventual development of multiple, malignant skin cancers. Patients are sensitive to light, tend to suffer from conjunctival inflammation, and sunburn easily. Some patients exhibit immunosuppression and neurological problems, especially in XPA and XPD. The intensity of symptoms varies by xeroderma pigmentosa class and exposure to ultraviolet light.

Screening and diagnosis: Clinical symptoms and family history are the first clues to xeroderma pigmentosa. Gene sequencing and other special tests are used to conclusively diagnose xeroderma pigmentosa.

Treatment and therapy: Avoiding exposure to ultraviolet light, using sunscreen, and aggressive monitoring for skin cancer are necessary. Experimental gene therapy for xeroderma pigmentosa is in clinical trials.

Prognosis, prevention, and outcomes: Because xeroderma pigmentosa is an inherited genetic disease, genetic counseling is encouraged before having children. Extreme measures are needed to protect the xeroderma pigmentosa patient from ultraviolet light from the sun or fluorescent lamps. Death from skin cancer is typically the outcome at an early age, usually in childhood or young adulthood.

Christopher Pung, B.S., C.L.Sp. (CG)

See also Childhood cancers; Eyelid cancer; Family history and risk assessment; Gene therapy; Genetic counseling; Genetics of cancer; Risks for cancer; Skin cancers; Sunscreens; Young adult cancers.

► Yolk sac carcinomas

Category: Diseases, symptoms, and conditions
Also known as: Endocervical sinus tumors, endodermal sinus tumors, orchidoblastomas

Related conditions: Testicular carcinomas

Definition: Yolk sac carcinomas are tumors that originate in the primitive germ tissue of humans, the cells of which resemble the yolk sac. The most common form of yolk sac carcinoma is testicular cancer in children, though the ovaries may also develop this form of disease. Yolk sac carcinomas are generally in a class known as nonseminomas, referring to the absence of sperm-producing cells.

Risk factors: Most men who develop testicular carcinomas have no known risk factors. However, cryptorchidism, a lack of descent of one or both testicles, is associated with an increased risk, accounting for 14 percent of testicular cancers. Lack of descent is not rare, with the testicles remaining in the groin region in some 3 percent of male children. Most cases of testicular cancer that do occur develop in the undescended testicle. The molecular basis for the association is unknown, but scientists believe the two conditions are the result of a similar genetic factor rather than that the direct result of the lack of descent. The condition can be corrected through surgery.

Etiology and the disease process: Most cancers that originate within the testicles are germ-cell tumors (GSTs), malignancies that develop in cells associated with sperm production. Most are seminomas, malignancies of sperm-producing cells, with the remainder nonseminomas, malignancies of other embryonal cell types.

Incidence: Malignant yolk sac tumors are rare in children and account for approximately 3 percent of childhood tumors. The incidence of malignant yolk sac carcinoma among the general population is less than 1 per 1 million. The actual chance of a man developing testicular cancer is low, with approximately 1 in 300 men at risk.

Symptoms: Nonseminomas such as yolk sac carcinomas release alpha-fetoprotein (AFP), which can be measured in blood samples. Alpha-fetoprotein is synthesized by the yolk sac during fetal development, and elevated levels may suggest a malignancy.

Screening and diagnosis: Diagnosis is based on biopsy of tissues, carried out in conjunction with the finding of elevated levels of alpha-fetoprotein.

Treatment and therapy: Surgical removal of the testicle is the treatment of choice. Chemotherapy may also be warranted depending on the extent of the disease and may include combinations of vincristine, actinomycin D, and cyclophosphamide.

Prognosis, prevention, and outcomes: Testicular carcinomas in children, when diagnosed early in their development, can usually be treated successfully. Similar malignancies developing in adults are more problematic, and prognosis depends on the stage of development and the types of cells associated with the tumor.

Richard Adler, Ph.D.

See also Alpha-fetoprotein (AFP) levels; Carcinomas; Cervical cancer; Childhood cancers; Cryptorchidism; Cyclophosphamide; Embryonal cell cancer; Germ-cell tumors; Teratocarcinomas; Testicular cancer.

► Young adult cancers

Category: Diseases, symptoms, and conditions
Also known as: Youth cancers, adolescent cancer, teen cancer

Definition: Young adult cancers are malignancies that occur in youth from their mid-teens through their twenties (ages fifteen through twenty-nine). Some sources include people in their thirties in this grouping as well.

Some common cancers diagnosed in young adults are as follows:
- Lymphoma: cancer of the lymph glands that help fight disease
- Melanoma: a malignant skin cancer
- Thyroid cancer: cancer in the butterfly-shaped endocrine gland in the front of the neck below the voice box that produces hormones to regulate growth, metabolism, and level of energy
- Leukemia: cancer of the blood and bone marrow
- Soft-tissue sarcoma: cancer in supportive or connective tissue; forms in muscle, nerves, tendons, blood vessels, fat, joints, and lymph nodes
- Germ-cell tumors: tumors of special cells that develop in an embryo that later become sexual organs, such as the male testes and female ovaries

Less common cancers in young adults include brain tumors, breast cancer, and colorectal cancer.

Risk factors: Researchers report no clear risk factors for cancer in young adults. Few studies have found any connection to environmental factors or inheritance. Most cases of young adult cancer appear sporadic and spontaneous with only 5 percent related to family history.

Cancers that may be connected to environmental factors include melanoma, cervical cancer, Kaposi sarcoma, non-Hodgkin lymphoma, Hodgkin disease, and Burkitt lymphoma. Having a cancer in childhood may increase the risk of developing a second cancer as a young adult.

Etiology and the disease process: Because increased cancer occurrence is usually noted in older adults, cancer is often regarded as a disease of the elderly. However, cancer occurs in people of all ages. Historically, minimal research has been directed toward cancer in young adults, ages fifteen through twenty-nine, but that is changing. In 2006, the National Cancer Institute joined with the Lance Armstrong Foundation to identify barriers that face young adults with cancer and to develop approaches that can improve outcomes for this age group.

Young adults with cancer face many challenges because of their age and developmental tasks. In the teenage years, young people try to achieve mature relationships with others of both sexes, establish gender role identities, learn to accept their bodies, achieve emotional independence from their parents, prepare for marriage, gain education for a career, acquire values that govern behaviors, and become socially responsible. In early adulthood, young adults select a mate, establish a home, start a family, struggle to establish their identity, complete their education and training to work and provide financial support, express independence, and become comfortable with their sexuality. These milestones may be difficult with a chronic disease process that threatens financial security and brings changes in body image, social relationships, and sexuality. The stresses of the young adult differ from those of children or older adults.

Incidence: Young adult cancers account for only about 2 percent of all invasive cancers (excluding skin cancer) in the United States. However, each year about 70,000 young adults in the second or third decade of their lives learn they have some form of cancer. Young adults between the ages of fifteen and twenty-nine are 2.7 times as likely to develop cancer as they were before they turned fifteen. Young men between the ages of fifteen and twenty-nine have a higher incidence and a poorer prognosis than young women in this age group. The incidence of young adult cancers has experienced a steady increase. In 2000, nearly 21,400 young adults between the ages of fifteen and twenty-nine were diagnosed with invasive cancer.

The United States Surveillance Epidemiology and End Results (SEER) report based on data from 1975 to 2000 provides the only treatise totally dedicated to young adults with cancer, ages fifteen through twenty-nine. SEER documented that the most common cancer in this age group is lymphoma, which accounts for 20 percent of young adult cancers; of these, 12 percent are Hodgkin disease. The next highest rate was skin cancer at 12 percent, with male genital system cancer equal to endocrine system cancer at 11 percent. Female genital cancers, primarily cervical and ovarian cancer, presented 9 percent of the cancer cases. Other young adult cancers were leukemia (6 percent); brain and spinal cord tumors (6 percent); breast cancer (5 percent); digestive tract cancers such as colon and liver (4 percent); soft-tissue sarcomas (3 percent); bone sarcomas such as Ewing sarcoma and osteosarcoma (3 percent); respiratory, oral, and urinary tract cancers (2 percent each); and germ-cell cancers (1 percent). The frequency of thyroid cancer is markedly higher in young women. Melanoma was fifth in frequency between the ages of fifteen and twenty-nine but moved up to first in the age group between twenty-five and twenty-nine.

Symptoms: Symptoms of young adult cancers are specific to the type cancer they have developed. The following are some common young adult cancers and symptoms:

Lymphoma symptoms include painless lumps in the neck, armpits, or groin; other possible signs are weight loss of up to 10 percent of total body weight, high infrequent fevers, loss of appetite, weakness and fatigue, generalized itchiness over the body, red irritated patches of skin, excessive sweating at night, and coughing or breathlessness with swelling of the face and neck.

Melanomas present in moles that change in size (become bigger), shape (especially with an irregular edge),

Estimated Incidence of Invasive Cancer in the United States, 2000

Age Group	Incidence per 1 Million People
Under 5	217
5-9	113
10-14	129
15-19	216
20-24	365
25-29	662
30-34	983
35-39	1,462
40-44	2,156

Source: Data from A. Bleyer et al., eds., *Cancer Epidemiology in Older Adolescents and Young Adults Fifteen to Twenty-nine Years of Age, Including SEER Incidence and Survival: 1975-2000* NIH Pub. No. 06-5767 (Bethesda, Md.: National Cancer Institute, 2006)

color (get darker or multicolored), become itchy or painful, bleed or become crusty, or appear inflamed or irritated.

Thyroid cancer symptoms are a lump or nodule on the neck; pain in the neck, jaw, and ear; difficulty swallowing; a tickle in the throat; or hoarseness.

Leukemia symptoms vary by type but most are vague and nonspecific, such as fatigue or general weakness; malaise (general uncomfortable feeling throughout the body); abnormal bleeding and excessive bruising; reduced tolerance for exercise; an enlarged spleen, liver, or lymph nodes; joint or bone pain; increased infection and fever; and abdominal pain or fullness. A blood test will most likely show anemia, leukopenia (low white cell count), and thrombocytopenia (low blood-clotting cell count).

Cervical cancer is a silent disease in its early stages, with later symptoms such as abnormal vaginal bleeding, heavy vaginal discharge, pelvic pain, pain during urination, or bleeding after intercourse, between menses, or after douching.

Brain tumors may present with signs of increased intracranial pressure such as headaches, vomiting especially on waking, mental changes such as drowsiness or sluggishness, seizures, and loss of coordination with clumsy movement. Depending on the tumor location, symptoms can also include buzzing or ringing in the ears, dizziness, blindness in one side, language disorders, loss of smell, or impaired vision.

Spinal cord tumors manifest with symptoms such as neck, arm, or leg pain; weakness; muscle wasting; spasms; sensory changes; or decrease in bowel and bladder control.

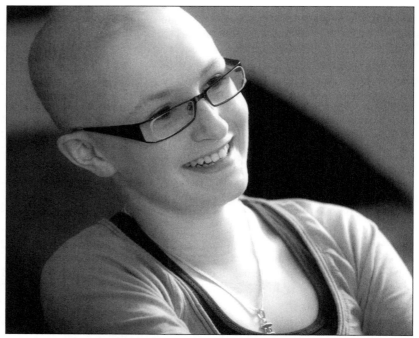

The risk factors for young adult cancer are not clear, as most cases appear sporadic and spontaneous, with only 5 percent related to family history. (©Steve Nagy/Design Pics/ Corbis)

Screening and diagnosis: Because young people are generally healthy, screening and diagnosis of cancer in young adults may be delayed. Young people may not recognize symptoms or may ignore their body's signs of illness. They may think that symptoms are related to their lifestyle choices. Most screening procedures are recommended for middle-age or older adults, not for young adults. Health care providers may overlook cancer as a possibility because of the person's youth and misdiagnose the disease.

Young adults in school or college may be covered by their parents' health insurance or have school health insurance with limited coverage; some may have no health insurance due to limited financial resources. They may delay dealing with symptoms because of the costs associated with health care providers, clinics, and testing. When they do seek help, they may encounter a complicated health care system and become frustrated with the process.

Treatment and therapy: Cancer treatment for young adults will be specific to the location, type, and stage of the cancer. If there is a malignant tumor or mass, surgery may be the best option. With or without surgery, chemotherapy (the use of drugs to kill cancer cells) may be used by the oncology physician to treat the cancer. Some cancers respond to radiation therapy, in which a high level of energy targets the cancer site to kill cancer cells. Immunotherapy may be used to stimulate the immune system to fight the cancer. Hormone therapy might be employed in certain cancers. Targeted therapy may be a treatment for metastasis of the cancer. A stem cell transplant might be useful in treatment. Joining a clinical trial directed to the young adult's specific cancer may prove beneficial.

Choosing a physician to provide cancer treatment and therapy is critical for young adults. The first consideration is to contact an oncologist, a doctor that specializes in cancer. Because cancer is less common in young adults, not all oncology physicians are familiar with this age-related specialty. They may not know about current treatment options and available support groups or resources for young adults. One example is that young adults with leukemia sometimes have better outcomes when treated with a regimen designed for children rather than the normal protocol for leukemia treatment in adults. Hence, young adults may need to consult specialists in pediatric oncology. However, practitioners who treat adults for cancers like breast, colon, or melanoma may provide the best treatment for young adults with these cancers.

Prognosis, prevention, and outcomes: The prognosis for young adults varies with their specific cancer. While overall survival rates for adults and children with cancer have improved over the past few years, the same is not true for young adults. The SEER report states that survival of a young person diagnosed with cancer today is worse than in the past. The SEER report documents no improvement in survival for cancer patients between the ages of twenty-five and thirty-five. The least improvement in survival for young women was demonstrated between the ages of twenty-five and twenty-nine. One study showed that poor survival rates for young adults may reflect a lack of participation in clinical trials. Some research has documented improved survival when young adults participate in clinical trials, such as the survival rate for young adults with Kaposi sarcoma.

Some studies suggest that young adult cancers can develop after previous childhood cancers. Research is currently examining lymphoma, leukemia, and testicular cancer, as these are diseases that affect children and young adults. Though no study has established why the second cancer occurs, some scientists believe that treatments such as chemotherapy and radiation therapy used to treat the first cancer may suppress the patient's immune systems as well as damage normal cells. Key to decreasing second cancers is determining the factors that might contribute and minimizing exposure.

One cancer on the rise among young adults is nonmelanoma skin cancers, which are preventable. Simple precautions can prevent skin cancer in young adults. The American Cancer Society has several recommendations to prevent skin cancer:

- Avoid extended exposure to sunlight from 10 A.M. to 4 P.M.
- Wear a hat, sunglasses, and clothes that cover the skin when in direct sunlight.
- Use sunscreen with a sun protection factor (SPF) of at least 15.

- Avoid tanning booths.
- Check skin often for any unusual moles, spots, or blemishes. Note any change in size, shape, or color.
- See a health care provider immediately if any suspicious spots or moles occur.

Marylane Wade Koch, M.S.N., R.N.

▶ **For Further Information**

Bleyer, A., M. O'Leary, R. Barr, and L. A. G. Ries, eds. *Cancer Epidemiology in Older Adolescents and Young Adults Fifteen to Twenty-nine Years of Age, Including SEER Incidence and Survival: 1975-2000.* Bethesda, Md.: National Cancer Institute, 2006.

Eden, T. O. B., et al., eds. *Cancer and the Adolescent.* 2d ed. Malden, Mass.: Blackwell, 2005.

Grinyer, Anne. *Cancer in Young Adults: Through Parents' Eyes.* Philadelphia: Open University Press, 2002.

▶ **Other Resources**

Cancer Planet
http://www.planetcancer.org/html/index.php

CancerCare
http://www.cancercare.org

Cancer.Net
Cancer in Young Adults
http://www.cancer.net/portal/site/patient/
menuitem.724de8b96edd64acfd748f68ee37a01d/
?vgnextoid=2ea803e8448d9010VgnVCM100000f27
30ad1RCRD

LiveStrong Young Adult Alliance
http://www.livestrong.org/site/c.jvKZLbMRIsG/
b.865471/k.B49/Young_Adult_Alliance.htm

M. D. Anderson Cancer Center
Adolescent and Young Adult Program
http://www.mdanderson.org/children/
display.cfm?id=51555960-bbea-11d4-
80fb00508b603a14&method=displayfull&pn=
38fff10f-474e-4506-9453cc8949d6732f

Young Survival Coalition
http://www.youngsurvival.org

See also Aging and cancer; Astrocytomas; Breast cancer in children and adolescents; Childhood cancers; Choriocarcinomas; Dioxins; Family history and risk assessment; Fibroadenomas; Juvenile polyposis syndrome; Pediatric oncology and hematology; Self-image and body image; Sexuality and cancer; Stress management.

► Zollinger-Ellison syndrome

Category: Diseases, symptoms, and conditions
Also known as: Z-E syndrome, gastrinoma, ZES

Related conditions: Gastroesophageal reflux disease (GERD), peptic ulcers, retained gastric antrum syndrome, antral G-cell syndrome

Definition: Zollinger-Ellison syndrome is a rare condition in which tumors in the pancreas or small intestine produce abnormally high levels of the hormone gastrin. Gastrin overproduction induces excessive secretion of stomach acid, which erodes the inner linings of the stomach and upper small intestine.

Risk factors: Some 25 percent of Zollinger-Ellison syndrome cases occur in people with multiple endocrine neoplasia type 1 (MEN 1), an autosomal dominant genetic condition characterized by pituitary and pancreatic endocrine tumors and overactivity of the parathyroid glands.

Etiology and the disease process: The inner linings of the stomach and small intestine (mucous membranes) are composed of several different cell types that work together to digest food. One of these cell types, G cells, resides in the mucous membranes that line the stomach and upper small intestine (duodenum) and produces a protein hormone called gastrin that is released into the bloodstream. Gastrin directly stimulates another group of cells in the stomach mucosa called parietal cells to secrete hydrochloric acid. The production of acid by the parietal cells is the main reason for the highly acidic environment in the stomach. Gastrin also signals to a third group of cells in the lining of the stomach called enterochromaffin-like (ECL) cells, which produce histamine in response to gastrin. Histamine is a powerful parietal cell-signaling molecule that causes parietal cells to make even more hydrochloric acid, which helps purge the stomach of most microorganisms, denatures proteins in foodstuffs, and activates the stomach-specific enzyme pepsin, which is secreted by the chief cells, a fourth type of cell found in the stomach mucosa. Pepsin secretion by the chief cells is also stimulated by gastrin.

Gastrin secretion is stimulated by the stretching of the stomach, activity of the vagus nerve, presence of digested proteins in the stomach, or high blood calcium levels. The presence of large amounts of stomach acid and hormones made by lower portions of the gastrointestinal tract inhibit gastrin release into the bloodstream.

Patients with Zollinger-Ellison syndrome have one or more typically small tumors (gastrinomas) in the pancreas or duodenum that produce excessive quantities of gastrin. Because these tumors do not reside in the stomach, the usual mechanisms that down-regulate gastrin production are not available. Continuous production of high blood gastrin levels constantly stimulates the parietal cells to overproduce hydrochloric acid, which erodes the stomach and duodenal mucous membranes.

Patients with multiple endocrine neoplasia type 1 (MEN 1) are at increased risk for Zollinger-Ellison syndrome. MEN 1 is also known as Wermer syndrome and is inherited as an autosomal dominant genetic condition that maps to chromosome 11. MEN 1 individuals also show a predisposition to develop pituitary, parathyroid, and pancreatic tumors.

Incidence: The average international incidence is approximately 1 per 1 million patients.

Symptoms: The most common symptoms are abdominal pain and diarrhea, usually experienced in combination, but not always. Other symptoms include heartburn, nausea, vomiting, gastrointestinal bleeding, and weight loss. People with MEN 1 also have a history of frequent kidney stones, excessive blood calcium (hypercalcemia), and pituitary disorders.

Screening and diagnosis: A blood test called a fasting gastrin test examines blood gastrin levels and is usually performed in combination with a gastric acid secretory test, which examines basic acid output (BAO). High blood gastrin levels and basic acid output are usually diagnostic for Zollinger-Ellison syndrome.

Provocative tests determine if gastrin production is subject to the normal control mechanisms. Typically blood gastrin levels are measured before and after the patient, who has fasted all night, is injected with secretin, an inhibitor of gastrin production. Large jumps in blood gastrin concentrations (above 200 nanograms per liter) are diagnostic for Zollinger-Ellison syndrome.

Imaging studies serve to detect the actual tumor and determine its location, size, and whether it has undergone metastasis. The imaging method of choice is somatostatin receptor scintigraphy (SRS). Somatostatin binds to any gastrin-producing cell, and during SRS, a radioactively labeled somatostatin-like molecule is injected into the patient. This molecule homes to the tumor and labels it, allowing it to be viewed. Computed tomography (CT) and magnetic resonance imaging (MRI) scans are also used, as is endoscopic ultrasound, which is more effective for detecting pancreatic gastrinomas. Esophagogastroduodenoscopy (EGD) is effective for visualizing the ulcerations present in the stomach and duodenum.

Treatment and therapy: Proton pump inhibitors are the drugs of choice to manage the excessive acid production.

These include omeprazole (Prilosec), pantoprazole (Protonix), esomeprazole (Nexium), and rabeprazole (Aciphex). Histamine-2 receptor antagonists (H2 blockers) such as cimetidine (Tagamet), famotidine (Pepcid), ranitidine (Zantac), or nizatidine (Azid) prevent reception of the histamine signal by the parietal cells and are much less effective for treating excessive acid production. In almost all cases, surgical removal of the tumors is highly recommended to prevent metastasis.

Prognosis, prevention, and outcomes: In patients without metastasis of the gastrinomas, prognosis is excellent. MEN 1 patients have a high frequency of recurrence. In those patients whose tumors have metastasized, the prognosis is rather poor.

Michael A. Buratovich, Ph.D.

▶ **For Further Information**

Fox, Stuart I. *Human Physiology*. 10th ed. New York: McGraw-Hill, 2007.

Miskovitz, Paul A., and Marian Betancourt. *The Doctor's Guide to Gastrointestinal Health*. Hoboken, N.J.: Wiley, 2005.

Parker, James N., and Philip M. Parker, eds. *The Official Patient's Sourcebook on Zollinger-Ellison Syndrome: A Revised and Updated Directory for the Internet Age*. San Diego, Calif.: Icon Health, 2002.

Piekin, Steven R. *Gastrointestinal Health: The Proven Nutritional Program to Prevent, Cure, or Alleviate Irritable Bowel Syndrome (IBS), Ulcers, Gas, Constipation, Heartburn, and Many Other Digestive Disorders*. 3d ed. Chino Hills, Calif.: Collins, 2005.

▶ **Other Resources**

MayoClinic.com
Zollinger-Ellison Syndrome
http://www.mayoclinic.com/health/
zollinger-ellison-syndrome/DS00461

National Digestive Diseases Information Clearinghouse
http://digestive.niddk.nih.gov/index.htm

See also Gastrinomas; Histamine 2 antagonists; Islet cell tumors; Neuroendocrine tumors; Pancreatic cancers; Small intestine cancer; Stomach cancers.

Appendixes

▶ Drugs by Generic Name

Generic Drug	Trade Name	Indicated For
abarelix	none	prostate cancer
absorbable gelatin sponge	Gelfoam	homeostasis
5-AC	Mylosar; Vidaza	myelodysplastic syndrome
acetylsalicylic acid	Aspergum; Ecotrin; Empirin; Entericin; Extren; Measurin	mild to moderate pain; fever; prevention of arterial and venous thrombosis
acitretin	Etretin; Soriatane	cutaneous T-cell lymphoma
acridinyl anisidide	Amsa P-D	leukemia
ACT-D	Cosmegen; Lyovac Cosmegen	Wilms' tumor; childhood rhabdomyosarcoma; Ewing sarcoma; testicular cancer; gestational trophoblastic neoplasia; choriocarcinoma; melanoma; neuroblastoma; retinoblastoma; uterine sarcomas; Kaposi sarcoma; sarcoma botryoides; soft-tissue sarcoma
actinomycin A IV	Cosmegen; Lyovac Cosmegen	Wilms' tumor; childhood rhabdomyosarcoma; Ewing sarcoma; testicular cancer; gestational trophoblastic neoplasia; choriocarcinoma; melanoma; neuroblastoma; retinoblastoma; uterine sarcomas; Kaposi sarcoma; sarcoma botryoides; soft-tissue sarcoma
actinomycin C1	Cosmegen; Lyovac Cosmegen	Wilms' tumor; childhood rhabdomyosarcoma; Ewing sarcoma; testicular cancer; gestational trophoblastic neoplasia; choriocarcinoma; melanoma; neuroblastoma; retinoblastoma; uterine sarcomas; Kaposi sarcoma; sarcoma botryoides; soft-tissue sarcoma
actinomycin D	Cosmegen; Lyovac Cosmegen	Wilms' tumor; childhood rhabdomyosarcoma; Ewing sarcoma; testicular cancer; gestational trophoblastic neoplasia; choriocarcinoma; melanoma; neuroblastoma; retinoblastoma; uterine sarcomas; Kaposi sarcoma; sarcoma botryoides; soft-tissue sarcoma
actinomycin I1	Cosmegen; Lyovac Cosmegen	Wilms' tumor; childhood rhabdomyosarcoma; Ewing sarcoma; testicular cancer; gestational trophoblastic neoplasia; choriocarcinoma; melanoma; neuroblastoma; retinoblastoma; uterine sarcomas; Kaposi sarcoma; sarcoma botryoides; soft-tissue sarcoma
actinomycin IV	Cosmegen; Lyovac Cosmegen	Wilms' tumor; childhood rhabdomyosarcoma; Ewing sarcoma; testicular cancer; gestational trophoblastic neoplasia; choriocarcinoma; melanoma; neuroblastoma; retinoblastoma; uterine sarcomas; Kaposi sarcoma; sarcoma botryoides; soft-tissue sarcoma
actinomycin X 1	Cosmegen; Lyovac Cosmegen	Wilms' tumor; childhood rhabdomyosarcoma; Ewing sarcoma; testicular cancer; gestational trophoblastic neoplasia; choriocarcinoma; melanoma; neuroblastoma; retinoblastoma; uterine sarcomas; Kaposi sarcoma; sarcoma botryoides; soft-tissue sarcoma

Generic Drug	Trade Name	Indicated For
actinomycin-[thr-val-pro-sar-meval]	Cosmegen; Lyovac Cosmegen	Wilms' tumor; childhood rhabdomyosarcoma; Ewing sarcoma; testicular cancer; gestational trophoblastic neoplasia; choriocarcinoma; melanoma; neuroblastoma; retinoblastoma; uterine sarcomas; Kaposi sarcoma; sarcoma botryoides; soft-tissue sarcoma
AD	Cosmegen; Lyovac Cosmegen	Wilms' tumor; childhood rhabdomyosarcoma; Ewing sarcoma; testicular cancer; gestational trophoblastic neoplasia; choriocarcinoma; melanoma; neuroblastoma; retinoblastoma; uterine sarcomas; Kaposi sarcoma; sarcoma botryoides; soft-tissue sarcoma
adefovir dipivoxil	Hepsera	chronic hepatitis B
adipogenesis inhibitory factor	Neumega	chemotherapy-related thrombocytopenia
ADM	Adriamycin	leukemias; Wilms' tumor; neuroblastoma; soft-tissue and bone sarcomas; small-cell carcinoma of the lung; lymphomas; multiple myeloma; mesotheliomas; germ-cell tumors of the ovary or testis
ADR	Adriamycin	leukemias; Wilms' tumor; neuroblastoma; soft-tissue and bone sarcomas; small-cell carcinoma of the lung; lymphomas; multiple myeloma; mesotheliomas; germ-cell tumors of the ovary or testis
adria	Adriamycin	leukemias; Wilms' tumor; neuroblastoma; soft-tissue and bone sarcomas; small-cell carcinoma of the lung; lymphomas; multiple myeloma; mesotheliomas; germ-cell tumors of the ovary or testis
alanine nitrogen mustard	Alkeran	breast cancer; neuroblastoma; palliative treatment of multiple myeloma and nonresectable epithelial ovarian carcinoma; rhabdomyosarcoma
albumin-stabilized nanoparticle paclitaxel	Taxol; Abraxane; Onxol	bladder cancer; breast cancer; adjuvant in breast cancer therapy; cervical cancer; endometrial adenocarcinoma; esophageal cancer; head and neck cancer; non-small-cell lung cancer; lymphoma; ovarian cancer; prostate cancer; testicular cancer; AIDS-related Kaposi sarcoma
aldesleukin	Proleukin	metastatic renal cell carcinoma; metastatic melanoma; stimulates the production of blood cells, especially platelets, during chemotherapy
alemtuzumab	Campath	B-cell chronic lymphocytic leukemia
alitretinoin	Panretin	topical treatment of cutaneous lesions in patients with AIDS-related Kaposi sarcoma
all-trans retinoic acid	Aberel; Aknoten; Avita; Renova; Retin-A; Retin-A MICRO; Vesanoid	(oral) acute promyelocytic leukemia (APL), characterized by the t(15;17) translocation or the PML/RARa gene; for patients refractory to or who have relapsed from anthracycline chemotherapy, or for where anthracycline-based chemotherapy is contraindicated; (topical) acne vulgaris; other dermatologic conditions; some skin cancers
all-trans retinol	Aquasol A; Del-Vi-A; Pedi-Vit-A	diminishing malignant cell growth; enhancing the immune system

Generic Drug	Trade Name	Indicated For
all-trans vitamin A acid	Aberel; Aknoten; Avita; Renova; Retin-A; Retin-A MICRO; Vesanoid	(oral) acute promyelocytic leukemia (APL), characterized by the t(15;17) translocation or the PML/RARa gene refractory, or for where anthracycline-based chemotherapy is contraindicated; (topical) acne vulgaris; other dermatologic conditions; some skin cancers
allopurinol	Zyloprim	treats high levels of uric acid in the body caused by certain cancer medications, especially for patients with leukemia, lymphoma, and solid-tumor malignancies
alpha-phthalimidoglutarimide	Synovir; Thalomid	Kaposi sarcoma; multiple myeloma; primary brain tumors
alprostadil	Caverject; MUSE	erectile dysfunction; patent ductus arteriosus
altretamine	Hexalen; Hexamethylmelamine	ovarian cancer
alum adjuvant	none	allergy; diagnosis
aluminum hydroxide	none	allergy; diagnosis
aluminum sulfate	none	allergy; diagnosis
amifostine trihydrate	Ethyol	cisplatin-induced nephrotoxicity; radiation-induced mucositis and xerostomia
aminobenzoate potassium	none	diseases involving fibrosis and nonsuppurative inflammation
aminoglutethimide	Cytadren	breast cancer; prostate cancer; decreases the production of sex hormones (estrogen in women or testosterone in men) and suppresses the growth of tumors that need sex hormones to grow
aminolevulinic acid	Levulan	photodynamic therapy to treat a skin condition called actinic keratosis
aminopropylaminoethylthio-phosphoric acid	Ethyol	cisplatin-induced nephrotoxicity; radiation-induced mucositis and xerostomia
amoxicillin-clavulanate potassium	Augmentin	various bacterial infections
amsacrine	Amsa P-D	leukemia
anagrelide	Agrylin	thrombocythemia secondary to myeloproliferative disorders; disrupts the postmitotic phase of megakaryocyte development
anastrozole	Arimidex	hormone receptor-positive early breast cancer
androfluorene	Android-F; Halodrin; Halotestin; Ora-Testryl; Ultandren; Androxy	certain types of breast cancer
androsterolo	Android-F; Halodrin; Halotestin; Ora-Testryl; Ultandren; Androxy	certain types of breast cancer
anidulafungin	Eraxis	candidemia
anti-B1; anti-B1 monoclonal antibody	Bexxar	CD20 positive follicular non-Hodgkin lymphoma refractory to rituximab
anti-CD20 antibody	Bexxar	CD20 positive follicular non-Hodgkin lymphoma refractory to rituximab

Generic Drug	Trade Name	Indicated For
anti-CD20 monoclonal antibody	Rituxan	diffuse large B-cell, CD20-positive, non-Hodgkin lymphoma
anti-CD52 monoclonal antibody	Campath	B-cell chronic lymphocytic leukemia
anti-c-erB-2; anti-c-erbB2 monoclonal antibody	Herceptin	breast cancer overexpressing HER2 protein; pancreatic cancer overexpressing p185HER2
anti-EGFR monoclonal antibody	Erbitux	advanced colorectal cancer; head and neck cancer
antiepidermal growth factor receptor monoclonal antibody	Erbitux	advanced colorectal cancer; head and neck cancer
anti-ERB-2; anti-erbB2 monoclonal antibody	Herceptin	breast cancer overexpressing HER2 protein; pancreatic cancer overexpressing p185HER2
anti-HER2/c-erbB2 monoclonal antibody	Herceptin	breast cancer overexpressing HER2 protein; pancreatic cancer overexpressing p185HER2
anti-infective vitamin	Aquasol A; Del-Vi-A; Pedi-Vit-A	diminishing malignant cell growth; enhancing the immune system
anti-p185-HER2	Herceptin	breast cancer overexpressing HER2 protein; pancreatic cancer overexpressing p185HER2
antithymocyte globulin	ATGAM; Thymoglobulin	heart and renal transplantation rejection; prophylaxis
anti-VEGF; anti-VEGF monoclonal antibody	Avastin	metastatic colorectal cancer, non-small-cell lung cancer
anti-VEGF humanized monoclonal antibody	Avastin	metastatic colorectal cancer, non-small-cell lung cancer
anti-VEGF RhuMAb	Avastin	metastatic colorectal cancer, non-small-cell lung cancer
antixerophthalmic vitamin	Aquasol A; Del-Vi-A; Pedi-Vit-A	diminishing malignant cell growth; enhancing the immune system
aprepitant	Emend	antiemetic (prevents vomiting)
arabinofuranosylcytosine	Cytosar-U; Tarabine PFS	acute nonlymphocytic leukemia; acute lymphocytic leukemia; chronic myelogenous leukemia; bone marrow transplantation; carcinomatous meningitis; Hodgkin disease; meningeal leukemia; myelodysplasic syndrome; non-Hodgkin lymphoma; ovarian cancer; retinoblastoma
arabinosylcytosine	Cytosar-U; Tarabine PFS	acute nonlymphocytic leukemia; acute lymphocytic leukemia; chronic myelogenous leukemia; bone marrow transplantation; carcinomatous meningitis; Hodgkin disease; meningeal leukemia; myelodysplasic syndrome; non-Hodgkin lymphoma; ovarian cancer; retinoblastoma
aracytidine	Cytosar-U; Tarabine PFS	acute nonlymphocytic leukemia; acute lymphocytic leukemia; chronic myelogenous leukemia; bone marrow transplantation; carcinomatous meningitis; Hodgkin disease; meningeal leukemia; myelodysplasic syndrome; non-Hodgkin lymphoma; ovarian cancer; retinoblastoma

Generic Drug	Trade Name	Indicated For
arsenic (III) oxide	Trisenox	myelodysplastic syndrome; multiple myeloma; chronic myeloid leukemia; acute myelocytic leukemia
arsenic sesquioxide	Trisenox	myelodysplastic syndrome; multiple myeloma; chronic myeloid leukemia; acute myelocytic leukemia
arsenic trioxide	Trisenox	myelodysplastic syndrome; multiple myeloma; chronic myeloid leukemia; acute myelocytic leukemia
arsenous acid	Trisenox	myelodysplastic syndrome; multiple myeloma; chronic myeloid leukemia; acute myelocytic leukemia
arsenous acid anhydride	Trisenox	myelodysplastic syndrome; multiple myeloma; chronic myeloid leukemia; acute myelocytic leukemia
arsenous oxide	Trisenox	myelodysplastic syndrome; multiple myeloma; chronic myeloid leukemia; acute myelocytic leukemia
ASNase	Elspar; Cristanaspase; L-Asnase	some blood cancers; acute lymphocytic leukemia; acute nonlymphocytic leukemia
ASP-1	Elspar; Cristanaspase; L-Asnase	some blood cancers; acute lymphocytic leukemia; acute nonlymphocytic leukemia
asparaginase; asparaginase II	Elspar; Cristanaspase; L-Asnase	some blood cancers; acute lymphocytic leukemia; acute nonlymphocytic leukemia
asparaginase erwinia	Elspar; Cristanaspase; L-Asnase	some blood cancers; acute lymphocytic leukemia; acute nonlymphocytic leukemia
aspirin	Aspergum; Ecotrin; Empirin; Entericin; Extren; Measurin	mild to moderate pain; fever; prevention of arterial and venous thrombosis
aureolic acid	Mithracin	testicular cancer
axerophthol	Aquasol A; Del-Vi-A; Pedi-Vit-A	diminishing malignant cell growth; enhancing the immune system
axerophtholum	Aquasol A; Del-Vi-A; Pedi-Vit-A	diminishing malignant cell growth; enhancing the immune system
azacitidine	Mylosar; Vidaza	myelodysplastic syndrome
azacytidine	Mylosar; Vidaza	myelodysplastic syndrome
5-azacytidine	Mylosar; Vidaza	myelodysplastic syndrome
5-aza-dCyd	Dacogen	myelodysplastic syndrome
azaepothilone B	Ixempra	metastatic or locally advanced breast cancer
azathioprine sodium	Imuran; Imurel	converted in vivo to its active metabolite 6-mercaptopurine (6-MP), which substitutes for the normal nucleoside and mistakenly gets incorporated into DNA sequences. This leads to inhibition of DNA, RNA, and protein synthesis. As a result, cell proliferation may be inhibited, particularly in lymphocytes and leukocytes
azathiopurine	Mercaptopurinum; Purinethol	acute lymphocytic leukemia; acute myelogenous leukemia; Crohn disease; Hodgkin disease in children; lymphoblastic lymphoma; ulcerative colitis
BAY 43-9006	Nexavar	advanced renal cell carcinoma; metastatic colorectal cancer

Generic Drug	Trade Name	Indicated For
BAY 43-9006 Tosylate Salt	Nexavar	advanced renal cell carcinoma; metastatic colorectal cancer
BCG	Immucyst	bladder cancer; malignant melanoma
bendamustine hydrochloride	Treanda	chronic lymphocytic leukemia
beta-carotene	Lumitene; Solatene	chemoprevention for cardiovascular disease and cancer
beta-cytosine arabinoside	Cytosar-U; Tarabine PFS	acute nonlymphocytic leukemia; acute lymphocytic leukemia; chronic myelogenous leukemia; bone marrow transplantation; carcinomatous meningitis; Hodgkin disease; meningeal leukemia; myelodysplasic syndrome; non-Hodgkin lymphoma; ovarian cancer; retinoblastoma
beta-retinoic acid	Aberel; Aknoten; Avita; Renova; Retin-A; Retin-A MICRO; Vesanoid	(oral) acute promyelocytic leukemia (APL), characterized by the t(15;17) translocation or the PML/RARa gene; for patients refractory to or who have relapsed from anthracycline chemotherapy, or for where anthracycline-based chemotherapy is contraindicated; (topical) acne vulgaris; other dermatologic conditions; some skin cancers
bevacizumab	Avastin	metastatic colorectal cancer, non-small-cell lung cancer
bexarotene	Targretin	oral or topical treatment of manifestations of cutaneous T-cell lymphoma
bicalutamide	Casodex	metastatic prostate cancer
biocarbazine	DTIC-Dome	carcinoid cancer; Hodgkin disease; islet cell carcinoma; melanoma; neuroblastoma; soft-tissue sarcoma
biosterol	Aquasol A; Del-Vi-A; Pedi-Vit-A	diminishing malignant cell growth; enhancing the immune system
bis(chloroethyl) nitrosourea	BiCNU; Becenum; Carmubris	cancerous brain tumors; colon cancer; lung cancer; Hodgkin disease; non-Hodgkin lymphomas; lymphomas; melanoma; multiple myeloma; mycosis fungoides
bis-chloronitrosourea	BiCNU; Becenum; Carmubris	cancerous brain tumors; colon cancer; lung cancer; Hodgkin disease; non-Hodgkin lymphomas; lymphomas; melanoma; multiple myeloma; mycosis fungoides
bleomycin	Blenoxane; bleomycin sulfate	skin cancer (squamous cell carcinoma) of the head, neck, penis, cervix, and vulva; lymphomas; testicular cancer; malignant pleural effusion
BMS-354825	Sprycel	chronic myeloid leukemia; Philadelphia chromosome-positive acute lymphoblastic leukemia
bortezomib	Velcade	multiple myeloma; advanced thyroid cancer
BSF	Busulfex; Mitosan; Myleran	bone marrow disorders; chronic myelogenous leukemia; palliative; neoadjuvant to allogeneic hematopoietic progenitor cell transplantation; neoplastic meningitis; primary brain malignancies
bupropion hydrochloride	Wellbutrin; Zyban	depression; smoking cessation
buserelin	Suprecur	breast cancer; contraception, female; endometriosis; infertility; in vitro fertilization; polycystic ovary syndrome; prostate cancer; uterine leiomyoma

Generic Drug	Trade Name	Indicated For
buspirone hydrochloride	Buspar	alcohol abuse; anxiety; depression; migraine prophylaxis; smoking cessation; panic disorder
bussulfam	Busulfex; Mitosan; Myleran	bone marrow disorders; chronic myelogenous leukemia; palliative; neoadjuvant to allogeneic hematopoietic progenitor cell transplantation; neoplastic meningitis; primary brain malignancies
busulfan; bunsulfanum	Busulfex; Mitosan; Myleran	bone marrow disorders; chronic myelogenous leukemia; palliative; neoadjuvant to allogeneic hematopoietic progenitor cell transplantation; neoplastic meningitis; primary brain malignancies
busulphan	Busulfex; Mitosan; Myleran	bone marrow disorders; chronic myelogenous leukemia; palliative; neoadjuvant to allogeneic hematopoietic progenitor cell transplantation; neoplastic meningitis; primary brain malignancies
C2B8 monoclonal antibody	Rituxan	diffuse large B-cell, CD20-positive, non-Hodgkin lymphoma
C225 monoclonal antibody	Erbitux	advanced colorectal cancer; head and neck cancer
cabergoline	Dostinex	pituitary tumors
CACP	Platinol; Platinol-AQ	metastatic testicular cancer; ovarian cancer; head and neck cancer; breast cancer; Hodgkin disease and non-Hodgkin lymphoma; myeloma and melanoma; advanced bladder cancer
Cain's acridine	Amsa P-D	leukemia
calcitriol	Rocaltrol	hyperparathyroidism; hypocalcemia
calcium carbonate	none	calcium deficiency, prophylaxis; hyperacidity; hyperphosphatemia; osteoporosis; rickets
calcium citrate	Acicontral; Citracal	calcium supplement; hypocalcemia; osteoporosis; rickets; tetany
calcium folinate	Wellcovorin	used to protect normal cells from high doses of the anticancer drug methotrexate; also used to increase the antitumor effects of fluorouracil and tegafur-uracil; megaloblastic anemia due to folate deficiency; enhanced fluorouracil inhibition of thymidylate synthase; reverse dihydrofolate reductase inhibition by methotrexate; folic acid antagonist overdose; nitrous oxide toxicity
calcium (6S)-folinate	Wellcovorin	used to protect normal cells from high doses of the anticancer drug methotrexate; also used to increase the antitumor effects of fluorouracil and tegafur-uracil; megaloblastic anemia due to folate deficiency; enhanced fluorouracil inhibition of thymidylate synthase; reverse dihydrofolate reductase inhibition by methotrexate; folic acid antagonist overdose; nitrous oxide toxicity
calcium gluconate	Calglucon	hyperkalemia; hypocalcemic tetany; magnesium intoxication
calicheamicin-conjugated humanized anti-CD33 monoclonal antibody	Mylotarg	acute myeloid leukemia
campath-1H	Campath	B-cell chronic lymphocytic leukemia
camptothecin-11	Camptosar	stage IVB cervical cancer; colorectal cancer; esophageal cancer; gastric cancer; non-small-cell lung cancer; small-cell lung cancer

Generic Drug	Trade Name	Indicated For
cannabinol	Marinol	antinausea
capecitabine	Xeloda	breast cancer; colorectal cancer; Stage III colon cancer
captopril	Capoten	hypertension; heart failure; left ventricular dysfunction; diabetic nephropathy
carbamazepine	Epitol; Tegretol	epilepsy
carbon-11 acetate	none	diagnostic imaging
carboplatin; carboplatin hexal	Paraplatin; Paraplat	ovarian cancer
carboplatino	Paraplatin; Paraplat	ovarian cancer
carmustin; carmustine	BiCNU; Becenum; Carmubris	cancerous brain tumors; colon cancer; lung cancer; Hodgkin disease; non-Hodgkin lymphomas; lymphomas; melanoma; multiple myeloma; mycosis fungoides
CBL	Ambochlorin; Amboclorin; Leukeran	chronic lymphocytic leukemia; malignant lymphomas
CDC-501	Revlimid	transfusion-dependent anemia due to low- or intermediate-1 risk myelodysplastic syndrome; multiple myeloma
cefepime hydrochloride	Maxipime	upper respiratory tract and urinary tract infections; febrile neutropenic conditions
celecoxib	Celebrex	familial adenomatous polyposis (inherited colorectal cancer syndrome)
cell cycle inhibitor 779	Torisel	renal cell carcinoma; advanced renal cell carcinoma
cetuximab	Erbitux	advanced colorectal cancer; head and neck cancer
cevimeline hydrochloride	Evoxac	Sjögren syndrome
CFR	Wellcovorin	used to protect normal cells from high doses of the anticancer drug methotrexate; also used to increase the antitumor effects of fluorouracil and tegafur-uracil; megaloblastic anemia due to folate deficiency; enhanced fluorouracil inhibition of thymidylate synthase; reverse dihydrofolate reductase inhibition by methotrexate; folic acid antagonist overdose; nitrous oxide toxicity
chimeric anti-EGFR monoclonal antibody	Erbitux	advanced colorectal cancer; head and neck cancer
chimeric monoclonal antibody C225	Erbitux	advanced colorectal cancer; head and neck cancer
chloditan; chlodithane	Lysodren	adrenal cortical carcinoma
chlorambucil; chlorambucilum	Ambochlorin; Amboclorin; Leukeran	chronic lymphocytic leukemia; malignant lymphomas
chloramin	Mustargen	bronchogenic carcinoma; chronic lymphocytic and myelcytic leukemia; Hodgkin disease, palliative; lymphosarcoma; mycosis fungoides; polycythemia vera
chloraminophen	Ambochlorin; Amboclorin; Leukeran	chronic lymphocytic leukemia; malignant lymphomas

Generic Drug	Trade Name	Indicated For
chlorbutin; chlorbutine	Ambochlorin; Amboclorin; Leukeran	chronic lymphocytic leukemia; malignant lymphomas
chlorbutinum	Ambochlorin; Amboclorin; Leukeran	chronic lymphocytic leukemia; malignant lymphomas
chlorethamine HCl; chlorethamine hydrochloride	Mustargen	bronchogenic carcinoma; chronic lymphocytic and myelcytic leukemia; Hodgkin disease, palliative; lymphosarcoma; mycosis fungoides; polycythemia vera
chlorethazine	Mustargen	bronchogenic carcinoma; chronic lymphocytic and myelcytic leukemia; Hodgkin disease, palliative; lymphosarcoma; mycosis fungoides; polycythemia vera
chlorethazine hydrochloride	Mustargen	bronchogenic carcinoma; chronic lymphocytic and myelcytic leukemia; Hodgkin disease, palliative; lymphosarcoma; mycosis fungoides; polycythemia vera
chlormethine	Mustargen	bronchogenic carcinoma; chronic lymphocytic and myelcytic leukemia; Hodgkin disease, palliative; lymphosarcoma; mycosis fungoides; polycythemia vera
chlormethine hydrochloride	Mustargen	bronchogenic carcinoma; chronic lymphocytic and myelcytic leukemia; Hodgkin disease, palliative; lymphosarcoma; mycosis fungoides; polycythemia vera
chloroambucil	Ambochlorin; Amboclorin; Leukeran	chronic lymphocytic leukemia; malignant lymphomas
chlorobutin; chlorobutine	Ambochlorin; Amboclorin; Leukeran	chronic lymphocytic leukemia; malignant lymphomas
2-chlorodeoxyadenosine	Leustatin	acute myeloid leukemia; chronic lymphocytic leukemia; cutaneous T-cell lymphoma; hairy cell leukemia; Langerhans cell histiocytosis; non-Hodgkin lymphoma; Waldenstrom macroglobulinemia
2-chloro-2-deoxyadenosine	Leustatin	acute myeloid leukemia; chronic lymphocytic leukemia; cutaneous T-cell lymphoma; hairy cell leukemia; Langerhans cell histiocytosis; non-Hodgkin lymphoma; Waldenström macroglobulinemia
chloromethine HCl	Mustargen	bronchogenic carcinoma; chronic lymphocytic and myelcytic leukemia; Hodgkin disease, palliative; lymphosarcoma; mycosis fungoides; polycythemia vera
ciclofosfamida; ciclofosfamide	Cytoxan; Clafen; Neosar	breast cancer; leukemias; lupus nephritis; lymphoma; multiple myeloma; neuroblastoma; nephrotic syndrome; ovarian cancer; retinoblastoma
cimetidine	Tagamet	gastrointestinal conditions; allergic reaction prevention; immune modulation
cinacalcet	Sensipar	treating an overactive parathyroid in dialysis patients with chronic kidney disease; also used to treat high blood calcium levels in patients with parathyroid cancer
ciprofloxacin	Cipro	inhaled anthrax, postexposure; susceptible infectious diseases

Generic Drug	Trade Name	Indicated For
cis-DDP	Platinol; Platinol-AQ	metastatic testicular cancer; ovarian cancer; head and neck cancer; breast cancer; Hodgkin disease and non-Hodgkin lymphoma; myeloma and melanoma; advanced bladder cancer
cis-diamminedichloro platinum (II)	Platinol; Platinol-AQ	metastatic testicular cancer; ovarian cancer; head and neck cancer; breast cancer; Hodgkin disease and non-Hodgkin lymphoma; myeloma and melanoma; advanced bladder cancer
cis-diamminedichloroplatinum	Platinol; Platinol-AQ	metastatic testicular cancer; ovarian cancer; head and neck cancer; breast cancer; Hodgkin disease and non-Hodgkin lymphoma; myeloma and melanoma; advanced bladder cancer
cis-dichloroammine platinum (II)	Platinol; Platinol-AQ	metastatic testicular cancer; ovarian cancer; head and neck cancer; breast cancer; Hodgkin disease and non-Hodgkin lymphoma; myeloma and melanoma; advanced bladder cancer
cis-platinous diamine dichloride	Platinol; Platinol-AQ	metastatic testicular cancer; ovarian cancer; head and neck cancer; breast cancer; Hodgkin disease and non-Hodgkin lymphoma; myeloma and melanoma; advanced bladder cancer
cis-platinum; cis-platinum II	Platinol; Platinol-AQ	metastatic testicular cancer; ovarian cancer; head and neck cancer; breast cancer; Hodgkin disease and non-Hodgkin lymphoma; myeloma and melanoma; advanced bladder cancer
cis-platinum II diamine dichloride	Platinol; Platinol-AQ	metastatic testicular cancer; ovarian cancer; head and neck cancer; breast cancer; Hodgkin disease and non-Hodgkin lymphoma; myeloma and melanoma; advanced bladder cancer
cismaplat	Platinol; Platinol-AQ	metastatic testicular cancer; ovarian cancer; head and neck cancer; breast cancer; Hodgkin disease and non-Hodgkin lymphoma; myeloma and melanoma; advanced bladder cancer
cisplatin; cisplatina	Platinol; Platinol-AQ	metastatic testicular cancer; ovarian cancer; head and neck cancer; breast cancer; Hodgkin disease and non-Hodgkin lymphoma; myeloma and melanoma; advanced bladder cancer
9-cis-retinoic acid	Panretin	topical treatment of cutaneous lesions in patients with AIDS-related Kaposi sarcoma
citrovorum factor	Wellcovorin	used to protect normal cells from high doses of the anticancer drug methotrexate; also used to increase the antitumor effects of fluorouracil and tegafur-uracil; megaloblastic anemia due to folate deficiency; enhanced fluorouracil inhibition of thymidylate synthase; reverse dihydrofolate reductase inhibition by methotrexate; folic acid antagonist overdose; nitrous oxide toxicity
cladribina; cladribine	Leustatin	acute myeloid leukemia; chronic lymphocytic leukemia; cutaneous T-cell lymphoma; hairy cell leukemia; Langerhans cell histiocytosis; non-Hodgkin lymphoma; Waldenström macroglobulinemia
claphene	Cytoxan; Clafen; Neosar	breast cancer; leukemias; lupus nephritis; lymphoma; multiple myeloma; neuroblastoma; nephrotic syndrome; ovarian cancer; retinoblastoma
clarithromycin	Abbott-56268; Biaxin	*H. pylori* infection; various bacterial infections
clobetasol propionate	Olux-E	psoriasis, eczema

Generic Drug	Trade Name	Indicated For
clodronate disodium	Clasteon; Difosfonal; Loron; Mebonat; Ossiten	adjuvant usage in bone metastasis of breast cancer
clofarabine	Clolar	accelerated approval (clinical benefit not established) for the treatment of pediatric patients one to twenty-one years old with relapsed or refractory acute lymphoblastic leukemia after at least two prior regimens
clopidogrel bisulfate	Plavix	thromboembolic disorders
cloridrato de daunorubicina	Cerubidine; Rubidomycin	acute lymphoblastic leukemia
co-codamol	Solpadol; Tylex; Kapake	painkiller
coenzyme Q10	Ubidecarenone; Ubiquinone 10	chronic heart failure; mitochondrial cytopathies
colaspase	Elspar; Cristanaspase; L-Asnase	some blood cancers; acute lymphocytic leukemia; acute nonlymphocytic leukemia
compound 112531	Eldisine	acute leukemia; lung cancer; carcinoma of the breast; squamous cell carcinoma of the esophagus, head, and neck; Hodgkin disease and non-Hodgkin lymphomas
conjugated estrogens	Femest; Premarin	advanced androgen-dependent prostate cancer, palliative; breast cancer, palliative
cordycepin	Kordicepin	TdT-positive acute lymphocytic leukemia
co-vidarabine	Nipent	chronic lymphocytic leukemia; cutaneous T-cell lymphoma; hairy cell leukemia
CP monohydrate	Cytoxan; Clafen; Neosar	breast cancer; leukemias; lupus nephritis; lymphoma; multiple myeloma; neuroblastoma; nephrotic syndrome; ovarian cancer; retinoblastoma
CPDD	Platinol; Platinol-AQ	metastatic testicular cancer; ovarian cancer; head and neck cancer; breast cancer; Hodgkin disease and non-Hodgkin lymphoma; myeloma and melanoma; advanced bladder cancer
CPM	Cytoxan; Clafen; Neosar	breast cancer; leukemias; lupus nephritis; lymphoma; multiple myeloma; neuroblastoma; nephrotic syndrome; ovarian cancer; retinoblastoma
cyclophospham	Cytoxan; Clafen; Neosar	breast cancer; leukemias; lupus nephritis; lymphoma; multiple myeloma; neuroblastoma; nephrotic syndrome; ovarian cancer; retinoblastoma
cyclophosphamid monohydrate	Cytoxan; Clafen; Neosar	breast cancer; leukemias; lupus nephritis; lymphoma; multiple myeloma; neuroblastoma; nephrotic syndrome; ovarian cancer; retinoblastoma
cyclophosphamide	Cytoxan; Clafen; Neosar	breast cancer; leukemias; lupus nephritis; lymphoma; multiple myeloma; neuroblastoma; nephrotic syndrome; ovarian cancer; retinoblastoma
cyclophosphamidum	Cytoxan; Clafen; Neosar	breast cancer; leukemias; lupus nephritis; lymphoma; multiple myeloma; neuroblastoma; nephrotic syndrome; ovarian cancer; retinoblastoma

Generic Drug	Trade Name	Indicated For
cyclophosphan; cyclophosphanum	Cytoxan; Clafen; Neosar	breast cancer; leukemias; lupus nephritis; lymphoma; multiple myeloma; neuroblastoma; nephrotic syndrome; ovarian cancer; retinoblastoma
cyclosporine	Neoral; Sandimmun; SangCya	allogenic transplants; prophylaxis of organ rejection in bone marrow; kidney; liver and heart transplants; psoriasis; rheumatoid arthritis; various diseases that involve autoimmune response
cyproheptadine hydrochloride	Periactin	hypersensitivity reactions
cyproterone acetate	Cyprostat	prostate cancer
cysplatyna	Platinol; Platinol-AQ	metastatic testicular cancer; ovarian cancer; head and neck cancer; breast cancer; Hodgkin disease and non-Hodgkin lymphoma; myeloma and melanoma; advanced bladder cancer
cytarabine	Cytosar-U; Tarabine PFS	acute nonlymphocytic leukemia; acute lymphocytic leukemia; chronic myelogenous leukemia; bone marrow transplantation; carcinomatous meningitis; Hodgkin disease; meningeal leukemia; lymphomatous meningitis; myelodysplasic syndrome; non-Hodgkin lymphoma; ovarian cancer; retinoblastoma
cytarabine hydrochloride	Cytosar-U; Tarabine PFS	acute nonlymphocytic leukemia; acute lymphocytic leukemia; chronic myelogenous leukemia; bone marrow transplantation; carcinomatous meningitis; Hodgkin disease; meningeal leukemia; lymphomatous meningitis; myelodysplasic syndrome; non-Hodgkin lymphoma; ovarian cancer; retinoblastoma
cytarabinum	Cytosar-U; Tarabine PFS	acute nonlymphocytic leukemia; acute lymphocytic leukemia; chronic myelogenous leukemia; bone marrow transplantation; carcinomatous meningitis; Hodgkin disease; meningeal leukemia; lymphomatous meningitis; myelodysplasic syndrome; non-Hodgkin lymphoma; ovarian cancer; retinoblastoma
cytophosphane	Cytoxan; Clafen; Neosar	breast cancer; leukemias; lupus nephritis; lymphoma; multiple myeloma; neuroblastoma; nephrotic syndrome; ovarian cancer; retinoblastoma
cytosine arabinoside	Cytosar-U; Tarabine PFS	acute nonlymphocytic leukemia; acute lymphocytic leukemia; chronic myelogenous leukemia; bone marrow transplantation; carcinomatous meningitis; Hodgkin disease; meningeal leukemia; lymphomatous meningitis; myelodysplasic syndrome; non-Hodgkin lymphoma; ovarian cancer; retinoblastoma
cytosine arabinosine hydrochloride	Cytosar-U; Tarabine PFS	acute nonlymphocytic leukemia; acute lymphocytic leukemia; chronic myelogenous leukemia; bone marrow transplantation; carcinomatous meningitis; Hodgkin disease; meningeal leukemia; lymphomatous meningitis; myelodysplasic syndrome; non-Hodgkin lymphoma; ovarian cancer; retinoblastoma
6-D-tryptophan-LH-RH	Decapeptyl	prostate carcinoma, palliative treatment
6-D-tryptophanluteinizing hormone-releasing factor	Decapeptyl	prostate carcinoma, palliative treatment
DAB389-IL2	Ontak	cutaneous T-cell lymphoma
DAB389 interleukin-2	Ontak	cutaneous T-cell lymphoma

Generic Drug	Trade Name	Indicated For
DAB389 interleukin-2 immunotoxin	Ontak	cutaneous T-cell lymphoma
dacarbazina	DTIC-Dome	carcinoid cancer; Hodgkin disease; islet cell carcinoma; melanoma; neuroblastoma; soft-tissue sarcoma
dacarbazina almirall	DTIC-Dome	carcinoid cancer; Hodgkin disease; islet cell carcinoma; melanoma; neuroblastoma; soft-tissue sarcoma
Dacarbazine; dacarbazine-DTIC	DTIC-Dome	carcinoid cancer; Hodgkin disease; islet cell carcinoma; melanoma; neuroblastoma; soft-tissue sarcoma
daclizumab	Zenapax	kidney transplant rejection, prevention
dactinomycin; dactinomycine	Cosmegen; Lyovac Cosmegen	Wilms' tumor; childhood rhabdomyosarcoma; Ewing sarcoma; testicular cancer; gestational trophoblastic neoplasia; choriocarcinoma; melanoma; neuroblastoma; retinoblastoma; uterine sarcomas; Kaposi sarcoma; sarcoma botryoides; soft-tissue sarcoma
dakarbazin	DTIC-Dome	carcinoid cancer; Hodgkin disease; islet cell carcinoma; melanoma; neuroblastoma; soft-tissue sarcoma
dalteparin	Fragmin	deep vein thrombosis, prophylaxis; ischemic complications in unstable angina and non-Q wave myocardial infarction, prophylaxis
dantrolene	Dantrium	treating episodes of severe high body temperature; also used to prevent or reduce the risk of severe high body temperature in certain patients before or after surgery or anesthesia
darbepoetin alfa	Aranesp	chemotherapy-induced anemia; chronic renal failure/insufficiency
dasatinib	Sprycel	chronic myeloid leukemia; Philadelphia chromosome-positive acute lymphoblastic leukemia
daunomycin	Cerubidine; Rubidomycin	acute lymphoblastic leukemia
daunomycin-HCL	Cerubidine; Rubidomycin	acute lymphoblastic leukemia
daunorubicin	Cerubidine; Rubidomycin	acute lymphoblastic leukemia
daunorubicin hydrochloride	Cerubidine; Rubidomycin	acute lymphoblastic leukemia
daunorubicin liposomal	DaunoXome	acute nonlymphocytic leukemia; acute lymphocytic leukemia; advanced HIV-associated Kaposi sarcoma
dauno-rubidomycine	Cerubidine; Rubidomycin	acute lymphoblastic leukemia
DDP	Platinol; Platinol-AQ	metastatic testicular cancer; ovarian cancer; head and neck cancer; breast cancer; Hodgkin disease and non-Hodgkin lymphoma; myeloma and melanoma; advanced bladder cancer
deacetyl vinblastine carboxamide	Eldisine	acute leukemia; lung cancer; carcinoma of the breast; squamous cell carcinoma of the esophagus, head, and neck; Hodgkin disease and non-Hodgkin lymphomas
decitabine	Dacogen	myelodysplastic syndrome
defibrotide	none	thrombotic thrombocytopenic purpura
delta 9-tetrahydrocannabinol	Marinol	antinausea

Generic Drug	Trade Name	Indicated For
deltacortisone	Delta-Dome; Deltasone; Liquid Pred; Lisacort; Meticorten; Orasone; Prednicen-M; Sk-Prednisone; Sterapred	inflammatory conditions; allergic conditions; hematologic conditions; neoplastic conditions; autoimmune conditions; replacement therapy in adrenal insufficiency
delta(1)-cortisone	Delta-Dome; Deltasone; Liquid Pred; Lisacort; Meticorten; Orasone; Prednicen-M; Sk-Prednisone; Sterapred	inflammatory conditions; allergic conditions; hematologic conditions; neoplastic conditions; autoimmune conditions; replacement therapy in adrenal insufficiency
deltadehydrocortisone	Delta-Dome; Deltasone; Liquid Pred; Lisacort; Meticorten; Orasone; Prednicen-M; Sk-Prednisone; Sterapred	inflammatory conditions; allergic conditions; hematologic conditions; neoplastic conditions; autoimmune conditions; replacement therapy in adrenal insufficiency
4-demethoxydaunomycin	Idamycin	acute myeloid leukemia (AML); acute nonlymphocytic leukemia
4-demethoxydaunorubicin	Idamycin	acute myeloid leukemia (AML); acute nonlymphocytic leukemia
demethyl epipodophyllotoxin ethylidine glucoside	VePesid; Lastet; Etopophos; Toposar	acute leukemia; adrenal cortical cancer; brain cancer; chronic lymphocytic leukemia; choriocarcinoma; esophageal cancer; Ewing sarcoma; gastric cancer; germ-cell cancer; gestational trophoblastic neoplasms; hepatocellular cancer; Hodgkin disease; hypereosinophilic syndrome; Kaposi sarcoma; testicular cancer; thymoma; thyroid cancer; uterine cancer; Wilms' tumor; Langerhans cell histiocytosis; mobilization of peripheral-blood progenitor cells; multiple myeloma; neuroblastoma; non-small-cell lung cancer; osteogenic sarcoma; ovarian cancer; retinoblastoma; small-cell lung cancer; soft-tissue sarcomas
denileukin diftitox	Ontak	cutaneous T-cell lymphoma
deoxyazacytidine	Dacogen	myelodysplastic syndrome
deoxycoformycin	Nipent	chronic lymphocytic leukemia; cutaneous T-cell lymphoma; hairy cell leukemia
2'-deoxycoformycin	Nipent	chronic lymphocytic leukemia; cutaneous T-cell lymphoma; hairy cell leukemia
desacetylvinblastine amide	Eldisine	acute leukemia; lung cancer; carcinoma of the breast; squamous cell carcinoma of the esophagus, head, and neck; Hodgkin disease and non-Hodgkin lymphomas
desamethasone	Aeroseb-Dex; Alba-Dex; Decaderm; Decadrol; Decadron; Decasone R.p.; Decaspray; Deenar; Deronil; Dex-4; Dexace; Dexameth; Dezone; Gammacorten; Hexadrol; Maxidex; Sk-Dexamethasone	antiemetic (prevents vomiting)
deslorelin	Ovuplant	central precocious puberty
detryptoreline	Decapeptyl	prostate carcinoma, palliative treatment

Generic Drug	Trade Name	Indicated For
dexamethasone; dexamethasonum	Aeroseb-Dex; Alba-Dex; Decaderm; Decadrol; Decadron; Decasone R.p.; Decaspray; Deenar; Deronil; Dex-4; Dexace; Dexameth; Dezone; Gammacorten; Hexadrol; Maxidex; Sk-Dexamethasone	antiemetic (prevents vomiting)
dexrazoxane hydrochloride	Totect; Zinecard	severe side effects caused by certain types of chemotherapy including extravasation; cardiac side effects by doxorubicin
dextroamphetamine-amphetamine	Adderall	attention deficit/hyperactivity disorder (ADHD); narcolepsy
dezocitidine	Dacogen	myelodysplastic syndrome
diaminocyclohexane oxalatoplatinum	Eloxatin	metastatic colorectal cancer; ovarian cancer
diazoxide	Proglycem	malignant hypertension
diethylstilbenediol	Acnestrol; Cyren A; Deladumone; Diastyl; Domestrol; Estrobene; Estrosyn; Fonatol; Makarol; Milestrol; Neo-Oestronol I; Oestrogenine; Oestromenin; Oestromon; Palestrol; Stilbestrol; Stilbetin; Stilboestroform; Stilboestrol; Synestrin; Synthoestrin; Vagestrol	breast cancer; prostate cancer
diethylstilbesterol	Acnestrol; Cyren A; Deladumone; Diastyl; Domestrol; Estrobene; Estrosyn; Fonatol; Makarol; Milestrol; Neo-Oestronol I; Oestrogenine; Oestromenin; Oestromon; Palestrol; Stilbestrol; Stilbetin; Stilboestroform; Stilboestrol; Synestrin; Synthoestrin; Vagestrol	breast cancer; prostate cancer
diethylstilbestrol dipropionate	Acnestrol; Cyren A; Deladumone; Diastyl; Domestrol; Estrobene; Estrosyn; Fonatol; Makarol; Milestrol; Neo-Oestronol I; Oestrogenine; Oestromenin; Oestromon; Palestrol; Stilbestrol; Stilbetin; Stilboestroform; Stilboestrol; Synestrin; Synthoestrin; Vagestrol	breast cancer; prostate cancer

Generic Drug	Trade Name	Indicated For
diethylstilbestrolum	Acnestrol; Cyren A; Deladumone; Diastyl; Domestrol; Estrobene; Estrosyn; Fonatol; Makarol; Milestrol; Neo-Oestronol I; Oestrogenine; Oestromenin; Oestromon; Palestrol; Stilbestrol; Stilbetin; Stilboestroform; Stilboestrol; Synestrin; Synthoestrin; Vagestrol	breast cancer; prostate cancer
diethylstilboestrol	Acnestrol; Cyren A; Deladumone; Diastyl; Domestrol; Estrobene; Estrosyn; Fonatol; Makarol; Milestrol; Neo-Oestronol I; Oestrogenine; Oestromenin; Oestromon; Palestrol; Stilbestrol; Stilbetin; Stilboestroform; Stilboestrol; Synestrin; Synthoestrin; Vagestrol	breast cancer; prostate cancer
difluorodeoxycytidine	Gemzar	bladder cancer; breast cancer; carcinoma of unknown primary origin; lung cancer; ovarian cancer; pancreatic cancer; renal cell carcinoma
dihematoporphyrin ether	Photofrin	photosensitizer; bladder, esophageal, gastric, lung, and rectal cancers
dihydroxyanthracenedione	Novantrone	acute leukemia; breast cancer; prostate cancer; non-Hodgkin lymphoma; multiple sclerosis
dihydroxyanthracenedione dihydrochloride	Novantrone	acute leukemia; breast cancer; prostate cancer; non-Hodgkin lymphoma; multiple sclerosis
dimesna	Mesna Disulfide; Tavocept	ifosfamide-induced hemorrhagic cystitis, prophylaxis
dimethyl triazeno imidazol carboxamide; dimethyl (triazeno) imidazolecarboxamide	DTIC-Dome	carcinoid cancer; Hodgkin disease; islet cell carcinoma; melanoma; neuroblastoma; soft-tissue sarcoma
disodium pamidronate	Aredia	myeloma, secondary breast cancer
DMDR	Idamycin	acute myeloid leukemia (AML); acute nonlymphocytic leukemia
docetaxel	Taxotere	breast cancer; esophageal cancer; gastric cancer; head/neck cancers; locally advanced or metastatic non-small-cell lung cancer; ovarian cancer; metastatic prostate cancer
dolasetron mesylate	Anzemet	nausea and vomiting prophylaxis, chemotherapy-induced and postoperative
donepezil hydrochloride	Aricept	Alzheimer's disease and opioid-induced sedation
doxercalciferol	Hectorol	secondary hyperparathyroidism in end-stage renal disease in patients on hemodialysis

Generic Drug	Trade Name	Indicated For
doxorubicin hydrochloride	Adriamycin	leukemias; Wilms' tumor; neuroblastoma; soft-tissue and bone sarcomas; small cell carcinoma of the lung; lymphomas; multiple myeloma; mesotheliomas; germ-cell tumors of the ovary or testis
doxorubicin hydrochloride liposome	Doxil; Dox-SL; Evacet; LipoDox	refractory metastatic carcinoma of the ovary; AIDS-related Kaposi sarcoma; breast cancer; relapsed/refractory multiple myeloma (with bortezomib)
dronabinol	Marinol	antinausea
D-TRP-6-LHRH	Decapeptyl	prostate carcinoma, palliative treatment
DXM	Aeroseb-Dex; Alba-Dex; Decaderm; Decadrol; Decadron; Decasone R.p.; Decaspray; Deenar; Deronil; Dex-4; Dexace; Dexameth; Dezone; Gammacorten; Hexadrol; Maxidex; Sk-Dexamethasone	antiemetic (prevents vomiting)
eculizumab	Alexion; Soliris	paroxysmal nocturnal hemoglobinuria
elcoril	Ambochlorin; Amboclorin; Leukeran	chronic lymphocytic leukemia; malignant lymphomas
Elliotts B solution	Elliotts B Solution	diluent for the intrathecal administration of methotrexate sodium and cytarabine for the prevention or treatment of meningeal leukemia or lymphocytic lymphoma
encapsulated cytarabine	DepoCyt; DepoFoam	lymphomatous meningitis
epi-ADR	Ellence	breast cancer; adjuvant in breast cancer therapy
4'-epiadriamycin	Ellence	breast cancer; adjuvant in breast cancer therapy
epidoxorubicin	Ellence	breast cancer; adjuvant in breast cancer therapy
4'-epidoxorubicin	Ellence	breast cancer; adjuvant in breast cancer therapy
4'-epi-doxorubicin HCl	Ellence	breast cancer; adjuvant in breast cancer therapy
epipodophyllotoxin	VePesid; Lastet; Etopophos; Toposar	acute leukemia; adrenal cortical cancer; brain cancer; chronic lymphocytic leukemia; choriocarcinoma; esophageal cancer; Ewing sarcoma; gastric cancer; germ-cell cancer; gestational trophoblastic neoplasms; hepatocellular cancer; Hodgkin disease; hypereosinophilic syndrome; Kaposi sarcoma; testicular cancer; thymoma; thyroid cancer; uterine cancer; Wilms' tumor; Langerhans cell histiocytosis; mobilization of peripheral-blood progenitor cells; multiple myeloma; neuroblastoma; non-small-cell lung cancer; osteogenic sarcoma; ovarian cancer; retinoblastoma; small-cell lung cancer; soft-tissue sarcomas
epirubicin	Ellence	breast cancer; adjuvant in breast cancer therapy
epoetin alfa	Epogen; Procrit	anemias associated with chronic renal failure, zidovudine (AZT) therapy, and cancer chemotherapy of nonmyeloid malignancies
epoetin beta	NeoRecormon	anemia associated with end-stage renal disease
epothilone-B BMS 247550	Ixempra	metastatic or locally advanced breast cancer

Generic Drug	Trade Name	Indicated For
epothilone B lactam	Ixempra	metastatic or locally advanced breast cancer
epratuzumab	LymphoCide; hLL2	systemic lupus erythematosus
erlotinib	Tarceva	malignant glioma; locally advanced or metastic non-small-cell lung carcinoma; locally advanced, unresectable or metastatic pancreatic carcinoma
erlotinib hydrochloride	Tarceva	malignant glioma; locally advanced or metastic non-small-cell lung carcinoma; locally advanced, unresectable or metastatic pancreatic carcinoma
erwinia asparaginase	Elspar; Cristanaspase; L-Asnase	some blood cancers; acute lymphocytic leukemia; acute nonlymphocytic leukemia
erythropoietin	Epogen; Procrit	anemias associated with chronic renal failure, zidovudine (AZT) therapy, and cancer chemotherapy of nonmyeloid malignancies
esterified estrogens	Menest; Estratab	breast cancer
estradiol	Clinagen LA 40; Dep Gynogen; Estrace; Estradiol Patch; Estragyn LA 5; Estro-Cyp; Estrogen Patches; Fempatch; Gynodiol, Gynogen LA 20; Menaval-20	breast cancer, palliative
estramustine phosphate	Emcyt	prostate neoplasm
estramustine phosphate sodium	Emcyt	prostate neoplasm
etanercept	Enbrel	juvenile arthritis; psoriatic arthritis; rheumatoid arthritis
ethinyl estradiol	Estinyl; Ethinoral; Eticylol; Feminone; Inestra; Lynoral; Orestralyn	advanced androgen-dependent prostate cancer, palliative; breast cancer, palliative; estrogen replacement; menopausal symptoms; postmenopausal osteoporosis
ethiodized oil	Ethiodol; Lipiodol	diagnostic imaging, hysterosalpingography and lymphography
ethiofos	Ethyol	cisplatin-induced nephrotoxicity; radiation-induced mucositis and xerostomia
etidronate	Didronel	treating adults with Paget disease; preventing and treating abnormal bone growth following hip replacement surgery or spinal cord injury
etoposide	VePesid; Lastet; Etopophos; Toposar	acute leukemia; adrenal cortical cancer; brain cancer; chronic lymphocytic leukemia; choriocarcinoma; esophageal cancer; Ewing sarcoma; gastric cancer; germ-cell cancer; gestational trophoblastic neoplasms; hepatocellular cancer; Hodgkin disease; hypereosinophilic syndrome; Kaposi sarcoma; testicular cancer; thymoma; thyroid cancer; uterine cancer; Wilms' tumor; Langerhans cell histiocytosis; mobilization of peripheral-blood progenitor cells; multiple myeloma; neuroblastoma; non-small-cell lung cancer; osteogenic sarcoma; ovarian cancer; retinoblastoma; small-cell lung cancer; soft-tissue sarcomas

Generic Drug	Trade Name	Indicated For
etoposide phosphate	Etopophos	acute leukemia; adrenal cortical cancer; brain cancer; chronic lymphocytic leukemia; choriocarcinoma; esophageal cancer; Ewing sarcoma; gastric cancer; germ-cell cancer; gestational trophoblastic neoplasms; hepatocellular cancer; Hodgkin disease; hypereosinophilic syndrome; Kaposi sarcoma; testicular cancer; thymoma; thyroid cancer; uterine cancer; Wilms' tumor; Langerhans cell histiocytosis; mobilization of peripheral-blood progenitor cells; multiple myeloma; neuroblastoma; non-small-cell lung cancer; osteogenic sarcoma; ovarian cancer; retinoblastoma; small-cell lung cancer; soft-tissue sarcomas
exemestane	Aromasin	estrogen receptor-positive early breast cancer
exisulind	Aptosyn; FGN-1; Sulindac sulfone	colonic adenomatous polyps in the inherited disease adenomatous polyposis coli, control and suppression
FdUrD	FUDF	gastrointestinal adenocarcinoma metastatic to the liver
fentanyl citrate	Actiq; Oralet; Sublimaze; Fentora	breakthrough pain in cancer patients
fibrin sealant	Beriplast P; TISSEEL	cardiovascular surgery; colostomy closure; congenital heart defects; coronary artery bypass grafting; mediastinal bleeding; microvascular bleeding; splenic trauma
filgrastim	Neupogen	bone marrow transplantation; cancer patients receiving myelosuppressive chemotherapy; neutropenia
filgrastim SD-01	Neulasta	chemotherapy-induced neutropenia
floxuridin	FUDF	gastrointestinal adenocarcinoma metastatic to the liver
floxuridine	FUDF	gastrointestinal adenocarcinoma metastatic to the liver
flucinom	Eulexin	prostate carcinoma; hirsutism
fluconazole	Diflucan	antifungal, prophylaxis in allogeneic bone marrow transplantation; candidiasis; cryptococcal meningitis
fludarabine phosphate	Fludara; Fludara Oral	chronic lymphocytic leukemia (CLL)
fludeoxyglucose F 18	FDG	radiopharmaceutical, cancer diagnostic
fludestrin	Teslac	advanced breast cancer in women, palliative
fludrocortisone	Florinef	breast cancer; adrenal cortical cancer
flugerel	Eulexin	prostate carcinoma; hirsutism
fluoro uracil	Adrucil; Efudex; Fluoroplex	palliative treatment for colorectal, breast, and pancreatic cancers; topical treatment for superficial basal cell carcinoma that cannot be treated with surgery, and actinic keratosis
fluorodeoxyuridine	FUDF	gastrointestinal adenocarcinoma metastatic to the liver
fluorouracil	Adrucil; Efudex; Fluoroplex	palliative treatment for colorectal, breast, and pancreatic cancers; topical treatment for superficial basal cell carcinoma that cannot be treated with surgery, and actinic keratosis
5-fluorouracil	Adrucil; Efudex; Fluoroplex	palliative treatment for colorectal, breast, and pancreatic cancers; topical treatment for superficial basal cell carcinoma that cannot be treated with surgery, and actinic keratosis

Generic Drug	Trade Name	Indicated For
fluorouridine deoxyribose	FUDF	gastrointestinal adenocarcinoma metastatic to the liver
fluouracil	Adrucil; Efudex; Fluoroplex	palliative treatment for colorectal, breast, and pancreatic cancers; topical treatment for superficial basal cell carcinoma that cannot be treated with surgery, and actinic keratosis
5-fluoracil	Adrucil; Efudex; Fluoroplex	palliative treatment for colorectal, breast, and pancreatic cancers; topical treatment for superficial basal cell carcinoma that cannot be treated with surgery, and actinic keratosis
fluoxymesterone	Android-F; Halodrin; Halotestin; Ora-Testryl; Ultandren; Androxy	certain types of breast cancer
flutamide	Eulexin	prostate carcinoma; hirsutism
folinate calcium	Wellcovorin	used to protect normal cells from high doses of the anticancer drug methotrexate; also used to increase the antitumor effects of fluorouracil and tegafur-uracil; megaloblastic anemia due to folate deficiency; enhanced fluorouracil inhibition of thymidylate synthase; reverse dihydrofolate reductase inhibition by methotrexate; folic acid antagonist overdose; nitrous oxide toxicity
folinic acid	Wellcovorin	used to protect normal cells from high doses of the anticancer drug methotrexate; also used to increase the antitumor effects of fluorouracil and tegafur-uracil; megaloblastic anemia due to folate deficiency; enhanced fluorouracil inhibition of thymidylate synthase; reverse dihydrofolate reductase inhibition by methotrexate; folic acid antagonist overdose; nitrous oxide toxicity
folinic acid calcium salt pentahydrate	Wellcovorin	used to protect normal cells from high doses of the anticancer drug methotrexate; also used to increase the antitumor effects of fluorouracil and tegafur-uracil; megaloblastic anemia due to folate deficiency; enhanced fluorouracil inhibition of thymidylate synthase; reverse dihydrofolate reductase inhibition by methotrexate; folic acid antagonist overdose; nitrous oxide toxicity
FU	Adrucil; Efudex; Fluoroplex	palliative treatment for colorectal, breast, and pancreatic cancers; topical treatment for superficial basal cell carcinoma that cannot be treated with surgery, and actinic keratosis
fulvestrant	Faslodex	hormone receptor-positive metastatic breast cancer
gabapentin	Neurontin	management of epilepsy; pain; mania; depression and anxiety disorders
gadopentetate dimeglumine	Gd-DTPA; Magnevist; MultiHance	angiography for leptomeningeal metastases and multiple sclerosis and magnetic resonance imaging for spine and brain
gammaphos	Ethyol	cisplatin-induced nephrotoxicity; radiation-induced mucositis and xerostomia
ganciclovir	Cymevan; DHPG; Nordeoxyguanosine; Virgan	cytomegalovirus (CMV) infections in immunocompromised patients
gefitinib	Iressa	non-small-cell lung carcinoma

Generic Drug	Trade Name	Indicated For
gemcitabine	Gemzar	bladder cancer; breast cancer; carcinoma of unknown primary origin; lung cancer; ovarian cancer; pancreatic cancer; renal cell carcinoma
gemcitabine hydrochloride	Gemzar	bladder cancer; breast cancer; carcinoma of unknown primary origin; lung cancer; ovarian cancer; pancreatic cancer; renal cell carcinoma
gemtuzumab ozogamicin	Mylotarg	acute myeloid leukemia
glutamine	Glutacerebro; Glutaven; L-Glutamine; Memoril; Nutrestore; Q. Levoglutamide	short bowel syndrome
glyzophrol	Busulfex; Mitosan; Myleran	bone marrow disorders; chronic myelogenous leukemia; palliative; neoadjuvant to allogeneic hematopoietic progenitor cell transplantation; neoplastic meningitis; primary brain malignancies
goserelin	Zoladex	breast cancer, palliative; prostate cancer
granisetron hydrochloride	Kytril	antinausea
granulocyte colony-stimulating factor	Neupogen	bone marrow transplantation; cancer patients receiving myelosuppressive chemotherapy; neutropenia
granulocyte macrophage colony-stimulating factor	Leukine; Prokine	melanoma; chemotherapy-induced neutropenia
haemophilus influenzae B vaccine	Hib TITER vaccine; HibTITER; PedvaxHIB	haemophilus influenzae B prophylaxis
halofuginone hydrobromide	Halofuginone IV (intravenous); RU 19110; Tempostatin	scleroderma and antiprotozoal; coccidiosis (vet)
hemel	Hexalen; Hexamethylmelamine	ovarian cancer
hexadecadrol	Aeroseb-Dex; Alba-Dex; Decaderm; Decadrol; Decadron; Decasone R.p.; Decaspray; Deenar; Deronil; Dex-4; Dexace; Dexameth; Dezone; Gammacorten; Hexadrol; Maxidex; Sk-Dexamethasone	antiemetic (prevents vomiting)
hexaloids	Hexalen; Hexamethylmelamine	ovarian cancer
histrelin acetate	Histrelin implant	palliative treatment of advanced prostate cancer
hP67.6-Calicheamicin	Mylotarg	acute myeloid leukemia
hycamptamine	Hycamtin	small cell lung carcinoma; cervical cancer
HYD	Hydrea, Droxia	chronic myelogenous leukemia; head and neck cancer; malignant melanoma; ovarian carcinoma; sickle cell anemia; adjuvant in retroviral therapy

Generic Drug	Trade Name	Indicated For
hydroxycarbamide	Hydrea, Droxia	chronic myelogenous leukemia; head and neck cancer; malignant melanoma; ovarian carcinoma; sickle cell anemia; adjuvant in retroviral therapy
hydroxychloroquine	none	malaria; rheumatoid arthritis
hydroxyurea	Hydrea, Droxia	chronic myelogenous leukemia; head and neck cancer; malignant melanoma; ovarian carcinoma; sickle cell anemia; adjuvant in retroviral therapy
hydurea	Hydrea, Droxia	chronic myelogenous leukemia; head and neck cancer; malignant melanoma; ovarian carcinoma; sickle cell anemia; adjuvant in retroviral therapy
hyperbaric oxygen	none	various diseases or injuries associated with hypoxia
131-I-anti-B1 antibody; 131-I-anti-B1 monoclonal antibody	Bexxar	CD-20-antigen-expressing, relapsed or refractory, low-grade, follicular, or transformed non-Hodgkin lymphoma
ibandronate sodium	Bondronate; Boniva	osteoporosis, treatment and prevention
ibenzmethyzin	Matulane	brain tumors; Hodgkin disease; non-Hodgkin lymphoma
ibenzmethyzin hydrochloride; ibenzmethyzine hydrochloride	Matulane	brain tumors; Hodgkin disease; non-Hodgkin lymphoma
ibritumomab (In2B8/Y2B8 radiolabeling kit)	Zevalin	non-Hodgkin lymphoma
ibritumomab tiuxetan	Zevalin	accelerated approval (clinical benefit not established) treatment of patients with relapsed or refractory low-grade, follicular, or transformed B-cell non-Hodgkin lymphoma, including patients with rituximab refractory follicular non-Hodgkin lymphoma
ibuprofen	none	painkiller
idarubicin	idamycin	acute myeloid leukemia (AML); acute nonlymphocytic leukemia
IDEC-C2B8 monoclonal antibody	Rituxan	diffuse large B-cell, CD20-positive, non-Hodgkin lymphoma
IDEC-Y2B8 monoclonal antibody	Zevalin	non-Hodgkin lymphoma
ifomide	Ifex; Cyfos; Ifosfamidum	breast cancer; gastric carcinoma; lung cancer; lymphocytic leukemias; Hodgkin disease and non-Hodgkin lymphoma; ovarian cancer; pancreatic carcinoma; sarcomas; testicular cancer
ifosfamide	Ifex; Cyfos; Ifosfamidum	breast cancer; gastric carcinoma; lung cancer; lymphocytic leukemias; Hodgkin disease and non-Hodgkin lymphoma; ovarian cancer; pancreatic carcinoma; sarcomas; testicular cancer
IFX	Ifex; Cyfos; Ifosfamidum	breast cancer; gastric carcinoma; lung cancer; lymphocytic leukemias; Hodgkin disease and non-Hodgkin lymphoma; ovarian cancer; pancreatic carcinoma; sarcomas; testicular cancer
IL-11	Neumega	chemotherapy-related thrombocytopenia

Generic Drug	Trade Name	Indicated For
imatinib mesylate	Gleevec	Philadelphia chromosome-positive chronic myeloid leukemia (CML); acute lymphocytic leukemia; gastrointestinal stromal tumor; hypereosinophillic syndrome; dermatofibrosarcoma protuberans; mutated-PDGFR myelodysplastic/myeloproliferative diseases
IMiD-1	Revlimid	transfusion-dependent anemia due to low- or intermediate-1 risk myelodysplastic syndrome; multiple myeloma
imidazole carboxamide	DTIC-Dome	carcinoid cancer; Hodgkin disease; islet cell carcinoma; melanoma; neuroblastoma; soft-tissue sarcoma
imidazole carboxamide dimethyltriazeno	DTIC-Dome	carcinoid cancer; Hodgkin disease; islet cell carcinoma; melanoma; neuroblastoma; soft-tissue sarcoma
imiquimod	Aldara	condyloma; superficial basal cell carcinoma; actinic keratosis
immunoglobulin G1	Erbitux	advanced colorectal cancer; head and neck cancer
immunoglobulin G1, anti-(human epidermal growth factor receptor) (human-mouse monoclonal C225 gamma1-chain), disulfide with human-mouse monoclonal C225 kappa-chain, dimer	Erbitux	advanced colorectal cancer; head and neck cancer
in 111 ibritumomab tiuxetan	IDEC In2B8	non-Hodgkin lymphoma
indomethacin	Indocin	dysmenorrhea; inflammatory disorders; pain
infliximab	Avakine; Remicade	ankylosis spondylitis; Crohn disease; plaque psoriasis; rheumatoid arthritis; sarcoidosis
interferon alfa-2a	Roferon-A	treating chronic hepatitis C and certain types of leukemia
interferon alfa-2b	Intron-A	certain types of leukemia, lymphoma, and hepatitis; certain AIDS-related illnesses (Kaposi sarcoma); and genital warts (condylomata acuminata); also used in addition to surgery to treat a certain type of skin cancer (malignant melanoma)
interferon beta-1b	Betaseron	treating relapsing forms of multiple sclerosis (MS) to reduce the number of flare-ups and slow down the development of physical disability associated with MS
interleukin; interleukin II	Proleukin	metastatic renal cell carcinoma; metastatic melanoma; stimulates the production of blood cells, especially platelets, during chemotherapy
interleukin-11	Neumega	chemotherapy-related thrombocytopenia
interleukin-2 fusion protein	Ontak	cutaneous T-cell lymphoma
interleukin-2 fusion toxin	Ontak	cutaneous T-cell lymphoma
iodine-131 anti-B1 antibody	Bexxar	CD-20-antigen-expressing, relapsed or refractory, low-grade, follicular, or transformed non-Hodgkin lymphoma
iodine-131 anti-CD20 monoclonal antibody	Bexxar	CD-20-antigen-expressing, relapsed or refractory, low-grade, follicular, or transformed non-Hodgkin lymphoma
iodine I 125	I-125	prostate cancer

Generic Drug	Trade Name	Indicated For
iodine I 131	I-131; Iodotope	hyperthyroidism
iodine I 131 metaiodobenzylguanidine	131 I-MIBG	diagnostic imaging
iodine I 131 MOAB anti-B1	Bexxar	CD-20-antigen-expressing, relapsed or refractory, low-grade, follicular, or transformed non-Hodgkin lymphoma
iodine I 131 monoclonal antibody anti-B1	Bexxar	CD-20-antigen-expressing, relapsed or refractory, low-grade, follicular, or transformed non-Hodgkin lymphoma
iodine I 131 tositumomab	Bexxar	CD-20-antigen-expressing, relapsed or refractory, low-grade, follicular, or transformed non-Hodgkin lymphoma
iphosphamid; iphosphamide	Ifex; Cyfos; Ifosfamidum	breast cancer; gastric carcinoma; lung cancer; lymphocytic leukemias; Hodgkin disease and non-Hodgkin lymphoma; ovarian cancer; pancreatic carcinoma; sarcomas; testicular cancer
IPP	Ifex; Cyfos; Ifosfamidum	breast cancer; gastric carcinoma; lung cancer; lymphocytic leukemias; Hodgkin disease and non-Hodgkin lymphoma; ovarian cancer; pancreatic carcinoma; sarcomas; testicular cancer
irinotecan	Camptosar	stage IVB cervical cancer; colorectal cancer; esophageal cancer; gastric cancer; non-small-cell lung cancer; small-cell lung cancer
irinotecan HCl; irinotecan hydrochloride	Camptosar	stage IVB cervical cancer; colorectal cancer; esophageal cancer; gastric cancer; non-small-cell lung cancer; small-cell lung cancer
iron sucrose injection	Venofer	treatment of iron deficiency for both dialysis and nondialysis patients with kidney disease, with or without concurrent erythropoietin therapy
isoendoxan	Ifex; Cyfos; Ifosfamidum	breast cancer; gastric carcinoma; lung cancer; lymphocytic leukemias; Hodgkin disease and non-Hodgkin lymphoma; ovarian cancer; pancreatic carcinoma; sarcomas; testicular cancer
isophosphamide	Ifex; Cyfos; Ifosfamidum	breast cancer; gastric carcinoma; lung cancer; lymphocytic leukemias; Hodgkin disease and non-Hodgkin lymphoma; ovarian cancer; pancreatic carcinoma; sarcomas; testicular cancer
isosulfan blue	Lymphazurin	diagnostic imaging
isotretinoin	Accutane	cutaneous T-cell lymphoma; juvenile metastatic neuroblastoma and leukemia
itraconazole	Sporanox	fungal infections
ixabepilone	Ixempra	metastatic or locally advanced breast cancer
juven	none	wasting syndrome, nutritional supplement
ketoconazole	Fungarest; Fungoral; Ketoderm; Ketoisdin; Nizoral; Orifungal M; Panfungol; R-41400; Xolegel	seborrheic dermatitis; prostate cancer
khloditan	Lysodren	adrenal cortical carcinoma
L-ASP	Elspar; Cristanaspase; L-Asnase	some blood cancers; acute lymphocytic leukemia; acute nonlymphocytic leukemia

Generic Drug	Trade Name	Indicated For
L-asparaginase	Elspar; Cristanaspase; L-Asnase	some blood cancers; acute lymphocytic leukemia; acute nonlymphocytic leukemia
L-asparaginase with polyethylene glycol	Oncaspar	acute lymphoblastic leukemia
L-asparagine amidohydrolase	Elspar; Cristanaspase; L-Asnase	some blood cancers; acute lymphocytic leukemia; acute nonlymphocytic leukemia
L-phenylalanine mustard	Alkeran	breast cancer; neuroblastoma; palliative treatment of multiple myeloma and nonresectable epithelial ovarian carcinoma; rhabdomyosarcoma
L-sarcolysin phenylalanine mustard	Alkeran	breast cancer; neuroblastoma; palliative treatment of multiple myeloma and nonresectable epithelial ovarian carcinoma; rhabdomyosarcoma
L-sarcolysine	Alkeran	breast cancer; neuroblastoma; palliative treatment of multiple myeloma and nonresectable epithelial ovarian carcinoma; rhabdomyosarcoma
ladakamycin	Mylosar; Vidaza	myelodysplastic syndrome
lamivudine	Epivir	chronic hepatitis B; HIV infection
lamotrigine	Lamictal	epilepsy
lanreotide	Somatuline	acromegaly
lapatinib	Tykerb	advanced or metastatic breast cancer
lapatinib ditosylate	Tykerb	advanced or metastatic breast cancer
lard-factor	Aquasol A; Del-Vi-A; Pedi-Vit-A	diminishing malignant cell growth; enhancing the immune system
LCR	Oncovin; Vincasar PFS	acute leukemia; brain tumors; chronic lymphocytic leukemia; gestational trophoblastic neoplasms; head and neck squamous cell carcinoma; Kaposi sarcoma; liver cancer; Hodgkin disease and non-Hodgkin lymphoma; malignant thymoma; multiple myeloma; osteogenic sarcoma; ovarian cancer; pheochromocytoma; retinoblastoma; rhabdomyosarcoma; soft-tissue sarcoma; testicular cancer; Wilms' tumor
lenalidomide	Revlimid	transfusion-dependent anemia due to low- or intermediate-1 risk myelodysplastic syndrome; multiple myeloma
lenograstim	Granocyte; Neutrogin	chemotherapy-induced neutropenia
letrozole	Femara	hormone receptor-positive early breast cancer; adjuvant in breast cancer therapy; endometrial cancer
leucovorin	Wellcovorin	used to protect normal cells from high doses of the anticancer drug methotrexate; also used to increase the antitumor effects of fluorouracil and tegafur-uracil; megaloblastic anemia due to folate deficiency; enhanced fluorouracil inhibition of thymidylate synthase; reverse dihydrofolate reductase inhibition by methotrexate; folic acid antagonist overdose; nitrous oxide toxicity

Generic Drug	Trade Name	Indicated For
leucovorin calcium	Wellcovorin	used to protect normal cells from high doses of the anticancer drug methotrexate; also used to increase the antitumor effects of fluorouracil and tegafur-uracil; megaloblastic anemia due to folate deficiency; enhanced fluorouracil inhibition of thymidylate synthase; reverse dihydrofolate reductase inhibition by methotrexate; folic acid antagonist overdose; nitrous oxide toxicity
leukersan	Ambochlorin; Amboclorin; Leukeran	chronic lymphocytic leukemia; malignant lymphomas
leukoran	Ambochlorin; Amboclorin; Leukeran	chronic lymphocytic leukemia; malignant lymphomas
leuprolide acetate	Lupron; Lupron Depot; Lupron Depot-3 Month; Lupron Depot-4 Month; Lupron Depot-Ped; Viadur	prostate cancer; uterine fibroid tumors
leuprorelin	Lupron; Lupron Depot; Lupron Depot-3 Month; Lupron Depot-4 Month; Lupron Depot-Ped; Viadur	prostate cancer; uterine fibroid tumors
leuprorelin acetate	Lupron; Lupron Depot; Lupron Depot-3 Month; Lupron Depot-4 Month; Lupron Depot-Ped; Viadur	prostate cancer; uterine fibroid tumors
leupurin	Mercaptopurinum; Purinethol	acute lymphocytic leukemia; acute myelogenous leukemia; Crohn disease; Hodgkin disease in children; lymphoblastic lymphoma; ulcerative colitis
leurocristine	Oncovin; Vincasar PFS	acute leukemia; brain tumors; chronic lymphocytic leukemia; gestational trophoblastic neoplasms; head and neck squamous cell carcinoma; Kaposi sarcoma; liver cancer; Hodgkin disease and non-Hodgkin lymphoma; malignant thymoma; multiple myeloma; osteogenic sarcoma; ovarian cancer; pheochromocytoma; retinoblastoma; rhabdomyosarcoma; soft-tissue sarcoma; testicular cancer; Wilms' tumor
leurocristine sulfate	Oncovin; Vincasar PFS	acute leukemia; brain tumors; chronic lymphocytic leukemia; gestational trophoblastic neoplasms; head and neck squamous cell carcinoma; Kaposi sarcoma; liver cancer; Hodgkin disease and non-Hodgkin lymphoma; malignant thymoma; multiple myeloma; osteogenic sarcoma; ovarian cancer; pheochromocytoma; retinoblastoma; rhabdomyosarcoma; soft-tissue sarcoma; testicular cancer; Wilms' tumor
levamisole	Ergamisol	colon cancer; nephrotic syndrome
levocarnitine	Carnitor	carnitine deficiency; end-stage renal disease
linfolizin	Ambochlorin; Amboclorin; Leukeran	chronic lymphocytic leukemia; malignant lymphomas
liposomal adriamycin	Doxil; Dox-SL; Evacet; LipoDox	refractory metastatic carcinoma of the ovary; AIDS-related Kaposi sarcoma; breast cancer; relapsed/refractory multiple myeloma (with bortezomib)

Generic Drug	Trade Name	Indicated For
liposomal cytarabine	DepoCyt; DepoFoam	lymphomatous meningitis
liposomal daunorubicin	DaunoXome	acute nonlymphocytic leukemia; acute lymphocytic leukemia; advanced HIV-associated Kaposi sarcoma
liposomal daunorubicin citrate	DaunoXome	acute nonlymphocytic leukemia; acute lymphocytic leukemia; advanced HIV-associated Kaposi sarcoma
liposomal doxorubicin	Doxil; Dox-SL; Evacet; LipoDox	refractory metastatic carcinoma of the ovary; AIDS-related Kaposi sarcoma; breast cancer; relapsed/refractory multiple myeloma (with bortezomib)
liposomal doxorubicin hydrochloride	Doxil; Dox-SL; Evacet; LipoDox	refractory metastatic carcinoma of the ovary; AIDS-related Kaposi sarcoma; breast cancer; relapsed/refractory multiple myeloma (with bortezomib)
liposome-encapsulated doxorubicin	Doxil; Dox-SL; Evacet; LipoDox	refractory metastatic carcinoma of the ovary; AIDS-related Kaposi sarcoma; breast cancer; relapsed/refractory multiple myeloma (with bortezomib)
lomustine; lomustinum	CeeNU; CCNU	brain tumors; Hodgkin disease
lovastatin	Mevacor; Mevinolin; Monacolin K	atherosclerosis; coronary heart disease, prevention; hypercholesterolemia
LV	Wellcovorin	used to protect normal cells from high doses of the anticancer drug methotrexate; also used to increase the antitumor effects of fluorouracil and tegafur-uracil; megaloblastic anemia due to folate deficiency; enhanced fluorouracil inhibition of thymidylate synthase; reverse dihydrofolate reductase inhibition by methotrexate; folic acid antagonist overdose; nitrous oxide toxicity
lymphocyte mitogenic factor	Proleukin	metastatic renal cell carcinoma; metastatic melanoma; stimulates the production of blood cells, especially platelets, during chemotherapy
lymphokine-activated killer cells	none	adoptive immunotherapy
lympholysin	Ambochlorin; Amboclorin; Leukeran	chronic lymphocytic leukemia; malignant lymphomas
mechlorethamine	Mustargen	bronchogenic carcinoma; chronic lymphocytic and myelcytic leukemia; Hodgkin disease, palliative; lymphosarcoma; mycosis fungoides; polycythemia vera
mechlorethamine HCl; mechlorethamine hydrochloride	Mustargen	bronchogenic carcinoma; chronic lymphocytic and myelcytic leukemia; Hodgkin disease, palliative; lymphosarcoma; mycosis fungoides; polycythemia vera
medroxyprogesterone	Curretab; Depo-Provera; Provera; Provera Dosepak	breast carcinoma; endometrial carcinoma; renal cell carcinoma
medroxyprogesterone acetate	Curretab; Depo-Provera; Provera; Provera Dosepak	breast carcinoma; endometrial carcinoma; renal cell carcinoma
megestrol acetate	Megace; Megace ES; Ovaban; Pallace	appetite enhancement, AIDS patients; breast cancer, palliative; endometrial carcinoma, palliative treatment

Generic Drug	Trade Name	Indicated For
melphalan	Alkeran	breast cancer; neuroblastoma; palliative treatment of multiple myeloma and nonresectable epithelial ovarian carcinoma; rhabdomyosarcoma
meractinomycin	Cosmegen; Lyovac Cosmegen	Wilms' tumor; childhood rhabdomyosarcoma; Ewing sarcoma; testicular cancer; gestational trophoblastic neoplasia; choriocarcinoma; melanoma; neuroblastoma; retinoblastoma; uterine sarcomas; Kaposi sarcoma; sarcoma botryoides; soft-tissue sarcoma
mercaptoethane sulfonate	Mesnex	helps protect the kidneys and bladder from the toxic effects of anticancer drugs such as ifosfamide and cyclophosphamide
mercaptopurine	Mercaptopurinum; Purinethol	acute lymphocytic leukemia; acute myelogenous leukemia; Crohn disease; Hodgkin disease in children; lymphoblastic lymphoma; ulcerative colitis
6-mercaptopurine	Mercaptopurinum; Purinethol	acute lymphocytic leukemia; acute myelogenous leukemia; Crohn disease; Hodgkin disease in children; lymphoblastic lymphoma; ulcerative colitis
6-mercaptopurine monohydrate	Mercaptopurinum; Purinethol	acute lymphocytic leukemia; acute myelogenous leukemia; Crohn disease; Hodgkin disease in children; lymphoblastic lymphoma; ulcerative colitis
mercapurin	Mercaptopurinum; Purinethol	acute lymphocytic leukemia; acute myelogenous leukemia; Crohn disease; Hodgkin disease in children; lymphoblastic lymphoma; ulcerative colitis
mern	Mercaptopurinum; Purinethol	acute lymphocytic leukemia; acute myelogenous leukemia; Crohn disease; Hodgkin disease in children; lymphoblastic lymphoma; ulcerative colitis
mesna	Mesnex	helps protect the kidneys and bladder from the toxic effects of anticancer drugs such as ifosfamide and cyclophosphamide
mesnum	Mesnex	helps protect the kidneys and bladder from the toxic effects of anticancer drugs such as ifosfamide and cyclophosphamide
metacortandracin	Delta-Dome; Deltasone; Liquid Pred; Lisacort; Meticorten; Orasone; Prednicen-M; Sk-Prednisone; Sterapred	inflammatory conditions; allergic conditions; hematologic conditions; neoplastic conditions; autoimmune conditions; replacement therapy in adrenal insufficiency
methanesulfonic acid tetramethylene ester	Busulfex; Mitosan; Myleran	bone marrow disorders; chronic myelogenous leukemia; palliative; neoadjuvant to allogeneic hematopoietic progenitor cell transplantation; neoplastic meningitis; primary brain malignancies
methionine C 11	none	PET radiopharmaceutical
methotrexate	Rheumatrex; Abitrexate; Folex; Folex PFS; Methotrexate LPF; Mexate; Mexate-AQ	bladder cancer; breast cancer; carcinomatous meningitis; chorioadenoma destruens; esophageal cancer; gestational choriocarcinoma; head/neck cancer; meningeal leukemia; lymphomas; Burkitt lymphoma; lung cancer; mycosis fungoides; osteosarcoma; Wegener granulomatosis
methoxsalen	Ammoidin; Oxsoralen; Oxsoralen-Ultra; Uvadex; Xanthotoxin	cutaneous T-cell lymphoma

Generic Drug	Trade Name	Indicated For
methoxy polyethylene glycol-beta	Mircera	anemia associated with chronic renal failure
methoxypsoralen	Ammoidin; Oxsoralen; Oxsoralen-Ultra; Uvadex; Xanthotoxin	cutaneous T-cell lymphoma
8-methoxypsoralen	Ammoidin; Oxsoralen; Oxsoralen-Ultra; Uvadex; Xanthotoxin	cutaneous T-cell lymphoma
3-methyl TTNEB	Targretin	oral or topical treatment of cutaneous manifestations of cutaneous T-cell lymphoma
methylchlorethamine	Mustargen	bronchogenic carcinoma; chronic lymphocytic and myelcytic leukemia; Hodgkin disease, palliative; lymphosarcoma; mycosis fungoides; polycythemia vera
methylene blue	CI Basic Blue 9; Collubleu; Desmoidpillen; Methylthioninium chloride; Schultz No. 1038; Tetramethylthionine Chloride Trihydrate; Urolene Blue; Vitableu	cyanide poisoning, antidote; diagnostic, indicator dye; genitourinary antiseptic; glutaricaciduria; methemoglobinemia; oxalate and phosphate urinary tract calculi, management
methylfluorprednisolone	Aeroseb-Dex; Alba-Dex; Decaderm; Decadrol; Decadron; Decasone R.p.; Decaspray; Deenar; Deronil; Dex-4; Dexace; Dexameth; Dezone; Gammacorten; Hexadrol; Maxidex; Sk-Dexamethasone	antiemetic (prevents vomiting)
methylphenidate hydrochloride	Concerta; Ritalin	attention deficit/hyperactivity disorder (ADHD); narcolepsy
methylprednisolone	Prednilen; Wyacort	adrenocortical insufficiency; conditions requiring immunosuppression; inflammatory conditions; multiple sclerosis; nephrotic syndrome
methyltestosterone	Android, Testred, Virilon	breast cancer, palliative
metoclopramide	Reglan; Octamide	antinausea
MIH	Matulane	brain tumors; Hodgkin disease; non-Hodgkin lymphoma
MIH hydrochloride	Matulane	brain tumors; Hodgkin disease; non-Hodgkin lymphoma
miltefosine	Miltex	skin metastasis of breast cancer
MITC	Mutamycin; Mitozytrex	gastric carcinoma; pancreatic adenocarcinoma
mithramycin	Mithracin	testicular cancer
mitocin-C	Mutamycin; Mitozytrex	gastric carcinoma; pancreatic adenocarcinoma
mitogenic factor	Proleukin	metastatic renal cell carcinoma; metastatic melanoma; stimulates the production of blood cells, especially platelets, during chemotherapy

Generic Drug	*Trade Name*	*Indicated For*
mitomycin C	Mutamycin; Mitozytrex	gastric carcinoma; pancreatic adenocarcinoma
mitotane	Lysodren	adrenal cortical carcinoma
mitoxan	Cytoxan; Clafen; Neosar	breast cancer; leukemias; lupus nephritis; lymphoma; multiple myeloma; neuroblastoma; nephrotic syndrome; ovarian cancer; retinoblastoma
mitoxantrone dihydrochloride	Novantrone	acute leukemia; breast cancer; prostate cancer; non-Hodgkin lymphoma; multiple sclerosis
mitoxantrone HCl; mitoxantrone hydrochloride	Novantrone	acute leukemia; breast cancer; prostate cancer; non-Hodgkin lymphoma; multiple sclerosis
mitoxantroni hydrochloridum	Novantrone	acute leukemia; breast cancer; prostate cancer; non-Hodgkin lymphoma; multiple sclerosis
mitozantrone	Novantrone	acute leukemia; breast cancer; prostate cancer; non-Hodgkin lymphoma; multiple sclerosis
modafinil	Provigil	narcolepsy
monobenzone	Benoquin	vitiligo
monoclonal antibody ABX-EGF	Vectibix	advanced stage colorectal cancer
monoclonal antibody C225	Erbitux	advanced colorectal cancer; head and neck cancer
monoclonal antibody campath-1H	Campath	B-cell chronic lymphocytic leukemia
monoclonal antibody CD52	Campath	B-cell chronic lymphocytic leukemia
monoclonal antibody c-erb-2	Herceptin	breast cancer overexpressing HER2 protein; pancreatic cancer overexpressing p185HER2
monoclonal antibody HER2	Herceptin	breast cancer overexpressing HER2 protein; pancreatic cancer overexpressing p185HER2
morphine	none	painkiller
moxifloxacin hydrochloride	Avelox; Viagmox	various bacterial infections
MTC	Mutamycin; Mitozytrex	gastric carcinoma; pancreatic adenocarcinoma
multitargeted antifolate	Alimta	malignant pleural mesothelioma; non-small-cell lung cancer
multivitamin	Geritol	vitamin supplement
muromonab-CD3	Orthoclone OKT3	allograft rejection
mustard	Mustargen	bronchogenic carcinoma; chronic lymphocytic and myelcytic leukemia; Hodgkin disease, palliative; lymphosarcoma; mycosis fungoides; polycythemia vera
mustargen HCl; mustargen hydrochloride	Mustargen	bronchogenic carcinoma; chronic lymphocytic and myelcytic leukemia; Hodgkin disease, palliative; lymphosarcoma; mycosis fungoides; polycythemia vera
mustine	Mustargen	bronchogenic carcinoma; chronic lymphocytic and myelcytic leukemia; Hodgkin disease, palliative; lymphosarcoma; mycosis fungoides; polycythemia vera

Generic Drug	Trade Name	Indicated For
mycophenolate mofetil	Cellcept	heart transplantation; kidney transplantation; liver transplantation; lupus nephritis
myeleukon	Busulfex; Mitosan; Myleran	bone marrow disorders; chronic myelogenous leukemia; palliative; neoadjuvant to allogeneic hematopoietic progenitor cell transplantation; neoplastic meningitis; primary brain malignancies
myeloleukon	Busulfex; Mitosan; Myleran	bone marrow disorders; chronic myelogenous leukemia; palliative; neoadjuvant to allogeneic hematopoietic progenitor cell transplantation; neoplastic meningitis; primary brain malignancies
myelosan	Busulfex; Mitosan; Myleran	bone marrow disorders; chronic myelogenous leukemia; palliative; neoadjuvant to allogeneic hematopoietic progenitor cell transplantation; neoplastic meningitis; primary brain malignancies
mylecytan	Busulfex; Mitosan; Myleran	bone marrow disorders; chronic myelogenous leukemia; palliative; neoadjuvant to allogeneic hematopoietic progenitor cell transplantation; neoplastic meningitis; primary brain malignancies
mytotan	Lysodren	adrenal cortical carcinoma
N-lost	Mustargen	bronchogenic carcinoma; chronic lymphocytic and myelcytic leukemia; Hodgkin disease, palliative; lymphosarcoma; mycosis fungoides; polycythemia vera
N-phthaloylglutamimide	Synovir; Thalomid	Kaposi sarcoma; multiple myeloma; primary brain tumors
N-phthalylglutamic acid imide	Synovir; Thalomid	Kaposi sarcoma; multiple myeloma; primary brain tumors
nab-paclitaxel	Taxol; Abraxane; Onxol	bladder cancer; breast cancer; adjuvant in breast cancer therapy; cervical cancer; endometrial adenocarcinoma; esophageal cancer; head and neck cancer; non-small-cell lung cancer; lymphoma; ovarian cancer; prostate cancer; testicular cancer; AIDS-related Kaposi sarcoma
nandrolone decanoate	Deca-Durabolin	anemia of renal insufficiency; metastatic breast cancer
nanoparticle paclitaxel	Taxol; Abraxane; Onxol	bladder cancer; breast cancer; adjuvant in breast cancer therapy; cervical cancer; endometrial adenocarcinoma; esophageal cancer; head and neck cancer; non-small-cell lung cancer; lymphoma; ovarian cancer; prostate cancer; testicular cancer; AIDS-related Kaposi sarcoma
navelbine ditartrate	Biovelbin; Eunades	non-small-cell lung cancer; metastatic breast cancer; uterine and cervical cancer; desmoid tumors; advanced Kaposi sarcoma
naxamide	Ifex; Cyfos; Ifosfamidum	breast cancer; gastric carcinoma; lung cancer; lymphocytic leukemias; Hodgkin disease and non-Hodgkin lymphoma; ovarian cancer; pancreatic carcinoma; sarcomas; testicular cancer
NDC-zoledronate	Zometa; Reclast	hypercalcemia of malignancy; multiple myeloma and metastatic bone lesions from solid tumors; Paget disease
nelarabine	Arranon	T-cell acute lymphoblastic leukemia; T-cell lymphoblastic lymphoma
NH-2	Mustargen	bronchogenic carcinoma; chronic lymphocytic and myelcytic leukemia; Hodgkin disease, palliative; lymphosarcoma; mycosis fungoides; polycythemia vera

Generic Drug	Trade Name	Indicated For
niacinamide	Nicamid; Nicosedine	pellagra, treatment and prophylaxis; various dermatologic conditions
nicotine	none	smoking cessation
niftolid	Eulexin	prostate carcinoma; hirsutism
nilotinib	Tasigna	chronic myeloid leukemia; Philadelphia chromosome-positive acute lymphoblastic leukemia
nilutamide	Nilandron	prostate cancer
nimotuzumab	Theraloc	glioma
nitrogen mustard	Mustargen	bronchogenic carcinoma; chronic lymphocytic and myelcytic leukemia; Hodgkin disease, palliative; lymphosarcoma; mycosis fungoides; polycythemia vera
nolatrexed dihydrochloride	Thymitaq	hepatocellular carcinoma
norgestrel	Neogest; Ovrette; Microlut	oral contraception
noscapine hydrochloride	none	cough
novaldex	Nolvadex; Soltamox	breast cancer, palliative; adjuvant in breast cancer therapy; endometrial cancer; gynecomastia; melanoma; ovarian cancer
novel erythropoiesis stimulating protein	Aranesp	chemotherapy-induced anemia; chronic renal failure/insufficiency
novo-levamisole	Ergamisol	colon cancer; nephrotic syndrome
octreotide acetate	Sandostatin; Longastatina; Samilstin	acromegaly; diarrhea
6-[O-(1,1-dimethylethyl)-D-serine]-10-deglycinamide luteinizing hormone-releasing factor (pig) 2-(aminocarbonyl)hydrazide	Zoladex	breast cancer, palliative; prostate cancer
ofloxacin	none	various bacterial infections
oleovitamin A	Aquasol A; Del-Vi-A; Pedi-Vit-A	diminishing malignant cell growth; enhancing the immune system
ondansetron	Zofran	nausea and vomiting prophylaxis, chemotherapy-induced and postoperative
o,p'-DDD	Lysodren	adrenal cortical carcinoma
ophthalamin	Aquasol A; Del-Vi-A; Pedi-Vit-A	diminishing malignant cell growth; enhancing the immune system
oprelvekin	Neumega	prevention of severe thrombocytopenia following myelosuppressive chemotherapy
oregovomab	OvaRex	epithelial ovarian cancer
ortho,para-DDD	Lysodren	adrenal cortical carcinoma
oxalatoplatin; oxalatoplatinum	Eloxatin	metastatic colorectal cancer; ovarian cancer
oxaliplatin	Eloxatin	metastatic colorectal cancer; ovarian cancer

Generic Drug	Trade Name	Indicated For
oxandrolone	Oxandrin	bone pain; Duchenne and Becker muscular dystrophy; HIV-associated muscle weakness; HIV-related wasting syndrome
paclitaxel	Taxol; Abraxane; Onxol	bladder cancer; breast cancer; adjuvant in breast cancer therapy; cervical cancer; endometrial adenocarcinoma; esophageal cancer; head and neck cancer; lung cancer; non-small cell; lymphoma; ovarian cancer; prostate cancer; testicular cancer; AIDS-related Kaposi sarcoma
paclitaxel protein-bound	Taxol; Abraxane; Onxol	bladder cancer; breast cancer; adjuvant in breast cancer therapy; cervical cancer; endometrial adenocarcinoma; esophageal cancer; head and neck cancer; lung cancer; non-small cell; lymphoma; ovarian cancer; prostate cancer; testicular cancer; AIDS-related Kaposi sarcoma
palifermin	Kepivance	decrease the incidence and duration of severe oral mucositis in patients with hematologic malignancies receiving myelotoxic therapy requiring hematopoetic stem cell support
palladium 103	none	early stage prostate cancer; localized tumors of the head, neck, lung, pancreas, breast, and uterus
palonosetron hydrochloride	Aloxi	antinausea; antiemetic (prevents vomiting)
pamidronate disodium	Aredia	hypercalcemia of malignancy; osteolytic bone lesions of multiple myeloma; osteolytic bone metastases of breast cancer; Paget disease
panitumumab	Vectibix	advanced stage colorectal cancer
papaverine	Cerespan; Pavabid; Pavatym; Cerebid; Pavacap; Unicelles; Vasal	ischemia, cerebral and peripheral
paracetamol	Panadol; Disprol	painkiller
paricalcitol	Zemplar	secondary hyperparathyroidism, prevention and treatment
paroxetine hydrochloride	Paxil	depression
PCB hydrochloride	Matulane	brain tumors; Hodgkin disease; non-Hodgkin lymphoma
PCZ	Matulane	brain tumors; Hodgkin disease; non-Hodgkin lymphoma
PDD	Platinol; Platinol-AQ	metastatic testicular cancer; ovarian cancer; head and neck cancer; breast cancer; Hodgkin disease and non-Hodgkin lymphoma; myeloma and melanoma; advanced bladder cancer
PEG-asparaginase	Oncaspar	acute lymphoblastic leukemia
PEG-interferon alfa-2a	PEGASYS	chronic hepatitis C; renal cell carcinoma; advanced melanoma; chronic myelogenous leukemia
PEG-interferon alfa-2b	PEG-Intron	chronic hepatitis C; renal cell carcinoma
PEG-L-asparaginase	Oncaspar	acute lymphoblastic leukemia
PEG-L-asparaginase(K-H)	Oncaspar	acute lymphoblastic leukemia
pegademase	Adagen	enzyme replacement therapy for patients with severe combined immunodeficiency as a result of adenosine deaminase deficiency
pegaspargase	Oncaspar	acute lymphoblastic leukemia

Generic Drug	Trade Name	Indicated For
pegfilgrastim	Neulasta	chemotherapy-induced neutropenia
pegylated doxorubicin HCl liposome	Doxil; Dox-SL; Evacet; LipoDox	refractory metastatic carcinoma of the ovary; AIDS-related Kaposi sarcoma; breast cancer; relapsed/refractory multiple myeloma (with bortezomib)
pegylated interferon alfa	PEG-interferon alfa	hepatitis C
pegylated liposomal doxorubicin	Doxil; Dox-SL; Evacet; LipoDox	refractory metastatic carcinoma of the ovary; AIDS-related Kaposi sarcoma; breast cancer; relapsed/refractory multiple myeloma (with bortezomib)
pegylated liposomal doxorubicin hydrochloride	DOXIL; Dox-SL; Evacet; LipoDox; CAELYX; Doxilen	refractory metastatic carcinoma of the ovary; AIDS-related Kaposi sarcoma; breast cancer; relapsed/refractory multiple myeloma (with bortezomib)
pemetrexed disodium	Alimta	malignant pleural mesothelioma; non-small-cell lung cancer
penicillamine	Cuprenil; Cuprimine; Depen; Perdolat; Sufortan; Atamir; Cupripen; Distamine; Kelatin; Mercaptyl; Metalcaptase; Pendramine; Trolovol	Wilson disease; heavy metal intoxication; cystinuria; rheumatoid arthritis; primary biliary cirrhosis; Felty syndrome; rheumatoid vasculitis
pentostatin	Nipent	chronic lymphocytic leukemia; cutaneous T-cell lymphoma; hairy cell leukemia
Peyrone's chloride	Platinol; Platinol-AQ	metastatic testicular cancer; ovarian cancer; head and neck cancer; breast cancer; Hodgkin disease and non-Hodgkin lymphoma; myeloma and melanoma; advanced bladder cancer
Peyrone's salt	Platinol; Platinol-AQ	metastatic testicular cancer; ovarian cancer; head and neck cancer; breast cancer; Hodgkin disease and non-Hodgkin lymphoma; myeloma and melanoma; advanced bladder cancer
phenobarbital	none	epilepsy
phentolamine mesylate	Regitine; Vasomax	dermal necrosis; hypertensive-associated episodes with pheochromocytoma, prevention or control
phenylalanine mustard	Alkeran	breast cancer; neuroblastoma; palliative treatment of multiple myeloma and nonresectable epithelial ovarian carcinoma; rhabdomyosarcoma
phenylalanine nitrogen mustard	Alkeran	breast cancer; neuroblastoma; palliative treatment of multiple myeloma and nonresectable epithelial ovarian carcinoma; rhabdomyosarcoma
phenylbutyric acid nitrogen mustard	Ambochlorin; Amboclorin; Leukeran	chronic lymphocytic leukemia; malignant lymphomas
photofrin II	Photofrin	photosensitizer; bladder, esophageal, gastric, lung, and rectal cancers
PI-88	none	malignant melanoma
pidorubicin	Ellence	breast cancer; adjuvant in breast cancer therapy
pipobroman	Vercyte	leukemias

Generic Drug	Trade Name	Indicated For
platinoxan	Platinol; Platinol-AQ	metastatic testicular cancer; ovarian cancer; head and neck cancer; breast cancer; Hodgkin disease and non-Hodgkin lymphoma; myeloma and melanoma; advanced bladder cancer
platinum diamminodichloride	Platinol; Platinol-AQ	metastatic testicular cancer; ovarian cancer; head and neck cancer; breast cancer; Hodgkin disease and non-Hodgkin lymphoma; myeloma and melanoma; advanced bladder cancer
plenaxis	none	prostate cancer
plicamycin	Mithracin	testicular cancer
polifeprosan 20 with carmustine implant	Gliadel wafer	malignant glioma, adjuvant to surgery and radiation; recurrent glioblastoma multiforme, adjuvant to surgery
polyethylene glycol-L-asparaginase	Oncaspar	acute lymphoblastic leukemia
porfimer	Photofrin	photosensitizer; bladder, esophageal, gastric, lung, and rectal cancers
porfimer sodium	Photofrin	photosensitizer; bladder, esophageal, gastric, lung, and rectal cancers
posaconazole	Noxafil	fungal infection prevention for immunocompromised host
potaba	none	diseases involving fibrosis and nonsuppurative inflammation
potassium p-aminobenzoate	none	diseases involving fibrosis and nonsuppurative inflammation
potassium para-aminobenzoate	none	diseases involving fibrosis and nonsuppurative inflammation
PRD	Delta-Dome; Deltasone; Liquid Pred; Lisacort; Meticorten; Orasone; Prednicen-M; Sk-Prednisone; Sterapred	inflammatory conditions; allergic conditions; hematologic conditions; neoplastic conditions; autoimmune conditions; replacement therapy in adrenal insufficiency
prednisolone	Cortalone; Delta-Cortef; Hydeltra; Hydeltrasol; Meti-derm; Prelone	inflammatory conditions; allergic conditions; hematologic conditions; neoplastic conditions; autoimmune conditions; replacement therapy in adrenal insufficiency
prednisone; prednisonum	Delta-Dome; Deltasone; Liquid Pred; Lisacort; Meticorten; Orasone; Prednicen-M; Sk-Prednisone; Sterapred	inflammatory conditions; allergic conditions; hematologic conditions; neoplastic conditions; autoimmune conditions; replacement therapy in adrenal insufficiency
procarbazin	Matulane	brain tumors; Hodgkin disease; non-Hodgkin lymphoma
procarbazine hydrochloride	Matulane	brain tumors; Hodgkin disease; non-Hodgkin lymphoma
prochlorperazine	Compazine	antinausea
purimethol	Mercaptopurinum; Purinethol	acute lymphocytic leukemia; acute myelogenous leukemia; Crohn disease; Hodgkin disease in children; lymphoblastic lymphoma; ulcerative colitis
6-purinethiol	Mercaptopurinum; Purinethol	acute lymphocytic leukemia; acute myelogenous leukemia; Crohn disease; Hodgkin disease in children; lymphoblastic lymphoma; ulcerative colitis

Generic Drug	Trade Name	Indicated For
raloxifene	Evista; Keoxifene	breast cancer; cardiovascular disease prophylaxis; osteoporosis
raltitrexed	Tomudex	advanced colorectal cancer
ranpirnase	Onconase	mesothelioma
rapamycin analog; rapamycin analog CCI-779	Torisel	renal cell carcinoma; advanced renal cell carcinoma
rasburicase	Elitek	chemotherapy-induced acute hyperuricemia, treatment and prophylaxis
recombinant adenovirus-p53	none	primary ovarian cancer
recombinant human interleukin-11	Neumega	chemotherapy-related thrombocytopenia
recombinant human papillomavirus 16 E6 peptide	none	cervical cancer vaccine (TA-HPV) component
recombinant humanized anti-VEGF monoclonal antibody	Avastin	metastatic colorectal cancer, non-small-cell lung cancer
recombinant humanized monoclonal antibody to vascular endothelial growth factor	Avastin	metastatic colorectal cancer, non-small-cell lung cancer
recombinant interferon alfa	Alferon N; Intron A; Roferon-A	used as antiviral and antitumor agents
recombinant interferon alpha-2a	Alferon; Roferon-A; Laroferon; Roceron; Roceron-A	chronic phase Philadelphia chromosome-positive chronic myelogenous leukemia; hairy cell leukemia; chronic hepatitis C; AIDS-related Kaposi sarcoma; bladder cancer; ovarian cancer; cervical cancer; non-Hodgkin lymphoma; renal cell carcinoma; melanoma
recombinant interferon beta	Betaseron; Rebif	multiple sclerosis
recombinant interferon gamma	Actimmune	chronic granulomatous disease; osteopetrosis
recombinant interleukin-2	Proleukin	metastatic renal cell carcinoma; metastatic melanoma; stimulates the production of blood cells, especially platelets, during chemotherapy
recombinant interleukin-11	Neumega	chemotherapy-related thrombocytopenia
recombinant methionyl human granulocyte colony stimulating factor	Neupogen	bone marrow transplantation; cancer patients receiving myelosuppressive chemotherapy; neutropenia
recombinant urate oxidase	Elitek	chemotherapy-induced acute hyperuricemia, treatment and prophylaxis
retinoic acid	Aberel; Aknoten; Avita; Renova; Retin-A; Retin-A MICRO; Vesanoid	(oral) acute promyelocytic leukemia (APL), characterized by the t(15;17) translocation or the PML/RARa gene; for patients refractory to or who have relapsed from anthracycline chemotherapy, or for where anthracycline-based chemotherapy is contraindicated; (topical) acne vulgaris; other dermatologic conditions; some skin cancers

Generic Drug	Trade Name	Indicated For
retinoicacid-9-cis	Panretin	topical treatment of cutaneous lesions in patients with AIDS-related Kaposi sarcoma
retinol	Aquasol A; Del-Vi-A; Pedi-Vit-A	diminishing malignant cell growth; enhancing the immune system
retinyl acetate	Retinol Acetate; vitamin A acetate	dietary supplement; vitamin A deficiency
r-HuEPO	Epogen; Procrit	anemias associated with chronic renal failure, zidovudine (AZT) therapy, and cancer chemotherapy of nonmyeloid malignancies
rhuMAb VEGF	Avastin	metastatic colorectal cancer, non-small-cell lung cancer
rifabutin	Mycobutin	prevention and treatment of *Mycobacterium avium* complex (MAC) and tuberculosis in patients with HIV infection
risedronate sodium	Actonel	osteoporosis, treatment and prevention; Paget disease
rituximab	Rituxan	diffuse large B-cell, CD20-positive, non-Hodgkin lymphoma
rofecoxib	Vioxx	pain; dysmenorrhea; osteoarthritis; rheumatoid arthritis
rosiglitazone maleate	Avandia	noninsulin-dependent diabetes mellitus and type II diabetes mellitus; type 2 diabetes
rubetican	Camptogen; Orathecin	AIDS, pediatric; HIV infection, pediatric
rubomycin C	Cerubidine; Rubidomycin	acute lymphoblastic leukemia
S-liposomal doxorubicin	Doxil; Dox-SL; Evacet; LipoDox	refractory metastatic carcinoma of the ovary; AIDS-related Kaposi sarcoma; breast cancer; relapsed/refractory multiple myeloma (with bortezomib)
samarium-153 EDTMP	Quadramet	pain due to bone cancer
samarium-153 ethylenediaminetetra-methylenephosphonate	Quadramet	pain due to bone cancer
samarium-153 ethylenediaminetetra-methylenephosphonic acid	Quadramet	pain due to bone cancer
samarium SM 153 lexidronam pentasodium	Quadramet	pain due to bone cancer
sarcoclorin	Alkeran	breast cancer; neuroblastoma; palliative treatment of multiple myeloma and nonresectable epithelial ovarian carcinoma; rhabdomyosarcoma
sargramostim	Leukine; Prokine	melanoma; chemotherapy-induced neutropenia
SD-01; SD-01 sustained duration G-CSF	Neulasta	chemotherapy-induced neutropenia
selenium	none	dandruff; psoriasis; seborrheic dermatitis; tinea capitis; tinea versicolor
sertraline hydrochloride	Zoloft	major depressive disorder; obsessive-compulsive disorder; panic disorder; posttraumatic stress disorder; premenstrual dysphoric disorder; social phobia

Generic Drug	Trade Name	Indicated For
sildenafil citrate	Viagra	erectile dysfunction
silymarin	none	nutritional supplement for liver damage induced by chemicals or toxins
sinestrol	Acnestrol; Cyren A; Deladumone; Diastyl; Domestrol; Estrobene; Estrosyn; Fonatol; Makarol; Milestrol; Neo-Oestronol I; Oestrogenine; Oestromenin; Oestromon; Palestrol; Stilbestrol; Stilbetin; Stilboestroform; Stilboestrol; Synestrin; Synthoestrin; Vagestrol	breast cancer; prostate cancer
siplizumab	none	T-cell lymphoma
sirolimus	Rapamune	kidney transplant rejection, prevention
sm-153 EDTMP	Quadramet	pain due to bone cancer
sodium clodronate	Bonefos, Loron	myeloma, secondary breast cancer
sodium iodide I 131	Iodotope	thyroid cancer
sodium phosphate P32	Sodium Phosphate P32 Solution	polycythemia vera; chronic myelocytic leukemia and chronic lymphocytic leukemia; multiple areas of skeletal metastases, palliative treatment
sodium salicylate	Disalcid	fever; inflammatory conditions; pain
sorafenib tosylate	Nexavar	advanced renal cell carcinoma; metastatic colorectal cancer
soy protein isolate	Revival	heart disease prevention; hyperlipidemia; menopausal symptoms
stealth liposomal doxorubicin	Doxil; Dox-SL; Evacet; LipoDox	refractory metastatic carcinoma of the ovary; AIDS-related Kaposi sarcoma; breast cancer; relapsed/refractory multiple myeloma (with bortezomib)
stilboestrol dipropionate	Acnestrol; Cyren A; Deladumone; Diastyl; Domestrol; Estrobene; Estrosyn; Fonatol; Makarol; Milestrol; Neo-Oestronol I; Oestrogenine; Oestromenin; Oestromon; Palestrol; Stilbestrol; Stilbetin; Stilboestroform; Stilboestrol; Synestrin; Synthoestrin; Vagestrol	breast cancer; prostate cancer
streptozocin	Zanosar	carcinoid tumor and syndrome; colorectal cancer, palliative; Hodgkin disease; metastatic islet cell carcinoma of the pancreas
streptozotocin	Zanosar	carcinoid tumor and syndrome; colorectal cancer, palliative; Hodgkin disease; metastatic islet cell carcinoma of the pancreas
strontium chloride Sr 89	Metastron	palliation of pain in bone metastases

Generic Drug	Trade Name	Indicated For
suberoylanilide hydroxamic acid	Zolinza	cutaneous T-cell lymphoma
sulfabutin	Busulfex; Mitosan; Myleran	bone marrow disorders; chronic myelogenous leukemia; palliative; neoadjuvant to allogeneic hematopoietic progenitor cell transplantation; neoplastic meningitis; primary brain malignancies
sulindac	Aflodac; Clinoril	arthritis; inflammatory conditions
sunitinib	Sutent	gastrointestinal stromal tumor; advanced metastatic renal cell carcinoma
sunitinib malate	Sutent	gastrointestinal stromal tumor; advanced metastatic renal cell carcinoma
suramin	309 F; Bayer 205; Fourneau 309; Germanin; Moranyl; Naganin; Naganine	trypanosomiasis; hormone-refractory prostate cancer
syklofosfamid	Cytoxan; Clafen; Neosar	breast cancer; leukemias; lupus nephritis; lymphoma; multiple myeloma; neuroblastoma; nephrotic syndrome; ovarian cancer; retinoblastoma
SZN	Zanosar	carcinoid tumor and syndrome; colorectal cancer, palliative; Hodgkin disease; metastatic islet cell carcinoma of the pancreas
T-cell growth factor	Proleukin	metastatic renal cell carcinoma; metastatic melanoma; stimulates the production of blood cells, especially platelets, during chemotherapy
tacrolimus	none	atopic dermatitis; kidney transplant rejection, prophylaxis; liver transplant rejection, prophylaxis
talc	Sclerosol Intrapleural Aerosol; Sterile Talc Powder; Steritalc	malignant pleural effusion; pneumothorax
tamoxifen	Nolvadex; Soltamox	breast cancer, palliative; adjuvant in breast cancer therapy; endometrial cancer; gynecomastia; melanoma; ovarian cancer
tamoxifen citrate	Nolvadex; Soltamox	breast cancer, palliative; adjuvant in breast cancer therapy; endometrial cancer; gynecomastia; melanoma; ovarian cancer
tamoxifeni citras	Nolvadex; Soltamox	breast cancer, palliative; adjuvant in breast cancer therapy; endometrial cancer; gynecomastia; melanoma; ovarian cancer
tamsulosin hydrochloride	Flomax	benign prostatic hyperplasia
tanespimycin	KOS-953	chronic myelogenous leukemia
tazarotene	Avage; Tazorac; Retisol-A; Stieva-A; Stieva-A Forte; Vitinoin	topical treatment of facial acne vulgaris; stable plaque psoriasis; mitigation (palliation) of facial fine wrinkling; facial mottled hyper- and hypopigmentation; benign facial lentigines
Tc 99m sulfur colloid	none	diagnostic imaging
TCGF	Proleukin	metastatic renal cell carcinoma; metastatic melanoma; stimulates the production of blood cells, especially platelets, during chemotherapy
technetium Tc 99m sulfur colloid	none	diagnostic imaging

Generic Drug	Trade Name	Indicated For
tegafur with uracil	Uftoral	bowel cancer
temozolomide	Methazolastone; Temodar	malignant glioma (anaplastic astrocytoma; anaplastic oligodendrogliomas; anaplastic oligoastrocytomas; glioblastoma multiforme); metastatic melanoma
temsirolimus	Torisel	renal cell carcinoma; advanced renal cell carcinoma
teniposide	Vumon	childhood acute lymphocytic leukemia
testolactone	Teslac	advanced breast cancer in women, palliative
testosterone	Andro LA 200; Andro-Cyp 100; Delatestryl; Delatest; Depandro 100; Depo-Testosterone; Testro; Testro AQ; Virilon IM; Depotest; Duratest; Durathate 200; Everone; FIRST-Testosterone; FIRST-Testosterone MC; Histerone; Meditest; Testamone-100; Testoderm; Testolin; Testopel; Testosterone Enanthate; Testostroval; Testostroval-PA; Testro AQ	breast cancer in women; delayed puberty in men; hypogonadism; metastatic mammary cancer
testosterone enanthate	Delatestryl; Testoderm; Testolin; Testostroval; Testostroval-PA; Testro AQ	delayed puberty, male; hypogonadism; metastatic mammary cancer
tetanus toxoid	none	tetanus prophylaxis
tetrahydrocannabinol	Marinol	antinausea
tetramethylene bis(methanesulfonate)	Busulfex; Mitosan; Myleran	bone marrow disorders; chronic myelogenous leukemia; palliative; neoadjuvant to allogeneic hematopoietic progenitor cell transplantation; neoplastic meningitis; primary brain malignancies
thalidomide	Synovir; Thalomid	Kaposi sarcoma; multiple myeloma; primary brain tumors
thenvlidene-lignan-P; thenylidene-lignan-P	Vumon	childhood acute lymphocytic leukemia
therapeutic dehydroepiandrosterone	Fidelin	adrenal insufficiency, replacement; systemic lupus erythematosus, treatment and steroid treatment reduction
therapeutic interleukin-11	Neumega	chemotherapy-related thrombocytopenia
therapeutic melatonin	Circadin	sleep disorders in blind people with no light perception
therapeutic progesterone	Colprosterone; Gesterol 100; Lipo-Lutin; Luteohormone; Progestin	amenorrhea; functional uterine bleeding; infertility; maintenance of pregnancy
therapeutic testolactone	Teslac	advanced breast cancer in women, palliative
therapeutic testosterone	Delatestryl; Testoderm; Testolin; Testostroval; Testostroval-PA; Testro AQ	delayed puberty, male; hypogonadism; metastatic mammary cancer

Generic Drug	Trade Name	Indicated For
thioguanine	Tabloid; Tabloid brand thioguanine; Tioguanine; Lanvis	acute nonlymphocytic leukemia
6 thiohypoxanthine	Mercaptopurinum; Purinethol	acute lymphocytic leukemia; acute myelogenous leukemia; Crohn disease; Hodgkin disease in children; lymphoblastic lymphoma; ulcerative colitis
thiophosphamide	Girostan; STEPA; TESPA; Thiofozil; Thioplex; Tifosyl	bladder cancer; breast cancer; ovarian cancer; Hodgkin disease; non-Hodgkin lymphoma
thiophosphoramide	Girostan; STEPA; TESPA; Thiofozil; Thioplex; Tifosyl	bladder cancer; breast cancer; ovarian cancer; Hodgkin disease; non-Hodgkin disease
6-thiopurine	Mercaptopurinum; Purinethol	acute lymphocytic leukemia; acute myelogenous leukemia; Crohn disease; Hodgkin disease in children; lymphoblastic lymphoma; ulcerative colitis
6-thioxopurine	Mercaptopurinum; Purinethol	acute lymphocytic leukemia; acute myelogenous leukemia; Crohn disease; Hodgkin disease in children; lymphoblastic lymphoma; ulcerative colitis
thiotepa	Girostan; STEPA; TESPA; Thiofozil; Thioplex; Tifosyl	bladder cancer; breast cancer; ovarian cancer; Hodgkin disease non-Hodgkin lymphoma
thymocyte stimulating factor	Proleukin	metastatic renal cell carcinoma; metastatic melanoma; stimulates the production of blood cells, especially platelets, during chemotherapy
thyrotropin alfa	Thyrogen	thyroid cancer
tinzaparin sodium	Innohep	treatment of acute symptomatic deep venous thrombosis (DVT) with or without a pulmonary embolism (PE), in conjunction with warfarin
TMQ	Neutrexin	head and neck cancer; metastatic colorectal adenocarcinoma; non-small-cell lung cancer; osteogenic sarcoma; pancreatic adenocarcinoma; pneumocystitis carinii pneumonia
topotecan hydrochloride	Hycamtin	small-cell lung carcinoma; cervical cancer
toremifene	Fareston	breast cancer; desmoid tumors
tositumomab	Bexxar	CD20 positive follicular non-Hodgkin lymphoma refractory to rituximab
TRA	Aberel; Aknoten; Avita; Renova; Retin-A; Retin-A MICRO; Vesanoid	(oral) acute promyelocytic leukemia (APL), characterized by the t(15;17) translocation or the PML/RARa gene refractory, or for where anthracycline-based chemotherapy is contraindicated; (topical) acne vulgaris; other dermatologic conditions; some skin cancers
trans retinoic acid	Aberel; Aknoten; Avita; Renova; Retin-A; Retin-A MICRO; Vesanoid	(oral) acute promyelocytic leukemia (APL), characterized by the t(15;17) translocation or the PML/RARa gene refractory, or for where anthracycline-based chemotherapy is contraindicated; (topical) acne vulgaris; other dermatologic conditions; some skin cancers
trans-testosterone	Delatestryl; Testoderm; Testolin; Testostroval; Testostroval-PA; Testro AQ	delayed puberty, male; hypogonadism; metastatic mammary cancer

Generic Drug	Trade Name	Indicated For
trans vitamin A acid	Aberel; Aknoten; Avita; Renova; Retin-A; Retin-A MICRO; Vesanoid	(oral) acute promyelocytic leukemia (APL), characterized by the t(15;17) translocation or the PML/RARa gene refractory, or for where anthracycline-based chemotherapy is contraindicated; (topical) acne vulgaris; other dermatologic conditions; some skin cancers
trastuzumab	Herceptin	breast cancer overexpressing HER2 protein; pancreatic cancer overexpressing p185HER2
treosulfan	none	ovarian cancer; leukemia
tretinoin; tretinoinum	Aberel; Aknoten; Avita; Renova; Retin-A; Retin-A MICRO; Vesanoid	(oral) acute promyelocytic leukemia (APL), characterized by the t(15;17) translocation or the PML/RARa gene refractory, or for where anthracycline-based chemotherapy is contraindicated; (topical) acne vulgaris; other dermatologic conditions; some skin cancers
triacetyluridine	none	mitochondrial disease
triethylene thiophosphoramide	Girostan; STEPA; TESPA; Thiofozil; Thioplex; Tifosyl	bladder cancer; breast cancer; ovarian cancer; Hodgkin disease; non-Hodgkin lymphoma
trimethoprim-sulfamethoxazole	Bactrim; Cotrim; Septra	pneumocystis carinii pneumonia; various bacterial infections
trimethylmethoxyphenyl-retinoic acid	Etretin; Soriatane	cutaneous T-cell lymphoma
trimetrexate glucuronate	Neutrexin	head and neck cancer; metastatic colorectal adenocarcinoma; non-small-cell lung cancer; osteogenic sarcoma; pancreatic adenocarcinoma; pneumocystitis carinii pneumonia
triptorelin	Decapeptyl	prostate carcinoma, palliative treatment
trivalent influenza vaccine	FluMist; Flushield; Fluvirin; Fluzone	influenza prophylaxis
tropisetron	Navoban	chemotherapy-induced nausea and vomiting
uracil mustard	Uracil Mustard Capsules	lymphomaûûnon-Hodgkin
urate oxidase	Elitek	chemotherapy-induced acute hyperuricemia, treatment and prophylaxis
ursodiol	Actigall; URSO; Deursil	gallstone dissolution; primary biliary cirrhosis
valdecoxib	Bextra	osteoarthritis; rheumatoid arthritis; dysmenorrhea
valganciclovir	Valcyte	cytomegalovirus retinitis
valproic acid	Depakene; Alti-Valproic; Ergenyl; Novo-Valproic	epilepsy; mania; migraine
valrubicin	Valstar	bladder cancer
vandetanib	Zactima	thyroid cancer
venlafaxine	Effexor	anxiety; depression
verteporfin	Visudyne	photosensitizer; subfoveal choroidal neovascularization

Generic Drug	Trade Name	Indicated For
vinblastine	Velban; Velsar	bladder cancer; breast cancer; choriocarcinoma; germ-cell tumors; idiopathic thrombocytopenic purpura; Kaposi sarcoma; Letterer-Siwe disease; various lymphomas; melanoma; mycosis fungoides; prostate cancer; testicular cancer
vincaleucoblastine	Velban; Velsar	bladder cancer; breast cancer; choriocarcinoma; germ-cell tumors; idiopathic thrombocytopenic purpura; Kaposi sarcoma; Letterer-Siwe disease; various lymphomas; melanoma; mycosis fungoides; prostate cancer; testicular cancer
vincasar	Oncovin; Vincasar PFS	acute leukemia; brain tumors; chronic lymphocytic leukemia; gestational trophoblastic neoplasms; head and neck squamous cell carcinoma; Kaposi sarcoma; liver cancer; Hodgkin disease and non-Hodgkin lymphoma; malignant thymoma; multiple myeloma; osteogenic sarcoma; ovarian cancer; pheochromocytoma; retinoblastoma; rhabdomyosarcoma; soft-tissue sarcoma; testicular cancer; Wilms' tumor
vincristine; vincrystine	Oncovin; Vincasar PFS	acute leukemia; brain tumors; chronic lymphocytic leukemia; gestational trophoblastic neoplasms; head and neck squamous cell carcinoma; Kaposi sarcoma; liver cancer; Hodgkin disease and non-Hodgkin lymphoma; malignant thymoma; multiple myeloma; osteogenic sarcoma; ovarian cancer; pheochromocytoma; retinoblastoma; rhabdomyosarcoma; soft-tissue sarcoma; testicular cancer; Wilms' tumor
vindesine	Eldisine	acute leukemia; lung cancer; carcinoma of the breast; squamous cell carcinoma of the esophagus, head, and neck; Hodgkin disease and non-Hodgkin lymphomas
vinorelbine ditartrate	Biovelbin; Eunades	non-small-cell lung cancer; metastatic breast cancer; uterine and cervical cancer; desmoid tumors; advanced Kaposi sarcoma
vinorelbine tartrate	Biovelbin; Eunades	non-small-cell lung cancer; metastatic breast cancer; uterine and cervical cancer; desmoid tumors; advanced Kaposi sarcoma
vitamin A	Aquasol A; Del-Vi-A; Pedi-Vit-A	diminishing malignant cell growth; enhancing the immune system
vitamin A acid	Aberel; Aknoten; Avita; Renova; Retin-A; Retin-A MICRO; Vesanoid	(oral) acute promyelocytic leukemia (APL), characterized by the t(15;17) translocation or the PML/RARa gene refractory, or for where anthracycline-based chemotherapy is contraindicated; (topical) acne vulgaris; other dermatologic conditions; some skin cancers
vitamin A alcohol	Aquasol A; Del-Vi-A; Pedi-Vit-A	diminishing malignant cell growth; enhancing the immune system
vitamin A compound	Aquasol A; Del-Vi-A; Pedi-Vit-A	diminishing malignant cell growth; enhancing the immune system
vitamin A USP	Aquasol A; Del-Vi-A; Pedi-Vit-A	diminishing malignant cell growth; enhancing the immune system
vitamin A1	Aquasol A; Del-Vi-A; Pedi-Vit-A	diminishing malignant cell growth; enhancing the immune system
vitamin E compound	none	vitamin E deficiency; used in cancer prevention

Generic Drug	Trade Name	Indicated For
vitaminum A	Aquasol A; Del-Vi-A; Pedi-Vit-A	diminishing malignant cell growth; enhancing the immune system
VM26	Vumon	childhood acute lymphocytic leukemia
voriconazole	none	aspergillosis, invasive; esophageal candidiasis; fungal infections, nonaspergillosis
vorinostat	Zolinza	cutaneous T-cell lymphoma
warfarin	Athrombin-K; Compound 42; Co-Rax; Coumadin; Panwarfin; Rodex; WARF Compound 42	pulmonary embolism and thromboembolic disorders, treatment and prophylaxis; venous thrombosis, prophylaxis and treatment
white arsenic	Trisenox	myelodysplastic syndrome; multiple myeloma; chronic myeloid leukemia; acute myelocytic leukemia
90Y ibritumomab tiuxetan	Zevalin	non-Hodgkin lymphoma
Y90-labeled ibritumomab tiuxetan	Zevalin	non-Hodgkin lymphoma
Y90 zevalin	Zevalin	non-Hodgkin lymphoma
YM177	Celebrex	familial adenomatous polyposis (inherited colorectal cancer syndrome)
yttrium-90 ibritumomab tiuxetan	Zevalin	non-Hodgkin lymphoma
yttrium Y 90 glass microspheres	TheraSphere	hepatocellular carcinoma, transarterial internal radiation
yttrium Y 90 ibritumomab tiuxetan	Zevalin	non-Hodgkin lymphoma
zidovudine	Retrovir; Aztec	AIDS-related complex; HIV infection; HIV transmission, prevention
zileuton	Zyflo	prevention and chronic treatment of asthma
zinc sulfate	none	common cold, symptoms; wound healing; zinc supplement
zoledronate	Zometa; Reclast	hypercalcemia of malignancy; multiple myeloma and metastatic bone lesions from solid tumors; Paget disease
zoledronic acid	Zometa; Reclast	hypercalcemia of malignancy; multiple myeloma and metastatic bone lesions from solid tumors; Paget disease
zytoxan	Cytoxan; Clafen; Neosar	breast cancer; leukemias; lupus nephritis; lymphoma; multiple myeloma; neuroblastoma; nephrotic syndrome; ovarian cancer; retinoblastoma

▶ Drugs by Trade Name

Trade Name	Generic Drug	Indicated For
Abbott-56268	clarithromycin	*H. pylori* infection; various bacterial infections
Aberel	tretinoin; all-trans retinoic acid; all-trans vitamin A acid; beta-retinoic acid; retinoic acid; TRA; trans retinoic acid; trans vitamin A acid; tretinoinum; vitamin A acid	(oral) acute promyelocytic leukemia (APL), characterized by the t(15;17) translocation or the PML/RARa gene; for patients refractory to or who have relapsed from anthracycline chemotherapy, or for where anthracycline-based chemotherapy is contraindicated; (topical) acne vulgaris; other dermatologic conditions; some skin cancers
Abitrexate	methotrexate	bladder cancer; breast cancer; carcinomatous; meningitis; chorioadenoma destruens; esophageal cancer; gestational choriocarcinoma; head/neck cancer; meningeal leukemia; lymphomas; Burkitt lymphoma; lung cancer; mycosis fungoides; osteosarcoma; Wegener granulomatosis
Abraxane	paclitaxel; paclitaxel protein-bound; albumin-stabilized nanoparticle paclitaxel; nab-paclitaxel; nanoparticle paclitaxel	bladder cancer; breast cancer; adjuvant in breast cancer therapy; cervical cancer; endometrial adenocarcinoma; esophageal cancer; head and neck cancer; non-small-cell lung cancer; lymphoma; ovarian cancer; prostate cancer; testicular cancer; AIDS-related Kaposi sarcoma
Accutane	isotretinoin	cutaneous T-cell lymphoma; juvenile metastatic neuroblastoma and leukemia
Acicontral	calcium citrate	calcium supplement; hypocalcemia; osteoporosis; rickets; tetany
Acnestrol	diethylstilbesterol; diethylstilbenediol; diethylstilbestrol dipropionate; diethylstilbestrolum; diethylstilboestrol; sinestrol; stilboestrol dipropionate	breast cancer; prostate cancer
Actigall	ursodiol	gallstone dissolution; primary biliary cirrhosis
Actimmune	recombinant interferon gamma	chronic granulomatous disease; osteopetrosis
Actiq	fentanyl citrate	breakthrough pain in cancer patients
Actonel	risedronate sodium	osteoporosis, treatment and prevention; Paget disease
Adagen	pegademase	enzyme replacement therapy for patients with severe combined immunodeficiency as a result of adenosine deaminase deficiency
Adderall	dextroamphetamine-amphetamine	attention deficit/hyperactivity disorder (ADHD); narcolepsy
Adriamycin	doxorubicin hydrochloride; ADM; ADR; adria	leukemias; Wilms' tumor; neuroblastoma; soft-tissue and bone sarcomas; small-cell carcinoma of the lung; lymphomas; multiple myeloma; mesotheliomas; germ-cell tumors of the ovary or testis
Adrucil	fluorouracil; 5-fluorouracil; 5-fluracil; fluoro uracil; fluouracil; FU	palliative treatment for colorectal, breast, and pancreatic cancers; topical treatment for superficial basal cell carcinoma that cannot be treated with surgery and actinic keratosis
Aeroseb-Dex	dexamethasone; desamethasone; dexamethasonum; DXM; hexadecadrol; methylfluorprednisolone	antiemetic (prevents vomiting)

Trade Name	Generic Drug	Indicated For
Aflodac	sulindac	arthritis; inflammatory conditions
Agrylin	anagrelide	thrombocythemia secondary to myeloproliferative disorders; disrupts the postmitotic phase of megakaryocyte development
Aknoten	tretinoin; all-trans retinoic acid; all-trans vitamin A acid; beta-retinoic acid; retinoic acid; TRA; trans retinoic acid; trans vitamin A acid; tretinoinum; vitamin A acid	(oral) acute promyelocytic leukemia (APL), characterized by the t(15;17) translocation or the PML/RARa gene; for patients refractory to or who have relapsed from anthracycline chemotherapy, or for where anthracycline-based chemotherapy is contraindicated; (topical) acne vulgaris; other dermatologic conditions; some skin cancers
Alba-Dex	dexamethasone; desamethasone; dexamethasonum; DXM; hexadecadrol; methylfluorprednisolone	antiemetic (prevents vomiting)
Aldara	imiquimod	condyloma; superficial basal cell carcinoma; actinic keratosis
Alexion	eculizumab	paroxysmal nocturnal hemoglobinuria
Alferon	recombinant interferon alpha-2a	chronic phase Philadelphia chromosome-positive chronic myelogenous leukemia; hairy cell leukemia; chronic hepatitis C; AIDS-related Kaposi sarcoma; bladder cancer; ovarian cancer; cervical cancer; non-Hodgkin lymphoma; renal-cell carcinoma; melanoma
Alferon N	recombinant interferon alfa	used as antiviral and antitumor agents
Alimta	pemetrexed disodium; multitargeted antifolate	malignant pleural mesothelioma; non-small-cell lung cancer
Alkeran	melphalan; alanine nitrogen mustard; L-phenylalanine mustard; L-sarcolysin; L-sarcolysin phenylalanine mustard; L-sarcolysine; phenylalanine mustard; phenylalanine nitrogen mustard; sarcoclorin	breast cancer; neuroblastoma; palliative treatment of multiple myeloma and nonresectable epithelial ovarian carcinoma; rhabdomyosarcoma
Aloxi	palonosetron hydrochloride	antinausea; antiemetic (prevents vomiting)
Alti-Valproic	valproic acid	epilepsy; mania; migraine
Ambochlorin	chlorambucil; CBL; chlorambucilum; chloraminophen; chlorbutin; chlorbutine; chlorbutinum; chloroambucil; chlorobutin; chlorobutine; elcoril; leukersan; leukoran; linfolizin; lympholysin; phenylbutyric acid nitrogen mustard	chronic lymphocytic leukemia; malignant lymphomas
Ammoidin	methoxsalen; 8-methoxypsoralen; methoxypsoralen	cutaneous T-cell lymphoma
Amsa P-D	amsacrine; acridinyl anisidide; Cain's acridine	leukemia

Trade Name	Generic Drug	Indicated For
Andro LA 200	testosterone	breast cancer in women, palliative
Andro-Cyp 100	testosterone	breast cancer in women, palliative
Android, Testred, Virilon	methyltestosterone	breast cancer, palliative
Android-F	fluoxymesterone; androfluorene; androsterolo	certain types of breast cancer
Androxy	fluoxymesterone; androfluorene; androsterolo	certain types of breast cancer
Anzemet	dolasetron mesylate	nausea and vomiting prophylaxis, chemotherapy-induced and postoperative
Aptosyn	exisulind	colonic adenomatous polyps in the inherited disease adenomatous polyposis coli, control and suppression
Aquasol A	vitamin A compound; all trans-retinol; anti-infective vitamin; antixerophthalmic vitamin; axerophthol; axeroptholum; biosterol; lard-factor; oleovitamin A; ophthalamin; retinol; vitamin A; vitamin A alcohol; vitamin A USP; vitamin A1; vitaminum A	diminishing malignant cell growth; enhancing the immune system
Aranesp	darbepoetin alfa; novel erythropoiesis stimulating protein	chemotherapy-induced anemia; chronic renal failure/insufficiency
Aredia	disodium pamidronate; pamidronate disodium	myeloma, secondary breast cancer; hypercalcemia of malignancy; osteolytic bone lesions of multiple myeloma; osteolytic bone metastases of breast cancer; Paget disease
Aricept	donepezil hydrochloride	Alzheimer's disease and opioid-induced sedation
Arimidex	anastrozole	hormone receptor-positive early breast cancer
Aromasin	exemestane	estrogen receptor-positive early breast cancer
Arranon	nelarabine	T-cell acute lymphoblastic leukemia; T-cell lymphoblastic lymphoma
Aspergum	acetylsalicylic acid; aspirin	mild to moderate pain; fever; prevention of arterial and venous thrombosis
Atamir	penicillamine	Wilson disease; heavy metal intoxication; cystinuria; rheumatoid arthritis; primary biliary cirrhosis; Felty syndrome; rheumatoid vasculitis
ATGAM	antithymocyte globulin	heart and renal transplantation rejection; prophylaxis
Athrombin-K	warfarin	pulmonary embolism and thromboembolic disorders, treatment and prophylaxis; venous thrombosis, prophylaxis and treatment
Augmentin	amoxicillin-clavulanate potassium	various bacterial infections
Avage	tazarotene	topical treatment of facial acne vulgaris; stable plaque psoriasis; mitigation (palliation) of facial fine wrinkling; facial mottled hyper- and hypopigmentation; benign facial lentigines

Trade Name	Generic Drug	Indicated For
Avakine	infliximab	ankylosis spondylitis; Crohn disease; plaque psoriasis; rheumatoid arthritis; sarcoidosis
Avandia	rosiglitazone maleate	noninsulin-dependent diabetes mellitus and type II diabetes mellitus; type 2 diabetes
Avastin	bevacizumab; anti-VEGF; anti-VEGF humanized monoclonal antibody; anti-VEGF monoclonal antibody; anti-VEGF RhuMAb; recombinant humanized anti-VEGF monoclonal antibody; recombinant humanized monoclonal antibody to vascular endothelial growth factor; rhuMAb VEGF	metastatic colorectal cancer, non-small-cell lung cancer
Avelox	moxifloxacin hydrochloride	various bacterial infections
Avita	tretinoin; all-trans retinoic acid; all-trans vitamin A acid; beta-retinoic acid; retinoic acid; TRA; trans retinoic acid; trans vitamin A acid; tretinoinum; vitamin A acid	(oral) acute promyelocytic leukemia (APL), characterized by the t(15;17) translocation or the PML/RARa gene; for patients refractory to or who have relapsed from anthracycline chemotherapy, or for where anthracycline-based chemotherapy is contraindicated; (topical) acne vulgaris; other dermatologic conditions; some skin cancers
Aztec	zidovudine	AIDS-related complex; HIV infection; HIV transmission, prevention
Bactrim	trimethoprim-sulfamethoxazole	*Pneumocystis carinii* pneumonia; various bacterial infections
Bayer 205	suramin	trypanosomiasis; hormone-refractory prostate cancer
Becenum	carmustine; bis(chloroethyl) nitrosourea; bis-chloronitrosourea; carmustin	cancerous brain tumors; colon cancer; lung cancer; Hodgkin disease; non-Hodgkin lymphomas; lymphomas; melanoma; multiple myeloma; mycosis fungoides
Benoquin	monobenzone	vitiligo
Beriplast P	fibrin sealant	cardiovascular surgery; colostomy closure; congenital heart defects; coronary artery bypass grafting; mediastinal bleeding; microvascular bleeding; splenic trauma
Betaseron	recombinant interferon beta; interferon beta-1b	multiple sclerosis (MS); treating relapsing forms of multiple sclerosis (MS) to reduce the number of flare-ups and slow down the development of physical disability associated with MS
Bextra	valdecoxib	osteoarthritis; rheumatoid arthritis; dysmenorrhea
Bexxar	iodine I 131 tositumomab; 131-I-anti-B1 antibody; 131-I-anti-B1 monoclonal antibody; iodine I 131 MOAB anti-B1; iodine I 131 monoclonal antibody anti-B1; iodine-131 anti-B1 antibody; iodine-131 anti-CD20 monoclonal antibody; tositumomab; anti-CD20 antibody	CD-20-antigen-expressing, relapsed or refractory, low-grade, follicular, or transformed non-Hodgkin lymphoma; CD20 positive follicular non-Hodgkin lymphoma refractory to rituximab

Trade Name	Generic Drug	Indicated For
Biaxin	clarithromycin	*H. pylori* infection; various bacterial infections
BiCNU	carmustine; bis(chloroethyl) nitrosourea; bis-chloronitrosourea; carmustin	cancerous brain tumors; colon cancer; lung cancer; Hodgkin disease; non-Hodgkin lymphomas; lymphomas; melanoma; multiple myeloma; mycosis fungoides
Biovelbin	vinorelbine ditartrate; navelbine ditartrate; vinorelbine tartrate	non-small-cell lung cancer; metastatic breast cancer; uterine and cervical cancer; desmoid tumors; advanced Kaposi sarcoma
Blenoxane	bleomycin	skin cancer (squamous cell carcinoma) of the head, neck, penis, cervix, and vulva; lymphomas; testicular cancer; malignant pleural effusion
Bondronate	ibandronate sodium	osteoporosis, treatment and prevention
Bonefos, Loron	sodium clodronate	myeloma, secondary breast cancer
Boniva	ibandronate sodium	osteoporosis, treatment and prevention
Buspar	buspirone hydrochloride	alcohol abuse; anxiety; depression; migraine prophylaxis; smoking cessation; panic disorder
Busulfex	busulfan; BSF; bussulfam; busulfanum; busulphan; glyzophrol; methanesulfonic acid tetramethylene ester; myelekon; myeloleukon; myelosan; mylecytan; sulfabutin; tetramethylene bis(methanesulfonate)	bone marrow disorders; chronic myelogenous leukemia; palliative; neoadjuvant to allogeneic hematopoietic progenitor cell transplantation; neoplastic meningitis; primary brain malignancies
CAELYX	pegylated liposomal doxorubicin hydrochloride	refractory metastatic carcinoma of the ovary; AIDS-related Kaposi sarcoma; breast cancer; relapsed/refractory multiple myeloma (with bortezomib)
Calglucon	calcium gluconate	hyperkalemia; hypocalcemic tetany; magnesium intoxication
Campath	alemtuzumab; anti-CD52 monoclonal antibody; Campath-1H; monoclonal antibody Campath-1H; monoclonal antibody CD52	B-cell chronic lymphocytic leukemia
Camptogen	rubetican	AIDS, pediatric; HIV infection, pediatric
Camptosar	irinotecan hydrochloride; camptothecin-11; irinotecan; irinotecan HCI	Stage IVB cervical cancer; colorectal cancer; esophageal cancer; gastric cancer; non-small-cell lung cancer; small-cell lung cancer
Capoten	captopril	hypertension; heart failure; left ventricular dysfunction; diabetic nephropathy
Carmubris	carmustine; bis(chloroethyl) nitrosourea; bis-chloronitrosourea; carmustin	cancerous brain tumors; colon cancer; lung cancer; Hodgkin disease; non-Hodgkin lymphomas; lymphomas; melanoma; multiple myeloma; mycosis fungoides
Carnitor	levocarnitine	carnitine deficiency; end-stage renal disease
Casodex	bicalutamide	metastatic prostate cancer
Caverject	alprostadil	erectile dysfunction; patent ductus arteriosus

Trade Name	Generic Drug	Indicated For
CCNU	lomustine; lomustinum	brain tumors; Hodgkin disease
CeeNU	lomustine; lomustinum	brain tumors; Hodgkin disease
Celebrex	celecoxib; YM177	familial adenomatous polyposis (inherited colorectal cancer syndrome)
Cellcept	mycophenolate mofetil	heart transplantation; kidney transplantation; liver transplantation; lupus nephritis
Cerebid	papaverine	ischemia, cerebral and peripheral
Cerespan	papaverine	ischemia, cerebral and peripheral
Cerubidine	daunorubicin hydrochloride; cloridrato de daunorubicina; daunomycin; daunomycin-HCL; daunorubicin; dauno-rubidomycine; rubomycin C	acute lymphoblastic leukemia
CI Basic Blue 9	methylene blue	cyanide poisoning, antidote; diagnostic, indicator dye; genitourinary antiseptic; glutaricaciduria; methemoglobinemia; oxalate and phosphate urinary tract calculi, management
Cipro	ciprofloxacin	inhaled anthrax, postexposure; susceptible infectious diseases
Circadin	therapeutic melatonin	sleep disorders in blind people with no light perception
Citracal	calcium citrate	calcium supplement; hypocalcemia; osteoporosis; rickets; tetany
Clafen	cyclophosphamide; ciclofosfamida; ciclofosfamide; claphene; CP monohydrate; CPM; cyclophospham; cyclophosphamid monohydrate; cyclophosphamidum; cyclophosphan; cyclophosphanum; cytophosphane; mitoxan; syklofosfamid; zytoxan	breast cancer; leukemias; lupus nephritis; lymphoma; multiple myeloma; neuroblastoma; nephrotic syndrome; ovarian cancer; retinoblastoma
Clasteon	clodronate disodium	adjuvant usage in bone metastasis of breast cancer
Clinagen LA 40	estradiol	breast cancer, palliative
Clinoril	sulindac	arthritis; inflammatory conditions
Clolar	clofarabine	accelerated approval (clinical benefit not established) for the treatment of pediatric patients one to twenty-one years old with relapsed or refractory acute lymphoblastic leukemia after at least two prior regimens
Collubleu	methylene blue	cyanide poisoning, antidote; diagnostic, indicator dye; genitourinary antiseptic; glutaricaciduria; methemoglobinemia; oxalate and phosphate urinary tract calculi, management
Colprosterone	therapeutic progesterone	amenorrhea; functional uterine bleeding; infertility; maintenance of pregnancy
Compazine	prochlorperazine	antinausea

Trade Name	Generic Drug	Indicated For
Compound 42	warfarin	pulmonary embolism and thromboembolic disorders, treatment and prophylaxis; venous thrombosis, prophylaxis and treatment
Concerta	methylphenidate hydrochloride	attention deficit/hyperactivity disorder (ADHD); narcolepsy
Co-Rax	warfarin	pulmonary embolism and thromboembolic disorders, treatment and prophylaxis; venous thrombosis, prophylaxis and treatment
Cortalone	prednisolone	inflammatory conditions; allergic conditions; hematologic conditions; neoplastic conditions; autoimmune conditions; replacement therapy in adrenal insufficiency
Cosmegen	dactinomycin; ACT-D; actinomycin A IV; actinomycin C1; actinomycin D; actinomycin I1; actinomycin IV; actinomycin X 1; actinomycin-[thr-val-pro-sar-meval]; AD; dactinomycine; meractinomycin	Wilms' tumor; childhood rhabdomyosarcoma; Ewing sarcoma; testicular cancer; gestational trophoblastic neoplasia; choriocarcinoma; melanoma; neuroblastoma; retinoblastoma; uterine sarcomas; Kaposi sarcoma; sarcoma botryoides; soft-tissue sarcoma
Cotrim	trimethoprim-sulfamethoxazole	*Pneumocystis carinii* pneumonia; various bacterial infections
Coumadin	warfarin	pulmonary embolism and thromboembolic disorders, treatment and prophylaxis; venous thrombosis, prophylaxis and treatment
Cristanaspase	asparaginase; ASNase; ASP-1; asparaginase erwinia; asparaginase II; colaspase; erwinia asparaginase; L-ASP; L-asparaginase; L-asparagine amidohydrolase	some blood cancers; acute lymphocytic leukemia; (acute nonlymphocytic leukemia)
Cuprenil	penicillamine	Wilson disease; heavy metal intoxication; cystinuria; rheumatoid arthritis; primary biliary cirrhosis; Felty syndrome; rheumatoid vasculitis
Cuprimine	penicillamine	Wilson disease; heavy metal intoxication; cystinuria; rheumatoid arthritis; primary biliary cirrhosis; Felty syndrome; rheumatoid vasculitis
Cupripen	penicillamine	Wilson disease; heavy metal intoxication; cystinuria; rheumatoid arthritis; primary biliary cirrhosis; Felty syndrome; rheumatoid vasculitis
Curretab	medroxyprogesterone; medroxyprogesterone acetate	breast carcinoma; endometrial carcinoma; renal cell carcinoma
Cyfos	ifosfamide; ifomide; IFX; iphosphamid; iphosphamide; IPP; isoendoxan; iso-endoxan; isophosphamide; naxamide	breast cancer; gastric carcinoma; lung cancer; lymphocytic leukemias; Hodgkin disease and non-Hodgkin lymphoma; ovarian cancer; pancreatic carcinoma; sarcomas; testicular cancer
Cymevan	ganciclovir	cytomegalovirus (CMV) infections in immunocompromised patients
Cyprostat	cyproterone acetate	prostate cancer

Trade Name	Generic Drug	Indicated For
Cyren A	diethylstilbesterol; diethylstilbenediol; diethylstilbestrol dipropionate; diethylstilbestrolum; diethylstilboestrol; sinestrol; stilboestrol dipropionate	breast cancer; prostate cancer
Cytadren	aminoglutethimide	breast cancer; prostate cancer; decreases the production of sex hormones (estrogen in women or testosterone in men) and suppresses the growth of tumors that need sex hormones to grow
Cytosar-U	cytarabine; arabinofuranosylcytosine; arabinosylcytosine; aracytidine; beta-cytosine arabinoside; cytarabine hydrochloride; cytarabinum; cytosine arabinoside; cytosine arabinosine hydrochloride	acute nonlymphocytic leukemia; acute lymphocytic leukemia; chronic myelogenous leukemia; bone marrow transplantation; carcinomatous meningitis; Hodgkin disease; meningeal leukemia; meningitis lymphomatous; myelodysplasic syndrome; non-Hodgkin lymphoma; ovarian cancer; retinoblastoma
Cytoxan	cyclophosphamide; ciclofosfamida; ciclofosfamide; claphene; CP monohydrate; CPM; cyclophospham; cyclophosphamid monohydrate; cyclophosphamidum; cyclophosphan; cyclophosphanum; cytophosphane; mitoxan; syklofosfamid; zytoxan	breast cancer; leukemias; lupus nephritis; lymphoma; multiple myeloma; neuroblastoma; nephrotic syndrome; ovarian cancer; retinoblastoma
Dacogen	decitabine; 5-aza-dCyd; deoxyazacytidine; dezocitidine	myelodysplastic syndrome
Dantrium	dantrolene	treating episodes of severe high body temperature; also used to prevent or reduce the risk of severe high body temperature in certain patients before or after surgery or anesthesia
DaunoXome	liposomal daunorubicin citrate; daunorubicin liposomal; liposomal daunorubicin	acute nonlymphocytic leukemia; acute lymphocytic leukemia; advanced HIV-associated Kaposi sarcoma
Decaderm	dexamethasone; desamethasone; dexamethasonum; DXM; hexadecadrol; methylfluorprednisolone	antiemetic (prevents vomiting)
Decadrol	dexamethasone; desamethasone; dexamethasonum; DXM; hexadecadrol; methylfluorprednisolone	antiemetic (prevents vomiting)
Decadron	dexamethasone; desamethasone; dexamethasonum; DXM; hexadecadrol; methylfluorprednisolone	antiemetic (prevents vomiting)
Deca-Durabolin	nandrolone decanoate	anemia of renal insufficiency; metastatic breast cancer

Trade Name	Generic Drug	Indicated For
Decapeptyl	triptorelin; 6-D-tryptophan-LH-RH; 6-D-tryptophanluteinizing hormone-releasing factor; detryptoreline; D-TRP-6-LHRH	prostate carcinoma, palliative treatment
Decasone R.p.	dexamethasone; desamethasone; dexamethasonum; DXM; hexadecadrol; methylfluorprednisolone	antiemetic (prevents vomiting)
Decaspray	dexamethasone; desamethasone; dexamethasonum; DXM; hexadecadrol; methylfluorprednisolone	antiemetic (prevents vomiting)
Deenar	dexamethasone; desamethasone; dexamethasonum; DXM; hexadecadrol; methylfluorprednisolone	antiemetic (prevents vomiting)
Deladumone	diethylstilbesterol; diethylstilbenediol; diethylstilbestrol dipropionate; diethylstilbestrolum; diethylstilboestrol; sinestrol; stilboestrol dipropionate	breast cancer; prostate cancer
Delatest	testosterone	breast cancer in women, palliative
Delatestryl	therapeutic testosterone; testosterone; testosterone enanthate; trans-testosterone	delayed puberty, male; hypogonadism; metastatic mammary cancer; breast cancer in women, palliative
Delta-Cortef	prednisolone	inflammatory conditions; allergic conditions; hematologic conditions; neoplastic conditions; autoimmune conditions; replacement therapy in adrenal insufficiency
Delta-Dome	prednisone; delta(1)-cortisone; deltacortisone; deltadehydrocortisone; metacortandracin; PRD; prednisonum	inflammatory conditions; allergic conditions; hematologic conditions; neoplastic conditions; autoimmune conditions; replacement therapy in adrenal insufficiency
Deltasone	prednisone; delta(1)-cortisone; deltacortisone; deltadehydrocortisone; metacortandracin; PRD; prednisonum	inflammatory conditions; allergic conditions; hematologic conditions; neoplastic conditions; autoimmune conditions; replacement therapy in adrenal insufficiency
Del-Vi-A	vitamin A compound; all trans retinol; anti-infective vitamin; antixerophthalmic vitamin; axerophthol; axeropthalum; biosterol; lard-factor; oleovitamin A; ophthalamin; retinol; vitamin A; vitamin A alcohol; vitamin A USP; vitamin A1; vitaminum A	diminishing malignant cell growth; enhancing the immune system

Trade Name	Generic Drug	Indicated For
Dep Gynogen	estradiol	breast cancer, palliative
Depakene	valproic acid	epilepsy; mania; migraine
Depandro 100	testosterone	breast cancer in women, palliative
Depen	penicillamine	Wilson disease; heavy metal intoxication; cystinuria; rheumatoid arthritis; primary biliary cirrhosis; Felty syndrome; rheumatoid vasculitis
DepoCyt	liposomal cytarabine; encapsulated cytarabine	lymphomatous meningitis
DepoFoam	liposomal cytarabine; encapsulated cytarabine	lymphomatous meningitis
Depo-Provera	medroxyprogesterone; medroxyprogesterone acetate	breast carcinoma; endometrial carcinoma; renal cell carcinoma
Depotest; Depo-Testosterone	testosterone	breast cancer in women, palliative
Deronil	dexamethasone; desamethasone; dexamethasonum; DXM; hexadecadrol; methylfluorprednisolone	antiemetic (prevents vomiting)
Desmoidpillen	methylene blue	cyanide poisoning, antidote; diagnostic, indicator dye; genitourinary antiseptic; glutaricaciduria; methemoglobinemia; oxalate and phosphate urinary tract calculi, management
Deursil	ursodiol	gallstone dissolution; primary biliary cirrhosis
Dex-4	dexamethasone; desamethasone; dexamethasonum; DXM; hexadecadrol; methylfluorprednisolone	antiemetic (prevents vomiting)
Dexace	dexamethasone; desamethasone; dexamethasonum; DXM; hexadecadrol; methylfluorprednisolone	antiemetic (prevents vomiting)
Dexameth	dexamethasone; desamethasone; dexamethasonum; DXM; hexadecadrol; methylfluorprednisolone	antiemetic (prevents vomiting)
Dezone	dexamethasone; desamethasone; dexamethasonum; DXM; hexadecadrol; methylfluorprednisolone	antiemetic (prevents vomiting)
DHPG	ganciclovir	cytomegalovirus (CMV) infections in immunocompromised patients

Trade Name	Generic Drug	Indicated For
Diastyl	diethylstilbesterol; diethylstilbenediol; diethylstilbestrol dipropionate; diethylstilbestrolum; diethylstilboestrol; sinestrol; stilboestrol dipropionate	breast cancer; prostate cancer
Didronel	etidronate	treating adults with Paget disease; preventing and treating abnormal bone growth following hip replacement surgery or spinal cord injury
Diflucan	fluconazole	antifungal, prophylaxis in allogeneic bone marrow transplantation; candidiasis; cryptococcal meningitis
Difosfonal	clodronate disodium	adjuvant usage in bone metastasis of breast cancer
Disalcid	sodium salicylate	fever; inflammatory conditions; pain
Disprol	paracetamol	painkiller
Distamine	penicillamine	Wilson disease; heavy metal intoxication; cystinuria; rheumatoid arthritis; primary biliary cirrhosis; Felty syndrome; rheumatoid vasculitis
Domestrol	diethylstilbesterol; diethylstilbenediol; diethylstilbestrol dipropionate; diethylstilbestrolum; diethylstilboestrol; sinestrol; stilboestrol dipropionate	breast cancer; prostate cancer
Dostinex	cabergoline	pituitary tumors
Doxil; DOXIL	doxorubicin hydrochloride liposome; doxorubicin hydrochloride liposome injection; liposomal adriamycin; liposomal doxorubicin; liposomal doxorubicin hydrochloride; liposome-encapsulated doxorubicin; pegylated doxorubicin HCl liposome; pegylated liposomal doxorubicin; pegylated liposomal doxorubicin hydrochloride; S-liposomal doxorubicin; stealth liposomal doxorubicin	refractory metastatic carcinoma of the ovary; AIDS-related Kaposi sarcoma; breast cancer; relapsed/refractory multiple myeloma (with bortezomib)
Doxilen	pegylated liposomal doxorubicin hydrochloride	refractory metastatic carcinoma of the ovary; AIDS-related Kaposi sarcoma; breast cancer; relapsed/refractory multiple myeloma (with bortezomib)

Trade Name	Generic Drug	Indicated For
Dox-SL	doxorubicin hydrochloride liposome; doxorubicin hydrochloride liposome injection; liposomal adriamycin; liposomal doxorubicin; liposomal doxorubicin hydrochloride; liposome-encapsulated doxorubicin; pegylated doxorubicin HCl liposome; pegylated liposomal doxorubicin; pegylated liposomal doxorubicin hydrochloride; S-liposomal doxorubicin; stealth liposomal doxorubicin	refractory metastatic carcinoma of the ovary; AIDS-related Kaposi sarcoma; breast cancer; relapsed/refractory multiple myeloma (with bortezomib)
DTIC-Dome	dacarbazine; biocarbazine; dacarbazina; dacarbazina almirall; dacarbazine-DTIC; dakarbazin; dimethyl (triazeno) imidazolecarboxamide; dimethyl triazeno imidazol carboxamide; dimethyl triazeno imidazole carboxamide; imidazole carboxamide; imidazole carboxamide dimethyltriazeno	carcinoid cancer; Hodgkin disease; islet cell carcinoma; melanoma; neuroblastoma; soft-tissue sarcoma
Duratest	testosterone	breast cancer in women, palliative
Durathate 200	testosterone	breast cancer in women, palliative
Ecotrin	acetylsalicylic acid; aspirin	mild to moderate pain; fever; prevention of arterial and venous thrombosis
Effexor	venlafaxine	anxiety; depression
Efudex	fluorouracil; 5-fluorouracil; 5-fluracil; fluoro uracil; fluouracil; FU	palliative treatment: colorectal cancer, breast cancer, stomach cancer, pancreatic cancer; topical treatment for the following: superficial basal cell carcinoma that cannot be treated with surgery, and actinic keratosis
Eldisine	vindesine; compound 112531; deacetyl vinblastine carboxamide; desacetylvinblastine amide	acute leukemia; lung cancer; carcinoma of the breast; squamous cell carcinoma of the esophagus, head, and neck; Hodgkin disease and non-Hodgkin lymphomas
Elitek	rasburicase; recombinant urate oxidase; urate oxidase	chemotherapy-induced acute hyperuricemia, treatment and prophylaxis
Ellence	epirubicin; 4'-epiadriamycin; 4'-epidoxorubicin; 4'-epi-doxorubicin Hcl; epi-ADR; epidoxorubicin; pidorubicin	breast cancer; adjuvant in breast cancer therapy
Elliott B Solution	Elliott B solution	diluent for the intrathecal administration of methotrexate sodium and cytarabine for the prevention or treatment of meningeal leukemia or lymphocytic lymphoma

Trade Name	Generic Drug	Indicated For
Eloxatin	oxaliplatin; diaminocyclohexane oxalatoplatinum; oxalatoplatin; oxalatoplatinum	metastatic colorectal cancer; ovarian cancer
Elspar	asparaginase; ASNase; ASP-1; asparaginase erwinia; asparaginase II; colaspase; erwinia asparaginase; L-ASP; L-asparaginase; L-asparagine amidohydrolase	some blood cancers; acute lymphocytic leukemia; acute nonlymphocytic leukemia
Emcyt	estramustine phosphate sodium; estramustine phosphate	prostate neoplasm
Emend	aprepitant	antiemetic (prevents vomiting)
Empirin	acetylsalicylic acid; aspirin	mild to moderate pain; fever; prevention of arterial and venous thrombosis
Enbrel	etanercept	juvenile arthritis; psoriatic arthritis; rheumatoid arthritis
Entericin	acetylsalicylic acid; aspirin	mild to moderate pain; fever; prevention of arterial and venous thrombosis
Epitol	carbamazepine	epilepsy
Epivir	lamivudine	chronic hepatitis B; HIV infection
Epogen	epoetin alfa; erythropoietin; r-HuEPO	anemias associated with chronic renal failure, zidovudine (AZT) therapy, and cancer chemotherapy of nonmyeloid malignancies
Eraxis	anidulafungin	candidemia
Erbitux	cetuximab; anti-EGFR monoclonal antibody; antiepidermal growth factor receptor monoclonal antibody; C225 monoclonal antibody; chimeric anti-EGFR monoclonal antibody; chimeric monoclonal antibody C225; immunoglobulin G1, anti-(human epidermal growth factor receptor) (human-mouse monoclonal C225 gamma1-chain), disulfide with human-mouse monoclonal C225 kappa-chain, dimer; monoclonal antibody C225	advanced colorectal cancer; head and neck cancer
Ergamisol	levamisole; novo-levamisole	colon cancer; nephrotic syndrome
Ergenyl	valproic acid	epilepsy; mania; migraine
Estinyl	ethinyl estradiol	advanced androgen-dependent prostate cancer, palliative; breast cancer, palliative; estrogen replacement; menopausal symptoms; postmenopausal osteoporosis
Estrace	estradiol	breast cancer, palliative
Estradiol Patch	estradiol	breast cancer, palliative

Trade Name	Generic Drug	Indicated For
Estragyn LA 5	estradiol	breast cancer, palliative
Estratab	esterified estrogens	breast cancer
Estrobene	diethylstilbesterol; diethylstilbenediol; diethylstilbestrol dipropionate; diethylstilbestrolum; diethylstilboestrol; sinestrol; stilboestrol dipropionate	breast cancer; prostate cancer
Estro-Cyp	estradiol	breast cancer, palliative
Estrogen Patches	estradiol	breast cancer, palliative
Estrosyn	diethylstilbesterol; diethylstilbenediol; diethylstilbestrol dipropionate; diethylstilbestrolum; diethylstilboestrol; sinestrol; stilboestrol dipropionate	breast cancer; prostate cancer
Ethinoral	ethinyl estradiol	advanced androgen-dependent prostate cancer, palliative; breast cancer, palliative; estrogen replacement; menopausal symptoms; postmenopausal osteoporosis
Ethiodol	ethiodized oil	diagnostic imaging, hysterosalpingography and lymphography
Ethyol	amifostine trihydrate; aminopropylaminoethylthiophosphoric acid; ethiofos; gammaphos	cisplatin-induced nephrotoxicity; radiation-induced mucositis and xerostomia
Eticylol	ethinyl estradiol	advanced androgen-dependent prostate cancer, palliative; breast cancer, palliative; estrogen replacement; menopausal symptoms; postmenopausal osteoporosis
Etopophos	etoposide phosphate; etoposide; demethyl epipodophyllotoxin ethylidine glucoside; epipodophyllotoxin	acute leukemia; adrenal cortical cancer; brain cancer; chronic lymphocytic leukemia; choriocarcinoma; esophageal cancer; Ewing sarcoma; gastric cancer; germ-cell cancer; gestational trophoblastic neoplasms; hepatocellular cancer; Hodgkin disease; hypereosinophilic syndrome; Kaposi sarcoma; testicular cancer; thymoma; thyroid cancer; uterine cancer; Wilms' tumor; Langerhans cell histiocytosis; mobilization of peripheral-blood progenitor cells; multiple myeloma; neuroblastoma; non-small-cell lung cancer; osteogenic sarcoma; ovarian cancer; retinoblastoma; small-cell lung cancer; soft-tissue sarcomas
Etretin	acitretin; trimethylmethoxyphenyl-retinoic acid	cutaneous T-cell lymphoma
Eulexin	flutamide; flucinom; flugerel; niftolid	prostate carcinoma; hirsutism
Eunades	vinorelbine ditartrate; navelbine ditartrate; vinorelbine tartrate	non-small-cell lung cancer; metastatic breast cancer; uterine and cervical cancer; desmoid tumors; advanced Kaposi sarcoma

Trade Name	Generic Drug	Indicated For
Evacet	doxorubicin hydrochloride liposome; doxorubicin hydrochloride liposome injection; liposomal adriamycin; liposomal doxorubicin; liposomal doxorubicin hydrochloride; liposome-encapsulated doxorubicin; pegylated doxorubicin HCl liposome; pegylated liposomal doxorubicin; pegylated liposomal doxorubicin hydrochloride; S-liposomal doxorubicin; stealth liposomal doxorubicin	refractory metastatic carcinoma of the ovary; AIDS-related Kaposi sarcoma; breast cancer; relapsed/refractory multiple myeloma (with bortezomib)
Everone	testosterone	breast cancer in women, palliative
Evista	raloxifene	breast cancer; cardiovascular disease prophylaxis; osteoporosis
Evoxac	cevimeline hydrochloride	Sjögren syndrome
Extren	acetylsalicylic acid; aspirin	mild to moderate pain; fever; prevention of arterial and venous thrombosis
Fareston	toremifene	breast cancer; desmoid tumors
Faslodex	fulvestrant	hormone receptor-positive metastatic breast cancer
FDG	fludeoxyglucose F 18	radiopharmaceutical, cancer diagnostic
Femara	letrozole	hormone receptor-positive early breast cancer; adjuvant in breast cancer therapy; endometrial cancer
Femest	conjugated estrogens	advanced androgen-dependent prostate cancer, palliative; breast cancer, palliative
Feminone	ethinyl estradiol	advanced androgen-dependent prostate cancer, palliative; breast cancer, palliative; estrogen replacement; menopausal symptoms; postmenopausal osteoporosis
Fempatch	estradiol	breast cancer, palliative
Fentora	fentanyl citrate	breakthrough pain in cancer patients
FGN-1	exisulind	colonic adenomatous polyps in the inherited disease adenomatous polyposis coli, control and suppression
Fidelin	therapeutic dehydroepiandrosterone	adrenal insufficiency, replacement; systemic lupus erythematosus, treatment and steroid treatment reduction
FIRST-Testosterone; FIRST-Testosterone MC	testosterone	breast cancer in women, palliative
Flomax	tamsulosin hydrochloride	benign prostatic hyperplasia
Florinef	fludrocortisone	breast cancer; adrenal cortical cancer
Fludara; Fludara Oral	fludarabine phosphate	chronic lymphocytic leukemia (CLL)
FluMist	trivalent influenza vaccine	influenza prophylaxis

Trade Name	Generic Drug	Indicated For
Fluoroplex	fluorouracil; 5-fluorouracil; 5-fluracil; fluoro uracil; fluouracil; FU	palliative treatment: colorectal cancer, breast cancer, stomach cancer, pancreatic cancer; topical treatment for the following: superficial basal cell carcinoma that cannot be treated with surgery, and actinic keratosis
Flushield	trivalent influenza vaccine	influenza prophylaxis
Fluvirin	trivalent influenza vaccine	influenza prophylaxis
Fluzone	trivalent influenza vaccine	influenza prophylaxis
Folex; Folex PFS	methotrexate	bladder cancer; breast cancer; carcinomatous meningitis; chorioadenoma destruens; esophageal cancer; gestational choriocarcinoma; head/neck cancer; meningeal leukemia; lymphomas; Burkitt lymphoma; lung cancer; mycosis fungoides; osteosarcoma; Wegener granulomatosis
Fonatol	diethylstilbesterol; diethylstilbenediol; diethylstilbestrol dipropionate; diethylstilbestrolum; diethylstilboestrol; sinestrol; stilboestrol dipropionate	breast cancer; prostate cancer
Fourneau 309	suramin	trypanosomiasis; hormone-refractory prostate cancer
Fragmin	dalteparin	deep vein thrombosis, prophylaxis; ischemic complications in unstable angina and non-Q wave myocardial infarction, prophylaxis
FUDF	floxuridine; FdUrD; floxuridin; fluorodeoxyuridine; fluorouridine deoxyribose; fluoruridine deoxyribose	gastrointestinal adenocarcinoma metastatic to the liver
Fungarest	ketoconazole	seborrheic dermatitis; prostate cancer
Fungoral	ketoconazole	seborrheic dermatitis; prostate cancer
Gammacorten	dexamethasone; desamethasone; dexamethasonum; DXM; hexadecadrol; methylfluorprednisolone	antiemetic (prevents vomiting)
Gd-DTPA	gadopentetate dimeglumine	angiography for leptomeningeal metastases and multiple sclerosis and magnetic resonance imaging for spine and brain
Gelfoam	absorbable gelatin sponge	homeostasis
Gemzar	gemcitabine hydrochloride; difluorodeoxycytidine; gemcitabine	bladder cancer; breast cancer; carcinoma of unknown primary origin; lung cancer; ovarian cancer; pancreatic cancer; renal cell carcinoma
Geritol	multivitamin	vitamin supplement
Germanin	suramin	trypanosomiasis; hormone-refractory prostate cancer
Gesterol 100	therapeutic progesterone	amenorrhea; functional uterine bleeding; infertility; maintenance of pregnancy

Trade Name	Generic Drug	Indicated For
Girostan	thiotepa; thiophosphamide; thiophosphoramide; triethylene thiophosphoramide	bladder cancer; breast cancer; ovarian cancer; Hodgkin disease; non-Hodgkin lymphoma
Gleevec	imatinib mesylate	Philadelphia chromosome-positive chronic myeloid leukemia (CML); acute lymphocytic leukemia; gastrointestinal stromal tumor; hypereosinophillic syndrome; dermatofibrosarcoma protuberans; mutated-PDGFR myelodysplastic/myeloproliferative diseases
Gliadel wafer	polifeprosan 20 with carmustine implant	malignant glioma, adjuvant to surgery and radiation; recurrent glioblastoma multiforme, adjuvant to surgery
Glutacerebro	glutamine	short bowel syndrome
Glutaven	glutamine	short bowel syndrome
Granocyte	lenograstim	chemotherapy-induced neutropenia
Gynodiol, Gynogen LA 20	estradiol	breast cancer, palliative
Halodrin	fluoxymesterone; androfluorene; androsterolo	certain types of breast cancer
Halofuginone IV (intravenous)	halofuginone hydrobromide	scleroderma and antiprotozoal; coccidiosis (vet)
Halotestin	fluoxymesterone; androfluorene; androsterolo	certain types of breast cancer
Hectorol	doxercalciferol	secondary hyperparathyroidism in end-stage renal disease in patients on hemodialysis
Hepsera	adefovir dipivoxil	chronic hepatitis B
Herceptin	trastuzumab; anti-c-erB-2; anti-c-erbB2 monoclonal antibody; anti-ERB-2; anti-erbB2 monoclonal antibody; anti-HER2/c-erbB2 monoclonal antibody; anti-p185-HER2; monoclonal antibody c-erb-2; monoclonal antibody HER2	breast cancer overexpressing HER2 protein; pancreatic cancer overexpressing p185HER2
Hexadrol	dexamethasone; desamethasone; dexamethasonum; DXM; hexadecadrol; methylfluorprednisolone	antiemetic (prevents vomiting)
Hexalen	altretamine; hemel; hexaloids	ovarian cancer
Hexamethylmelamine	altretamine; hemel; hexaloids	ovarian cancer
Hib TITER vaccine	haemophilus influenzae B vaccine	haemophilus influenzae B prophylaxis
Histerone	testosterone	breast cancer in women, palliative
Histrelin implant	histrelin acetate	palliative treatment of advanced prostate cancer
hLL2	epratuzumab	systemic lupus erythematosus

Trade Name	Generic Drug	Indicated For
Hycamtin	topotecan hydrochloride; hycamptamine	small-cell lung carcinoma; cervical cancer
Hydeltra	prednisolone	inflammatory conditions; allergic conditions; hematologic conditions; neoplastic conditions; autoimmune conditions; replacement therapy in adrenal insufficiency
Hydeltrasol	prednisolone	inflammatory conditions; allergic conditions; hematologic conditions; neoplastic conditions; autoimmune conditions; replacement therapy in adrenal insufficiency
Hydrea, Droxia	hydroxyurea; HYD; hydroxycarbamide; hydurea	chronic myelogenous leukemia; head and neck cancer; malignant melanoma; ovarian carcinoma; sickle cell anemia; adjuvant in retroviral therapy
I-125	iodine I 125	prostate cancer
I-131	iodine I 131	hyperthyroidism
Idamycin	Idarubicin; 4-demethoxydaunomycin; 4-demethoxydaunorubicin; DMDR	acute myeloid leukemia (AML); acute nonlymphocytic leukemia
IDEC in2B8	in 111 ibritumomab tiuxetan	non-Hodgkin lymphoma
Ifex	ifosfamide; ifomide; IFX; iphosphamid; iphosphamide; IPP; isoendoxan; iso-endoxan; isophosphamide; naxamide	breast cancer; gastric carcinoma; lung cancer; lymphocytic leukemias; Hodgkin disease and non-Hodgkin lymphoma; ovarian cancer; pancreatic carcinoma; sarcomas; testicular cancer
Ifosfamidum	ifosfamide; ifomide; IFX; iphosphamid; iphosphamide; IPP; isoendoxan; iso-endoxan; isophosphamide; naxamide	breast cancer; gastric carcinoma; lung cancer; lymphocytic leukemias; Hodgkin disease and non-Hodgkin lymphoma; ovarian cancer; pancreatic carcinoma; sarcomas; testicular cancer
131 I-MIBG	iodine I 131 metaiodobenzylguanidine	diagnostic imaging
Immucyst	BCG	bladder cancer; malignant melanoma
Imuran	azathioprine sodium	converted in vivo to its active metabolite 6-mercaptopurine (6-MP), which substitutes for the normal nucleoside and mistakenly gets incorporated into DNA sequences. This leads to inhibition of DNA, RNA, and protein synthesis. As a result, cell proliferation may be inhibited, particularly in lymphocytes and leukocytes
Imurel	azathioprine sodium	converted in vivo to its active metabolite 6-mercaptopurine (6-MP), which substitutes for the normal nucleoside and mistakenly gets incorporated into DNA sequences. This leads to inhibition of DNA, RNA, and protein synthesis. As a result, cell proliferation may be inhibited, particularly in lymphocytes and leukocytes
Indocin	indomethacin	dysmenorrhea; inflammatory disorders; pain
Inestra	ethinyl estradiol	advanced androgen-dependent prostate cancer, palliative; breast cancer, palliative; estrogen replacement; menopausal symptoms; postmenopausal osteoporosis

Trade Name	Generic Drug	Indicated For
Innohep	tinzaparin sodium	treatment of acute symptomatic deep venous thrombosis (DVT) with or without a pulmonary embolism (PE), in conjunction with warfarin
Intron-A	interferon alfa-2b; recombinant interferon alfa	certain types of leukemia, lymphoma, and hepatitis; certain AIDS-related illnesses (Kaposi sarcoma); and genital warts (condylomata acuminata); also used in addition to surgery to treat a certain type of skin cancer (malignant melanoma)
Iodotope	sodium iodide I 131; iodine I 131	thyroid cancer; hyperthyroidism
Iressa	gefitinib	non-small-cell lung carcinoma
Ixempra	ixabepilone; azaepothilone B; epothilone B lactam; epothilone-B BMS 247550	metastatic or locally advanced breast cancer
Kapake	co-codamol	painkiller
Kelatin	penicillamine	Wilson disease; heavy metal intoxication; cystinuria; rheumatoid arthritis; primary biliary cirrhosis; Felty syndrome; rheumatoid vasculitis
Keoxifene	raloxifene	breast cancer; cardiovascular disease prophylaxis; osteoporosis
Kepivance	palifermin	decrease the incidence and duration of severe oral mucositis in patients with hematologic malignancies receiving myelotoxic therapy requiring hematopoetic stem cell support
Ketoderm	ketoconazole	seborrheic dermatitis; prostate cancer
Ketoisdin	ketoconazole	seborrheic dermatitis; prostate cancer
Kordicepin	cordycepin	TdT-positive acute lymphocytic leukemia
KOS-953	tanespimycin	chronic myelogenous leukemia
Kytril	granisetron hydrochloride	antinausea
L-Asnase	asparaginase; ASNase; ASP-1; asparaginase erwinia; asparaginase II; colaspase; erwinia asparaginase; L-ASP; L-asparaginase; L-asparagine amidohydrolase	some blood cancers; acute lymphocytic leukemia; acute nonlymphocytic leukemia
Lamictal	lamotrigine	epilepsy
Lanvis	thioguanine	acute nonlymphocytic leukemia
Laroferon	recombinant interferon alfa	used as antiviral and antitumor agents

Trade Name	Generic Drug	Indicated For
Lastet	etoposide; demethyl epipodophyllotoxin ethylidine glucoside; epipodophyllotoxin	acute leukemia; adrenal cortical cancer; brain cancer; chronic lymphocytic leukemia; choriocarcinoma; esophageal cancer; Ewing sarcoma; gastric cancer; germ-cell cancer; gestational trophoblastic neoplasms; hepatocellular cancer; Hodgkin disease; hypereosinophilic syndrome; Kaposi sarcoma; testicular cancer; thymoma; thyroid cancer; uterine cancer; Wilms' tumor; Langerhans cell histiocytosis; mobilization of peripheral-blood progenitor cells; multiple myeloma; neuroblastoma; non-small-cell lung cancer; osteogenic sarcoma; ovarian cancer; retinoblastoma; small-cell lung cancer; soft-tissue sarcomas
Leukeran	chlorambucil; CBL; chlorambucilum; chloraminophen; chlorbutin; chlorbutine; chlorbutinum; chloroambucil; chlorobutin; chlorobutine; elcoril; leukersan; leukoran; linfolizin; lympholysin; phenylbutyric acid nitrogen mustard	chronic lymphocytic leukemia; malignant lymphomas
Leukine	sargramostim; granulocyte macrophage colony-stimulating factor	melanoma; chemotherapy-induced neutropenia
Leustatin	Cladribine; 2-chloro-2-deoxyadenosine; 2-chlorodeoxyadenosine; cladribina	acute myeloid leukemia; chronic lymphocytic leukemia; cutaneous T-cell lymphoma; hairy cell leukemia; Langerhans cell histiocytosis; non-Hodgkin lymphoma; Waldenström macroglobulinemia
Levulan	aminolevulinic acid	photodynamic therapy to treat a skin condition called actinic keratosis
L-Glutamine	glutamine	short bowel syndrome
Lipiodol	ethiodized oil	diagnostic imaging, hysterosalpingography and lymphography
LipoDox	doxorubicin hydrochloride liposome; doxorubicin hydrochloride liposome injection; liposomal adriamycin; liposomal doxorubicin; liposomal doxorubicin hydrochloride; liposome-encapsulated doxorubicin; pegylated doxorubicin HCl liposome; pegylated liposomal doxorubicin; pegylated liposomal doxorubicin hydrochloride; S-liposomal doxorubicin; stealth liposomal doxorubicin	refractory metastatic carcinoma of the ovary; AIDS-related Kaposi sarcoma; breast cancer; relapsed/refractory multiple myeloma (with bortezomib)
Lipo-Lutin	therapeutic progesterone	amenorrhea; functional uterine bleeding; infertility; maintenance of pregnancy

Trade Name	Generic Drug	Indicated For
Liquid Pred	prednisone; delta(1)-cortisone; deltacortisone; deltadehydrocortisone; metacortandracin; PRD; prednisonum	inflammatory conditions; allergic conditions; hematologic conditions; neoplastic conditions; autoimmune conditions; replacement therapy in adrenal insufficiency
Lisacort	prednisone; delta(1)-cortisone; deltacortisone; deltadehydrocortisone; metacortandracin; PRD; prednisonum	inflammatory conditions; allergic conditions; hematologic conditions; neoplastic conditions; autoimmune conditions; replacement therapy in adrenal insufficiency
Longastatina	octreotide acetate	acromegaly; diarrhea
Loron	clodronate disodium	adjuvant usage in bone metastasis of breast cancer
Lumitene	beta carotene	chemoprevention for cardiovascular disease and cancer
Lupron	leuprolide acetate; leuprorelin; leuprorelin acetate	prostate cancer; uterine fibroid tumors
Lupron Depot; Lupron Depot-3 Month; -4 Month	leuprolide acetate; leuprorelin; leuprorelin acetate	prostate cancer; uterine fibroid tumors
Lupron Depot-Ped	leuprolide acetate; leuprorelin; leuprorelin acetate	prostate cancer; uterine fibroid tumors
Luteohormone	therapeutic progesterone	amenorrhea; functional uterine bleeding; infertility; maintenance of pregnancy
Lymphazurin	isosulfan blue	diagnostic imaging
LymphoCide	epratuzumab	systemic lupus erythematosus
Lynoral	ethinyl estradiol	advanced androgen-dependent prostate cancer, palliative; breast cancer, palliative; estrogen replacement; menopausal symptoms; postmenopausal osteoporosis
Lyovac Cosmegen	dactinomycin; ACT-D; actinomycin A IV; actinomycin C1; actinomycin D; actinomycin I1; actinomycin IV; actinomycin X 1; actinomycin-[thr-val-pro-sar-meval]; AD; dactinomycine; meractinomycin	Wilms' tumor; childhood rhabdomyosarcoma; Ewing sarcoma; testicular cancer; gestational trophoblastic neoplasia; choriocarcinoma; melanoma; neuroblastoma; retinoblastoma; uterine sarcomas; Kaposi sarcoma; sarcoma botryoides; soft-tissue sarcoma
Lysodren	mitotane; chloditan; chlodithane; khloditan; mytotan; o,p'-DDD; ortho,para-DDD	adrenal cortical carcinoma
Magnevist	gadopentetate dimeglumine	angiography for leptomeningeal metastases and multiple sclerosis and magnetic resonance imaging for spine and brain
Makarol	diethylstilbesterol; diethylstilbenediol; diethylstilbestrol dipropionate; diethylstilbestrolum; diethylstilboestrol; sinestrol; stilboestrol dipropionate	breast cancer; prostate cancer

Trade Name	Generic Drug	Indicated For
Marinol	dronabinol; cannabinol; delta 9-tetrahydrocannabinol; tetrahydrocannabinol	antinausea
Matulane	procarbazine hydrochloride; ibenzmethyzin; ibenzmethyzin hydrochloride; ibenzmethyzine hydrochloride; MIH; MIH hydrochloride; PCB hydrochloride; PCZ; procarbazin	brain tumors; Hodgkin disease; non-Hodgkin lymphoma
Maxidex	dexamethasone; desamethasone; dexamethasonum; DXM; hexadecadrol; methylfluorprednisolone	antiemetic (prevents vomiting)
Maxipime	cefepime hydrochloride	upper respiratory tract and urinary tract infections; febrile neutropenic conditions
Measurin	acetylsalicylic acid; aspirin	mild to moderate pain; fever; prevention of arterial and venous thrombosis
Mebonat	clodronate disodium	adjuvant usage in bone metastasis of breast cancer
Meditest	testosterone	breast cancer in women, palliative
Megace; Megace ES	megestrol acetate	appetite enhancement, AIDS patients; breast cancer, palliative; endometrial carcinoma, palliative treatment
Memoril	glutamine	short bowel syndrome
Menaval-20	estradiol	breast cancer, palliative
Menest	esterified estrogens	breast cancer
Mercaptopurinum	Mercaptopurine; 6-thiohypoxanthine; 6-mercaptopurine; 6-mercaptopurine monohydrate; 6-purinethiol; 6-thiopurine; 6-thioxopurine; azathiopurine; leupurin; mercapurin; mern; purimethol	acute lymphocytic leukemia; acute myelogenous leukemia; Crohn disease; Hodgkin disease in children; lymphoblastic lymphoma; ulcerative colitis
Mercaptyl	penicillamine	Wilson disease; heavy metal intoxication; cystinuria; rheumatoid arthritis; primary biliary cirrhosis; Felty syndrome; rheumatoid vasculitis
Mesna Disulfide	dimesna	ifosfamide-induced hemorrhagic cystitis, prophylaxis
Mesnex	mesna; mercaptoethane sulfonate; mesnum	helps protect the kidneys and bladder from the toxic effects of anticancer drugs such as ifosfamide and cyclophosphamide
Metalcaptase	penicillamine	Wilson disease; heavy metal intoxication; cystinuria; rheumatoid arthritis; primary biliary cirrhosis; Felty syndrome; rheumatoid vasculitis
Metastron	strontium chloride Sr 89	palliation of pain in bone metastases

Trade Name	Generic Drug	Indicated For
Methazolastone	temozolomide	malignant glioma (anaplastic astrocytoma; anaplastic oligodendrogliomas; anaplastic oligoastrocytomas; glioblastoma multiforme); metastatic melanoma
Methotrexate LPF	methotrexate	bladder cancer; breast cancer; carcinomatous; meningitis; chorioadenoma destruens; esophageal cancer; gestational choriocarcinoma; head/neck cancer; meningeal leukemia; lymphomas; Burkitt lymphoma; lung cancer; mycosis fungoides; osteosarcoma; Wegener granulomatosis
Methylthioninium chloride	methylene blue	cyanide poisoning, antidote; diagnostic, indicator dye; genitourinary antiseptic; glutaricaciduria; methemoglobinemia; oxalate and phosphate urinary tract calculi, management
Meticorten	prednisone; delta(1)-cortisone; deltacortisone; deltadehydrocortisone; metacortandracin; PRD; prednisonum	inflammatory conditions; allergic conditions; hematologic conditions; neoplastic conditions; autoimmune conditions; replacement therapy in adrenal insufficiency
Meti-derm	prednisolone	inflammatory conditions; allergic conditions; hematologic conditions; neoplastic conditions; autoimmune conditions; replacement therapy in adrenal insufficiency
Mevacor	lovastatin	atherosclerosis; coronary heart disease, prevention; hypercholesterolemia
Mevinolin	lovastatin	atherosclerosis; coronary heart disease, prevention; hypercholesterolemia
Mexate; Mexate-AQ	methotrexate	bladder cancer; breast cancer; carcinomatous; meningitis; chorioadenoma destruens; esophageal cancer; gestational choriocarcinoma; head/neck cancer; meningeal leukemia; lymphomas; Burkitt lymphoma; lung cancer; mycosis fungoides; osteosarcoma; Wegener granulomatosis
Microlut	norgestrel	oral contraception
Milestrol	diethylstilbesterol; diethylstilbenediol; diethylstilbestrol dipropionate; diethylstilbestrolum; diethylstilboestrol; sinestrol; stilboestrol dipropionate	breast cancer; prostate cancer
Miltex	Miltefosine	skin metastasis of breast cancer
Mircera	methoxy polyethylene glycol-beta	anemia associated with chronic renal failure
Mithracin	plicamycin; aureolic acid; mithramycin	testicular cancer

Trade Name	Generic Drug	Indicated For
Mitosan	busulfan; BSF; bussulfam; busulfanum; busulphan; glyzophrol; methanesulfonic acid tetramethylene ester; myeleukon; myeloleukon; myelosan; mylecytan; sulfabutin; tetramethylene bis(methanesulfonate)	bone marrow disorders; chronic myelogenous leukemia; palliative; neoadjuvant to allogeneic hematopoietic progenitor cell transplantation; neoplastic meningitis; primary brain malignancies
Mitozytrex	mitomycin C; MITC; mitocin-C; MTC	gastric carcinoma; pancreatic adenocarcinoma
Monacolin K	lovastatin	atherosclerosis; coronary heart disease, prevention; hypercholesterolemia
Moranyl	suramin	trypanosomiasis; hormone-refractory prostate cancer
MultiHance	gadopentetate dimeglumine	angiography for leptomeningeal metastases and multiple sclerosis and magnetic resonance imaging for spine and brain
MUSE	alprostadil	erectile dysfunction; patent ductus arteriosus
Mustargen	mechlorethamine hydrochloride; chloramin; chlorethamine HCl; chlorethamine hydrochloride; chlorethazine; chlorethazine hydrochloride; chlormethine; chlormethine hydrochloride; chloromethine HCl; mechlorethamine; mechlorethamine HCl; methylchlorethamine; mustard; mustargen HCl; mustargen hydrochloride; mustine; NH-2; nitrogen mustard; N-lost	bronchogenic carcinoma; chronic lymphocytic and myelcytic leukemia; Hodgkin disease, palliative; lymphosarcoma; mycosis fungoides; polycythemia vera
Mutamycin	mitomycin C; MITC; mitocin-C; MTC	gastric carcinoma; pancreatic adenocarcinoma
Mycobutin	rifabutin	prevention and treatment of *Mycobacterium avium* complex (MAC) and tuberculosis in patients with HIV infection
Myleran	busulfan; BSF; bussulfam; busulfanum; busulphan; glyzophrol; methanesulfonic acid tetramethylene ester; myeleukon; myeloleukon; myelosan; mylecytan; sulfabutin; tetramethylene bis(methanesulfonate)	bone marrow disorders; chronic myelogenous leukemia; palliative; neoadjuvant to allogeneic hematopoietic progenitor cell transplantation; neoplastic meningitis; primary brain malignancies
Mylosar	azacitidine; 5-AC; 5-azacytidine; azacytidine; ladakamycin	myelodysplastic syndrome

Trade Name	Generic Drug	Indicated For
Mylotarg	gemtuzumab ozogamicin; calicheamicin-conjugated humanized anti-CD33 monoclonal antibody; hP67.6-calicheamicin	acute myeloid leukemia
Naganin; Naganine	suramin	trypanosomiasis; hormone-refractory prostate cancer
Navoban	tropisetron	chemotherapy-induced nausea and vomiting
Neo-Oestronol I	diethylstilbesterol; diethylstilbenediol; diethylstilbestrol dipropionate; diethylstilbestrolum; diethylstilboestrol; sinestrol; stilboestrol dipropionate	breast cancer; prostate cancer
Neogest	norgestrel	oral contraception
Neoral	cyclosporine	allogenic transplants; prophylaxis of organ rejection in bone marrow; kidney; liver and heart transplants; psoriasis; rheumatoid arthritis; various diseases that involve autoimmune response
NeoRecormon	epoetin beta	anemia associated with end-stage renal disease
Neosar	cyclophosphamide; ciclofosfamida; ciclofosfamide; claphene; CP monohydrate; CPM; cyclophospham; cyclophosphamid monohydrate; cyclophosphamidum; cyclophosphan; cyclophosphanum; cytophosphane; mitoxan; syklofosfamid; zytoxan	breast cancer; leukemias; lupus nephritis; lymphoma; multiple myeloma; neuroblastoma; nephrotic syndrome; ovarian cancer; retinoblastoma
Neulasta	pegfilgrastim; filgrastim SD-01; SD-01; SD-01 sustained duration G-CSF	chemotherapy-induced neutropenia
Neumega	recombinant interleukin-11; adipogenesis inhibitory factor; IL-11; interleukin-11; oprelvekin; recombinant human interleukin-11; therapeutic interleukin-11	chemotherapy-related thrombocytopenia; prevention of severe thrombocytopenia following myelosuppressive chemotherapy
Neupogen	filgrastim; granulocyte colony-stimulating factor; recombinant methionyl human granulocyte colony stimulating factor	bone marrow transplantation; cancer patients receiving myelosuppressive chemotherapy; neutropenia
Neurontin	gabapentin	management of epilepsy; pain; mania; depression and anxiety disorders
Neutrexin	trimetrexate glucuronate; TMQ	head and neck cancer; metastatic colorectal adenocarcinoma; non-small-cell lung cancer; osteogenic sarcoma; pancreatic adenocarcinoma; pneumocystitis carinii pneumonia

Trade Name	Generic Drug	Indicated For
Neutrogin	lenograstim	chemotherapy-induced neutropenia
Nexavar	sorafenib tosylate; BAY 43-9006; BAY 43-9006 tosylate salt	advanced renal cell carcinoma; metastatic colorectal cancer
Nicamid	niacinamide	pellagra, treatment and prophylaxis; various dermatologic conditions
Nicosedine	niacinamide	pellagra, treatment and prophylaxis; various dermatologic conditions
Nilandron	nilutamide	prostate cancer
Nipent	pentostatin; 2′-deoxycoformycin; co-vidarabine; deoxycoformycin; pentostatine	chronic lymphocytic leukemia; cutaneous T-cell lymphoma; hairy cell leukemia
Nizoral	ketoconazole	seborrheic dermatitis; prostate cancer
Nolvadex	tamoxifen citrate; novaldex; tamoxifen; tamoxifeni citras	breast cancer, palliative; adjuvant in breast cancer therapy; endometrial cancer; gynecomastia; melanoma; ovarian cancer
Nordeoxyguanosine	ganciclovir	cytomegalovirus (CMV) infections in immunocompromised patients
Novantrone	mitoxantrone hydrochloride; dihydroxyanthracenedione; dihydroxyanthracenedione dihydrochloride; mitoxantrone dihydrochloride; mitoxantrone HCl; mitoxantroni hydrochloridum; mitozantrone	acute leukemia; breast cancer; prostate cancer; non-Hodgkin lymphoma; multiple sclerosis
Novo-Valproic	valproic acid	epilepsy; mania; migraine
Noxafil	posaconazole	fungal infection prevention for immunocompromised host
Nutrestore	glutamine	short bowel syndrome
Octamide	metoclopramide	antinausea
Oestrogenine	diethylstilbesterol; diethylstilbenediol; diethylstilbestrol dipropionate; diethylstilbestrolum; diethylstilboestrol; sinestrol; stilboestrol dipropionate	breast cancer; prostate cancer
Oestromenin	diethylstilbesterol; diethylstilbenediol; diethylstilbestrol dipropionate; diethylstilbestrolum; diethylstilboestrol; sinestrol; stilboestrol dipropionate	breast cancer; prostate cancer
Oestromon	diethylstilbesterol; diethylstilbenediol; diethylstilbestrol dipropionate; diethylstilbestrolum; diethylstilboestrol; sinestrol; stilboestrol dipropionate	breast cancer; prostate cancer

Trade Name	Generic Drug	Indicated For
Olux-E	clobetasol propionate	psoriasis, eczema
Oncaspar	pegaspargase; L-Asparaginase with polyethylene glycol; PEG-asparaginase; PEG-L-asparaginase; PEG-L-asparaginase(K-H); polyethylene glycol-L-asparaginase	acute lymphoblastic leukemia
Onconase	ranpirnase	mesothelioma
Oncovin	vincristine; LCR; leurocristine; leurocristine sulfate; vincasar; vincrystine	acute leukemia; brain tumors; chronic lymphocytic leukemia; gestational trophoblastic neoplasms; head and neck squamous cell carcinoma; Kaposi sarcoma; liver cancer; Hodgkin disease and non-Hodgkin lymphoma; malignant thymoma; multiple myeloma; osteogenic sarcoma; ovarian cancer; pheochromocytoma; retinoblastoma; rhabdomyosarcoma; soft-tissue sarcoma; testicular cancer; Wilms' tumor
Ontak	denileukin diftitox; DAB(389)-interleukin-2; DAB389 interleukin-2; DAB389 interleukin-2 immunotoxin; DAB389-IL2; interleukin-2 fusion protein; interleukin-2 fusion toxin	cutaneous T-cell lymphoma
Onxol	paclitaxel; paclitaxel protein-bound; albumin-stabilized nanoparticle paclitaxel; nab-paclitaxel; nanoparticle paclitaxel	bladder cancer; breast cancer; adjuvant in breast cancer therapy; cervical cancer; endometrial adenocarcinoma; esophageal cancer; head and neck cancer; non-small-cell lung cancer; lymphoma; ovarian cancer; prostate cancer; testicular cancer; AIDS-related Kaposi sarcoma
Oralet	fentanyl citrate	breakthrough pain in cancer patients
Orasone	prednisone; delta(1)-cortisone; deltacortisone; deltadehydrocortisone; metacortandracin; PRD; prednisonum	inflammatory conditions; allergic conditions; hematologic conditions; neoplastic conditions; autoimmune conditions; replacement therapy in adrenal insufficiency
Ora-Testryl	fluoxymesterone; androfluorene; androsterolo	certain types of breast cancer
Orathecin	rubetican	AIDS, pediatric; HIV infection, pediatric
Orestralyn	ethinyl estradiol	advanced androgen-dependent prostate cancer, palliative; breast cancer, palliative; estrogen replacement; menopausal symptoms; postmenopausal osteoporosis
Orifungal M	ketoconazole	seborrheic dermatitis; prostate cancer
Orthoclone OKT3	muromonab-CD3	allograft rejection
Ossiten	clodronate disodium	adjuvant usage in bone metastasis of breast cancer
Ovaban	megestrol acetate	appetite enhancement, AIDS patients; breast cancer, palliative; endometrial carcinoma, palliative treatment

Trade Name	Generic Drug	Indicated For
OvaRex	oregovomab	epithelial ovarian cancer
Ovrette	norgestrel	oral contraception
Ovuplant	deslorelin	central precocious puberty
Oxandrin	oxandrolone	bone pain; Duchenne and Becker muscular dystrophy; HIV-associated muscle weakness; HIV-related wasting syndrome
Oxsoralen; Oxsoralen-Ultra	methoxsalen; 8-methoxypsoralen; methoxypsoralen	cutaneous T-cell lymphoma
Palestrol	diethylstilbesterol; diethylstilbenediol; diethylstilbestrol dipropionate; diethylstilbestrolum; diethylstilboestrol; sinestrol; stilboestrol dipropionate	breast cancer; prostate cancer
Pallace	megestrol acetate	appetite enhancement, AIDS patients; breast cancer, palliative; endometrial carcinoma, palliative treatment
Panadol	paracetamol	painkiller
Panfungol	ketoconazole	seborrheic dermatitis; prostate cancer
Panretin	alitretinoin; 9-cis-retinoic acid; retinoicacid-9-cis	topical treatment of cutaneous lesions in patients with AIDS-related Kaposi sarcoma
Panwarfin	warfarin	pulmonary embolism and thromboembolic disorders, treatment and prophylaxis; venous thrombosis, prophylaxis and treatment
Paraplat	carboplatin; carboplatin hexal; carboplatino	ovarian cancer
Paraplatin	carboplatin; carboplatin hexal; carboplatino	ovarian cancer
Pavabid	papaverine	ischemia, cerebral and peripheral
Pavacap	papaverine	ischemia, cerebral and peripheral
Pavatym	papaverine	ischemia, cerebral and peripheral
Paxil	paroxetine hydrochloride	depression
Pedi-Vit-A	vitamin A compound; all trans retinol; anti-infective vitamin; antixerophthalmic vitamin; axerophthol; axeroptholum; biosterol; lard-factor; oleovitamin A; ophthalamin; retinol; vitamin A; vitamin A alcohol; vitamin A USP; vitamin A1; vitaminum A	diminishing malignant cell growth; enhancing the immune system
PedvaxHIB	haemophilus influenzae B vaccine	haemophilus influenzae B prophylaxis
PEGASYS	PEG-interferon alfa-2a	chronic hepatitis C; renal cell carcinoma; advanced melanoma; chronic myelogenous leukemia

Trade Name	Generic Drug	Indicated For
PEG-Interferon Alfa	pegylated interferon alfa	hepatitis C
PEG-Intron	PEG-interferon alfa-2b	chronic hepatitis C; renal cell carcinoma
Pendramine	penicillamine	Wilson disease; heavy metal intoxication; cystinuria; rheumatoid arthritis; primary biliary cirrhosis; Felty syndrome; rheumatoid vasculitis
Perdolat	penicillamine	Wilson disease; heavy metal intoxication; cystinuria; rheumatoid arthritis; primary biliary cirrhosis; Felty syndrome; rheumatoid vasculitis
Periactin	cyproheptadine hydrochloride	hypersensitivity reactions
Photofrin	porfimer sodium; dihematoporphyrin ether; photofrin II; porfimer	photosensitizer; bladder, esophageal, gastric, lung, and rectal cancers
Platinol; Platinol-AQ	cisplatin; CACP; cis-DDP; cis-diamminedichloro platinum (II); cis-diamminedichloroplatinum; cis-dichloroammine platinum (II); cismaplat; cisplatina; cis-platinous diamine dichloride; cis-platinum; cis-platinum II; cis-platinum II diamine dichloride; CPDD; cysplatyna; DDP; PDD; Peyrone's chloride; Peyrone's salt; platinoxan; platinum diamminodichloride	metastatic testicular cancer; ovarian cancer; head and neck cancer; breast cancer; Hodgkin disease and non-Hodgkin lymphoma; myeloma and melanoma; advanced bladder cancer
Plavix	clopidogrel bisulfate	thromboembolic disorders
Prednicen-M	prednisone; delta(1)-cortisone; deltacortisone; deltadehydrocortisone; metacortandracin; PRD; prednisonum	inflammatory conditions; allergic conditions; hematologic conditions; neoplastic conditions; autoimmune conditions; replacement therapy in adrenal insufficiency
Prednilen	methylprednisolone	adrenocortical insufficiency; conditions requiring immunosuppression; inflammatory conditions; multiple sclerosis; nephrotic syndrome
Prelone	prednisolone	inflammatory conditions; allergic conditions; hematologic conditions; neoplastic conditions; autoimmune conditions; replacement therapy in adrenal insufficiency
Premarin	conjugated estrogens	advanced androgen-dependent prostate cancer, palliative; breast cancer, palliative
Procrit	epoetin alfa; erythropoietin; r-HuEPO	anemias associated with chronic renal failure, zidovudine (AZT) therapy, and cancer chemotherapy of nonmyeloid malignancies
Progestin	therapeutic progesterone	amenorrhea; functional uterine bleeding; infertility; maintenance of pregnancy
Proglycem	diazoxide	malignant hypertension

Trade Name	Generic Drug	Indicated For
Prokine	sargramostim; granulocyte macrophage colony-stimulating factor	melanoma; chemotherapy-induced neutropenia
Proleukin	aldesleukin; interleukin II; interleukin-2; lymphocyte mitogenic factor; mitogenic factor; recombinant interleukin-2; T-cell growth factor; TCGF, interleukin; thymocyte stimulating factor	metastatic renal cell carcinoma; metastatic melanoma; stimulates the production of blood cells, especially platelets, during chemotherapy
Provera; Provera Dosepak	medroxyprogesterone; medroxyprogesterone acetate	breast carcinoma; endometrial carcinoma; renal cell carcinoma
Provigil	modafinil	narcolepsy
Purinethol	Mercaptopurine; 6 thiohypoxanthine; 6-mercaptopurine; 6-mercaptopurine monohydrate; 6-purinethiol; 6-thiopurine; 6-thioxopurine; azathiopurine; leupurin; mercapurin; mern; purimethol	acute lymphocytic leukemia; acute myelogenous leukemia; Crohn disease; Hodgkin disease in children; lymphoblastic lymphoma; ulcerative colitis
Q. Levoglutamide	glutamine	short bowel syndrome
Quadramet	samarium SM 153 lexidronam pentasodium; samarium-153 EDTMP; samarium-153 ethylenediaminetetramethylenephosphonate; samarium-153 ethylenediaminetetramethylenephosphonic acid; Sm-153 EDTMP	pain due to bone cancer
R-41400	ketoconazole	seborrheic dermatitis; prostate cancer
Rapamune	sirolimus	kidney transplant rejection, prevention
Rebif	interferon beta-1b	treating relapsing forms of multiple sclerosis (MS) to reduce the number of flare-ups and slow down the development of physical disability associated with MS
Reclast	zoledronic acid; NDC-zoledronate; zoledronate	hypercalcemia of malignancy; multiple myeloma and metastatic bone lesions from solid tumors; Paget disease
Regitine	phentolamine mesylate	dermal necrosis; hypertensive-associated episodes with pheochromocytoma, prevention or control
Reglan	metoclopramide	antinausea
Remicade	infliximab	ankylosis spondylitis; Crohn disease; plaque psoriasis; rheumatoid arthritis; sarcoidosis

Trade Name	Generic Drug	Indicated For
Renova	tretinoin; all-trans retinoic acid; all-trans vitamin A acid; beta-retinoic acid; retinoic acid; TRA; trans retinoic acid; trans vitamin A acid; tretinoinum; vitamin A acid	(oral) acute promyelocytic leukemia (APL), characterized by the t(15;17) translocation or the PML/RARa gene; for patients refractory to or who have relapsed from anthracycline chemotherapy, or for where anthracycline-based chemotherapy is contraindicated; (topical) acne vulgaris; other dermatologic conditions; some skin cancers
Retin-A; Retin-A MICRO	tretinoin; all-trans retinoic acid; all-trans vitamin A acid; beta-retinoic acid; retinoic acid; TRA; trans retinoic acid; trans vitamin A acid; tretinoinum; vitamin A acid	(oral) acute promyelocytic leukemia (APL), characterized by the t(15;17) translocation or the PML/RARa gene; for patients refractory to or who have relapsed from anthracycline chemotherapy, or for where anthracycline-based chemotherapy is contraindicated; (topical) acne vulgaris; other dermatologic conditions; some skin cancers
Retinol Acetate	retinyl acetate	dietary supplement; vitamin A deficiency
Retisol-A	tazarotene	topical treatment of facial acne vulgaris; stable plaque psoriasis; mitigation (palliation) of facial fine wrinkling; facial mottled hyper- and hypopigmentation; benign facial lentigines
Retrovir	zidovudine	AIDS-related complex; HIV infection; HIV transmission, prevention
Revival	soy protein isolate	heart disease prevention; hyperlipidemia; menopausal symptoms
Revlimid	lenalidomide; CDC-501; IMiD-1	transfusion-dependent anemia due to low- or intermediate-1 risk myelodysplastic syndrome; multiple myeloma
Rheumatrex	methotrexate	bladder cancer; breast cancer; carcinomatous; meningitis; chorioadenoma destruens; esophageal cancer; gestational choriocarcinoma; head/neck cancer; meningeal leukemia; lymphomas; Burkitt lymphoma; lung cancer; mycosis fungoides; osteosarcoma; Wegener granulomatosis
Ritalin	methylphenidate hydrochloride	attention deficit/hyperactivity disorder (ADHD); narcolepsy
Rituxan	rituximab; anti-CD20 monoclonal antibody; C2B8 monoclonal antibody; IDEC-C2B8 monoclonal antibody	diffuse large B-cell, CD20-positive, non-Hodgkin lymphoma
Rocaltrol	calcitriol	hyperparathyroidism; hypocalcemia
Roceron; Roceron-A	recombinant interferon alfa	used as antiviral and antitumor agents
Rodex	warfarin	pulmonary embolism and thromboembolic disorders, treatment and prophylaxis; venous thrombosis, prophylaxis and treatment
Roferon-A	interferon alfa-2a; recombinant interferon alfa	treating chronic hepatitis C and certain types of leukemia; used as antiviral and antitumor agents
RU 19110	halofuginone hydrobromide	scleroderma and antiprotozoal; coccidiosis (vet)
Rubidomycin	daunorubicin hydrochloride; cloridrato de daunorubicina; daunomycin; daunomycin-HCL; daunorubicin; dauno-rubidomycine; rubomycin C	acute lymphoblastic leukemia
Samilstin	octreotide acetate	acromegaly; diarrhea

Trade Name	Generic Drug	Indicated For
Sandimmun	cyclosporine	allogenic transplants; prophylaxis of organ rejection in bone marrow; kidney; liver and heart transplants; psoriasis; rheumatoid arthritis; various diseases that involve autoimmune response
Sandostatin	octreotide acetate	acromegaly; diarrhea
SangCya	cyclosporine	allogenic transplants; prophylaxis of organ rejection in bone marrow; kidney; liver and heart transplants; psoriasis; rheumatoid arthritis; various diseases that involve autoimmune response
Schultz No. 1038	methylene blue	cyanide poisoning, antidote; diagnostic, indicator dye; genitourinary antiseptic; glutaricaciduria; methemoglobinemia; oxalate and phosphate urinary tract calculi, management
Sclerosol Intrapleural Aerosol	talc	malignant pleural effusion; pneumothorax
Sensipar	cinacalcet	treating an overactive parathyroid in dialysis patients with chronic kidney disease; also used to treat high blood calcium levels in patients with parathyroid cancer.
Septra	trimethoprim-sulfamethoxazole	*Pneumocystis carinii* pneumonia; various bacterial infections
Sk-Dexamethasone	dexamethasone; desamethasone; dexamethasonum; DXM; hexadecadrol; methylfluorprednisolone	antiemetic (prevents vomiting)
Sk-Prednisone	prednisone; delta(1)-cortisone; deltacortisone; deltadehydrocortisone; metacortandracin; PRD; prednisonum	inflammatory conditions; allergic conditions; hematologic conditions; neoplastic conditions; autoimmune conditions; replacement therapy in adrenal insufficiency
Sodium Phosphate P32 Solution	sodium phosphate P32	polycythemia vera; chronic myelocytic leukemia and chronic lymphocytic leukemia; multiple areas of skeletal metastases, palliative treatment
Solatene	beta-carotene	chemoprevention for cardiovascular disease and cancer
Soliris	eculizumab	paroxysmal nocturnal hemoglobinuria
Solpadol	co-codamol	painkiller
Soltamox	tamoxifen citrate; novaldex; tamoxifen; tamoxifeni citras	breast cancer, palliative; adjuvant in breast cancer therapy; endometrial cancer; gynecomastia; melanoma; ovarian cancer
Somatuline	lanreotide	acromegaly
Soriatane	acitretin; trimethylmethoxyphenyl-retinoic acid	cutaneous T-cell lymphoma
Sporanox	itraconazole	fungal infections
Sprycel	dasatinib; BMS-354825	chronic myeloid leukemia; Philadelphia chromosome-positive acute lymphoblastic leukemia
STEPA	thiotepa; thiophosphamide; thiophosphoramide; triethylene thiophosphoramide	bladder cancer; breast cancer; ovarian cancer; Hodgkin disease; non-Hodgkin lymphoma

Trade Name	Generic Drug	Indicated For
Sterapred	prednisone; delta(1)-cortisone; deltacortisone; deltadehydrocortisone; metacortandracin; PRD; prednisonum	inflammatory conditions; allergic conditions; hematologic conditions; neoplastic conditions; autoimmune conditions; replacement therapy in adrenal insufficiency
Sterile Talc Powder	talc	malignant pleural effusion; pneumothorax
Steritalc	talc	malignant pleural effusion; pneumothorax
Stieva-A; Stieva-A Forte	tazarotene	topical treatment of facial acne vulgaris; stable plaque psoriasis; mitigation (palliation) of facial fine wrinkling; facial mottled hyper- and hypopigmentation; benign facial lentigines
Stilbestrol; Stilboestrol	diethylstilbesterol; diethylstilbenediol; diethylstilbestrol dipropionate; diethylstilbestrolum; diethylstilboestrol; sinestrol; stilboestrol dipropionate	breast cancer; prostate cancer
Stilbetin	diethylstilbesterol; diethylstilbenediol; diethylstilbestrol dipropionate; diethylstilbestrolum; diethylstilboestrol; sinestrol; stilboestrol dipropionate	breast cancer; prostate cancer
Stilboestroform	diethylstilbesterol; diethylstilbenediol; diethylstilbestrol dipropionate; diethylstilbestrolum; diethylstilboestrol; sinestrol; stilboestrol dipropionate	breast cancer; prostate cancer
Sublimaze	fentanyl citrate	breakthrough pain in cancer patients
Sufortan	penicillamine	Wilson disease; heavy metal intoxication; cystinuria; rheumatoid arthritis; primary biliary cirrhosis; Felty syndrome; rheumatoid vasculitis
Sulindac sulfone	exisulind	colonic adenomatous polyps in the inherited disease adenomatous polyposis coli, control and suppression
Suprecur	buserelin	breast cancer; contraception, female; endometriosis; infertility; in vitro fertilization; polycystic ovary syndrome; prostate cancer; uterine leiomyoma
Sutent	sunitinib malate; sunitinib	gastrointestinal stromal tumor; advanced metastatic renal cell carcinoma
Synestrin	diethylstilbesterol; diethylstilbenediol; diethylstilbestrol dipropionate; diethylstilbestrolum; diethylstilboestrol; sinestrol; stilboestrol dipropionate	breast cancer; prostate cancer

Trade Name	Generic Drug	Indicated For
Synovir	thalidomide; alpha-phthalimidoglutarimide; N-phthaloylglutamimide; N-phthalylglutamic acid imide	Kaposi sarcoma; multiple myeloma; primary brain tumors
Synthoestrin	diethylstilbesterol; diethylstilbenediol; diethylstilbestrol dipropionate; diethylstilbestrolum; diethylstilboestrol; sinestrol; stilboestrol dipropionate	breast cancer; prostate cancer
Tabloid	thioguanine	acute nonlymphocytic leukemia
Tagamet	cimetidine	gastrointestinal conditions; allergic reaction prevention; immune modulation
Tarabine PFS	cytarabine; arabinofuranosylcytosine; arabinosylcytosine; aracytidine; beta-cytosine arabinoside; cytarabine hydrochloride; cytarabinum; cytosine arabinoside; cytosine arabinosine hydrochloride	acute nonlymphocytic leukemia; acute lymphocytic leukemia; chronic myelogenous leukemia; bone marrow transplantation; carcinomatous meningitis; Hodgkin disease; meningeal leukemia; meningitis lymphomatous; myelodysplasic syndrome; non-Hodgkin lymphoma; ovarian cancer; retinoblastoma
Tarceva	erlotinib hydrochloride; erlotinib	malignant glioma; locally advanced or metastic non-small-cell lung carcinoma; locally advanced, unresectable or metastatic pancreatic carcinoma
Targretin	bexarotene; 3-methyl TTNEB	oral or topical treatment of manifestations of cutaneous T-cell lymphoma
Tasigna	nilotinib	chronic myeloid leukemia; Philadelphia chromosome-positive acute lymphoblastic leukemia
Tavocept	dimesna	ifosfamide-induced hemorrhagic cystitis, prophylaxis
Taxol	paclitaxel; paclitaxel protein-bound; albumin-stabilized nanoparticle paclitaxel; nab-paclitaxel; nanoparticle paclitaxel	bladder cancer; breast cancer; adjuvant in breast cancer therapy; cervical cancer; endometrial adenocarcinoma; esophageal cancer; head and neck cancer; non-small-cell lung cancer; lymphoma; ovarian cancer; prostate cancer; testicular cancer; AIDS-related Kaposi sarcoma
Taxotere	docetaxel	breast cancer; esophageal cancer; gastric cancer; head/neck cancers; locally advanced or metastatic non-small-cell lung cancer; ovarian cancer; metastatic prostate cancer
Tazorac	tazarotene	topical treatment of facial acne vulgaris; stable plaque psoriasis; mitigation (palliation) of facial fine wrinkling; facial mottled hyper- and hypopigmentation; benign facial lentigines
Tegretol	carbamazepine	epilepsy
Temodar	temozolomide	malignant glioma (anaplastic astrocytoma; anaplastic oligodendrogliomas; anaplastic oligoastrocytomas; glioblastoma multiforme); metastatic melanoma
Tempostatin	halofuginone hydrobromide	scleroderma and antiprotozoal; coccidiosis (vet)

Trade Name	Generic Drug	Indicated For
Teslac	testolactone; fludestrin; therapeutic testolactone	advanced breast cancer in women, palliative
TESPA	thiotepa; thiophosphamide; thiophosphoramide; triethylene thiophosphoramide	bladder cancer; breast cancer; ovarian cancer; Hodgkin disease; non-Hodgkin lymphoma
Testamone-100	testosterone	breast cancer in women, palliative
Testoderm	therapeutic testosterone; testosterone; testosterone enanthate; trans-testosterone	delayed puberty, male; hypogonadism; metastatic mammary cancer; breast cancer in women, palliative
Testolin	therapeutic testosterone; testosterone; testosterone enanthate; trans-testosterone	delayed puberty, male; hypogonadism; metastatic mammary cancer; breast cancer in women, palliative
Testopel	testosterone	breast cancer in women, palliative
Testosterone Enanthate	testosterone	breast cancer in women, palliative
Testostroval; Testostroval-PA	therapeutic testosterone; testosterone; testosterone enanthate; Trans-Testosterone	delayed puberty, male; hypogonadism; metastatic mammary cancer
Testro; Testro AQ	therapeutic testosterone; testosterone; testosterone enanthate; Trans-Testosterone	delayed puberty, male; hypogonadism; metastatic mammary cancer; breast cancer in women, palliative
Tetramethylthionine Chloride Trihydrate	methylene blue	cyanide poisoning, antidote; diagnostic, indicator dye; genitourinary antiseptic; glutaricaciduria; methemoglobinemia; oxalate and phosphate urinary tract calculi, management
Thalomid	thalidomide; alpha-phthalimidoglutarimide; N-phthaloylglutamimide; N-phthalylglutamic acid imide	Kaposi sarcoma; multiple myeloma; primary brain tumors
Theraloc	nimotuzumab	glioma
TheraSphere	yttrium Y 90 glass microspheres	hepatocellular carcinoma, transarterial internal radiation
Thiofozil	thiotepa; thiophosphamide; thiophosphoramide; triethylene thiophosphoramide	bladder cancer; breast cancer; ovarian cancer; Hodgkin disease; non-Hodgkin lymphoma
Thioplex	thiotepa; thiophosphamide; thiophosphoramide; triethylene thiophosphoramide	bladder cancer; breast cancer; ovarian cancer; Hodgkin disease; non-Hodgkin lymphoma
309 F	suramin	trypanosomiasis; hormone-refractory prostate cancer
Thymitaq	nolatrexed dihydrochloride	hepatocellular carcinoma
Thymoglobulin	antithymocyte globulin	heart and renal transplantation rejection; prophylaxis
Thyrogen	thyrotropin alfa	thyroid cancer
Tifosyl	thiotepa; thiophosphamide; thiophosphoramide; triethylene thiophosphoramide	bladder cancer; breast cancer; ovarian cancer; Hodgkin disease; non-Hodgkin lymphoma

Trade Name	Generic Drug	Indicated For
Tioguanine	thioguanine	acute nonlymphocytic leukemia
TISSEEL	fibrin sealant	cardiovascular surgery; colostomy closure; congenital heart defects; coronary artery bypass grafting; mediastinal bleeding; microvascular bleeding; splenic trauma
Tomudex	raltitrexed	advanced colorectal cancer
Toposar	etoposide; demethyl epipodophyllotoxin ethylidine glucoside; epipodophyllotoxin	acute leukemia; adrenal cortical cancer; brain cancer; chronic lymphocytic leukemia; choriocarcinoma; esophageal cancer; Ewing sarcoma; gastric cancer; germ-cell cancer; gestational trophoblastic neoplasms; hepatocellular cancer; Hodgkin disease; hypereosinophilic syndrome; Kaposi sarcoma; testicular cancer; thymoma; thyroid cancer; uterine cancer; Wilms' tumor; Langerhans cell histiocytosis; mobilization of peripheral-blood progenitor cells; multiple myeloma; neuroblastoma; non-small-cell lung cancer; osteogenic sarcoma; ovarian cancer; retinoblastoma; small-cell lung cancer; soft-tissue sarcomas
Torisel	temsirolimus; cell cycle inhibitor 779; rapamycin analog; rapamycin analog CCI-779	renal cell carcinoma; advanced renal cell carcinoma
Totect	dexrazoxane hydrochloride	severe side effects caused by certain types of chemotherapy including extravasation; cardiac side effects by doxorubicin
Treanda	bendamustine hydrochloride	chronic lymphocytic leukemia
Trisenox	arsenic trioxide; arsenic (III) oxide; arsenic sesquioxide; arsenous acid; arsenous acid anhydride; arsenous oxide; white arsenic	myelodysplastic syndrome; multiple myeloma; chronic myeloid leukemia; acute myelocytic leukemia
Trolovol	penicillamine	Wilson disease; heavy metal intoxication; cystinuria; rheumatoid arthritis; primary biliary cirrhosis; Felty syndrome; rheumatoid vasculitis
Tykerb	lapatinib ditosylate; lapatinib	advanced or metastatic breast cancer
Tylex	co-codamol	painkiller
Ubidecarenone	coenzyme Q10	chronic heart failure; mitochondrial cytopathies
Ubiquinone 10	coenzyme Q10	chronic heart failure; mitochondrial cytopathies
Uftoral	tegafur with uracil	bowel cancer
Ultandren	fluoxymesterone; androfluorene; androsterolo	certain types of breast cancer
Unicelles	papaverine	ischemia, cerebral and peripheral
Uracil Mustard Capsules	uracil mustard	non-Hodgkin lymphoma
Urolene Blue	methylene blue	cyanide poisoning, antidote; diagnostic, indicator dye; genitourinary antiseptic; glutaricaciduria; methemoglobinemia; oxalate and phosphate urinary tract calculi, management
URSO	ursodiol	gallstone dissolution; primary biliary cirrhosis

Trade Name	Generic Drug	Indicated For
Uvadex	methoxsalen; 8-methoxypsoralen; methoxypsoralen	cutaneous T-cell lymphoma
Vagestrol	diethylstilbesterol; diethylstilbenediol; diethylstilbestrol dipropionate; diethylstilbestrolum; diethylstilboestrol; sinestrol; stilboestrol dipropionate	breast cancer; prostate cancer
Valcyte	valganciclovir	cytomegalovirus retinitis
Valstar	valrubicin	bladder cancer
Vasal	papaverine	ischemia, cerebral and peripheral
Vasomax	phentolamine mesylate	dermal necrosis; hypertensive-associated episodes with pheochromocytoma, prevention or control
Vectibix	panitumumab; monoclonal antibody ABX-EGF	advanced stage colorectal cancer
Velban	vinblastine; vincaleucoblastine	bladder cancer; breast cancer; choriocarcinoma; germ-cell tumors; idiopathic thrombocytopenic purpura; Kaposi sarcoma; Letterer-Siwe disease; various lymphomas; melanoma; mycosis fungoides; prostate cancer; testicular cancer
Velcade	bortezomib	multiple myeloma; advanced thyroid cancer
Velsar	vinblastine; vincaleucoblastine	bladder cancer; breast cancer; choriocarcinoma; germ-cell tumors; idiopathic thrombocytopenic purpura; Kaposi sarcoma; Letterer-Siwe disease; various lymphomas; melanoma; mycosis fungoides; prostate cancer; testicular cancer
Venofer	iron sucrose injection	treatment of iron deficiency for both dialysis and nondialysis patients with kidney disease, with or without concurrent erythropoietin therapy
VePesid	etoposide; demethyl epipodophyllotoxin ethylidine glucoside; epipodophyllotoxin	acute leukemia; adrenal cortical cancer; brain cancer; chronic lymphocytic leukemia; choriocarcinoma; esophageal cancer; Ewing sarcoma; gastric cancer; germ-cell cancer; gestational trophoblastic neoplasms; hepatocellular cancer; Hodgkin disease; hypereosinophilic syndrome; Kaposi sarcoma; testicular cancer; thymoma; thyroid cancer; uterine cancer; Wilms' tumor; Langerhans cell histiocytosis; mobilization of peripheral-blood progenitor cells; multiple myeloma; neuroblastoma; non-small-cell lung cancer; osteogenic sarcoma; ovarian cancer; retinoblastoma; small-cell lung cancer; soft-tissue sarcomas
Vercyte	pipobroman	leukemias
Vesanoid	tretinoin; all-trans retinoic acid; all-trans vitamin A acid; beta-retinoic acid; retinoic acid; TRA; trans retinoic acid; trans vitamin A acid; tretinoinum; vitamin A acid	(oral) acute promyelocytic leukemia (APL), characterized by the t(15;17) translocation or the PML/RARa gene refractory to or have relapsed from anthracycline chemotherapy, or for where anthracycline-based chemotherapy is contraindicated; (topical) acne vulgaris; other dermatologic conditions; some skin cancers
Viadur	leuprolide acetate; leuprorelin; leuprorelin acetate	prostate cancer; uterine fibroid tumors

Trade Name	Generic Drug	Indicated For
Viagmox	moxifloxacin hydrochloride	various bacterial infections
Viagra	sildenafil citrate	erectile dysfunction
Vidaza	azacitidine; 5-AC; 5-azacytidine; azacytidine; ladakamycin	myelodysplastic syndrome
Vincasar PFS	vincristine; LCR; leurocristine; leurocristine sulfate; vincasar; vincrystine	acute leukemia; brain tumors; chronic lymphocytic leukemia; gestational trophoblastic neoplasms; head and neck squamous cell carcinoma; Kaposi sarcoma; liver cancer; Hodgkin disease and non-Hodgkin lymphoma; malignant thymoma; multiple myeloma; osteogenic sarcoma; ovarian cancer; pheochromocytoma; retinoblastoma; rhabdomyosarcoma; soft-tissue sarcoma; testicular cancer; Wilms' tumor
Vioxx	rofecoxib	pain; dysmenorrhea; osteoarthritis; rheumatoid arthritis
Virgan	ganciclovir	cytomegalovirus (CMV) infections in immunocompromised patients
Virilon IM	testosterone	breast cancer in women, palliative
Visudyne	verteporfin	photosensitizer; subfoveal choroidal neovascularization
Vitableu	methylene blue	cyanide poisoning, antidote; diagnostic, indicator dye; genitourinary antiseptic; glutaricaciduria; methemoglobinemia; oxalate and phosphate urinary tract calculi, management
Vitinoin	tazarotene	topical treatment of facial acne vulgaris; stable plaque psoriasis; mitigation (palliation) of facial fine wrinkling; facial mottled hyper- and hypopigmentation; benign facial lentigines
Vumon	teniposide; thenvlidene-lignan-P; thenylidene-lignan-P; VM26	childhood acute lymphocytic leukemia
WARF Compound 42	warfarin	pulmonary embolism and thromboembolic disorders, treatment and prophylaxis; venous thrombosis, prophylaxis and treatment
Wellbutrin	bupropion hydrochloride	depression; smoking cessation
Wellcovorin	leucovorin calcium; calcium (6S)-folinate; calcium folinate; CFR; citrovorum factor; folinate calcium; folinic acid; folinic acid calcium salt pentahydrate; leucovorin; LV	used to protect normal cells from high doses of the anticancer drug methotrexate; also used to increase the antitumor effects of fluorouracil and tegafur-uracil; megaloblastic anemia due to folate deficiency; enhanced fluorouracil inhibition of thymidylate synthase; reverse dihydrofolate reductase inhibition by methotrexate; folic acid antagonist overdose; nitrous oxide toxicity
Wyacort	methylprednisolone	adrenocortical insufficiency; conditions requiring immunosuppression; inflammatory conditions; multiple sclerosis; nephrotic syndrome
Xanthotoxin	methoxsalen; 8-methoxypsoralen; methoxypsoralen	cutaneous T-cell lymphoma
Xeloda	capecitabine	breast cancer; colorectal cancer; Stage III colon cancer
Xolegel	ketoconazole	seborrheic dermatitis; prostate cancer
Zactima	vandetanib	thyroid cancer

Trade Name	Generic Drug	Indicated For
Zanosar	streptozocin; streptozotocin; SZN	carcinoid tumor and syndrome; colorectal cancer, palliative; Hodgkin disease; metastatic islet cell carcinoma of the pancreas
Zemplar	paricalcitol	secondary hyperparathyroidism, prevention and treatment
Zenapax	daclizumab	kidney transplant rejection, prevention
Zevalin	yttrium Y 90 ibritumomab tiuxetan; 90Y ibritumomab tiuxetan; ibritumomab (In2B8/ Y2B8 radiolabeling kit); ibritumomab tiuxetan; IDEC-Y2B8 monoclonal antibody; Y90 zevalin; Y90-labeled ibritumomab tiuxetan; yttrium-90 ibritumomab tiuxetan	accelerated approval (clinical benefit not established) treatment of patients with relapsed or refractory low-grade, follicular, or transformed B-cell non-Hodgkin lymphoma, including patients with rituximab refractory follicular non-Hodgkin lymphoma
Zinecard	dexrazoxane hydrochloride	severe side effects caused by certain types of chemotherapy including extravasation; cardiac side effects by doxorubicin
Zofran	ondansetron	nausea and vomiting prophylaxis, chemotherapy-induced and postoperative
Zoladex	goserelin; 6-[O-(1,1-dimethylethyl)-D-serine]-10-deglycinamide luteinizing hormone-releasing factor (pig) 2-(aminocarbonyl)hydrazide	breast cancer, palliative; prostate cancer
Zolinza	vorinostat; suberoylanilide hydroxamic acid	cutaneous T-cell lymphoma
Zoloft	sertraline hydrochloride	major depressive disorder; obsessive-compulsive disorder; panic disorder; posttraumatic stress disorder; premenstrual dysphoric disorder; social phobia
Zometa	zoledronic acid; NDC-zoledronate; zoledronate	hypercalcemia of malignancy; multiple myeloma and metastatic bone lesions from solid tumors; Paget disease
Zyban	bupropion hydrochloride	depression; smoking cessation
Zyflo	zileuton	prevention and chronic treatment of asthma
Zyloprim	allopurinol	treats high levels of uric acid in the body caused by certain cancer medications, especially for patients with leukemia, lymphoma, and solid-tumor malignancies

► Associations and Agencies

American Association for Cancer Research

http://www.aacr.org

Provides programs and services that promote the exchange of knowledge and new ideas among cancer research scientists; provides training opportunities for upcoming cancer researchers and promotes public education about cancer.

American Cancer Society

http://www.cancer.org

Nonprofit organization providing the largest private source of cancer research funds in the United States. Offers prevention and early detection information in addition to a wide variety of patient services programs.

American Lung Association

http://www.lungusa.org

Provides educational materials on treatments and research related to lung cancer, as well as information on the dangers of smoking and secondhand smoke. Offers smoking-cessation support programs.

American Society of Clinical Oncology (ASCO)

http://www.asco.org; http://www.Cancer.Net

A nonprofit organization consisting of more than twenty-five thousand oncology practitioners who conduct clinical cancer research and treat cancer patients. Primary Web site provides news releases, cancer research articles, and new drug information. ASCO also manages a Web site called Cancer.Net (formerly People Living with Cancer), which provides information on different types of cancer, discusses clinical trials, offers suggestions for managing side effects, and features an oncologist database.

Association of American Cancer Institutes (AACI)

http://www.aaci.org

Comprises ninety-one U.S. cancer research centers; promotes cancer research, prevention, treatment, and patient care; provides research news and a list of member cancer centers.

Blue Faery: The Adrienne Wilson Liver Cancer Association

http://www.bluefaery.org

Dedicated to increasing research, education, and advocacy for the prevention, treatment, and cure of primary liver cancer, specifically hepatocellular carcinoma. Web site provides liver cancer information and latest news updates.

Breast Cancer Action

http://www.bcaction.org

Advocates for policy changes related to breast cancer issues and educates people about breast cancer and related topics. Provides a booklet for newly diagnosed breast cancer patients, monthly e-alerts with important breast cancer news, and a bimonthly newsletter called *The Source*. Web site offers recent breast cancer news and downloadable flyers and fact sheets.

The Breast Cancer Fund

http://www.breastcancerfund.org

Identifies environmental and other preventable contributors to breast cancer and advocates for their elimination. Educates the public about cancer prevention. Web site offers a monthly e-newsletter and fact sheets.

The Breast Cancer Research Foundation

http://www.bcrfcure.org

Raises funds for breast cancer research and increases awareness of good breast health. Provides a biannual newsletter.

C3: Colorectal Cancer Coalition

http://www.fightcolorectalcancer.org

Advocates to promote colorectal cancer research, policy, and awareness in an effort to improve screening, diagnosis, and treatment of colorectal cancer. Provides a monthly e-newsletter and a quarterly print newsletter called *Momentum*. Offers information on treatment options and clinical trials.

Canadian Cancer Society

http://www.cancer.ca

A Canadian, community-based organization of volunteers that provides information about cancer, prevention, research, support services, and publications. Web site provides information by province/territory in English and French.

Centers for Disease Control and Prevention (CDC)

http://www.cdc.gov

Web site offers information on cancer, provides statistical information on cancer diagnosis in the United States, discusses smoking-cessation programs, and provides educational materials on cancer treatment and awareness. It also hosts a cancer survivorship issues page.

Children's Cause for Cancer Advocacy

http://www.childrenscause.org

Works with leading medical, scientific, and public policy experts to advance cancer research and treatment and to provide services for childhood cancer patients, survivors, and families. Web site offers information on Rise to Action Survivors Program and the opportunity to sign up for their newsletter, *The Next Step*.

CureSearch

http://www.curesearch.org

Unites Children's Oncology Group and National Childhood Cancer Foundation in their efforts to cure and prevent pediatric cancer. Web site provides information about types of pediatric cancers, treatment options available, risks and benefits of different treatment methods, prevention of and preparation for side effects, and ways to maintain a healthy lifestyle after treatment.

Esophageal Cancer Awareness Association (ECAA)

http://www.ecaware.org

Dedicated to helping patients, survivors, and caregivers deal more effectively with the uncertainties and consequences of esophageal cancer. Web site provides information about esophageal cancer and its diagnosis, staging, and treatments, as well as their newsletter, *Swallow Tales*, and contact information for members willing to offer support and advice.

Food and Drug Administration (FDA)

http://www.fda.gov

Web site provides information on clinical trials, discusses clinical trial regulations, and provides consumer education information. The FDA's Cancer Liaison Program provides answers to questions about therapies asked by cancer patients and patient advocates; its Drug Development Patient Consultant Program allows cancer patient advocates to participate in the FDA drug review regulatory process; and its Cancer Patient Representative Program recruits, assesses, and selects patient representatives to serve as members of advisory committees.

Friends of Cancer Research

http://www.focr.org

Pioneers public-private partnerships in research and clinical trials, organizes public policy forums, educates public about prevention, detection, and treatment of cancers, and collaborates with media and the motion picture industry to promote cancer research and education. Web site offers news and events articles related to cancer and a monthly newsletter.

Hurricane Voices

http://www.hurricanevoices.org

Organizes public awareness campaigns and educational programs and provides grants and sponsorships in support of breast cancer programs. Web site provides news articles about breast cancer and a list of books suggested for families affected by breast cancer.

Inflammatory Breast Cancer Association

http://www.ibchelp.org

Educates people about inflammatory breast cancer (IBC). Web site provides information about signs and symptoms, screening methods, and treatments of IBC, news reports and videos about IBC, an IBC forum and registries, as well as survivors' stories.

Inflammatory Breast Cancer Research Foundation

http://www.ibcresearch.org

Educates people about inflammatory breast cancer. Advocates for advancement of research and raises awareness of the symptoms associated with the disease, to aid in early detection. Web site offers educational materials, e-mail discussion lists, and a newsletter.

Institute of Medicine (IOM)

http://www.iom.edu

Consists of volunteer scientists and laypeople not employed by the U.S. government who provide analysis and guidance on important health issues. Web site provides reports on cancer research, survivorship, and palliative care.

Intercultural Cancer Council

http://iccnetwork.org

Advocates for programs, policies, partnerships, and research aimed at eliminating cancer within racial and ethnic minorities and medically underserved populations in the United States. Sponsors biennial symposia. Web site provides cancer fact sheets and a quarterly newsletter called *The Voice*.

International Agency for Research on Cancer (IARC)

http://www.iarc.fr

Part of the World Health Organization, IARC coordinates and conducts cancer research, including monitoring global cancer occurrence, identifying causes of cancer and the mechanisms of carcinogenesis, and developing scientific strategies for cancer control; also distributes scientific information through publications, meetings, courses, and fellowships.

International Union Against Cancer

http://www.uicc.org

A global association of cancer-fighting organizations that educates people about cancer prevention and control worldwide. Offers fellowship and training opportunities for scientists. Publishes the *International Journal of Cancer.* Web site provides press releases, newsletters, publications, and a list of suggested books.

Joan Scarangello Foundation to Conquer Lung Cancer

http://www.joanslegacy.org

Increases awareness about lung cancer and raises money to provide research grants. The Joanie Award recognizes journalists who focus on the problem of lung cancer. Web site offers information on lung cancer and a list of patient resources.

Kidney Cancer Association

http://kidneycancer.org

Provides information on kidney cancer, treatment options, and clinical trials. Funds research, advocates on behalf of patients, and distributes the *Kidney Cancer Journal.* Web site provides links to a forum, calendar of events, online store, and the Fourth Angel Caregiver Mentoring Program.

Leukemia and Lymphoma Society

http://www.leukemia-lymphoma.org

Provides information on blood cancers such as leukemia, lymphoma, Hodgkin disease, and myeloma. Funds blood cancer research, education, and patient services. Web site offers information on blood cancers, newsletters, a First Connection (peer-to-peer) program, education programs, calendar of events, and a call center.

Multiple Myeloma Research Foundation (MMRF)

http://www.multiplemyeloma.org

Provides research grants and advocates for myeloma research. Web site offers information about the disease, treatment options, and clinical trials, in addition to news and events.

National Asian Women's Health Organization (NAWHO)

http://www.nawho.org

Raises awareness about the health issues facing Asian American women, including breast cancer and cervical cancer, and provides a list of Asian-language informational resources.

National Breast Cancer Coalition (NBCC)

http://www.natlbcc.org

Promotes breast cancer research and works toward improving access for all women to high-quality breast cancer screening, diagnosis, treatment, and care; informs and trains breast cancer survivors and others in effective advocacy efforts aimed at eradicating breast cancer. Web site provides breast cancer information, latest news, and sign-up for their e-newsletter.

National Cancer Institute (NCI)

http://www.cancer.gov

Part of the medical research agency of the U.S. government, NCI conducts and supports research, training, and information distribution regarding the cause, diagnosis, prevention and treatment of cancer, rehabilitation from cancer, and the continuing care of cancer patients. Web site offers fact sheets, a dictionary of cancer terms, a dictionary of drug names, suggestions on coping with cancer, research news, and information on cancer prevention and screening, clinical trials, statistics, research funding, and complementary and alternative medicine.

National Cancer Institute of Canada (NCIC)

http://www.ncic.cancer.ca

Provides support for cancer research and related programs undertaken at Canadian universities, hospitals, and other research institutions. Web site offers video of commonly asked questions about cancer, information about program project grants, and an e-newsletter for cancer researchers.

National Cancer Institute of Canada Clinical Trials Group (NCIC CTG)

http://www.ctg.queensu.ca

Conducts clinical trials related to cancer therapy and prevention. Web site provides a list of publications and descriptions of clinical trials.

National Cervical Cancer Coalition (NCCC)

http://www.nccc-online.org

Educates people about cervical cancer and the importance of early detection, advocates for quality patient care, and provides support through its Phone Pals and E-Pals programs, which match women with cervical cancer survivors. Web site provides links to many resources related to cervical cancer, the NCCC Store, latest news, and its newsletter *Extraordinary Moments.*

National Comprehensive Cancer Network (NCCN)

http://www.nccn.org

A not-for-profit alliance of leading cancer centers. Web site provides information on treatment guidelines and supportive care, clinical trials, and member centers for people looking for physicians, pediatric cancer treatment, and genetic testing or screening.

National Institute of Environmental Health Sciences (NIEHS)

http://www.niehs.nih.gov

Part of the medical research agency of the U.S. government, the institute studies how environmental factors affect a person's chances of developing certain diseases, including cancers. Web site offers a library of resources, such as fact sheets, research reports, and a peer-reviewed journal called *Environmental Health Perspectives*. NIEHS performs a long-term study, called the Sister Study, of women whose sisters had breast cancer in an effort to learn how environment and genes affect a woman's chances of developing breast cancer.

National Library of Medicine

http://www.nlm.nih.gov

World's largest medical library offering a link to *PubMed*, an online searchable database of biomedical journal literature, and a link to MedlinePlus, an online searchable database of health and drug information for patients and loved ones, as well as links to many NLM databases and electronic resources.

National Ovarian Cancer Coalition (NOCC)

http://www.ovarian.org

Raises awareness and promotes education about ovarian cancer. Web site lists state chapters, support groups and services, and clinical trials, in addition to providing latest news, NOCC newsletter, and medical information about ovarian cancer.

Ovarian Cancer National Alliance (OCNA)

http://www.ovariancancer.org

An alliance of seven ovarian cancer groups that advocate for ovarian cancer education, policy, and research issues with national policy makers and women's health care leaders. Web site provides educational resources, support services, latest news, and clinical trials.

Prevent Cancer Foundation

http://www.preventcancer.org

Attempts to prevent cancer by funding research, educating people about prevention, and reaching out to communities through events and partnerships with other organizations.

Sarcoma Foundation of America

http://www.curesarcoma.org

Advocates for increased sarcoma research, raises funds to provide research grants to sarcoma researchers, and works to raise awareness of the treatment needs of sarcoma patients.

Skin Cancer Foundation

http://www.skincancer.org

Provides educational material about skin cancer prevention and detection. Web site provides information about different types of skin cancer, an Ask the Expert feature, a link to the SCF Store, and a Physician Finder database.

WebMD

http://www.webmd.com/cancer

An online cancer health center that provides timely reports about medical research and other cancer issues. Web site includes links to top cancer news articles, information about common cancers and treatments, current clinical trials and research, blogs, message boards, Ask the Experts resource, drug information, a database for finding a doctor, WebMD video library, sign-up for WebMD newsletter, a symptom checker, and much more.

► Cancer Centers and Hospitals

Abramson Cancer Center of the University of Pennsylvania

http://www.penncancer.org

A National Cancer Institute (NCI)-designated comprehensive cancer center in Philadelphia that is part of a network of hospitals throughout Pennsylvania and New Jersey dedicated to providing state-of-the-art cancer care, research, and education.

Arizona Cancer Center at the University of Arizona

http://www.azcc.arizona.edu

An NCI-designated comprehensive cancer center in Tucson, Arizona. Offers specialized care to each patient through research, outreach, education, and information programs (including a patient education library), and support groups as well as social services and interpreters, and leading-edge clinical care.

Barbara Ann Karmanos Cancer Institute/Meyer L. Prentis Comprehensive Cancer Center of Metropolitan Detroit

http://www.karmanos.org

An NCI-designated comprehensive cancer center based in Detroit, Michigan. Videoconferencing and physician-to-physician communication throughout the Karmanos affiliate network allows for leading-edge patient care, cancer research, clinical trials, and education statewide.

Cancer Institute of New Jersey (CINJ) at Robert Wood Johnson Medical School

http://www.cinj.org

An NCI-designated comprehensive cancer center based in New Brunswick, New Jersey, consisting of a statewide network of sixteen hospitals. Provides cancer research, clinical trials, patient care, support groups, and education. Produces publications useful to patients and their families, including its quarterly newsletter *Oncolyte*.

Cancer Treatment Centers of America (CTCA)

http://www.cancercenter.com

Uses aggressive research and innovative new techniques to provide personalized medical, nutritional, physical, psychological, and spiritual therapies to fight cancer. Several locations nationwide. Web site offers many survivor stories, CTCA news releases, media coverage, brochures, and treatment diagrams.

Case Comprehensive Cancer Center

http://cancer.case.edu

An NCI-designated comprehensive cancer center based in Cleveland, Ohio, in partnership with University Hospitals of Cleveland and the Cleveland Clinic. Uses coordinated interdisciplinary clinical research to improve cancer diagnosis, treatment, prevention, and control.

Chao Family Comprehensive Cancer Center at the University of California, Irvine

http://www.ucihs.uci.edu/cancer

An NCI-designated comprehensive cancer center located in Irvine, California, that integrates research, prevention, diagnostic, treatment, and rehabilitation programs to provide patient-centered care for patients and families coping with cancer.

City of Hope

http://www.cityofhope.org

A biomedical research, treatment, and educational institution in Duarte, California, and an NCI-designated comprehensive cancer center dedicated to the prevention and cure of cancer and other life-threatening diseases. Mission follows a compassionate patient-centered philosophy. Supported by a national foundation of humanitarian philanthropy.

Dana-Farber Cancer Institute, Brigham and Women's Hospital, and Massachusetts General Hospital

http://www.cancercare.harvard.edu

Teaching affiliates of Harvard Medical School and founding members of Dana-Farber/Harvard Cancer Center, an NCI-designated comprehensive cancer center, in Boston. Develops and provides comprehensive, multidisciplinary care plans for cancer patients. A major leader in cancer research.

Duke Comprehensive Cancer Center

http://www.cancer.duke.edu

An NCI-designated comprehensive cancer center in Durham, North Carolina, that strives to provide cutting-edge research and compassionate care. Web site provides a tumor registry detailing cancer incidence seen at Duke.

Fox Chase Cancer Center

http://www.fccc.edu

An NCI-designated comprehensive cancer center in Philadelphia that provides basic, clinical, and prevention research in addition to programs for detection and treatment of cancer and community outreach services.

Fred Hutchinson Cancer Research Center (Seattle Cancer Care Alliance)

http://www.fhcrc.org (http://www.seattlecca.org)

An NCI-designated comprehensive cancer center in Seattle, Washington. Has pioneered new diagnostic and treatment techniques. Web site offers a Patient Guide to Clinical Trials and information on its Survivorship Program.

H. Lee Moffitt Cancer Center and Research Institute at the University of South Florida

http://www.moffitt.org

A nonprofit, NCI-designated comprehensive cancer center in Tampa, Florida, that provides rapid translation of scientific research discoveries to patient care, a blood and marrow transplant program, outpatient treatment programs, and a lifetime cancer screening program.

Herbert Irving Comprehensive Cancer Center at Columbia University

http://www.ccc.columbia.edu

An NCI-designated comprehensive cancer center in New York, in partnership with New York Presbyterian Hospital, that provides patient care, clinical trials, research, and education.

Holden Comprehensive Cancer Center at the University of Iowa

http://www.uihealthcare.com/depts/cancercenter

An NCI-designated comprehensive cancer center in Iowa City, Iowa, that provides cancer-related research, clinical trials, education, and patient care throughout many departments in the University of Iowa and its hospitals and clinics.

Huntsman Cancer Institute at the University of Utah

http://www.huntsmancancer.org

An NCI-designated cancer center in Salt Lake City, Utah, that consists of scientists, physicians, and health educators working to prevent, diagnose, and treat cancers. Web site offers a link to the Huntsman Online Patient Education (HOPE) Guide.

Indiana University Melvin and Bren Simon Cancer Center

http://iucc.iu.edu

An NCI-designated cancer center in Indianapolis, Indiana, that consists of a partnership between the Indiana University School of Medicine and Clarian Health. Provides quality patient care, research, clinical trials, and educational programs.

John Wayne Cancer Institute at St. John's Health Center

http://www.jwci.org

A cancer research institute in Santa Monica, California, that conducts multidisciplinary basic, clinical translational research, focusing mainly on melanoma, sarcoma, breast cancer, prostate cancer, and colon cancer.

Jonsson Comprehensive Cancer Center

http://www.cancer.mednet.ucla.edu

An NCI-designated comprehensive cancer center at the University of California, Los Angeles, that provides interdisciplinary, team-oriented care for cancer patients. Provides information on research advances in the laboratory, clinical trials, Food and Drug Administration-approved treatments, and psychosocial and supportive care for cancer patients and their families, including people at high risk of cancer due to family histories or inherited genetic mutations.

Kimmel Cancer Center at Thomas Jefferson University Hospital

http://www.kimmelcancercenter.org

An NCI-designated comprehensive cancer center in Philadelphia. Translates latest research discoveries and clinical trials into high-quality patient care, provides patient education and support programs, and maintains a cancer registry.

Lineberger Comprehensive Cancer Center at University of North Carolina

http://cancer.med.unc.edu

A comprehensive cancer center at Chapel Hill's School of Medicine. A member of the Lance Armstrong Foundation Survivorship Network, the center provides multidisciplinary teams, patient and family support, research, clinical trials, survivor services, and an NC Cancer Hospital oncology newsletter.

Lombardi Comprehensive Cancer Center, Georgetown University Medical Center

http://lombardi.georgetown.edu

An NCI-designated comprehensive cancer center in Washington, D.C., that provides comprehensive patient care, research, clinical trials, and community outreach. The center also provides the Lombardi Cancerline to answer questions confidentially.

M. D. Anderson Cancer Center

http://www.mdanderson.org

In association with Children's Cancer Hospital, a comprehensive cancer center in Houston, Texas, that provides integrated programs in cancer treatment, clinical trials, education programs and cancer prevention.

Mayo Clinic Cancer Center

http://mayoresearch.mayo.edu/mayo/research/
cancercenter

An NCI-designated comprehensive cancer center with three campuses nationwide. Offers research, clinical trials, patient care, and outreach programs, including Outreach to American Indians and Alaska Natives.

Memorial Sloan-Kettering Cancer Center

http://www.mskcc.org

Close collaboration between scientists and physicians underlines this NCI-designated comprehensive cancer center's commitment to exceptional patient care, research, and educational programs. Located in New York.

Norris Cotton Cancer Center at Dartmouth-Hitchcock Medical Center

http://www.cancer.dartmouth.edu/index.shtml

An NCI-designated comprehensive cancer center in Lebanon, New Hampshire. Multidisciplinary teams work to provide the best treatment, cure, and recovery environment possible for patients through research, clinical trials, support groups, and education.

NYU Cancer Institute

http://www.med.nyu.edu/nyuci

Part of the New York University Medical Center in New York, it provides programs in patient care, research, prevention, and community outreach and education dealing with cancer.

Ohio State University Comprehensive Cancer Center

http://www.OSUCCC.osu.edu

An NCI-designated comprehensive cancer center in Columbus, Ohio, that translates research into high-quality patient care by offering educational programs, individualized treatments and preventive strategies designed to meet unique personal health care needs.

Rebecca and John Moores University of California, San Diego, Cancer Center

http://cancer.ucsd.edu

An NCI-designated comprehensive cancer center in San Diego, California, dedicated to translating research into promising new treatments and to providing community outreach to educate the public, especially underserved populations, about prevention studies and cancer information.

Robert H. Lurie Comprehensive Cancer Center of Northwestern University

http://www.cancer.northwestern.edu

An NCI-designated comprehensive cancer center in Chicago that performs laboratory and clinical cancer research and offers innovative cancer treatments involving clinical trials, cancer prevention and control programs, training and education of health care professionals, cancer information services, and community outreach and education.

Roswell Park Cancer Institute

http://www.roswellpark.org

America's first cancer center, now an NCI-designated comprehensive cancer center in Buffalo, New York, includes a comprehensive diagnostic and treatment center and a medical research complex.

St. Jude Children's Research Hospital

http://www.stjude.org

A comprehensive pediatric cancer center in Memphis, Tennessee, St. Jude is America's third-largest health care charity. Concentrates its efforts on researching and curing childhood cancers and diseases, becoming pioneers in unique procedures and cures.

The Sidney Kimmel Comprehensive Cancer Center at Johns Hopkins

http://www.hopkinskimmelcancercenter.org

An NCI-designated comprehensive cancer center in Baltimore, Maryland, dedicated to finding more effective cancer treatments through programs in clinical and laboratory research, education, community outreach, and prevention and control. Offers counseling, survivors and palliative care programs, and two residences for out-of-town patients.

Siteman Cancer Center at Barnes-Jewish Hospital and Washington University School of Medicine

http://www.siteman.wustl.edu

An NCI-designated comprehensive cancer center in St. Louis, Missouri, that provides expertise of research scientists and physicians, advanced diagnostic and treatment services, and an active outreach program of cancer screening and education.

Stanford Cancer Center

http://cancer.stanford.edu

An NCI-designated cancer center in Stanford, California, that uses the latest detection, diagnosis, treatment, and prevention discoveries with comprehensive support services to provide the most advanced patient care available.

UC Davis Cancer Center

http://www.ucdmc.ucdavis.edu/cancer

An NCI-designated cancer center in Sacramento, California, that provides multidisciplinary teams for patient care, clinical trials, and support groups and services, including the Triumph Fitness Program and the Writing as Healing Program. Web site provides survivor stories, news releases, and a link to its biannual magazine called *Synthesis*.

UCSF Helen Diller Family Comprehensive Cancer Center

http://cancer.ucsf.edu

An NCI-designated comprehensive cancer center in San Francisco that combines basic science, clinical research, population science, epidemiology/cancer control, and patient care.

University of Alabama at Birmingham Comprehensive Cancer Center

http://www3.ccc.uab.edu

An NCI-designated comprehensive cancer center in Birmingham, Alabama, that includes a large patient resource library, a preventive care program for women's cancers, many support groups, and its magazine called *Crossroads*.

University of Colorado Cancer Center

http://www.uccc.info

An NCI-designated comprehensive cancer center in Aurora, Colorado, that provides a multidisciplinary team approach to patient care. Web site offers information on support groups, patient programs and classes, spiritual counseling, and palliative care.

University of Michigan Comprehensive Cancer Center

http://www.mcancer.org

An NCI-designated comprehensive cancer center in Ann Arbor, Michigan, that provides research, patient care, a patient education resource center, complementary therapies, nutrition counseling, child and family life services, art therapy, and social work services.

University of Minnesota Cancer Center

http://www.cancer.umn.edu

An NCI-designated comprehensive cancer center in Minneapolis that strives to enhance knowledge of the prevention, causes, detection, and treatment of cancer to improve quality of life for patients and survivors through research, clinical trials, and education. Web site offers access to cancer center stories, news, and publications.

University of Nebraska Medical Center Eppley Cancer Center

http://www.unmc.edu:80/cancercenter

A comprehensive cancer center in Omaha, Nebraska, that performs cancer research and provides patient care and educational programs.

University of New Mexico Cancer Center

http://cancer.unm.edu

An NCI-designated cancer center in Albuquerque, New Mexico, integrates research, clinical trials, patient care, support services, and community outreach to serve its region's multiethnic populations.

University of Pittsburgh Cancer Institute

http://www.upci.upmc.edu

An NCI-designated comprehensive cancer center in Pittsburgh, Pennsylvania. Provides research, clinical trials, patient care, and education. Web site offers links to a variety of cancer-related publications.

University of Tennessee Cancer Institute

http://www.utcancer.com

A partnership between the University of Tennessee Health Science Center and Boston Baskin Cancer Group in Memphis, this institute provides surgical oncology, radiation oncology, gynecologic oncology, genetic counseling, multidisciplinary clinics, and cancer prevention and supportive care programs.

University of Virginia Health System Cancer Center

http://www.healthsystem.virginia.edu/internet/cancer

An NCI-designated cancer center in Charlottesville, Virginia, that provides cancer care teams, research, clinical trials, and support services.

University of Wisconsin Paul P. Carbone Comprehensive Cancer Center

http://www.cancer.wisc.edu

An NCI-designated comprehensive cancer center in Madison, Wisconsin, that provides research, clinical trials, patient care, and outreach. Web site provides information on news articles and outreach programs, including tobacco cessation and quality of life/pain and symptom management.

USC/Norris Comprehensive Cancer Center

http://ccnt.hsc.usc.edu

An NCI-designated comprehensive cancer center in Los Angeles that provides inpatient and outpatient care in its affiliated hospitals and outpatient clinics, conducts research and clinical trials, and translates that research into new patient therapies.

Vanderbilt-Ingram Cancer Center

http://www.vicc.org

An NCI-designated comprehensive cancer center in Nashville, Tennessee, that performs research and clinical trials and uses an interdisciplinary team approach to patient care; also provides childhood cancer programs.

Vermont Cancer Center at the University of Vermont

http://www.vermontcancer.org

An NCI-designated comprehensive cancer center in Burlington, Vermont, that provides interdisciplinary approaches to cancer research, prevention, patient care, and community education. Web site provides cancer, information, news, and information about support groups and services.

Wake Forest University Baptist Medical Center

http://www1.wfubmc.edu/cancer

An NCI-designated comprehensive cancer center in Winston-Salem, North Carolina, that provides patient care, clinical trials, research, pastoral care, support groups, and education. Web site provides drug interaction information, health encyclopedia, nutrition center, alternative and complementary medicine information, and a physician directory.

Yale Cancer Center at Yale University School of Medicine

http://yalecancercenter.org

An NCI-designated comprehensive cancer center in New Haven, Connecticut, that provides specialized team care, customized treatment plans, many support services, and a weekly informative radio show called *Yale Cancer Center Answers*. Web site offers an alphabetical list of cancer information and information on clinical trials and research.

▶ Cancer Support Groups

Adenoid Cystic Carcinoma Organization International

http://www.accoi.org

Provides information about adenoid cystic carcinoma. Offers support services in several different languages. Web site provides information on treatment options, research, clinical trials, the ACC tumor registry, and financial resources.

American Cancer Society

http://www.cancer.org

Educates the public about cancer, raises funds for cancer research, and runs support groups across the country. Web site provides links to a variety of support groups.

Association of Cancer Online Resources

http://www.acor.org

Provides links to more than one hundred mailing lists and support resources.

BC Cancer Agency

http://www.bccancer.bc.ca

Educates people of British Columbia and the Yukon about cancer, including prevention, screening, early detection, and treatment options, as well as alternative therapies. Offers one-on-one support services and support groups.

The Brain Tumor Society

http://www.tbts.org

Provides educational material and support services, including a newsletter called *Heads Up,* a monthly e-newsletter called *Head Lines,* and a comprehensive resource guide called *Color Me Hope.* Its COPE (Connection of Personal Experiences) program provides sharing of mutual experiences via e-mail and telephone conversations.

Breast Cancer Network of Strength

http://www.networkofstrength.org

Provides support services and resources for people affected by breast cancer and offers a twenty-four-hour breast cancer hotline with interpreters in 150 languages.

Cancer Hope Network

http://www.cancerhopenetwork.org

Provides free, confidential one-on-one support to those affected by cancer by specially trained cancer survivor volunteers.

CancerCare

http://www.cancercare.org

Provides free counseling and support, online and by telephone, in English and Spanish, by trained oncology social workers. Also provides financial assistance to those in need and affected by cancer.

The Carcinoid Cancer Foundation

http://www.carcinoid.org

Provides information on carcinoid cancer, treatment options, and clinical trials. Web site offers a list of doctors in the United States and Canada who specialize in treating carcinoid cancer, a list of carcinoid cancer support groups, resources for medical professionals, financial assistance resources, and archived articles.

The Childhood Brain Tumor Foundation

http://www.childhoodbraintumor.org

Provides information about brain tumors and cancer research, especially that related to childhood brain tumors. Offers the Childhood Cancer Ombudsman Program, which helps families with health insurance analysis and applications and with employment and educational difficulties that may arise during or after treatment.

Children's Cancer Association

http://www.childrenscancerassociation.org

Provides many resources and support services to help children and their families cope with cancer, including the DreamCatcher Wish program, the CCA Caring Cabin, and the Kids' Cancer Pages.

Colon Cancer Alliance

http://www.ccalliance.org

Provides support and educational resources for newly diagnosed colon cancer patients. Web site lists organizations and programs that may help with the financial issues related to medical treatment.

Colorectal Cancer Network

http://clickonium.com/colorectal-cancer.net/html

Provides a support network, including support groups, listserves, chat rooms, and a system of matching long-term survivors with newly diagnosed patients. Web site provides information about prevention and screening, treatment options, advocacy, and resources for newly diagnosed colon cancer patients.

Corporate Angel Network

http://www.corpangelnetwork.org

Arranges free travel on corporate jets, using empty seats on routine business flights, for cancer patients, bone marrow donors, and bone marrow recipients who are traveling to cancer treatment centers.

Florida Prostate Cancer Network

http://www.charityadvantage.com/www.florida-prostate-cancer.org/HomePage.asp

Educates men of Florida about the risks of developing prostate cancer. Supports research and promotes legislation to increase health insurance coverage of prostate cancer screenings. Web site offers information about early detection, support organizations, clinical trials, and current treatment options.

Gilda's Club Worldwide

http://www.gildasclub.org

Provides lectures, workshops, and support groups for those people whose lives have been touched by cancer, including a support program called *Noogieland* for children and teens. Web site lists Gilda's Clubhouse locations across the United States.

The Gynecologic Cancer Foundation

http://www.thegcf.org

Provides brochures and educational materials about gynecologic cancer. Supports research and training related to gynecologic cancers and organizes annual ovarian cancer survivor's courses.

International Myeloma Foundation

http://www.myeloma.org

Provides comprehensive information on myeloma treatment options, disease management, and programs and services for patients, family members, and health care professionals. Resources are available in fourteen languages. Web site offers educational resources, webcasts, a newsletter, and a toll-free hotline.

Lance Armstrong Foundation

http://www.livestrong.org

Provides survivorship education and resources, national advocacy initiatives, community programs, and scientific and clinical research grants. Web site provides information on LiveStrong SurvivorCare, a LiveStrong blog, a LiveStrong survivorship notebook, many cancer survivor brochures, sign-up for the LiveStrong Newsletter, and a link to the LiveStrong Store, where LiveStrong apparel and accessories can be purchased, the proceeds of which help support LiveStrong programs and services.

Leukemia and Lymphoma Society

http://www.leukemia-lymphoma.org

Provides information on leukemia, lymphoma, myeloma, and other blood cancers and support services for newly diagnosed and long-term survivors. Also supports research on blood cancers and pursues advocacy aimed at

governmental decision makers. Web site hosts several discussion boards and offers medical news, event listings, and treatment information. Informational booklets are published in English, Spanish, and French.

Linda Creed Breast Cancer Foundation

http://www.lindacreed.org

Provides educational materials about the detection, treatment, and survivorship of breast cancer; offers access to detection and treatment resources; provides financial assistance to women in the Philadelphia area receiving breast cancer treatment; and advocates for critical cancer legislation and governmental funding for breast cancer research.

Living Beyond Breast Cancer

http://www.lbbc.org

Provides educational programs and services to women affected by breast cancer, including a toll-free Survivors' Helpline, a quarterly newsletter called *Insight,* publications for African American and Latina women, current information about treatment options, and networking programs for women of color and young survivors.

Lung Cancer Alliance

http://www.lungcanceralliance.org

Provides support and advocacy for people at risk for and those living with lung cancer. Offers a peer-to-peer support network, toll-free information and referral services, and a quarterly newsletter called *Spirit and Breath.*

Lustgarten Foundation for Pancreatic Cancer Research

http://www.lustgarten.org/LUS/CDA/HomePage.jsp

Provides research grants to support pancreatic cancer research, information on clinical trials, and patient and caregiver support services. Web site provides information on selecting a treatment provider, an Ask an Expert series, research news, and information on legal, insurance, and benefits assistance.

Lymphoma Research Foundation

http://www.lymphoma.org

Raises funds for lymphoma research; provides educational materials on Hodgkin disease and non-Hodgkin lymphoma; provides information on diagnostic techniques, treatment options, and clinical trials; offers support for people living with lymphoma; sponsors lectures for scientists who conduct lymphoma research; and matches patients with peer support through its Lymphoma Support Network. Web site provides lymphoma news and features, fact sheets and booklets, and access to webcasts and podcasts.

Marti Nelson Cancer Foundation/ CancerActionNow.org

http://www.canceractionnow.org

Advocates for different options for cancer patients when standard treatments have not helped by providing information on nonstandard cancer treatment options, clinical trials, and experimental drugs.

Mautner Project, the National Lesbian Health Organization

http://www.mautnerproject.org

Offers support, advocacy, and educational information for lesbian, bisexual, and transgender women and their families, especially those living with cancer.

Melanoma International Foundation

http://www.melanomainternational.org

Provides melanoma facts, and tips on coping with a melanoma diagnosis. Web site provides an extensive list of melanoma treatment centers, forums, blogs, message boards, the latest news, and upcoming events.

National Brain Tumor Foundation

http://www.braintumor.org

Provides information about types of brain tumors, treatments, treatment centers, financial assistance, support services, and upcoming events as well as survivor stories and the latest news.

National Breast Cancer Coalition

http://www.natlbcc.org

Promotes breast cancer research and works toward improving access for all women to high-quality breast cancer screening, diagnosis, treatment, and care; informs and trains breast cancer survivors and others in effective advocacy efforts aimed at eradicating breast cancer. Web site provides breast cancer information, the latest news, and an e-newsletter.

National Cervical Cancer Coalition

http://www.nccc-online.org

Educates people about cervical cancer and the importance of early detection, advocates for quality patient care, and provides support through its Phone Pals and E-Pals programs. Web site provides links to many resources related to cervical cancer, the NCCC Store, and sign-up for its newsletter *Extraordinary Moments*.

National Coalition for Cancer Survivorship

http://www.canceradvocacy.org

Raises awareness about cancer survivorship issues, self-advocacy, and public advocacy, and provides resources for cancer patients, including information on types of cancer, treatment issues, side effects, financial advice,

and other cancer-related topics. Web site offers sign-up for online newsletter called *InterAction* and a Cancer Survival Toolbox.

National Lymphedema Network

http://www.lymphnet.org

Provides information about lymphedema and news about medical and scientific developments, sponsors a national conference and a patient summit, supports research into causes and possible alternative treatments, and advocates to standardize quality treatment for lymphedema patients. Web site lists treatment centers, health care professionals, and support groups.

National Ovarian Cancer Coalition

http://www.ovarian.org

Raises awareness and promotes education about ovarian cancer. Web site lists state chapters, support groups and services, and clinical trials, and provides the latest news, an NOCC newsletter, and medical information about ovarian cancer.

Native American Cancer Research

http://natamcancer.org

Provides culturally sensitive information and support to Native Americans living with cancer. Web site provides information on clinical trials, treatment, the Native American Cancer Survivors Network, and printable handouts.

Native People's Circle of Hope

http://www.nativepeoplescoh.org

A coalition of Native American cancer support groups in which Native American cancer survivors offer culturally sensitive support and counseling for newly diagnosed Native American cancer patients.

Oklahoma Brain Tumor Foundation

http://www.okbtf.org

Provides education, support groups, advocacy, and financial assistance for people in Oklahoma affected by primary brain or central nervous system tumors. Web site provides information about tumors, treatments, clinical trials, and area oncologists.

Oncolink

http://www.oncolink.com

Online cancer resource Web site operated by the University of Pennsylvania with an Ask the Experts page. Includes links to OncoLife, which offers an individualized survivorship care plan created on the basis of answers provided in a questionnaire; OncoTip of the Day; OncoPilot, a guide for navigating the cancer journey; and *OncoLink eNews*, a monthly newsletter.

Ovarian Cancer Canada

http://www.ovariancancercanada.ca

Provides ovarian cancer education, support, a quarterly newsletter, and other resources to Canadian residents. All services are available in English and French.

Ovarian Cancer Research Fund

http://www.ocrf.org

Promotes and raises funds for ovarian cancer research and its early diagnosis, and provides support and information to patients and loved ones, including an informational hotline mainly staffed by ovarian cancer survivor volunteers.

Pediatric Brain Tumor Foundation

http://www.pbtfus.org

Offers educational materials and support to children with brain tumors and their parents, and raises money for pediatric brain tumor research, awareness, and detection.

The Prostate Net

http://www.prostate-online.org

Provides information, support, and resources to simplify the treatment decision-making process.

Research Advocacy Network

http://www.researchadvocacy.org

Provides education, support, and advocacy by working with all participants in the medical research process to improve patient care.

Sarcoma Alliance

http://www.sarcomaalliance.org

Provides guidance, education, and support to those people whose lives have been affected by sarcoma. Web site provides information on services, programs, survivor and caregiver support groups, and an assistance fund developed to help sarcoma patients obtain second opinions from sarcoma specialists across the country.

SHARE: Self-help for Women with Breast or Ovarian Cancer

http://www.sharecancersupport.org

Trained breast or ovarian cancer survivors staff nationwide hotlines and run support groups and educational programs for women with breast or ovarian cancer in the New York metropolitan area.

Sisters Network

http://www.sistersnetworkinc.org

A national African American breast cancer survivorship organization that provides African American women with educational materials about breast cancer risk, symptoms, and treatment, as well as support services.

Skin Cancer Foundation

http://www.skincancer.org

Provides educational material about skin cancer prevention and detection. Web site provides information about different types of skin cancer, an Ask the Expert feature, and a physician finder database.

Support for People with Oral and Head and Neck Cancer

http://www.spohnc.org

Provides information and support groups for people living with oral cancer and cancers of the head and neck. Web site provides educational resources, information on clinical trials, and news releases.

Susan G. Komen for the Cure

http://www.komen.org

Funds research grants; provides breast cancer education; gives information about screening, treatment options, and community support groups; and provides a national toll-free helpline, which is available in English and Spanish.

ThyCa: Thyroid Cancer Survivors' Association

http://www.thyca.org

Provides information and support services for people living with thyroid cancer and hosts survivor workshops and an annual conference. Web site provides access to a new-patient packet, resource list, low iodine cookbook, and an online newsletter.

The Ulman Cancer Fund for Young Adults

http://www.ulmanfund.org

Provides educational programs and support groups for teens and young adults facing the challenges of cancer, and conducts community outreach programs as well as maintains a scholarship fund for young people who are facing or who have overcome cancer.

Us TOO International

http://www.ustoo.com

Provides prostate cancer education and a support network with hundreds of support groups across the United States, and advocates for increased funding for prostate cancer detection, diagnosis, treatment, and research. Web site provides a list of clinical trials, publications, informational newsletters, and a resource kit for newly diagnosed patients.

The Wellness Community

http://www.thewellnesscommunity.org

Provides online support groups in English and Spanish, as well as an online resource guide with information about various types of cancer, clinical trials, and advice on managing treatment side effects.

Wisconsin Multiple Myeloma Support Group

http://www.madison.com/communities/
multiplemyeloma

Hosts monthly support meetings and publishes a monthly newsletter that provides a resource list and notes on new research.

Young Survival Coalition

http://www.youngsurvival.org

Provides educational and support services that are unique to young women and breast cancer. Web site provides information about research, clinical trials, and programs; informational brochures; a quarterly newsletter; and an online bulletin board.

► Carcinogens

The following list of carcinogens is based on the National Toxicology Program's *Report on Carcinogens* (RoC, 11th ed.). Human carcinogens that are both "known" and "reasonably anticipated" are listed here, with a summary of each carcinogen along with its status (K for "known" or RA for "reasonably anticipated") according to the *ROC*. The *ROC* can be fully accessed as a PDF file for more in-depth technical description from the home page of the National Toxicology Program, http://ntp.niehs.nih.gov.

acetaldehyde: RA. Primarily used in the production of a variety of chemicals. Also found in tobacco, ripe fruit, wine, and other alcoholic beverages. Produced by plants as part of their normal life cycle. Main source of human exposure is through the metabolism of alcohol. Other sources include food, beverages, and, to a lesser extent, the air. Studies indicate an increased incidence of squamous cell carcinomas and adenocarcinomas in exposed laboratory animals; inadequate evidence to evaluate the carcinogenicity in humans.

2-acetylaminofluorene: RA. Used as a positive control by toxicologists. Potential human exposure includes inhalation and skin contact. Resulting cancers in laboratory animals include carcinomas of the urinary bladder and the liver and subcutaneous carcinomas on the face; no adequate data are available to evaluate the carcinogenicity in humans.

acrylamide: RA. Used in treating municipal drinking water and wastewater. Also found in home appliances, building materials, automotive parts, cosmetics, soaps, and lotions. Can be absorbed through unbroken skin, mucous membranes, lungs, and the gastrointestinal tract. Resulting cancers in laboratory animals; no adequate data are available to evaluate the carcinogenicity in humans.

acrylonitrile: RA. Used extensively in the manufacture of synthetic fibers, resins, plastics, elastomers, and rubber for consumer goods such as textiles, dinnerware, food containers, toys, luggage, automotive parts, small appliances, and telephones. A variety of cancers have developed in laboratory animals. Studies have indicated an increased risk of lung cancer in textile plant workers exposed to acrylonitrile.

Adriamycin (doxorubicin hydrochloride): RA. An antibiotic used in antimitotic chemotherapy to treat various neoplastic diseases; human exposure routes include injection, skin contact, and inhalation. Cancers that developed in laboratory animals include mammary tumors, bladder papillomas, urinary bladder tumors, and local sarcomas near injection sites. Although no adequate data are available to evaluate the carcinogenicity in humans, in a study of cancer patients receiving Adriamycin in combination with alkylating agents and radiotherapy, patients developed leukemia and bone cancer.

aflatoxins: K. Toxins produced by *Aspergillus* fungi that grow naturally on grains and other agricultural crops. Exposure occurs by eating contaminated foods or by inhalation of dust containing aflatoxins. Studies have confirmed carcinogenicity in humans resulting in liver cancer (hepatocellular carcinoma and primary liver-cell cancer).

alcoholic beverage consumption: K. Known or suspected as human carcinogens, include acetaldehyde, nitrosamines, aflatoxins, ethyl carbamate (urethane), asbestos, and arsenic compounds. Studies have indicated an increased risk of cancers of the mouth, pharynx, larynx, and esophagus with increased alcoholic beverage consumption, especially when combined with smoking.

2-aminoanthraquinone: RA. Used in the production of anthraquinone dyes, which are used in automotive paints, high-quality paints and enamels, textile dyes, plastics, rubber, and printing inks. Hepatocellular carcinomas, neoplastic nodules, and lymphomas have resulted in laboratory animals that have ingested 2-aminoanthraquinone; however, potential human exposure is through skin contact, and no adequate data are available to evaluate the carcinogenicity in humans.

o-**aminoazotoluene: RA.** Used in coloring oils, fats, waxes, and medicine, and in the production of the dyes Solvent Red 24 and Acid Red 115. Cancers of the liver, lungs, and urinary bladder have resulted in laboratory animals that have ingested *o*-aminoazotoluene; potential human exposure is through skin contact and inhalation and no adequate data are available to evaluate the carcinogenicity in humans.

4-aminobiphenyl: K. Previously used commercially as a rubber antioxidant, as a dye intermediate, and in the detection of sulfates; later used only in laboratory research because of sufficient evidence for carcinogenicity in humans.

1-amino-2,4-dibromoanthraquinone: RA. Used in the production of dyes, especially those used in textiles. Tumors in various sites have been reported in laboratory animals in which 1-amino-2,4-dibromoanthraquinone had been orally administered; however, no adequate data are available to evaluate the carcinogenicity in humans. Human exposure is primarily through skin contact.

1-amino-2-methylanthraquinone: RA. Was used in the production of dyes for synthetic fibers, furs, and thermoplastic resins, specifically for the dyes Solvent Blue 13 and Acid Blue 47. No longer commercially produced in the United States. Liver and kidney cancer have occurred in exposed laboratory animals; no adequate data are available to evaluate the carcinogenicity in humans. Human exposure would be primarily through skin contact and inhalation.

amitrole: RA. Widely used as an herbicide on annual and perennial broadleaf and grass-type weeds, on noncrop land prior to sowing, and as control of pondweeds. When administered in the diet of laboratory animals, increased incidence of tumors in the liver and thyroid occurred. No adequate data are available to evaluate the carcinogenicity in humans. Human exposure is through inhalation and skin contact or ingestion of contaminated food or drinking water.

o-**anisidine hydrochloride: RA.** Used in the production of dyes and pharmaceuticals, as a corrosion inhibitor for steel, and as an antioxidant for polymercaptan resins. Tumors of the urinary bladder, the renal pelvis, and the thyroid occurred in laboratory animals. No adequate data are available to evaluate the carcinogenicity in humans. Human exposure is through inhalation and skin contact; the general population may be exposed to the chemical as an environmental pollutant or through cigarette smoke.

arsenic compounds, inorganic: K. Used in a variety of substances ranging from pesticides to medicines; later more commonly used in pressure-treated wood. Effective December 31, 2003, a voluntary phaseout in wood for residential uses began. Also used in the production of lead alloys. Sufficient evidence confirms that humans exposed to arsenic compounds have increased risks of cancers of the skin, lung, digestive tract, liver, bladder, kidney, and lymphatic and hematopoietic systems. Occupational exposure includes inhalation and skin contact. For the general population, exposure is primarily through the ingestion of foods or by inhalation of contaminated air.

asbestos: K. Has been used in roofing, flooring, thermal and electrical insulation, cement pipe and sheets, friction materials, gaskets, coatings, plastics, textiles, paper, and other products. Banned in general-use garments, but it may be used in firefighting garments. Human exposure is primarily through inhalation and ingestion. Although the potential for exposure is widespread be-

cause of its previous extensive use, the potential for exposure continues to decline because of the elimination of asbestos products from the market. Sufficient evidence confirms that asbestos exposure in humans causes respiratory-tract cancer, pleural and peritoneal mesothelioma, lung cancer, laryngeal cancer, cancer of the digestive tract, and other cancers.

azacitidine: RA. Has been used in treatment of acute myeloblastic anemia, acute lymphoblastic leukemia, and myelodysplastic syndromes. Has been used in combination with other antineoplastic agents in cancer treatment trial protocols, as well as in clinical trials for beta thalassemia, acute myeloid leukemia, myelodysplastic syndrome, advanced or metastatic solid tumors, non-Hodgkin lymphoma, multiple myeloma, non-small-cell lung cancer, and prostate cancer. Malignant tumor formation at multiple tissue sites occurred in laboratory animals when administered by injection. No adequate data are available to evaluate the carcinogenicity in humans.

azathioprine: K. Used as an immunosuppressive agent, usually in combination with a corticosteroid, to prevent rejection following transplant surgery and to manage severe cases of rheumatoid arthritis in adults, and as a second-line treatment for some immunological diseases. A high occurrence of cancers in patients and others routinely treated with azathioprine confirms carcinogenicity in humans.

benzene: K. Used primarily as a solvent in the chemical and pharmaceutical industries, in the synthesis of numerous chemicals, and in gasoline. Also used in the production of styrene, phenol, acetone, cyclohexane, nitrobenzene, detergent alkylate, and chlorobenzenes. Benzene is known to cause leukemia.

benzidine and dyes metabolized to benzidine: K. Has been used in the production of azo dyes, fast-color salts, naphthols, sulfur dyes, and other dyeing compounds. Also used in clinical laboratories for detection of blood, as a rubber-compounding agent, in the manufacture of plastic films, for detection of hydrogen peroxide in milk, and for quantitative determination of nicotine. Most of these uses have been discontinued because of concerns about potential carcinogenicity. Although potential for exposure is low, human exposure may occur through inhalation, ingestion, or skin contact. Liver cancer has been reported in association with occupational exposure to benzidine, and limited evidence has associated it with a variety of other cancers.

benzotrichloride: RA. Used as a chemical intermediate to stabilize plastics in the presence of ultraviolet light, in the preparation of specific dyes and pigments, and to make benzotrifluoride, hydroxybenzophenone, antiseptics, and antimicrobial agents. Human exposure is through inhalation, ingestion, and skin contact. A variety of cancers have developed in laboratory animals exposed to benzotrichloride. Increased risk of respiratory cancer has been reported in humans involved in the production of chlorinated toluenes, which involves potential exposure to benzotrichloride and other chemicals; otherwise, no data are available to evaluate the carcinogenicity in humans.

beryllium and beryllium compounds: K. Used as an alloy, metal, and oxide in electrical components and in aerospace and defense applications. Also used in molds for injection-molded plastics, computers, home appliances, telecommunications devices, dental applications, bicycle frames, golf clubs, and many other applications. Inhalation of dusts and fumes is the primary route of human exposure, but it may also be ingested in drinking water or food. Studies showing an increased risk of lung cancer in occupational groups exposed to beryllium or beryllium compounds provide sufficient evidence of carcinogenicity in humans.

bromodichloromethane: RA. Used in the synthesis of organic chemicals and as a reagent in laboratory research. Also has been used to separate minerals and salts, as a flame retardant, and in fire extinguishers. It is also formed as a result of the chlorination treatment of drinking, waste, or cooling water. Human exposure is through the consumption of contaminated drinking water, beverages, and food products, and inhalation of contaminated ambient air. Tumors in the kidney, intestine, and liver have been reported in laboratory animals when administered by stomach tube. Sufficient data are not available to evaluate the carcinogenic effects in humans.

2,2-bis-(bromoethyl)-1,3-propanediol (technical grade): RA. Used as a flame retardant, especially in unsaturated polyester resins, molded products, and rigid polyurethane foam. Tumor formation at multiple tissue sites and leukemia occurred in laboratory animals. No data are available to evaluate the carcinogenicity in humans. Contamination occurs in the environment as dust and through wastewater; therefore, human exposure is through inhalation and skin contact.

1,3-butadiene: K. Used in a variety of rubber products. Also used in a number of industrial chemicals and in the manufacture of fungicides. Also found in gasoline, automobile exhausts, and cigarette smoke. Human exposure is primarily through inhalation; some exposure may occur from ingesting contaminated food or water, or through skin contact. Lymphatic and hematopoietic cancers have been reported in humans who have been exposed to 1,3-butadiene.

1,4-butanediol dimethanesulfonate (Myleran): K. Used in chemotherapeutic treatment by ingestion or intravenous administration to treat some forms of leukemia. Also may be used in combination with cyclophosphamide before bone marrow transplants for chronic myelogenous leukemia. Cancer at different tissue sites has been reported among leukemia patients receiving 1,4-butanediol dimethanesulfonate. Also, leukemia was reported in a follow-up study of bronchial cancer patients treated with 1,4-butanediol dimethanesulfonate.

butylated hydroxyanisole (BHA): RA. Used primarily as an antioxidant and preservative in an extensive list of foods (especially those containing vegetable oils and animal fats), food packaging, animal feed, and cosmetics, and in rubber and petroleum products. Administration in the diet induced tumors in the forestomach of laboratory animals. No data are available to evaluate the carcinogenicity in humans. Human exposure is through ingestion and skin contact.

cadmium and cadmium compounds: K. Used primarily in batteries. Cadmium compounds are used in analytical chemistry, calico printing, dyeing, mirrors, electron-beam-pumped lasers, electroplating, fluorescent screens, lubricants, nuclear reactors, photocopying, photographic emulsions, radiation detectors, smoke detectors, solar cells, thin-film transistors and diodes, phosphors, photomultipliers, and vacuum tubes. Also used as a fungicide, nematocide, or ascaricide; to color glass and porcelain; and in the production of cadmium-containing stabilizers and pigments for paints, glass, ceramics, plastics, textiles, paper, and fireworks. Human exposure is through ingestion of contaminated food, drinking water, soil, and dust, and inhalation of particles of cadmium from ambient air or cigarette smoke. The largest intake of cadmium is estimated to come from cereal grain products, potatoes, and other vegetables. Studies have confirmed that exposure to various cadmium compounds increases the risk of lung cancer. Evidence also suggests an increased risk of prostate, kidney, and bladder cancer.

carbon tetrachloride: RA. Used primarily in the production of Freon 11 and 12. Human exposure is through inhalation, ingestion, and skin contact. The general population is most likely exposed through air and drinking water. Liver tumors occurred in laboratory animals exposed to carbon tetrachloride. Although no adequate data are available to evaluate the carcinogenicity in humans, liver tumors, respiratory cancers, and leukemia have been reported in humans exposed to carbon tetrachloride.

ceramic fibers (respirable size): RA. Used as insulation materials, primarily for lining furnaces and kilns and as replacement for asbestos. Products produced using ceramic fibers are blankets, boards, bulk fibers, felts, vacuum-formed or cast shapes, paper, and textile products. Human exposure is through inhalation, mainly in the manufacturing environment, during installation, and during removal. Tumors of the lung occurred in laboratory animals. No adequate studies have confirmed carcinogenicity in humans.

chlorambucil: K. Used primarily in the treatment of chronic lymphocytic leukemia and primary (Waldenström) macroglobulinemia. Also used as an immunosuppressive agent in the treatment of systemic lupus erythematosus, acute and chronic glomerular nephritis, nephrotic syndrome, chronic active hepatitis, cold agglutinic disease, psoriasis, and Wegener granulomatosis. Human exposure is through ingestion, inhalation, and skin contact. Increased risk of cancers, especially acute nonlymphocytic leukemia, has been reported with exposure to chlorambucil.

chloramphenicol: RA. An antimicrobial agent used to combat serious infections; has restricted use because it causes blood dyscrasia. Human exposure is primarily by the oral or topical route through its use as a drug; exposure also may occur through inhalation, ingestion, skin contact, or contact with contaminated water or soil. Although no adequate studies have confirmed cancers in laboratory animals exposed to chloramphenicol, many human case reports have implicated chloramphenicol as a cause of aplastic anemia and an increased risk of leukemia.

chlorendic acid: RA. Used primarily as a flame retardant in polyester resins and coatings, epoxy resins, and polyurethane foams. Also used in the manufacture of corrosion-resistant polyester resins, oil-modified paints and coatings, flame-retardant additives, extreme pressure lubricants, and epoxy resins used in printed circuit boards. Human exposure is primarily through skin contact; small exposure may occur through inhalation. Tumors of the liver, pancreas, lung, and preputial gland occurred in laboratory animals in which chlorendic acid was administered in the diet. No data are available to evaluate the carcinogenicity in humans.

chlorinated paraffins (C_{12}, 60 percent chlorine): RA. Used primarily as extreme-pressure lubricant additives in metalworking and in flame retardants and plasticizers for plastics. Also used in rubber, paints, adhe-

sives, caulks, and sealants, and as a plasticizer in inks, paper and textile coatings, and flexible polyvinyl chloride. Tumors of the liver, kidney, and thyroid gland, as well as leukemia, occurred in laboratory animals in which chlorinated paraffins were administered by stomach tube. No data are available to evaluate the carcinogenicity in humans.

1-(2-chloroethyl)-3-cyclohexyl-1-nitrosourea (CCNU): RA. Has limited use in the treatment of Hodgkin disease, brain tumors, colorectal tumors, and specific pulmonary malignancies. Human exposure is through ingestion, inhalation, and skin contact. Tumors of the lung and lymphosarcomas occurred in laboratory animals in which CCNU was administered by injection. No adequate data are available to evaluate the carcinogenicity in humans; however, cases of leukemia have been reported in cancer patients who have received CCNU.

1-(2-chloroethyl)-3-(4-methylcyclohexyl)-1-nitrosourea (methyl-CCNU): K. Used an investigational drug in the treatment of several types of cancers. Clinical trials in which cancer patients were given adjuvant treatment with methyl-CCNU showed an increased risk of developing leukemia and preleukemia.

bis(chloroethyl) nitrosourea (BCNU): RA. Used in the treatment of Hodgkin disease, multiple myeloma, and brain tumors. Human exposure is through injection, inhalation, and skin contact. Tumors of the lung and peritoneal cavity have occurred in laboratory animals administered BCNU by injection. Limited evidence of carcinogenicity in humans is available in that BCNU is associated with acute nonlymphocytic leukemia following its use with other anticancer therapies in the treatment of previously existing cancer.

chloroform: RA. Primarily used to produce hydrochlorofluorocarbon-22; also used as a solvent and in certain medical procedures. Human exposure is through inhalation, skin contact with water, and ingestion, primarily drinking water. Tumors of the kidney and liver occurred in laboratory animals that were exposed to chloroform. There is no adequate evidence of carcinogenicity in humans; however, some studies indicate that there is an association between cancer of the large intestine, rectum, and urinary bladder and the components of chlorinated water.

bis(chloromethyl) ether (BCME) and technical-grade chloromethyl methyl ether (CMME): K. Used primarily as chemical intermediates and alkylating agents. Human exposure is through inhalation and skin contact; however, probability of exposure is very low. Potential for exposure is greatest for chemical plant workers, ion-exchange resin makers, laboratory workers, and polymer makers. Studies have demonstrated that occupational exposure causes lung cancer.

3-chloro-2-methylpropene: RA. Used primarily in the production of carbofuran, an insecticide used mostly on corn. Also used in the production of plastics, pharmaceuticals, herbicides, and other organic chemicals; as a textile additive; and as a perfume additive. Human exposure is through inhalation, ingestion, and skin contact. Tumors of the forestomach occurred in laboratory animals when administered by stomach tube. No data are available to evaluate the carcinogenicity in humans.

4-chloro-*o*-phenylenediamine: RA. Patented as a hair dye component and used in the production of a photographic chemical, as a curing agent for epoxy resins, and as a reagent in gas chromatography. Human exposure is through ingestion, inhalation, and skin contact. Little exposure is expected in the general population due to its limited use in consumer products. Tumors of the urinary bladder and liver occurred in laboratory animals when administered in the diet. No data are available to evaluate the carcinogenicity in humans.

chloroprene: RA. Used in the production of neoprene, a synthetic rubber used in the production of automotive and mechanical rubber goods, adhesives, caulks, construction goods, fiber binding, footwear, flame-resistant cushioning, fabric coatings, roof coatings, and sealants for dams or locks in waterways. Human exposure is through inhalation. Inhalation exposure in laboratory animals induced tumor formation at multiple tissue sites. Limited data demonstrating that occupational exposure to chloroprene increases the risk for various tumors may suggest carcinogenicity in humans.

***p*-chloro-*o*-toluidine and *p*-chloro-*o*-toluidine hydrochloride: RA.** Has been used to produce azo dyes for cotton, silk, acetate, and nylon, and to produce Pigment Red 7 and Pigment Yellow 49, as well as in the manufacture of the pesticide chlordimeform. Human exposure is through inhalation, ingestion, and skin contact. Increased incidences of urinary bladder tumors have been documented in workers exposed to *p*-chloro-*o*-toluidine; however, as they were also exposed to numerous other compounds, this provides limited evidence of carcinogenicity in humans. Increased incidence of tumors occurred in laboratory animals exposed to *p*-chloro-*o*-toluidine hydrochloride.

chlorozotocin: RA. Used in the investigational treatment of various cancers. Human exposure is through intravenous administration. An increased incidence of sarcoma and mesothelioma in the peritoneal cavity, and tumors of the nervous system, lungs, and forestomach, occurred in laboratory animals in which chlorozotocin was administered. No adequate data are available to evaluate the carcinogenicity in humans.

chromium hexavalent compounds: K. Used as corrosion inhibitors, in wood preservatives, in leather tanning, in metal finishing and chrome plating, in stainless-steel production, and in the manufacture of pigments. Also used in textile dyeing processes, printing inks, drilling muds, pyrotechnics, water treatment, and chemical synthesis. Residential uses as wood preservatives are expected to decrease because of a voluntary phase-out that went into effect December 31, 2003. Exposure for the general population is through inhalation of the ambient air, ingestion of water, or skin contact. Increased risks of lung cancer and a rare cancer of the sinonasal cavity among workers engaged in chromate production, chromate pigment production, and chromium plating have been reported. Other studies suggest that exposure to chromium may also be associated with cancer at other tissue sites, including leukemia and bone cancer.

C.I. Basic Red 9 monohydrochloride: RA. Used primarily in a nutrient agar for bacterium identification; as a biological stain; in a commercial magenta dye used for coloring textiles, china clay products, leather, and printing inks; and as a filter dye in photography. Also used in tinting automobile antifreeze solutions and toilet sanitary preparations. Human exposure is primarily through skin contact. A variety of tumors have occurred in laboratory animals exposed to the compound. An increase in urinary bladder tumors in workers involved in the manufacture of magenta dye has been reported; however, inadequate evidence is available to determine if this is attributable to exposure to the magenta or to other intermediates and impurities.

cisplatin: RA. Used in the treatment of various malignancies, often in combination with other cancer treatments. Human exposure is not only through treatment but also through skin absorption and inhalation. Significant increases in the incidence and number of lung adenomas and skin papillomas, as well as leukemia, occurred in laboratory animals in which cisplatin was administered by injection. No adequate data are available to evaluate the carcinogenicity in humans.

coal tars and coal tar pitches: K. Used primarily for the production of refined chemicals and coal tar products. Have also been used in surface-coating formulations, pesticides, and epoxy-resin surface coatings, and as fuel in open-hearth furnaces and blast furnaces in the steel industry. U.S. pharmacopeia-grade coal tar is used in denatured alcohol and in preparations used to treat various skin conditions. Coal tar pitches are used primarily as the binder for aluminum-smelting electrodes and in roofing materials, refractory brick, and surface coatings; as a binder for foundry cores; and to produce pitch coke. Also used for road paving and construction, as well as in the production of naphthalene, recovery of benzene, production of anthracene paste, briquetting of smokeless solid fuel, impregnation of electrodes and fibers, and manufacture of electrodes and graphite. Human exposure is through inhalation, ingestion, and skin contact. Increased incidences of leukemia and a variety of other cancers have occurred in humans exposed to coal tars or coal tar pitches. Coal tars and coal tar pitches contain known and potential carcinogens, such as benzene, naphthalene, and other polycyclic aromatic hydrocarbons.

cobalt sulfate: **RA.** Used in the electrochemical and electroplating industries; as a drier in lithographic inks, varnishes, paints, and linoleum; and in storage batteries, ceramics, enamels, glazes, and porcelain. Has been used in animal feeds as a mineral supplement and on pastures to supplement forage with cobalt, as well as in beers and to treat anemia in people not responsive to other treatments. Human exposure is through inhalation of ambient air and ingestion of food or drinking water. Occupational exposure also includes skin contact. Tumors of the lung and adrenal gland occurred in laboratory animals when administered by inhalation. No significant data are available to evaluate the carcinogenicity in humans.

coke oven emissions: **K.** Used in iron-making blast furnaces, to synthesize calcium carbide, and to manufacture graphite and electrodes. Coke oven gas is used as a fuel. Coke by-products may be refined into commodity chemicals, such as benzene, toluene, naphthalene, sulfur, and ammonium sulfate. Human exposure to coke oven emissions is through inhalation and skin contact. A variety of cancers have been reported in humans exposed to coke oven emissions.

p-cresidine: **RA.** Used exclusively in the production of azo dyes and pigments—such as Direct Orange 72, FD&C Red 40, and Direct Violet 9—to be used in the textile industry. Human exposure is through inhalation and skin contact. Increased incidences of urinary bladder cancer, liver cancer, and olfactory neuroblastomas occurred in laboratory animals when administered in the diet. No adequate data are available to evaluate the carcinogenicity in humans.

cupferron: **RA.** Used to separate and precipitate metals such as copper, iron, vanadium, and thorium; also used in analytical laboratories. Human exposure is through ingestion and inhalation of dust from the dry salt, and through skin contact. Hemangiosarcomas and a variety of tumors have occurred in laboratory animals when administered in the diet. No data are available to evaluate the carcinogenicity in humans.

cyclophosphamide: **K.** Used to treat a variety of cancers; also used as an immunosuppressive agent following organ transplants or to treat autoimmune disorders. Exposure for the general population is through medical treatment; occupational exposure is through skin contact or inhalation of dust. Bladder cancer and leukemia have been reported in patients administered cyclophosphamide.

cyclosporin A: **K.** Used as an immunosuppressive agent in the prevention and treatment of graft-versus-host reactions in bone marrow transplantation and for the prevention of rejection of organ transplants. Has also been tested for the treatment of a variety of diseases. Human exposure is through intravenous and oral administration. Lymphoma and skin cancer have been reported in transplant recipients, psoriasis patients, and rheumatoid arthritis patients treated with cyclosporin A.

dacarbazine: **RA.** Used in the treatment of Hodgkin disease, malignant melanomas, neuroblastomas, osteogenic sarcomas, and soft-tissue sarcomas, and occasionally in the therapy for other neoplastic diseases that have become resistant to alternative treatment. Human exposure is through injection, inhalation, and skin contact. A variety of cancers have resulted in laboratory animals when administered dacarbazine. No adequate data are available to evaluate the carcinogenicity in humans.

danthron (1,8-dihydroxyanthraquinone): **RA.** Used in synthetic lubricants, experimental antitumor agents, a fungicide used to control powdery mildew, and certain dyes. Tumors of the colon, cecum, and liver occurred in laboratory animals when administered in the diet. No adequate data are available to evaluate the carcinogenicity in humans.

2,4-diaminoanisole sulfate: **RA.** Used primarily in hair and fur dyes; also used in production of C.I. Basic Brown 2, which is used to dye clothing and is also an ingredient in shoe polishes. Human exposure is through skin contact and inhalation. Tumors at various tissue sites occurred in laboratory animals when administered in the diet. No adequate data are available to evaluate the carcinogenicity in humans.

2,4-diaminotoluene: **RA.** Used primarily in the production of toluene diisocyanate, which is used to produce polyurethane. Also used to produce dyes for biological stains, furs, leathers, textiles, and wood. Human exposure is through skin contact and inhalation. Tumors of the liver and mammary gland and lymphomas occurred in laboratory animals when administered in the diet, and local tumors occurred when injected. No adequate data are available to evaluate the carcinogenicity in humans.

diazoaminobenzene (DAAB): RA. Used in organic synthesis and in the manufacture of insecticides and dyes, particularly D&C Red no. 33, FD&C Yellow no. 5 (tartrazine), and FD&C Yellow no. 6, which are used in drugs and cosmetics; the latter two are allowed in food. Human exposure is through ingestion of products containing those dyes or skin contact with these products. DAAB is metabolized to benzene, a known human carcinogen that causes leukemia; evidence also shows that DAAB causes genetic damage.

1,2-dibromo-3-chloropropane: RA. Before being banned by the Environmental Protection Agency in 1985, 1,2-dibromo-3-chloropropane was used as a pesticide; later used only for research purposes. Human exposure is probably minimal; however, ingestion of previously contaminated drinking water and food may occur. A variety of cancers have resulted in laboratory animals when exposed to 1,2-dibromo-3-chloropropane. There is inadequate evidence for the carcinogenicity in humans.

1,2-dibromoethane (ethylene dibromide): RA. Used to make vinyl bromide, a flame retardant in modacrylic fibers. Also used as a nonflammable solvent for resins, gums, and waxes, and used in the preparation of dyes and pharmaceuticals. Formerly used in lead gasoline and as a pesticide, it is still detected in ambient air, soil, groundwater, and food. Major source of human exposure is through the ingestion of contaminated drinking water. A variety of cancers have resulted in laboratory animals when exposed to 1,2-dibromoethane. There is inadequate evidence for the carcinogenicity in humans.

2,3-dibromo-1-propanol (DBP): RA. Used in the production of flame retardants, insecticides, and pharmaceuticals. Human exposure is through inhalation and skin contact. A variety of tumors have occurred in laboratory animals when painted onto the skin for numerous weeks. There is inadequate evidence for the carcinogenicity in humans.

tris(2,3-dibromopropyl) phosphate: RA. Previously used as a flame-retardant additive for textiles and plastics. It was banned in 1977 for use in children's clothing and in any textiles intended for use in clothing and is no longer used in the United States; however, in 1978, the Consumer Product Safety Commission identified twenty-

two products containing the compound that were still commercially available. Human exposure is through inhalation, skin contact, and ingestion. A variety of cancers have resulted in laboratory animals exposed to tris(2,3-dibromopropyl) phosphate. There is inadequate evidence for the carcinogenicity in humans.

1,4-dichlorobenzene: RA. Used primarily as a space deodorant and as an insecticide fumigant for moth control. Also used in the production of polyphenylene sulfide and in the production of 1,2,4-trichlorobenzene; yellow, red, and orange pigments; air deodorizers; dyes; pharmaceuticals; and resin-bonded abrasives. Also used as a germicide/disinfectant, soil fumigant, insecticide, pesticide, animal repellent, and an agent to control mold and mildew growth. Human exposure is primarily through inhalation; skin contact and ingestion are also routes of potential exposure. Tumors of the kidney and liver occurred in laboratory animals when administered by stomach tube. No adequate data are available to evaluate the carcinogenicity in humans.

3,3′-dichlorobenzidine and 3,3′-dichlorobenzidine dihydrochloride: RA. Used primarily in the manufacture of pigments for printing ink, paint, paper, plastics, rubber, and textiles, and as a curing agent for isocyanate-containing polymers and solid urethane plastics. Human exposure is through inhalation of airborne dust, ingestion of contaminated well water near hazardous waste sites, and skin contact. Tumors at multiple tissue sites and leukemia occurred in laboratory animals administered the compound. No adequate data are available to evaluate the carcinogenicity in humans.

dichlorodiphenyltrichloroethane (DDT): RA. Used extensively as an insecticide until 1972, when it was banned for the majority of uses in the United States. Later used only under official supervision for public health emergencies or for health quarantine. Although residue levels have been declining, DDT is still being detected in air, soil, rain, water, animal and plant tissues, food, and the work environment, and can be ingested in small amounts from some foods. Tumors at multiple tissue sites occurred in laboratory animals administered DDT. There is inadequate evidence for the carcinogenicity in humans.

1,2-dichloroethane (ethylene dichloride): RA. Used primarily to produce vinyl chloride, although it has been used as a solvent, degreaser, insect fumigant, and general anesthetic, among other uses. Human exposure is through inhalation, ingestion, and skin contact. Tumors at multiple tissue sites occurred in laboratory animals administered 1,2-dichloroethane. No adequate data are available to evaluate carcinogenicity in humans.

dichloromethane (methylene chloride): RA. Used primarily as a solvent in paint removers. Used also as an aerosol propellant; as a processing solvent in the manufacture of steroids, antibiotics, vitamins, and tablet coatings; as a degreasing agent; in electronics manufacturing, and as a polyurethane foam blowing agent. Also used in spray shoe polish, water repellents, spot removers, cleaners, glues, adhesive removers, and lubricants, among other products. Human exposure is through inhalation, ingestion, and, to a limited degree, skin absorption. Increased incidences of alveolar/bronchiolar neoplasms, hepatocellular neoplasms, and fibroadenoma of the mammary gland occurred in laboratory animals when administered by inhalation. No adequate data are available to evaluate the carcinogenicity in humans.

1,3-dichloropropene (technical grade): RA. Used in the manufacture of 3,3-dichloro-1-propene and other pesticides, such as Telone II, a widely used agricultural soil fumigant for parasitic nematodes. Human exposure is through inhalation of vapors, ingestion of contaminated foods and water, and skin contact. A variety of tumors occurred in laboratory animals when Telone II was administered by stomach tube, and injection-site fibrosarcomas occurred when administered by injection. No adequate data are available to evaluate the carcinogenicity in humans.

diepoxybutane: RA. Not produced commercially in the United States since 1978; however, may be used in small quantities for research, as a curing agent for polymers, in textile fabrics, and to synthesize erythritol and other pharmaceuticals. Human exposure is through inhalation and skin contact. Skin cancer occurred in laboratory animals when applied topically; local fibrosarcomas and lung tumors occurred when administered by injection. No adequate data are available to evaluate the carcinogenicity in humans.

diesel exhaust particulates: RA. Come from vehicles, oil and gas production facilities, stationary engines, repair yards, chemical manufacturing, and electric utilities. The type and condition of the engine, fuel composition and additives, operating conditions, and emission control devices determine the composition and quantity of the emissions from an engine. Limited evidence of increased risk for lung cancer has been found in human studies.

diethyl sulfate: RA. Used primarily in dyes, pigments, textiles, and carbonless papers. Also used in cosmetics, household products, pharmaceuticals, agricultural chemicals, and some laboratory chemical processes. Human exposure is through inhalation and skin con-

tact. Administration by injection induced local sarcomas in laboratory animals and tumors of the nervous system in their offspring; tumors of the forestomach occurred when administered by stomach tube. Limited evidence is available for the carcinogenicity in humans; a study found excess mortality from laryngeal cancer in workers exposed to high concentrations of diethyl sulfate.

diethylstilbestrol: K. Originally used as synthetic estrogen, and then widely prescribed for other uses in human medicine. Its use has since been reduced because of its cardiovascular toxicity and its link to a rare vaginal cancer in female offspring and possibly to testicular cancer among male offspring when given to pregnant mothers. Used in clinical trials for treatment of prostate and breast cancer and in biochemical research.

diglycidyl resorcinol ether: RA. Used as a liquid spray epoxy resin and in other epoxy resins used in electrical, tooling, adhesive, and laminating applications. Also used in polysulfide rubber and in certain pavements, and as a coating for metal. Human exposure is through inhalation and skin contact. Tumors of the forestomach of laboratory animals occurred when administered by stomach tube. No adequate data is available to evaluate the carcinogenicity in humans.

3,3′-dimethoxybenzidine and dyes metabolized to 3,3′-dimethoxybenzidine: RA. Used in production of dyes and pigments, as well as in the production of *o*-dianisidine diisocyanate for use in adhesives and as a component of polyurethanes. Human exposure is through inhalation and skin contact. Tumors at multiple tissue sites occurred in laboratory animals when administered 3,3′-dimethoxybenzidine. No adequate data are available to evaluate the carcinogenicity in humans.

4-dimethylaminoazobenzene: RA. No longer produced or used commercially in the United States; previously used to color polishes and other wax products, polystyrene, and soap. Human exposure is through inhalation and skin contact. Tumors at multiple tissue sites occurred in laboratory animals when administered 4-dimethylaminoazobenzene. No adequate data are available to evaluate the carcinogenicity in humans.

3,3′-dimethylbenzidine and dyes metabolized to 3,3′-dimethylbenzidine: RA. Used in production of dyes and pigments, as well as in the production of polyurethane-based high-strength elastomers, coatings, and rigid plastics. Also used in clinical laboratories in test tapes for the detection of blood and by water companies and swimming pool owners to test for chlorine in water or air. Human exposure is through inhalation, ingestion, and skin contact. Tumors at multiple tissue sites occurred in laboratory animals when administered 3,3′-dimethylbenzidine. No adequate data are available to evaluate the carcinogenicity in humans.

dimethylcarbamoyl chloride: RA. Used primarily in the production of dyes, pharmaceuticals, and pesticides. Human exposure is through inhalation and skin contact. Skin cancer was induced in laboratory animals when applied topically, local sarcomas when injected, and tumors of the nasal tract when inhaled. No adequate data are available to evaluate the carcinogenicity in humans.

1,1-dimethylhydrazine: RA. Used primarily as a component of jet and rocket fuels. Also used in organic peroxide fuel additives, in photography, as an absorbent for acid gases, and as a plant growth control agent. Human exposure is through inhalation, ingestion, and skin contact. Increased incidences of lung tumors occurred in laboratory animals when administered by stomach tube, and angiosarcomas in various organs and tumors of the kidneys, lungs, and liver when administered in drinking water. No adequate data are available to evaluate the carcinogenicity in humans.

dimethyl sulfate: RA. Used in the manufacture of dyes, drugs, perfumes, pesticides, phenol derivatives, and other organic chemicals. Also used in polyurethane-based adhesives, in the analysis of auto fluids, and as a solvent for the separation of mineral oils. Human exposure is through inhalation and skin contact. Squamous cell carcinomas of the nasal cavity occurred in laboratory animals when administered by inhalation, local sarcomas when administered by injection, and tumors of the nervous system in offspring when administered by intravenous injection to pregnant animals. There is inadequate evidence for the carcinogenicity in humans; however, cases of bronchial carcinoma, pulmonary carcinoma, and choroidal melanoma have been reported in some humans exposed to dimethyl sulfate.

dimethylvinyl chloride: RA. Not used commercially; only for research. Human exposure is through inhalation. Cancers of the nasal cavity, oral cavity, esophagus, and forestomach have occurred in laboratory animals when administered by stomach tube. No data are available to evaluate the carcinogenicity in humans.

1,6-dinitropyrene: RA. Not used commercially; available for research purposes. Found in particulate emissions from combustion sources, especially diesel exhaust. Studies have determined malignant tumor formation at multiple sites in laboratory animals when exposed to 1,6-dinitropyrene by multiple routes. Human studies show limited evidence of increased risk for lung cancer

when exposed to diesel exhaust particulates; however, it has not been determined whether 1,6-dinitropyrene is responsible.

1,8-dinitropyrene: RA. Not used commercially; available for research purposes. Found in particulate emissions from combustion sources, especially diesel exhaust. Human studies show limited evidence of increased risk for lung cancer when exposed to diesel exhaust particulates; however, it has not been determined whether 1,8-dinitropyrene is responsible. Studies have determined malignant tumor formation at multiple sites in laboratory animals when exposed to 1,8-dinitropyrene by multiple routes.

1,4-dioxane: RA. Used primarily as a stabilizer in chlorinated solvents; also used as a solvent, in textile processing, and in laboratory research and testing. Human exposure is through inhalation, ingestion, and skin contact. Increased incidence of cancers of the nasal turbinates, liver, gallbladder, lung, and skin occurred in laboratory animals exposed to 1,4-dioxane. Inadequate evidence for the carcinogenicity in humans.

Disperse Blue 1: RA. An anthraquinone dye used in hair color formulations and in coloring fabrics and plastics. Human exposure is through inhalation and skin contact. Tumor development in the urinary bladder and liver occurred in laboratory animals exposed to Disperse Blue 1. There is inadequate evidence for the carcinogenicity in humans.

epichlorohydrin: RA. Used in the production of epoxy resins, synthetic glycerin, elastomers, and other synthetic materials. Has also been used to cure propylene-base rubbers, as a solvent for cellulose esters and ethers, and in resins for the paper industry; also widely used as a stabilizer. Human exposure is through ingestion, inhalation, and skin contact. Tumors of the forestomach occurred in laboratory animals when administered by stomach tube, tumors of the nasal cavity when administered by inhalation, and local sarcomas when administered by injection. There is inadequate evidence for the carcinogenicity in humans.

erionite: K. Belonging to a group of minerals called zeolites, erionite is no longer mined or marketed for commercial purposes. Domestic uses for natural zeolite are pet litter, animal feed, horticultural applications, oil absorbent, odor control, desiccant, pesticide carrier, water purification, aquaculture, wastewater cleanup, gas absorbent, and other miscellaneous applications. The use of other zeolites may result in potential human exposure to erionite. Deposits of fibrous erionite are found in Arizona, Nevada, Oregon, and Utah, and erionite fibers have been detected in road dust in Nevada, potentially exposing humans to erionite in ambient air. Mesothelioma and lung cancer have been linked to erionite exposure.

estrogens, steroidal: K. Most commonly used for estrogen replacement therapy or in combination with a progestogen for hormone replacement therapy. Also used in oral contraceptives; to treat breast cancer, prostate cancer, and other medical conditions; and for biomedical research. Unopposed estrogens have been shown to cause uterine endometrial cancer; however, addition of a progestogen greatly diminishes that risk. Some evidence also suggests an increased risk of breast cancer.

ethylene oxide: K. Used primarily in the production of several industrial chemicals, such as ethylene glycol (antifreeze), nonionic surfactants (detergents and dishwashing formulations), glycol ethers (solvents), ethanolamines (used in soaps, detergents, and textile chemicals), diethylene glycol (used in resins, plasticizers, and acrylate), triethylene glycol (used in dehydration of natural gas), polyethylene glycol (osmotic laxative), urethane polyols, fumigants, sterilizing agents, disinfectants, and insecticides. Human exposure is through inhalation and ingestion; very low risk of exposure from skin contact. An association between exposure to ethylene oxide and an increased risk of leukemia, stomach cancer, breast cancer, and lymphatic and hematopoietic cancers has been reported.

ethylene thiourea: RA. Used primarily in neoprene and polyacrylate rubbers. Also used in pesticides, dyes, pharmaceuticals, and synthetic resins, and in electroplating baths and antioxidant production. Human exposure is through inhalation, ingestion, and skin contact. Cancer of the thyroid, liver, and pituitary gland occurred in laboratory animals exposed to ethylene thiourea.

di(2-ethylhexyl) phthalate: RA. Used as a plasticizer in polyvinyl chloride (PVC) resins for fabricating flexible vinyl products; also used to manufacture non-PVC plasticizer. A variety of miscellaneous uses for di(2-ethylhexyl) phthalate exist. Human exposure is through inhalation, ingestion, and skin contact, and through medical procedures. Tumors of the liver occurred in laboratory animals when administered in the diet. No adequate data are available to evaluate the carcinogenicity in humans.

ethyl methanesulfonate: RA. Used in laboratory research; not produced commercially in the United States. Tumors of the lung and kidney occurred in laboratory animals exposed to ethyl methanesulfonate. No adequate data are available to evaluate the carcinogenicity in humans.

formaldehyde (gas): RA. Used primarily for the production of urea-formaldehyde and phenolic resins (adhesives in pressed-wood products and building materials); also used to make other chemicals, household products, preservatives, permanent press fabrics, and paper product coatings. Human exposure is through inhalation and skin contact. Some studies have shown excess incidences of nasopharyngeal cancers in humans exposed to formaldehyde (gas).

furan: RA. Used primarily in the production of tetrahydrofuran (solvent), pyrrole, and thiophene. Also used in the formation of lacquers, as a solvent for resins, and in the production of agricultural chemicals (insecticides), pharmaceuticals, and stabilizers. Human exposure is through inhalation. Liver cancers and leukemia occurred in laboratory animals when administered by stomach tube. No adequate data are available to evaluate the carcinogenicity in humans.

glass wool (respirable size): RA. Used primarily in acoustical, electrical, and thermal insulation; filtration media; and weatherproofing. Human exposure is through inhalation and skin or eye contact. Various tumors and mesotheliomas occurred in laboratory animals when exposed to glass wool. There is inadequate evidence for the carcinogenicity in humans.

glycidol: RA. Used in many pharmaceutical and fine chemical applications, in the manufacture of vinyl polymers and natural oils, and in the synthesis of glycerol, glycidyl ethers, and amines. Also used as an alkylating agent, as a demulsifer, as a dye-leveling agent, and for sterilizing milk of magnesia. Human exposure is through inhalation, skin and eye contact, and ingestion. Tumors at multiple sites occurred in laboratory animals when administered by stomach tube. No adequate data are available to evaluate the carcinogenicity in humans.

hepatitis B virus (HBV): K. A virus that infects liver cells, causing acute or chronic hepatitis B. May be transmitted via injection or transfusion, via sexual contact, from mother to infant at time of birth, and through health care practices. Studies have demonstrated that chronic HBV infection causes liver cancer.

hepatitis C virus (HCV): K. A virus that causes most non-B viral hepatitis, acute or chronic. May be transmitted via injection (intravenous drug use), transfusion, or sexual contact; from mother to infant at time of birth; and through health care practices. Studies have demonstrated that chronic HCV infection causes malignant tumors of the liver.

heterocyclic amines (2-amino-3,4-dimethylimidazo-[4,5-*f*]quinoline (MeIQ), 2-amino-3,8-dimethylimidazo-[4,5-*f*]quinoxaline (MeIQx), 2-amino-3-methylimidazo [4,5-*f*]quinoline (IQ), 2-amino-1-methyl-6-phenylimidazo[4,5-*b*]pyridine (PhIP)): RA. Formed naturally when muscle-derived foods (meat and fish) are browned during cooking. Sufficient evidence of carcinogenicity in experimental animals exists, with tumors resulting at multiple tissue sites; however, no adequate epidemiology studies have been reported that indicate a human cancer risk.

hexachlorobenzene: RA. Has not been produced commercially in the United States since the late 1970's; however, it is produced as a by-product or impurity during the synthesis of several chlorinated solvents and pesticides. Human exposure is through ingestion, inhalation, and skin contact. Tumors of the liver and thyroid occurred in laboratory animals when administered in the diet. There is inadequate evidence for the carcinogenicity in humans.

hexachloroethane: RA. Used to improve the quality of various metals and alloys, as an ignition suppressant, by the military for smoke munitions, and in various other applications. Human exposure is through inhalation, ingestion of contaminated drinking water or fish, and skin absorption. Increased incidences of tumors of the kidney, adrenal gland, and liver occurred in laboratory animals when administered by stomach tube. Few data are available to evaluate the carcinogenicity in humans.

hexamethylphosphoramide: RA. Used as a solvent, a polymerization catalyst, a stabilizer against thermal degradation in polystyrene, an additive to resins to protect against degradation by ultraviolet light, a de-icing additive for jet fuels, and a rodenticide. Human exposure is through inhalation, ingestion, and skin contact. Nasal tumors occurred in laboratory animals when administered by inhalation. There is inadequate evidence for the carcinogenicity in humans.

human papillomaviruses (HPV), some genital-mucosal types: K. Viruses that infect the genital skin and genital and nongenital mucosa; transmitted primarily through sexual contact. Low-risk HPV viruses can cause genital warts or cervical abnormalities; high-risk HPV viruses can cause cervical cancer. Evidence also suggests associations between HPV infection and cancer of the vulva, as well as some cancers of the head and neck, especially, the oropharynx (the soft palate, tonsils, and back of the tongue and throat).

hydrazine and hydrazine sulfate: RA. Used primarily to produce agricultural chemicals, spandex fibers, and antioxidants. Also used as rocket fuel, a water treatment chemical, a polymerization catalyst, a reducing agent, and a blowing agent. Additionally used for plating metals on glass and plastics and in fuel cells, solder fluxes, photographic chemicals, pharmaceuticals, textile dyes, and various other products. Human exposure is through ingestion, inhalation, and skin contact. Potential for general population exposure is low. A variety of tumors occurred when administered to laboratory animals. There is inadequate evidence for the carcinogenicity in humans.

hydrazobenzene: RA. Used primarily in the dye manufacturing industry; also used in the manufacture of pharmaceuticals and hydrogen peroxide, in the reclamation of rubber, as an additive in motor oil, as a desuckering agent for tobacco plants, in resin compositions, and in polymerization reactions. Human exposure is through inhalation, ingestion, and skin contact. A variety of tumors occurred in laboratory animals exposed to hydrazobenzene.

iron dextran complex: RA. Used to treat iron-deficiency anemia when oral treatment has failed; also used in veterinary medicine to treat baby pigs. Human exposure is through inhalation, skin contact, and treatment by injection. Local tumors occurred in laboratory animals when administered by injection. There is inadequate evidence for the carcinogenicity in humans; however, tumors at probable sites of injection in humans have been reported.

isoprene: RA. Used primarily to produce cis-1,4-polyisoprene (rubber); also used to produce butyl rubber (isobutene-isoprene copolymer) and thermoplastic, elastomeric co-block (SIS) polymers. Isoprene is emitted through human breath, from tobacco smoke, and from plants and trees, resulting in low concentrations in the environment. A variety of tumors occurred in laboratory animals when exposed to isoprene through inhalation. There is inadequate evidence for the carcinogenicity in humans.

Kepone (chlordecone): RA. No longer used in the United States; used until 1978 as an insecticide for leaf-eating insects, ants, and cockroaches, and as a larvicide for flies. Human exposure is through inhalation, ingestion, and skin contact. Tumors of the liver occurred in laboratory animals when administered in the diet. There is inadequate evidence for the carcinogenicity in humans.

lead and lead compounds: RA. Lead is used largely in lead-acid storage batteries for motor vehicles and general industry; also used for ammunition, cable covering, piping, brass and bronze, bearing metals for machinery, and sheet lead. There are many lead compounds (soluble, insoluble, and organic) with many and varied uses, such as in water repellant, cotton dyes, varnishes, chrome pigments, asbestos clutch or brake linings, flame retardants, matches, explosives, paints, rubber, and plastics. Human exposure is through inhalation, ingestion, and skin contact. Tumors of the kidney, brain, hematopoietic system, and lung were reported in laboratory animals exposed to lead; lead exposure has been associated with an increased risk of lung, stomach, and bladder cancer in humans.

lindane and other hexachlorocyclohexane isomers: RA. Used primarily as an insecticidal treatment for hardwood logs and lumber, seed grains, and livestock. Also used as an insecticide for fruit and vegetable crops, and as a scabicide and pediculicide for humans in the form of a lotion, cream, or shampoo. Human exposure is through ingestion, inhalation, and skin contact. Tumors of the liver and thyroid occurred in laboratory animals when administered in the diet. There is inadequate evidence for the carcinogenicity in humans.

melphalan: K. Used to treat cancer and other medical conditions; also used as an insect chemosterilant. Studies have found that patients treated with melphalan for bone marrow cancer, breast cancer, and ovarian cancer have an increased risk of leukemia.

methoxsalen with ultraviolet A therapy (PUVA): K. Used to treat alopecia areata, atopic dermatitis, cutaneous T-cell lymphoma, lichen planus, mycosis fungoides, severe psoriasis, urticaria pigmentosa, vitiligo, and some forms of photosensitivity. Human exposure is through skin contact and ingestion. Studies have found that patients treated with PUVA have an increased risk of skin cancer.

2-methylaziridine (propylenimine): RA. Used in the adhesive, oil-additive, paper, pharmaceutical, rubber, and textile industries. Human exposure is through inhalation, ingestion, and skin contact. Leukemia and a variety of tumors have occurred in laboratory animals when administered by stomach tube or in the diet. No adequate data are available to evaluate the carcinogenicity in humans.

4,4′-methylenebis(2-chloroaniline): RA. Used primarily in the manufacture of castable urethane rubber products; has also been used in the laboratory as a model compound for studying carcinogens. Human exposure is through inhalation, skin contact, and ingestion. Liver cancer and a variety of tumors have occurred in laboratory animals exposed to 4,4′-methylenebis-(2-chloroaniline). There is inadequate evidence for the carcinogenicity in humans.

4-4′-methylenebis(*N,N*-dimethyl)benzenamine: RA. Used in manufacture of dyes, including basic yellow 2, basic orange 14, and solvent yellow 34; also used to process hydrochloride salt and as an analytical reagent for lead. Human exposure is through inhalation and skin contact. Tumors of the liver and thyroid occurred in laboratory animals when administered in the diet. No adequate data are available to evaluate the carcinogenicity in humans.

4,4′-methylenedianiline and its dihydrochloride salt: RA. 4,4′-Methylenedianiline is used in the production of 4,4′-methylenedianiline diisocyanate and polyisocyanates, which are used to produce a variety of polymers and resins. Dihydrochloride is used as a research chemical. Human exposure is through inhalation and skin contact. Increased incidences of tumors of the thyroid, liver, and adrenal gland occurred in laboratory animals when administered methylenedianiline dihydrochloride in the drinking water. No adequate data are available to evaluate the carcinogenicity in humans.

methyleugenol: RA. Used as a flavoring agent in jellies, baked goods, candy, chewing gum, nonalcoholic beverages, pudding, relish, and ice cream. Has also been used as an anesthetic in rodents and as an insect attractant in combination with insecticides. Human exposure is through ingestion and inhalation. A variety of tumors occurred in laboratory animals when administered orally. No adequate data are available to evaluate the carcinogenicity in humans.

methyl methanesulfonate: RA. Used experimentally as a research chemical and in the manufacturing of synthetic chemicals. Has been tested as a cancer treatment; potentially could be used to control insect populations and as a human male contraceptive. Human exposure is limited to laboratory research personnel. Studies have determined malignant tumor formation at multiple sites in laboratory animals exposed to methyl methanesulfonate by multiple routes. No adequate data are available to evaluate the carcinogenicity in humans.

***N*-methyl-*N*-nitro-*N*-nitrosoguanidine (MNNG): RA.** Has no known commercial use; it is used as a research chemical. Human exposure is most likely limited to research scientists. Studies have determined malignant tumor formation at multiple sites in laboratory animals exposed to MNNG by multiple routes. There is inadequate evidence available to evaluate the carcinogenicity in humans.

metronidazole: RA. Used primarily for the treatment of infections due to protozoan parasites; has also been used to treat Vincent's infection, acne rosacea, invasive intestinal amoebiasis, and amoebic hepatic abscess. Human exposure is through ingestion or topical application when used in medical treatment. Lymphomas as well as lung, mammary, pituitary, testicular, and liver tumors occurred in laboratory animals when administered orally. There is inadequate evidence available to evaluate the carcinogenicity in humans.

Michler's ketone [4,4′-(dimethylamino)benzophenone]: RA. Used in the production of at least thirteen dyes and pigments used to dye paper, leather, and textiles; one is also used as an antiseptic fungicide. Human exposure is through inhalation and skin contact. Increased incidences of liver tumors and hemangiosarcomas occurred in laboratory animals when administered orally in the diet. No adequate data are available to evaluate the carcinogenicity in humans.

mineral oils (untreated and mildly treated): K. Used primarily as lubricant base oils to produce further refined oil products used in the manufacturing, automotive, mining, construction, and other miscellaneous industries. Human exposure is through inhalation, ingestion, and skin contact. Exposure to mineral oils is strongly associated with a variety of cancers.

mirex: RA. All uses of mirex were suspended in 1977. Its primary use was as a fire-retardant additive under the name Dechlorane; it was also used as an insecticide to control fire ants in southeastern states. Mirex is very persistent in the environment and highly resistant to degradation; therefore, potential exposure to low concentrations still exists. Human exposure is through ingestion of fish caught from contaminated water, and for populations that live near a former manufacturing or waste disposal site, or live in areas where mirex was extensively used to control fire ants. Increased incidences of liver cancer, tumors of the adrenal gland, and leukemia occurred in laboratory animals when administered by stomach tube and then in the diet. No adequate data are available to evaluate the carcinogenicity in humans.

mustard gas: K. A blister-inducing agent that has been used in chemical warfare; used in research. Human exposure is through inhalation and skin contact, with military personnel being at the greatest risk. Mustard gas is associated with an increased risk of lung, laryngeal, pharyngeal, and upper respiratory tract cancers.

naphthalene: RA. Used in the production of insect repellents, phthalate plasticizers, pharmaceuticals, and other materials. Has also been used in the production of 1-naphthyl-*N*-methylcarbamate insecticides, beta-naphthol, moth repellents, surfactants, synthetic leather tanning chemicals, and toilet bowl deodorants. Human exposure is through inhalation and skin contact. Nasal tumors, neuroblastomas in the brain, and lung tumors occurred in laboratory animals when administered by inhalation. No adequate data are available to evaluate the carcinogenicity in humans.

2-naphthylamine: K. Used only in laboratory research; formerly used in the manufacture of dyes, rubber, and 2-chloronaphthylamine. Potential for human exposure is low; however, may occur through inhalation of emissions from sources where nitrogen-containing organic matter is burned, such as coal furnaces and cigarettes. Studies have shown that 2-naphthylamine causes bladder cancer.

neutrons: K. Used medically in external beam therapy, in boron neutron capture therapy, and to make radioisotopes. Also used in oil-well logging, nuclear reactors, neutron activation analysis and radiography, sterilization of materials, radiometric dating of rocks, and scientific and engineering research. Human exposure occurs naturally from cosmic radiation originating from outer space; however, additional exposure occurs in cancer patients receiving radiation therapy, nuclear-industry workers, airline crews and passengers, and survivors of atomic bomb blasts. Studies show that neutron radiation induces chromosomal aberrations, mutations, deoxytibonucleic acid (DNA) damage, and many various tumors.

nickel compounds: K. Includes stainless steel, copper–nickel alloys, and other corrosion-resistant alloys. Human exposure occurs through inhalation, ingestion, and skin contact. Studies have shown an increased risk of death from lung cancer and nasal cancer.

nickel (metallic): RA. Used in alkaline batteries, coins, electrical contacts and electrodes, electroplating, machinery parts, magnets, spark plugs, surgical and dental prostheses, and welding products. Human exposure occurs through inhalation, ingestion, and skin contact. An increased incidence of malignant tumors at multiple tissue sites occurred in laboratory animals exposed to metallic nickel powder. No adequate data are available to evaluate the carcinogenicity in humans.

nitrilotriacetic acid: RA. Used primarily as a chelating agent and as a laundry detergent builder. Also used in water and textile treatment, metal plating and cleaning, pulp and paper processing, leather tanning, the manufacture of pharmaceuticals, photographic development, synthetic rubber production, and herbicide formulations and micronutrient solutions in agriculture. Human exposure is through inhalation, ingestion, and skin contact. Tumors of the kidney, ureter, urinary bladder, adrenal gland, and liver occurred in laboratory animals when administered in the diet. No adequate data are available to evaluate the carcinogenicity in humans.

o-**nitroanisole: RA.** Used primarily in the synthesis of azo dyes; has also been used in the pharmaceutical industry. Human exposure is through skin contact, ingestion, and inhalation. Leukemia and tumors of the urinary bladder, kidney, large intestine, and liver occurred in laboratory animals when administered in the diet. No adequate data are available to evaluate the carcinogenicity in humans.

nitrobenzene: RA. Used primarily in the manufacture of aniline; also used in the manufacture of azobenzene, benzidine, dyes, isocyanates, lubricating oils, pesticides, pharmaceuticals, pyroxylin compounds, quinoline, rubber chemicals, soaps, and shoe and metal polishes. Human exposure is through inhalation, ingestion, and skin contact. Increased incidences of tumors at multiple tissue sites occurred in laboratory animals when administered by inhalation. No adequate data are available to evaluate the carcinogenicity in humans.

6-nitrochrysene: RA. Not used commercially; available for research purposes. Found in particulate emissions from combustion sources, especially diesel exhaust. Limited evidence of increased risk for lung cancer when exposed to diesel exhaust particulates has been found in human studies. Studies have determined malignant tumor formation at multiple sites in laboratory animals exposed to 6-nitrochrysene.

nitrofen (2,4-dichlorophenyl-*p*-nitrophenyl ether): RA. No longer used commercially; was used as an herbicide to control annual grasses and broadleaf weeds on various food and ornamental crops. Human exposure is through inhalation, skin contact, and ingestion. Tumors of the liver, spleen, and pancreas occurred in laboratory animals when administered in the diet. No adequate data are available to evaluate the carcinogenicity in humans.

nitrogen mustard hydrochloride: RA. Used to treat neoplastic diseases; also used to control pleural, peritoneal, and pericardial effusions caused by metastatic tumors, and has been used in clinical trials for rheumatoid arthritis, in tissue transplantation studies, and for other nonmalignant diseases. Human exposure is through injection, inhalation, and skin contact. Tumors in various organs occurred in laboratory animals exposed to nitrogen mustard hydrochloride. There is limited evidence of carcinogenicity in humans, including skin cancer, leukemia, and various other malignant tumors.

nitromethane: RA. Used primarily in the making of nitromethane derivatives, which are used as agricul-

tural soil fumigants, industrial antimicrobials, and pharmaceuticals. Also used as a fuel or fuel additive. Human exposure is through inhalation, especially of motor vehicle exhaust and cigarette smoke; ingestion of contaminated water; and skin contact. Tumors of the harderian gland, lung, liver, and mammary gland occurred in laboratory animals when administered by inhalation. No adequate data are available to evaluate the carcinogenicity in humans.

2-nitropropane: RA. Used primarily as a solvent in adhesives, inks, paints, polymers, varnishes, and synthetic materials, and used in the manufacture of 2-nitro-2-methyl-1-propanol and 2-amino-2-methyl-1-propanol. Also used in explosives and propellants, and in fuels for internal combustion engines. Human exposure is through inhalation, ingestion, and skin contact. Liver cancer occurred in laboratory animals when administered by inhalation. No adequate data are available to evaluate the carcinogenicity in humans.

1-nitropyrene: RA. Limited use in the production of 1-azidopyrene, which is used in photosensitive printing; available for research purposes in the United States. Found in particulate emissions from combustion sources, especially diesel exhaust. Limited evidence of increased risk for lung cancer when exposed to diesel exhaust particulates has been found in human studies; however, it has not been determined whether 1-nitropyrene is responsible. Studies have determined malignant tumor formation at multiple sites in laboratory animals exposed to 1-nitropyrene by multiple routes.

4-nitropyrene: RA. Used only as a laboratory chemical. Found in particulate emissions from combustion sources, especially diesel exhaust. Limited evidence of increased risk for lung cancer when exposed to diesel exhaust particulates has been found in human studies; however, it has not been determined whether 4-nitropyrene is responsible. Studies have determined malignant tumor formation at multiple sites in laboratory animals exposed to 1-nitropyrene.

N-**nitrosodi-*n*-butylamine: RA.** Used primarily as a research chemical; once used in the synthesis of di-*n*-butylhydrazine. Human exposure is through ingestion, inhalation, and skin contact. Leukemia and a variety of tumors occurred in laboratory animals exposed to *N*-nitrosodi-*n*-butylamine. No adequate data are available to evaluate the carcinogenicity in humans.

N-**nitrosodiethanolamine: RA.** No longer used commercially; however, it is widespread in the environment; used as a research chemical. Human exposure is through skin contact, ingestion, and inhalation. Nitrosodiethanolamine is a known contaminant of antifreeze, cosmetics, lotions, cutting fluids, shampoos, some pesticides, and tobacco. Tumors of the liver and kidney occurred in laboratory animals when administered in the drinking water, and tumors of the nasal cavity, trachea, liver, and injection site occurred when administered by injection. No adequate data are available to evaluate the carcinogenicity in humans.

N-nitrosodiethylamine: RA. Used primarily as a research chemical. Also used as an antioxidant, copolymer softener, gasoline and lubricant additive, fiber industry solvent, and stabilizer in plastics, and in the synthesis of 1,1-diethylhydrazine. Human exposure is through ingestion, inhalation, and skin contact. A variety of tumors occurred in laboratory animals exposed to N-nitrosodiethylamine. No adequate data are available to evaluate the carcinogenicity in humans.

N-nitrosodimethylamine: RA. Used primarily as a research chemical; also used to control nematodes (worms) and inhibit nitrification in soil. Used in rubber and acrylonitrile polymers, fluoride polymers, copolymers, high-energy batteries, and lubricants; as a solvent in the fiber and plastics industry; and as an antioxidant. Human exposure is through ingestion, inhalation, and skin contact. A variety of tumors occurred in animals exposed to N-nitrosodimethylamine. No adequate data are available to evaluate the carcinogenicity in humans.

N-nitrosodi-*n*-propylamine: RA. Not used commercially; used in laboratory research. Human exposure is through ingestion, inhalation, and skin contact. A variety of tumors occurred in laboratory animals exposed to N-nitrosodi-*n*-propylamine. No adequate data are available to evaluate the carcinogenicity in humans.

N-nitroso-N-ethylurea: RA. Used to synthesize diazoethane in the laboratory. Human exposure is limited; however, occupational exposure may occur through inhalation or skin contact. Leukemia and tumors at multiple sites occurred in laboratory animals when exposed to N-nitroso-N-ethylurea. No adequate data are available to evaluate the carcinogenicity in humans.

4-(N-nitrosomethylamino)-1-(3-pyridyl)-1-butanone (NNK): RA. Used as a laboratory chemical. Human exposure is through the inhalation of tobacco smoke or during tobacco chewing or oral snuff use. Tumors of the nasal cavity, lung, liver, and trachea occurred in laboratory animals when exposed to NNK. No adequate data are available to evaluate the carcinogenicity in humans.

N-nitroso-N-methylurea: RA. Used in research; has been used to synthesize diazomethane in the laboratory and has been studied as a chemotherapeutic agent in cancer treatment. Human exposure is limited; however,

occupational exposure may occur through inhalation or skin contact. Leukemia and tumors at multiple sites occurred in laboratory animals when exposed to N-nitroso-N-methylurea. No adequate data are available to evaluate the carcinogenicity in humans.

N-nitrosomethylvinylamine: RA. Used as a research chemical. Human exposure is primarily limited to researchers; however, N-nitroso compounds have been identified in a variety of food products and can therefore be ingested. Tumors of the esophagus, tongue, pharynx, nasal cavity, and skin have occurred in laboratory animals when exposed to N-nitrosomethylvinylamine. No adequate data are available to evaluate the carcinogenicity in humans.

N-nitrosomorpholine: RA. Not used commercially; however, patents have been issued for its use in the production of N-aminomorpholine and as a solvent for polyacrylonitrile. A variety of tumors occurred in laboratory animals exposed to N-nitrosomorpholine. No adequate data are available to evaluate the carcinogenicity in humans.

N-nitrosonornicotine: RA. Used as a research chemical. Human exposure is through the use of tobacco products or the inhalation of sidestream smoke. Tumors of the esophagus, nasal cavity, trachea, and lung occurred in laboratory animals exposed to N-nitrosonornicotine. No adequate data are available to evaluate the carcinogenicity in humans.

N-nitrosopiperidine: RA. Used as a research chemical. Human exposure is limited; however, exposure may occur from cigarette smoke and certain meats and fish. A variety of tumors occurred in animals exposed to N-nitrosopiperidine. No adequate data are available to evaluate the carcinogenicity in humans.

N-nitrosopyrrolidine: RA. Used primarily as a research chemical; not used commercially. N-nitrosopyrrolidine is produced when foods preserved or contaminated with nitrites, especially fatty foods, are heat prepared; human exposure occurs through ingestion of these foods or inhalation of vapors released during cooking. Leukemia and a variety of tumors occurred in laboratory animals when administered in the drinking water. No adequate data are available to evaluate the carcinogenicity in humans.

N-nitrososarcosine: RA. Not used commercially; has limited use in research. Human exposure is through inhalation, ingestion, and skin contact. Skin cancer of the nasal region and tumors of the esophagus and liver occurred in laboratory animals when exposed to N-nitrososarcosine. No adequate data are available to evaluate the carcinogenicity in humans.

norethisterone: RA. Used primarily as the progestin in progestin-estrogen combination oral contraceptives. Also used in medicines used to treat amenorrhea, dysmenorrhea, dysfunctional uterine bleeding, endometriosis, premenstrual tension, and inoperable malignant tumors of the breast. Human exposure is through ingestion, skin contact, and inhalation. Tumors of the pituitary, mammary gland, and ovaries occurred in laboratory animals when exposed to norethisterone. No adequate data are available to evaluate the carcinogenicity in humans.

ochratoxin A: RA. Not used commercially; it is an experimental teratogen and carcinogen. Human exposure is probably widespread through ingestion of food and handling of animal feed since ochratoxin A is a naturally occurring mycotoxin. Tumors of the liver, kidney, and mammary gland occurred in laboratory animals exposed to ochratoxin A. No adequate data are available to evaluate the carcinogenicity in humans.

4,4′-oxydianiline: RA. Used in the production of polyimide and poly(ester)imide resins, which are used in the manufacture of temperature-resistant products (such as wire enamels, coatings, and adhesives). Human exposure is through inhalation and through eye and skin contact. Tumors of the harderian gland, liver, and thyroid occurred in laboratory animals exposed to 4,4′-oxydianiline. No adequate data are available to evaluate the carcinogenicity in humans.

oxymetholone: RA. A steroid hormone used to treat many conditions, including hypogonadism, delayed puberty, hereditary angioneurotic edema, and carcinoma of the breast. Also used to stimulate the formation of red blood cells (especially to treat anemias), to promote a positive nitrogen balance following surgery or injury, and to counteract weakness and promote weight gain during debilitating diseases. Human exposure is through ingestion and skin contact. Increased incidences of liver tumors occurred in laboratory animals when exposed to oxymetholone. Cases of liver tumors have been reported in patients treated for long periods with oxymetholone; however, a causal relationship cannot be established.

phenacetin: RA. Was used as an analgesic and fever-reducing drug until it was implicated in kidney disease and withdrawn from the U.S. market in 1983; it was also once used in hair-bleaching preparations. Human exposure was through ingestion, with occupational exposure through inhalation and skin contact. Tumors of the urinary tract and nasal cavity occurred in laboratory animals when phenacetin was administered in the diet.

There is limited evidence for the carcinogenicity in humans because phenacetin was usually taken mixed with other drugs.

phenacetin-containing analgesic mixtures: K. Was used as an analgesic and fever-reducing drug until it was implicated in kidney disease and withdrawn from the U.S. market in 1983; cancers of the urinary tract, renal pelvis, and bladder have also been reported in patients using large amounts of phenacetin-containing analgesic mixtures.

phenazopyridine hydrochloride: RA. Has been used as an analgesic drug to reduce pain associated with urinary tract infections or irritation; often combined with sulfonamides and antibiotics. Human exposure is through ingestion, with occupational exposure through inhalation and skin contact. Tumors of the liver, colon, and rectum occurred in laboratory animals when administered in the diet. There is inadequate evidence for the carcinogenicity in humans.

phenolphthalein: RA. Used in various ingested products, including laxatives, as well as in some scientific applications. Human exposure is through ingestion, skin contact, and inhalation. Increased incidences of tumors in multiple tissue sites occurred in laboratory animals when exposed to phenolphthalein. There is inadequate evidence for the carcinogenicity in humans.

phenoxybenzamine hydrochloride: RA. Used primarily to treat hypertension caused by pheochromocytoma; also used to treat benign prostatic hypertrophy under certain conditions. Has been used to treat peripheral vascular disorders, hypertension, and shock. Human exposure is through ingestion during its medical use and skin contact during its production. Peritoneal tumors and lung tumors occurred in laboratory animals when administered by injection. No adequate data are available to evaluate the carcinogenicity in humans.

phenytoin: RA. An anticonvulsant drug used to treat grand mal epileptic patients with focal and psychomotor seizures; has been used to treat varous other conditions. Also used to control seizures occurring during neurosurgery, to prevent postcountershock arrhythmias in digitalized patients, and to reverse digitalis-induced arrhythmias. Human exposure is through injection, ingestion, inhalation, and skin contact. Thymic, generalized, and mesenteric lymphomas; liver tumors; and leukemias occurred in laboratory animals exposed to phenytoin. There is inadequate evidence for the carcinogenicity in humans; however, there is limited evidence suggesting that phenytoin may be a transplacental carcinogen in humans.

polybrominated biphenyls (PBBs): RA. Used as flame-retardant additives in synthetic fibers and molded plastics. Human exposure is through ingestion, inhalation, and skin contact. Liver tumors occurred in laboratory animals when exposed to a PBB. No adequate data are available to evaluate the carcinogenicity in humans.

polychlorinated biphenyls (PCBs): RA. Uses are confined to closed systems, such as electrical capacitors, gas-transmission turbines, and vacuum pumps; exemptions are granted to individual petitioners for use as a mounting medium in microscopy, an immersion oil in low fluorescence microscopy, or an optical liquid, and for research and development. Human exposure is through ingestion, inhalation, and skin contact. Liver tumors occurred in laboratory animals when exposed to Aroclor 1260, Aroclor 1254, and Kanechlor 500 (all PCBs). There is inadequate evidence for the carcinogenicity in humans; however, an increase in the incidence of cancer, particularly skin cancer and cancers of the digestive system and of the lymphatic and hematopoietic tissues, has been reported in men exposed to PCBs.

polycyclic aromatic hydrocarbons (PAHs) (benz[*a*]anthracene, benzo[*b*]fluoranthene, benzo[*j*]fluoranthene, benzo[*k*]fluoranthene, benzo[*a*]pyrene, dibenz[*a,h*]acridine, dibenz[*a,j*]acridine, dibenz[*a,h*]anthracene, 7*H*-dibenzo[*c,g*]carbazole, dibenzo[*a,e*]pyrene, dibenzo[*a,h*]pyrene, dibenzo[*a,i*]pyrene, dibenzo[*a,l*]pyrene, indeno[1,2,3-*cd*]pyrene, 5-methylchrysene): RA. Other than dibenzo[*a,h*]pyrene, dibenzo[*a,i*]pyrene, and 5-methylchrysene, which have no known uses, the other PAHs are used only in biomedical, biochemical, laboratory, and cancer research. At least eight of those are found in coal tar and coal tar products, which include coal tar pitch and creosote. Human exposure is through inhalation of contaminated air, tobacco smoke, and wood smoke, and ingestion of contaminated water and foods, especially smoked, barbecued, and charcoal-broiled foods. Studies have determined malignant tumor formation at multiple sites in laboratory animals exposed to PAHs by multiple routes. There is inadequate evidence for the carcinogenicity in humans; however, many studies show increased incidences of cancer, including lung, skin, and genitourinary cancers, in humans exposed to mixtures of PAHs.

procarbazine hydrochloride: RA. Used in combination with other anticancer medications to treat Hodgkin disease, non-Hodgkin lymphoma, malignant melanoma, and small-cell carcinomas of the lung. Human exposure is through ingestion, inhalation, and skin contact. Leukemia, lymphomas, hemangiosarcomas, and tumors at multiple sites occurred in laboratory animals when

exposed to procarbazine hydrochloride. There is inadequate evidence for the carcinogenicity in humans; however, the use of procarbazine hydrochloride in combination with other chemotherapeutic medications for the treatment of Hodgkin disease has repeatedly been shown to lead to the appearance of acute nonlymphocytic leukemia.

progesterone: RA. A naturally occurring steroidal hormone secreted by female ovaries, the placenta in pregnant females, and the adrenal cortex; used as a contraception and to treat secondary amenorrhea and dysfunctional uterine bleeding. Has also been used to treat dysmenorrhea and premenstrual tension, habitual and threatened abortion, preeclampsia and toxemia of pregnancy, female hypogonadism, mastodynia, uterine fibroma, and tumors of the breast and endometrium. Human exposure is through ingestion, injection, implantation, skin contact, and inhalation. Cancers of the breast, ovaries, endometrium, cervix, vagina, and genital tract occurred in female laboratory animals, including neonatal and newborn animals, when exposed to progesterone through injections and implants. No adequate data are available to evaluate the carcinogenicity in humans.

1,3-propane sultone: RA. Used in the production of fungicides, insecticides, some resins, dyes, detergents, lathering agents, bacteriostats, a variety of other chemicals, and untempered steel. Human exposure is through ingestion and inhalation. Brain tumors, breast tumors, and increased incidences of leukemia, tumors of the small intestine, and skin cancer of the ear occurred in laboratory animals when administered by stomach tube, and injection site tumors occurred when administered by injection. No adequate data are available to evaluate the carcinogenicity in humans.

β-propiolactone: RA. Has been used to sterilize blood plasma, vaccines, tissue grafts, surgical instruments, and enzymes; to kill spores of vegetative bacteria, pathogenic fungi, and viruses; and to manufacture acrylic acid and esters. Has also been used as a vapor-phase disinfectant in enclosed spaces, and in organic synthesis. Human exposure is limited because it is no longer used as a sterilant in medical procedures or in food; however, occupational exposure may occur through inhalation and skin contact when used as a chemical intermediate in industrial facilities. Tumors of the forestomach and skin cancer occurred in laboratory animals exposed to β-propiolactone. No adequate data are available to evaluate the carcinogenicity in humans.

propylene oxide: RA. Used primarily in the production of polyurethane polyols (used to make polyurethane foams), propylene glycols (used to make polyester resins for the textile and construction industries, as well as in drugs, cosmetics, solvents and emollients in food, plasticizers, heat transfer and hydraulic fluids, and antifreezes), glycol ethers, and specialty chemicals, including pesticides. May also be used in fumigation chambers for the sterilization of packaged foods. Human exposure is through ingestion; inhalation, and skin contact. Tumors of the nasal cavity, adrenal gland, and peritoneum occurred in laboratory animals when administered by inhalation; local tumors and tumors of the forestomach when administered by stomach tube; and local tumors when administered by injection. No adequate data are available to evaluate the carcinogenicity in humans.

propylthiouracil: RA. Used as an antithyroid agent for the treatment of hyperthyroidism. Human exposure is primarily through ingestion as a drug. Tumors of the pituitary gland and thyroid occurred in laboratory animals when ingested. No adequate data are available to evaluate the carcinogenicity in humans.

radon: K. Used primarily for research; however, it is produced in nature by radioactive decay of radium and is released from soil into the air and groundwater. Human exposure is through inhalation and ingestion. An increased risk of lung cancer, as well as tracheal and bronchial cancer, is associated with exposure to radon.

reserpine: RA. A naturally occurring alkaloid used to lower blood pressure and reduce the heart rate and as a tranquilizer and sedative. Human exposure is through ingestion and skin contact. Tumors of the adrenal gland, breast, and seminal vesicles occurred in laboratory animals when reserpine was administered in the diet and by injection. No adequate data are available to evaluate the carcinogenicity in humans.

safrole: RA. Has been used in drugs, beverages, foods, soap, and perfumes, and in the manufacture of heliotropin and piperonyl butoxide. Human exposure is through ingestion and skin contact. Liver tumors and lung tumors occurred in laboratory animals when administered safrole. No adequate data are available to evaluate the carcinogenicity in humans.

selenium sulfide: RA. Used in antidandruff shampoos and fungicides. Human exposure is through skin contact and inhalation. Liver tumors and alveolar/bronchiolar tumors occurred in laboratory animals when administered by stomach tube. No adequate data are available to evaluate the carcinogenicity in humans.

silica, crystalline (respirable size): K. Used in the production of quartzite, tripoli, gannister, chert, and novaculite; occurs naturally as agate, amethyst, chalcedony, cristobalite, flint, quartz, tridymite, and sand. Sand is used in the manufacture of glass, ceramics, foundry castings, abrasives, sandblasting materials, silicon, and ferrosilicon metals; as a filter in municipal water and sewage treatment plants; and in hydraulic fracturing in oil and gas recovery. Human exposure is through inhalation and ingestion. An increased risk of lung cancer is associated with exposure to respirable crystalline silica.

solar radiation: K. Emitted by the sun; has been determined to cause skin cancer and may also cause melanoma of the eye and non-Hodgkin lymphoma.

soots: K. Unwanted by-products of the incomplete combustion or burning of organic materials; have been used as fertilizer to provide small amounts of nitrogen and essential trace metals to plants, as a slug deterrent, as a soil conditioner, and in the recovery of trace metals in the metallurgical industry. Human exposure is through inhalation, ingestion, and skin contact. Increased risks, of scrotal cancer, lung cancer, and leukemia, as well as total lymphatic and hematopoietic cancer and cancer of the esophagus, liver, prostate, and bladder, are associated with exposure to soots.

streptozotocin: RA. Used in the treatment of metastasizing pancreatic islet cell tumors and malignant carcinoid tumors. Tumors of the kidney, lung, uterus, pancreas, liver, peritoneum, and bile ducts occurred in laboratory animals when exposed to streptozotocin. No adequate data are available to evaluate the carcinogenicity in humans.

strong inorganic acid mists containing sulfuric acid: K. Produced during the manufacture or use of sulfuric acid, sulfur trioxide, or oleum. The following industries use sulfuric acid: fertilizer, mining and metallurgy, ore processing, petroleum refining, inorganic and organic chemicals, cellulose fibers and films, inorganic pigments and paints, synthetic rubber and plastics, pulp and paper, soap and detergents, and water treatment. Lead-acid batteries are the primary consumer products containing sulfuric acid, which is also used as a general purpose food additive. Human exposure is through inhalation, ingestion, and skin contact. Exposure to strong inorganic acid mists containing sulfuric acid is associated with laryngeal and lung cancer in humans.

styrene-7,8-oxide: RA. Used in the production of styrene glycol and its derivatives, cosmetics, surface coatings, agricultural and biological chemicals, epoxy resins, and cross-linked polyesters and polyurethanes. Has also been used in the production of 2-phenylethanol used in perfumes, in the treatment of fibers and textiles, and in hydraulic fluids, chlorinated cleaning compositions, petroleum distillates, dielectric fluids, and acid-sensitive polymers and copolymers. Human exposure is through contact with contaminated air or water. Tumors of the forestomach and liver occurred in laboratory animals when administered by stomach tube. No adequate data are available to evaluate the carcinogenicity in humans.

sulfallate: RA. Was used as an herbicide to control particular annual grasses and broadleaf weeds around vegetable and fruit crops; however, manufacture of sulfallate products was discontinued in the early 1990's. Potential for further human exposure is low. Tumors of the breast, forestomach, and lung occurred in laboratory animals when administered in the diet. No adequate data are available to evaluate the carcinogenicity in humans.

sunlamps or sun beds, exposure to: K. Emit primarily ultraviolet A (UVA) and ultraviolet B (UVB) radiation; have been determined to increase risk of skin cancer.

tamoxifen: K. Used primarily in the treatment of breast cancer; has also been tested as a possible treatment for other cancers. Human exposure is through ingestion and inhalation. An increased risk of endometrial cancer (cancer of the uterus) has been associated with exposure to tamoxifen.

2,3,7,8-tetrachlorodibenzo-*p*-dioxin (TCDD); "Dioxin": K. Used as a research chemical. Has no known commercial applications; however, is inadvertently produced by incineration of municipal, toxic, and hospital wastes; by paper and pulp bleaching; in PCB-filled electrical transformer fires; in smelters; and during production of chlorophenoxy herbicides. Human exposure is through inhalation, ingestion (especially of meat, fish, and dairy products), and skin contact. Studies have determined that a significant increased risk for all cancers combined, lung cancer, and non-Hodgkin lymphoma is associated with exposure to TCDD.

tetrachloroethylene (perchloroethylene): RA. Used primarily as a cleaning solvent (especially in the dry cleaning industry) and as a chemical precursor for fluorocarbons. Also used as an insulating fluid and cooling gas in electrical transformers; in adhesive formulations, leather treatments, paint removers, printing inks, and paper coatings; in aerosol formulations such as water repellants, automotive cleaners, spot removers, and silicone lubricants; as an extractant for pharmaceuticals; and as an agent that kills parasitic worms. As tetrachloroethylene is widely distributed in the environment, human exposure is through inhalation and ingestion of contaminated water or food; skin contact may also occur. Leukemia and tumors of the liver and kidney occurred in laboratory animals exposed to tetrachloroethylene. There is limited evidence for the carcinogenicity in humans. Studies have reported increased incidences of lymphosarcomas, leukemias, and cancers of the skin, colon, lung, urogenital tract, larynx, and urinary bladder in laundry and dry cleaning workers, however, these workers are also exposed to petroleum solvents and other dry cleaning agents. There is evidence as well for consistent positive associations between tetrachloroethylene exposure and non-Hodgkin lymphoma and esophageal and cervical cancer.

tetrafluoroethylene (TFE): RA. Used primarily in the synthesis of polytetrafluoroethylene; also used to produce copolymers with monomers such as ethylene and hexafluoropropylene. Human exposure is primarily through inhalation. Leukemia and tumors of the liver and kidney occurred in laboratory animals when administered by inhalation. No adequate data are available to evaluate the carcinogenicity in humans.

tetranitromethane: RA. Used in rocket propellants, explosives, and diesel fuel, and as an organic reagent. Human exposure is through inhalation. A dose-related increase in alveolar/bronchiolar tumors occurred in laboratory animals when administered by inhalation. No adequate data are available to evaluate the carcinogenicity in humans.

thioacetamide: RA. Used as a replacement for hydrogen sulfide in qualitative analyses; has also been used as an organic solvent. Human exposure is through inhalation and skin contact. Tumors of the liver and bile duct have occurred in laboratory animals. No adequate data are available to evaluate the carcinogenicity in humans.

4,4′-thiodianaline: RA. Was used in the production of C.I. Mordant Yellow 16 dye, Milling Red G dye, and Milling Red FR dye; however, has not been used since the early 1990's. Human exposure may have been through skin contact, accidental ingestion, and inhalation. Tumors of the liver, thyroid, Zymbal gland, uterus, and colon occurred in laboratory animals when exposed to 4,4′-thiodianaline. No adequate data are available to evaluate the carcinogenicity in humans.

thiotepa: K. Used to treat a variety of cancers, including bladder, brain, breast, ovarian, and lung, and lymphomas. Studies have determined that patients treated with thiotepa are at increased risk to develop secondary leukemia.

thiourea: RA. Has been used in the synthesis of pharmaceuticals and insecticides, in boiler water treatment, as a photographic toning agent, as a dry cleaning agent, in hair preparations, and as a reagent for bismuth and selenite. Human exposure is through inhalation and skin contact. No adequate data are available to evaluate the carcinogenicity in humans.

thorium dioxide: K. Used in high-temperature ceramics, gas mantles, crucibles, nuclear fuel, flame spraying, medicines, nonsilica optical glass, and thoriated tungsten filaments. Concerns over its naturally occurring radioactivity have led to its substantially decreased use. Human exposure is through inhalation, intravenous injection, ingestion, and skin contact. Studies have determined a significantly increased risk of liver tumors, leukemia, and bone cancer for those exposed to thorium dioxide.

tobacco, smokeless: K. Main forms are chewing tobacco and snuff. Has been determined to cause tumors of the oral cavity, especially at the site of placement.

tobacco, smoking: K. Used in cigarettes, pipes, cigars, and bidis. Has been determined to cause cancer of the lung, urinary bladder, renal pelvis, oral cavity, pharynx, larynx, esophagus, lip, and pancreas. Sufficient evidence exists for the carcinogenicity of cigarette smoking and cancers of the nasal cavities and nasal sinus, stomach, liver, kidney, and uterine cervix, as well as myeloid leukemia.

tobacco smoke, environmental: K. Passive exposure (sidestream smoke) produced from tobacco products (cigarettes, pipes, cigars, and bidis) has been determined to cause lung cancer and cancers of the nasal cavity.

toluene diisocyanate: RA. Used primarily in the synthesis of polyurethane foams, which are used in furniture, bedding, and insulation. Also used in floor finishes, wood finishes, paints, concrete sealants, adhesive and sealant compounds, automobile parts, shoe soles, roller skate wheels, pond liners, and blood bags, and in oil fields and mines. Human exposure is through inhalation and skin contact. Tumors at multiple sites occurred in laboratory animals exposed to toluene diisocyanate. No adequate data are available to evaluate the carcinogenicity in humans.

***o*-toluidine and *o*-toluidine hydrochloride: RA.** Used primarily in the manufacture of dyes and pigments; also used in the manufacture of synthetic rubber, rubber vulcanizing chemicals, pharmaceuticals, and pesticides, as well as in organic synthesis and glucose analysis. Human exposure is through inhalation and skin contact. Tumors at multiple sites occurred in laboratory animals when administered in the diet. There is limited evidence for the carcinogenicity in humans. An excess of bladder cancers has been reported in workers exposed to *o*-toluidine; however, they were also exposed to other potential bladder carcinogens at the same time.

toxaphene: RA. Was used primarily as a pesticide, especially on cotton crops, until it was banned in the United States in 1990; was also used to control insect pests on livestock and poultry. Human exposure is through ingestion of contaminated food and water, skin contact, and inhalation. Tumors of the liver and thyroid occurred in laboratory animals when administered in the diet. No adequate data are available to evaluate the carcinogenicity in humans.

trichloroethylene (TCE): RA. Used primarily as a degreaser for metal parts, mainly by industries that manufacture furniture and fixtures, fabricated metal products, electrical and electronic equipment, transport equipment, and other miscellaneous products; it is also used in adhesives, lubricants, paint strippers, paints, varnishes, pesticides, and cold metal cleaners. Human exposure is through ingestion of food and water and through inhalation. Malignant tumor formation at multiple sites occurred in laboratory animals when exposed to TCE. There is limited evidence for the carcinogenicity in humans; studies have consistently showed an increased risk for kidney cancer, liver cancer, Hodgkin disease, non-Hodgkin lymphoma, and cervical cancer with occupational exposure to TCE.

2,4,6-trichlorophenol: RA. Has been used primarily in pesticides and wood preservatives; has also been used in fungicides, glue preservatives, insecticides, bactericides, and antimildew agents for textiles; however, most uses have been discontinued in the United States except in fungicides. Human exposure is through ingestion of contaminated food and water, inhalation of contaminated air, and skin contact. Increased incidences of leukemias, lymphomas, and liver cancer occurred in laboratory animals when administered in the diet. There is limited evidence for the carcinogenicity in humans, including soft-tissue sarcomas and non-Hodgkin lymphomas, when exposed to chlorophenols, which contain 2,4,6-trichlorophenol as well as tetrachlorodibenzo-*p*-dioxin (TCDD), which is a known carcinogen.

1,2,3-trichloropropane: RA. Used in the production of polysulfone liquid polymers and dichloropropene, and in the synthesis of hexafluoropropylene and polysulfides; it also was used as a solvent and extractive agent, and in the manufacture of a soil fumigant. Human exposure is through inhalation of vapors, skin contact, and ingestion of contaminated water. Malignant tumor formation at multiple sites occurred in laboratory animals when administered by stomach tube. No adequate data are available to evaluate the carcinogenicity in humans.

ultraviolet A radiation (UVA), ultraviolet B radiation (UVB), and ultraviolet C radiation (UVC): RA. All are components of broad-spectrum ultraviolet radiation (UVR); exposure is through solar radiation (except for UVC, which is absorbed by the ozone layer) and artificial devices emitting broad-spectrum UVR, such as sunlamps and sun beds. Exposure to each of these components induced skin tumors in laboratory animals; limited evidence shows that each of these components causes DNA damage in human tissue, which may lead to skin cancer.

ultraviolet radiation (UVR), broad spectrum: K. Exposure is through solar radiation and artificial devices emitting broad-spectrum UVR, such as sunlamps and sun beds. Has been determined to cause skin cancer.

urethane: RA. Used in the preparation of amino resins, which are used in permanent press textiles; also used in the manufacture of pesticides, fumigants, cosmetics, and pharmaceuticals, and in biochemical research. Human exposure is through inhalation, ingestion, and skin contact. Leukemias and tumors at multiple sites occurred in laboratory animals when exposed to urethane. No adequate data are available to evaluate the carcinogenicity in humans.

vinyl bromide: RA. Used primarily in the production of polymers and copolymers, which are used as flame retardants, and in the production of carpet-backing material, fabrics, home furnishings, granular products, films, laminated fibers, and rubber substitutes; also used in leather and fabricated metal products and in the production of pharmaceuticals and fumigants. Human exposure is through inhalation and skin contact. Tumors of the liver and Zymbal gland occurred in laboratory animals when vinyl bromide was administered by inhalation. No adequate data are available to evaluate the carcinogenicity in humans.

vinyl chloride: K. Used mainly by the plastics industry to produce polyvinyl chloride (PVC) and copolymers. Common items containing PVC include automotive parts and accessories, battery cell separators, containers, credit cards, electrical insulation, flooring, furniture, medical supplies, windows, wrapping film, and videodiscs. Vinyl chloride-vinyl acetate copolymers are used to produce films and resins. Human exposure is through inhalation of contaminated air, ingestion of contaminated foods and water, and skin contact. Studies indicate that vinyl chloride causes a rare tumor of the liver (angiosarcoma), as well as other tumors.

4-vinyl-1-cyclohexene diepoxide: RA. Used to dilute other diepoxides and for epoxy resins. Exposure is through inhalation and especially through skin contact. Skin cancer at the site of application and tumors of the ovary occurred in laboratory animals when exposed to 4-vinyl-1-cyclohexene diepoxide. No adequate data are available to evaluate the carcinogenicity in humans.

vinyl fluoride: RA. Used primarily in the production of polyvinyl fluoride and other fluoropolymers, which are commonly used as building materials. Human exposure is primarily by inhalation, but skin and eye contact may also occur. A variety of tumors have occurred in laboratory animals when administered by inhalation. No adequate data are available to evaluate the carcinogenicity in humans.

wood dust: K. Usually produced as a by-product of manufacturing wood products; commercially used in wood composts. Human exposure is through inhalation. Studies have determined that cancer of the nasal cavities and paranasal sinuses is associated with wood dust exposure, with limited evidence for cancer of the nasopharynx and larynx and Hodgkin disease.

X radiation and gamma radiation: K. Used in medicine (radiotherapy, computed tomography, positron emission tomography), the nuclear power industry, the military (nuclear weapons), scientific research, industry (well logging, sterilizing products, irradiating foods), and various consumer products (smoke detectors, televisions, radioluminescent clocks and watches, self-luminous signs). Exposure to X radiation and gamma radiation is strongly associated with leukemia and cancer of the thyroid, breast, and lung; cancer of the bladder, central nervous system, colon, salivary glands, skin, stomach, and ovary have also been reported.

▶ Glossary

ABCD rating: A system used to describe the stages of prostate cancer, with "A" and "B" describing cancer that is confined to the prostate, "C" for cancer that has grown out of the prostate but has not metastasized or spread to lymph nodes, and "D" for cancer that has metastasized or spread to lymph nodes.

ablation: The removal, destruction, or severing of diseased or damaged tissue, body part, or its functionality through surgery, drugs, heat, hormones, radiofrequency, or other means.

abscess: A pus-filled cavity that is usually swollen and inflamed and is a result of bacterial infection.

acquired immunodeficiency syndrome (AIDS): A disease of the immune system, caused by the human immunodeficiency virus (HIV), that causes a substantially increased risk for developing certain cancers and infections.

acromegaly: A rare disorder of adults in which an overproduction of growth hormones causes an enlargement of the bones of the hands, feet, nose, jaw, and head, as well as various other signs and symptoms.

actinic keratosis: Precancerous patches of skin that are thick and scaly. (Also called solar keratosis and senile keratosis.)

acute: That which begins and worsens quickly.

adeno-: Referring to a gland.

adenoma: A tumor of glandular origin or of a glandular structure that is not cancerous.

adenopathy: Swollen or large lymph glands.

adenosine triphosphate (ATP): The chemical compound in all living cells that provides the energy needed for metabolic processes.

adenosquamous carcinoma: A malignant tumor that contains both glandular cells and squamous cells.

adjunct therapy: Another treatment used in addition to a primary treatment to aid the primary treatment and increase the chance for a cure, such as chemotherapy used in addition to surgery.

adnexal mass: A growth of tissue in the uterine adnexa, usually in the ovary or Fallopian tube; it includes ovarian cysts, benign or malignant tumors, and ectopic (tubal) pregnancies.

adrenal glands: Small endocrine glands located on top of both kidneys that make and secrete adrenaline and noradrenaline, the steroid hormones that help control heart rate, blood pressure, and other body functions. (Also called suprarenal glands.)

adrenalectomy: Surgical removal of one or both adrenal glands.

adrenocortical: Pertaining to the outer layer of the adrenal gland.

adult T-cell leukemia/lymphoma (ATLL): A fast-growing T-cell non-Hodgkin lymphoma, which is a cancer of the immune system's T cells; it is believed to be caused by the human T-cell leukemia/lymphotropic virus type 1 (HTLV-1).

aggravating factor: Something that makes a medical condition worse, more serious, or more severe.

aggressive: That which grows, develops, or spreads quickly.

agnogenic myeloid metaplasia (AMM): A slow-developing, long-term disease that occurs when bone marrow is replaced by fibrous tissue, making the bone marrow unable to manufacture blood cells properly and creating a condition in which blood is then made in organs such as the liver and the spleen; this may lead to the enlargement of these organs and progressive anemia.

AIDS: *See* aquired immunodeficiency syndrome.

AJCC staging system: Developed by the American Joint Committee on Cancer, this system describes the extent of cancer in a patient's body using T to describe the size of the tumor and if it has invaded nearby tissue, N to describe any nearby lymph nodes that are involved, and M to describe distant metastasis (spread of the cancer to another part of the body).

alanine aminopeptidase (AAP): An enzyme that is used as a biomarker to detect kidney damage and that can be used to help diagnose certain kidney disorders; high levels occur in the urine when there are problems with the kidney.

alanine transferase: An enzyme found in the liver and various bodily tissues and which, when present in abnormally high levels in the blood, may be a sign of liver damage, cancer, or other diseases.

allogeneic bone marrow transplantation: A procedure in which stem cells derived from the bone marrow are transferred to the cancer patient from a genetically similar but not identical donor, such as a brother or sister.

allogeneic stem cell transplantation: A procedure in which blood-forming stem cells are transferred to the cancer patient from a genetically similar but not identical donor, such as a brother or sister.

allopathic medicine: *See* conventional medicine.

amelanotic melanoma: A cancerous skin lesion that has little or no color, although it may appear red, pink, or white, and has an asymmetrical shape with an irregular faintly pigmented border that may be light brown, tan, or gray.

ampullary cancer: Cancer of the ampulla of Vater, which is the area where the pancreatic duct and the common bile duct (from the liver) join together and enter the small intestine.

analgesic: A drug, such as aspirin, acetaminophen, and ibuprofen, that reduces pain.

anaphylactic shock: The most severe and sometimes life-threatening whole-body allergic reaction during which a person may experience itchy skin, edema, collapsed blood vessels, fainting, difficulty in breathing, and then death if medical treatment is not received promptly.

anaplastic: Rapidly dividing cancer cells with an abnormal appearance.

anaplastic large cell lymphoma (ALCL): A fast-growing non-Hodgkin lymphoma, that is usually a cancer of the immune system's T cells and that may occur in the lymph nodes of the neck, armpit, or groin, as well as in the bones, liver, lungs, soft tissues, or skin.

anaplastic thyroid cancer: A rare and aggressive thyroid cancer consisting of abnormal-looking cancer cells.

anastomosis: A surgical procedure in which healthy sections of tubular structures in the body are connected together after a diseased portion has been surgically removed.

androblastoma: A rare ovarian tumor that secretes a male sex hormone, usually causing physical characteristics of men to appear in women.

anesthetic: A medical substance that puts the patient to sleep, causing a loss of feeling and awareness when administered systemically (general anesthetics) or causing a loss of feeling in only part of the body when applied locally.

angioimmunoblastic T-cell lymphoma: A fast-growing T-cell non-Hodgkin lymphoma that causes enlarged lymph nodes and increased antibodies in the blood, and may also cause a skin rash, fever, weight loss, and night sweats.

angiomyolipoma: A benign tumor of fat and muscle tissue usually found in the kidney and that may bleed or grow painfully large enough to cause kidney failure but otherwise rarely causes any symptoms.

anorexia: An abnormal loss of appetite.

anterior mediastinotomy: A procedure in which a tube is inserted through an incision next the breastbone to view the tissues and organs in the area between the breastbone and heart and between the lungs.

anterior pelvic exenteration: The surgical removal of the uterus, cervix, vagina, urethra, lower part of the ureters, and bladder.

anterior urethral cancer: Cancer of the part of the urethra (the tube that carries urine from the bladder to the outside of the body) that is closest to the outside of the body.

antiangiogenic: That which reduces the growth of new blood vessels.

antibody: A specific type of protein created by plasma cells (white blood cells) as an immune response to a specific antigen (foreign substance, such as a virus or bacterium) that may be a threat to the body, to neutralize or destroy that antigen. (Also called an immunoglobulin.)

antibody therapy: A medical treatment that uses an antibody to kill specific tumor cells, either directly or by stimulating the immune system to kill the tumor cells.

anticoagulant: A drug used to aid in the prevention of blood clots. (Also called a blood thinner.)

antiemetic: A drug used to prevent or reduce nausea and vomiting.

antigen: A substance that stimulates a specific immune response, namely the production of antibodies.

antiglobulin test: A laboratory test used to determine blood type and to diagnose blood disorders in which antibodies are produced that destroy a patient's own red blood cells or platelets.

antimitotic agent: A drug used to treat cancer by stopping cell division (mitosis) and thereby blocking cell growth.

apheresis: A procedure in which blood is withdrawn from a patient or donor, the blood is passed through an apparatus that separates out one or more components from the blood, and then the remaining blood is transfused back into the patient or donor.

aromatase inhibitor: A drug that interferes with the role of the aromatase enzyme in the production of estradiol, a female hormone; it is used as hormone therapy for postmenopausal women who have hormone-dependent breast cancer.

arterial access device: A semipermanent implantable device, such as a port, chemo-port, port-a-cath, or PICC line, that allows a medical professional direct access to an artery without having to put a needle into the artery every time treatment is given, making administration of chemotherapy easier and reducing the risk of certain chemotherapy-related complications.

arteriogram: An X ray of arteries taken after the injection into the arteries of a special dye.

aspiration: The removal of a sample of tissue or fluid for examination by suctioning through a needle attached to a syringe, or the accidental inhalation of a foreign substance into the lungs.

assay: A laboratory test that finds and measures the quantity of one or more components within a specific substance.

ataxia: Loss of the ability to coordinate voluntary muscle movements.

atypical teratoid/rhabdoid tumor: An aggressive and rare pediatric cancer involving the central nervous system, kidney, or liver.

autoimmune hemolytic anemia: A condition in which the body's immune system interferes with the formation of red blood cells; it may occur in patients with chronic lymphocytic leukemia (CLL).

autologous bone marrow transplantation: A procedure in which a patient's own bone marrow is removed, stored, and then returned back to that person's body after intensive treatment, such as high-dose chemotherapy.

autologous stem cell transplantation: A procedure in which a patient's own blood-forming stem cells are removed, stored, and then returned back to that person's body.

autonomic nervous system (ANS): The part of the nervous system that controls muscles of internal organs (such as the blood vessels, heart, lungs, intestines, and stomach) and glands (such as sweat glands and salivary glands) and affects involuntary, reflexive functions, such as heart rate, respiration rate, digestion, perspiration, and salivation. It consists of three parts: the parasympathetic nervous system, which induces fight-or-flight responses in emergencies or stressful situations; the sympathetic nervous system, which allows the body to rest and digest; and the enteric nervous system, which controls the gastrointestinal system.

B cell: A white blood cell that makes antibodies and helps fight infections.

B-cell acute lymphocytic leukemia: With this leukemia, the most common type of acute lymphoblastic leukemia (ALL), abnormal immature white blood cells (B-cell lymphoblasts) crowd out the normal white blood cells, red blood cells, and platelets the body needs. (Also called B-cell acute lymphoblastic leukemia and precursor B-lymphoblastic leukemia.)

B-cell lymphoma: A type of non-Hodgkin lymphoma that affects B cells (immature white blood cells) and may be either slow-growing or fast-growing; there are many types of B-cell lymphomas.

barbiturate: A drug that depresses the central nervous system, causing a sedative effect that can be used to relieve anxiety before surgery and to treat insomnia, seizures, and convulsions.

barium swallow: *See* esophagram.

Bellini duct carcinoma (BDC): A rare, fast-growing, and fast-spreading kidney cancer that begins in the duct of Bellini in the kidney.

Bench Jones protein: A protein produced by plasma cells that is found in the urine of patients with certain diseases, especially multiple myeloma.

benign: Not cancerous.

Biafine cream: A cream applied topically by patients receiving radiation treatment to reduce the risk of and to treat skin reactions to the radiation.

bilateral cancer: Cancer that occurs in both the left and right organs, such as both breasts or both ovaries.

biliary: Pertaining to the liver, bile ducts, and gallbladder.

biological response modifier (BRM) therapy: A treatment that uses monoclonal antibodies, growth factors, and vaccines to enhance or restore the immune system's ability to fight infections, cancer, and other diseases, as well as to reduce certain side effects that may be caused by some cancer treatments.

biomedicine: *See* conventional medicine.

biopsy: The removal of cells, tissues, or entire lumps or suspicious areas for microscopic examination by a pathologist.

blood-brain barrier (BBB): A network of blood vessels with closely spaced cells that prevents many potentially toxic substances, including anticancer drugs, from leaving the bloodstream and crossing the protective blood vessel walls into the brain tissues.

blood-brain barrier disruption (BBBD): The use of drugs to create gaps between the cells of the barrier so that anticancer drugs may be delivered to a brain tumor via an artery that goes into the brain.

blood cell count: *See* complete blood count (CBC).

blood thinner: *See* anticoagulant.

blood urea nitrogen (BUN): A substance in the blood that occurs naturally as a result of the breakdown of protein in liver and that is usually filtered out of the blood and into the urine by the kidneys; a high level of urea nitrogen in the blood may indicate a kidney problem.

bolus infusion: A single dose of drug given quickly by intravenous injection.

bone metastasis: Cancer that has spread to the bone from the original tumor.

bone-seeking radioisotope: A substance that gives off low-level radiation, which kills cancer cells; it is administered through a vein, then collects in bone cells and tumor cells that have spread to the bone.

brain stem gliomas: Tumors of the brain stem (the part of the brain that connects to the spinal cord).

breast-conserving surgery: The surgical removal of the breast cancer without removing all of the breast. The surgery may involve the removal of the lump (lumpectomy); the removal of one quarter, or quadrant, of the breast (quadrantectomy); or the removal of the tumor and some of the breast tissue around the tumor, as well as the lining over the chest muscles below the tumor (segmental mastectomy). (Also called breast-sparing surgery.)

breast duct endoscopy: A procedure in which a thin, flexible tube attached to a camera is inserted through the nipple and into the breast ducts deep into the breast to look for abnormal tissue in the lining of the breast ducts; samples of tissue and fluid may be removed during the procedure.

bronchogenic carcinoma: Lung cancer that begins in the lining of the airways of the lungs (bronchi) and includes small-cell and non-small cell lung cancer.

bronchoscopy: A procedure in which a thin, flexible tube with a light and lens is inserted through the nose or mouth and into the trachea, bronchi (airways of the lungs), and lungs to look for signs of cancer, remove tissue for microscopic examination by a pathologist, or perform treatment procedures.

Burkitt lymphoma: A rare, aggressive leukemia (cancer of the blood) in which an excess of white blood cells (B lymphocytes) forms in the blood and bone marrow; it has been linked to infection with the Epstein-Barr virus.

cancer: A group of diseases in which abnormal cells divide without control and then can invade nearby tissues and may even spread to other locations in the body via the blood and lymph systems.

cancer of the adrenal cortex: A rare cancer of the outer part of the adrenal gland that may or may not make more than a normal amount of certain hormones (aldosterone, cortisol, estrogen, or testosterone).

carbogen: A mixture of oxygen and carbon dioxide that is inhaled and induces an increased sensitivity of tumor cells to the effects of radiation therapy.

carcinogen: A substance that causes cancer.

carcinogenesis: The process in which normal cells are transformed into cancer cells.

carcinoma: A malignant tumor that begins in the skin or in the tissues that line or cover the internal organs (epithelial tissue).

carcinoma of unknown primary origin (CUP): A cancer in which cancer cells have spread and been found in the body; however, the initial location where the cells first started growing cannot be established.

carcinosarcoma: A malignant tumor containing both epithelial tissue (such as skin or tissue that lines or covers internal organs) and connective tissue (such as bone, cartilage, or fat).

cardiac sarcoma: A rare cancer in heart tissue. (Also called heart cancer.)

catheter: A flexible tube used to inject or withdraw fluids from the body.

cauterize: To destroy tissue by using extreme heat or cold, an electric current, or caustic chemicals.

CBC: *See* complete blood count (CBC).

cellular adoptive immunotherapy: A treatment in which the T cells (white blood cells) of a cancer patient are collected, grown, and multiplied in number in the laboratory, then given back to the patient to help the patient's immune system fight the cancer.

central nervous system primitive neuroectodermal tumor: A cancer that originates from a particular type of cell in the brain or spinal cord.

central nervous system prophylaxis: A preventive medical treatment in which chemotherapy or radiation is administered to the central nervous system to kill cancer cells that may be undetectable in the brain and spinal cord.

cerebellar hemangioblastoma: A benign, slow-growing tumor in the posterior part of the brain (cerebellum).

cervical intraepithelial neoplasia (CIN): The formation of abnormal cells on the surface of the cervix.

chemoimmunotherapy: The use of chemotherapy to kill or slow cancer cell growth, combined with immunotherapy to restore the immune system's ability to fight cancer.

chemoprotective agent: A drug used to protect healthy tissues in the body from the toxic effects of anticancer drugs.

chemoradiation: A medical treatment that combines chemotherapy and radiation therapy.

chemotherapy: A drug treatment used to kill cancer cells.

chloroma: *See* granulocytic sarcoma.

cholangiocarcinoma: A rare cancer that occurs in the lining of the bile ducts in the liver.

cholangiosarcoma: A tumor of the connective tissues of the bile ducts in the liver.

chondrosarcoma: A cancer that forms in cartilage.

chorioadenoma destruens: A cancer that typically forms after fertilization of an egg and that grows into the muscular wall of the uterus.

choroid plexus tumor: A rare cancer that develops in the ventricles of the brain and usually occurs in children younger than two years old.

chronic: A disease or condition that continues, slowly progresses, or returns, often over a long period of time.

clear cell adenocarcinoma: A rare tumor, especially of the female genital tract, that contains cells that look clear inside when viewed under a microscope.

clinical resistance: An unsuccessful reduction in the amount of a cancer after treatment.

colorectal: Pertaining to the colon and the rectum.

complete blood count (CBC): A laboratory test that determines the number of red blood cells, white blood cells, and platelets in a sample of blood. (Also called blood cell count.)

complete hysterectomy: The surgical removal of the uterus and the cervix.

complete metastasectomy: The surgical removal of all tumors formed from cancerous cells that have spread from the original tumor.

complete remission: A period during which any clinical signs of a disease disappear in response to a treatment; however, this does not necessarily mean that the disease has been cured.

computed tomography (CT) scan: A series of detailed pictures of structures within the body, created by a computer that takes the data from multiple X-ray images taken from different angles and turns them into pictures on a screen. (Also called computerized axial tomography scan, tomography scan, computerized tomography, and CAT scan.)

concurrent therapy: A medical treatment given at the same time as another.

congenital mesoblastic nephroma: A kidney tumor, containing connective tissue cells, that may spread to nearby tissue or the other kidney and that is found in a fetus before birth or in an infant within the first three months of life.

consolidation therapy: A high-dose chemotherapy given after induction therapy as the second phase of a cancer treatment regimen, to help further reduce the presence of cancer cells in the body. (Also called intensification therapy.)

contraindication: Something, such as a medical condition or a symptom, that makes a particular treatment inadvisable because of the increased likelihood of a bad reaction.

contrast material: A dye or other substance that is given to a patient by intravenous injection, enema, or mouth and used with X rays, computed tomography (CT) scans, magnetic resonance imaging (MRI), or other imaging tests to show abnormal areas inside the body.

conventional medicine: A system of medicine in which symptoms and diseases are treated using drugs, radiation, or surgery by medical doctors with the assistance of other health care professionals, such as nurses, pharmacists, and therapists. (Also called allopathic medicine and biomedicine.)

CT scan: *See* computed tomography (CT) scan.

cystoprostatectomy: The surgical removal of the bladder and the prostate; the seminal vesicles are also removed in a radical cystoprostatectomy.

cystosarcoma phyllodes (CSP): Tumors that occur in breast tissue and are usually benign but may be malignant.

cystourethrectomy: The surgical removal of the bladder and the urethra.

cytopenia: A deficiency of blood cells.

debulking: Surgically removing as much of a tumor as possible.

desmoplastic melanoma: A rare form of skin cancer, specifically a variant of malignant melanoma, that is characterized by nonpigmented lesions on sun-exposed areas of the body, especially on the head and neck.

diffuse hyperplastic perilobar nephroblastomatosis (DHPLN): Abnormal tissue growth on the outer part of one or both kidneys that occurs during childhood and that may develop into Wilms' tumor (childhood kidney cancer) if not treated.

diffuse large B-cell lymphoma: A fast-growing cancer of the immune system (a non-Hodgkin lymphoma) that is characterized by tumors in the lymph nodes, bone marrow, liver, spleen, and other organs, as well as fever, night sweats, and weight loss.

distant metastasis: The spread of cancer from the original site to distant organs or distant lymph nodes.

donor lymphocyte infusion: A therapy in which lymphocytes (a type of white blood cell) are taken from the blood of the stem cell transplant donor and given to the recipient patient to kill remaining cancer cells.

ductal carcinoma: Cancer that begins in the cells that line the milk ducts in the breast, which is the most common type of breast cancer.

durable power of attorney: A legal document that gives one person the authority to make medical, legal, or financial decisions for another person until that person dies or cancels it; it may go into effect immediately or when that person is incapable of making those decisions.

early-stage cancer: Cancer that is in the beginning stage of its growth and has not spread to other parts of the body.

ectomesenchymoma: A rare, fast-growing tumor of the nervous system or soft tissue that may form in the abdomen, head, neck, limbs, perineum, or scrotum in children and young adults.

-ectomy: Surgical removal.

endocrine: Pertaining to tissues, such as the pituitary, thyroid, and adrenal glands, which make hormones and release them throughout the body via the bloodstream; these hormones control the actions of other cells or organs.

endoscopic ultrasound (EUS): A procedure in which a thin, tubelike instrument (an endoscope) is inserted into the body and a probe at the end of the endoscope uses high-energy sound waves (ultrasound) to make a picture (sonogram) of internal organs. (Also called endosonography.)

epithelial carcinoma: Cancer that originates in the cells that line an organ.

epithelial ovarian cancer: Cancer that occurs in the cells on the outside of the ovary.

erythrocyte sedimentation rate (ESR): The distance red blood cells travel in one hour in a sample of blood as they settle to the bottom of a test tube; this rate increases when inflammation, infection, cancer, diseases of the blood and bone marrow, and rheumatic diseases are present.

erythroleukemia: Cancer of the blood-forming tissues in which an excess of immature, abnormal red blood cells is found in the blood and bone marrow.

erythroleukoplakia: Potentially cancerous patches of red and white tissue that form on mucous membranes in the mouth; alcohol and tobacco (smoking or chewing) increase the risk of erythroleukoplakia.

esophageal stent: A metal mesh, plastic, or silicone tube that is placed in the esophagus to keep a blocked area open so that the patient can swallow soft food and liquids; it may be used in the treatment of esophageal cancer.

esophagram: A series of X rays of the esophagus taken after the patient drinks a barium solution. (Also called barium swallow and upper GI series.)

Ewing family of tumors (EFTs): A group of tumors that all come from the same type of stem cell and include Ewing tumor of bone (ETB or Ewing sarcoma of bone), extraosseous Ewing (EOE) tumors, Askin tumors (PNET of the chest wall), and primitive neuroectodermal tumors (PNET or peripheral neuroepithelioma).

excision: Removal by surgery.

excisional biopsy: The surgical removal of a lump or suspicious area for microscopic examination by a pathologist.

excisional skin surgery: The surgical removal of cysts, moles, other skin growths, and skin cancer (including some of the healthy tissue around it) using local anesthesia.

extracranial germ-cell tumor: A rare cancer that originates in reproductive cells (germ cells) in the ovary or testicle, or in germ cells that have traveled to areas of the body other than the brain, such as the abdomen, chest, or tailbone.

extrahepatic bile duct cancer: A rare cancer that occurs in the part of the bile duct that is outside the liver.

extrapleural pneumonectomy: The surgical removal of a diseased lung, part of the membrane covering the heart (pericardium), part of the muscle between the lungs and the abdomen (diaphragm), and part of the membrane lining the chest (parietal pleura); this surgery is often used to treat malignant mesothelioma.

familial adenomatous polyposis (FAP): An inherited condition in which many growths (polyps) form on the inside walls of the colon and rectum; this condition increases the risk for colorectal cancer.

familial dysplastic nevi: A hereditary condition in which at least two members of a family have atypical moles (dysplastic nevi) and are at very high risk for developing melanoma.

familial isolated hyperparathyroidism (FIHP): A rare inherited condition characterized by a loss of calcium in the bones, an elevated calcium level in the blood (hypercalcemia), and an excessive amount of parathyroid hormone (PTH) being produced because of one or more tumors in the parathyroid glands.

familial medullary thyroid cancer: An inherited form of cancer that develops in the cells of the thyroid that make the hormone calcitonin.

fast-neutron beam radiation: A type of radiation therapy in which a machine (a cyclotron) focuses a beam of high-energy neutrons to kill cancer cells.

fibroid: A benign smooth-muscle tumor most often found in the uterus or gastrointestinal tract. (Also called leiomyoma.)

fibromatosis: A condition in which many benign tumors grow in connective tissues.

fine needle aspiration (FNA) biopsy: The removal of a sample of tissue or fluid for examination under a microscope by suctioning through a thin needle attached to a syringe.

fluoroscopy: An imaging technique that allows a physician to see internal organs in motion by the use of a fluoroscope (a machine that transmits an X-ray beam through a patient so that it strikes a fluorescent plate that is attached to a television camera, causing the images to be visible live on a television monitor); this technique is often used to observe the digestive tract.

FOLFOX: A chemotherapy drug combination of folinic acid (leucovorin), fluorouracil, and oxaliplatin that is used to treat colorectal cancer.

follicular large-cell lymphoma: A rare, slow-growing cancer of the lymphatic system (a non-Hodgkin lymphoma) with large cancer cells.

follicular lymphoma: A cancer of the immune system (a B-cell non-Hodgkin lymphoma) in which tumor cells grow as groups to form nodules.

follicular mixed-cell lymphoma: A slow-growing cancer of the lymphatic system (a B-cell non-Hodgkin lymphoma) with both large and small cancer cells.

follicular thyroid cancer: A slow-growing, highly treatable cancer of the follicular cells in the thyroid.

functional magnetic resonance imaging (fMRI): A noninvasive diagnostic tool that uses a powerful magnetic field, radio waves, and a computer to produce detailed pictures of the brain, spinal cord, or other organs and allows physicians to measure the metabolic changes that are taking place by detecting changes in blood flow and blood oxygenation.

fungating lesion: A type of skin lesion that develops when an underlying malignant tumor increases in size and extends through the epithelium, leaving a visible ulceration with tissue necrosis (death of living tissue), infection, and odor, and that may occur in many types of cancer, especially in advanced disease.

gamma irradiation: A type of radiation therapy that uses a high-energy radiation different from X rays called gamma radiation.

gastrectomy: Surgical removal of all or part of the stomach.

gastroscopy: Examination of the inside of the stomach by passing a thin, tubelike instrument with a light and lens for viewing through the mouth and esophagus into the stomach. (Also called upper endoscopy.)

germinoma: A germ-cell tumor that is most often found in the brain.

glial tumors: Tumors of the central nervous system, which include astrocytomas, ependymal tumors, glioblastoma multiforme, and primitive neuroectodermal tumors.

glucagonoma: A fast-growing tumor of the central nervous system originating in the glial tissue of the brain and spinal cord.

graft-versus-host (GVD) disease: An antitumor effect in which immune system cells in transplanted tissue from a donor (for example, bone marrow or peripheral blood) attack and help eliminate the recipient patient's tumor cells.

granulocytic sarcoma: A malignant, green-colored tumor composed of immature white blood cells (myeloblasts) and often associated with myelogenous leukemia. (Also called chloroma.)

health care proxy (HCP): A legal document that gives one person the authority to make health care decisions for another person when that person loses the ability to make those decisions.

heart cancer: *See* cardiac sarcoma.

hematoma: A mass of clotted or partially clotted blood that forms in a tissue, an organ, or a body space as a result of a broken blood vessel.

hematopoiesis: The production of new blood cells.

hemilaryngectomy: The surgical removal of one side of the larynx (voice box).

hemorrhage: Extensive blood loss from damaged blood vessels, usually within a short amount of time.

hepatectomy: Surgical removal of all or part of the liver.

hepatic: Pertaining to the liver.

hepatic arterial occlusion: A blockage in the blood flow to the liver; can be caused intentionally using drugs or other agents to help kill cancer cells growing in the liver or inadvertently while providing chemotherapy through a catheter in the hepatic artery.

hepatic veno-occlusive disease: A blockage in some of the veins in the liver, which is a common complication of high-dose chemotherapy given before a bone marrow transplant and which causes increases in weight, liver size, and blood levels of bilirubin.

hepatobiliary: Pertaining to the liver, bile ducts, and gallbladder.

hepatoblastoma: A malignant liver tumor of infants and young children.

hepatocellular carcinoma: The most common type of liver tumor; it originates in the hepatocytes, the major type of cell in the liver, and is usually caused by cirrhosis (scarring of the liver).

hepatoma: A tumor of the liver.

hereditary nonpolyposis colorectal cancer (HNPCC): An inherited cancer syndrome in which a person has a very high risk of developing colorectal cancer and an above-normal risk of other cancers, including uterus, ovary, stomach, small intestine, biliary system, urinary tract, brain, and skin. (Also called Lynch syndrome.)

high-dose chemotherapy: An intensive anticancer drug treatment that also destroys bone marrow and may cause other severe side effects; bone marrow or stem cell transplantation to rebuild the bone marrow usually follows this type of chemotherapy.

high-dose radiation (HDR) therapy: A greater amount of radiation than in typical radiation therapy is directed precisely at the tumor, so as to kill more cancer cells in fewer treatments without damaging healthy tissue.

high dose rate remote radiation therapy: A radiation treatment that involves placing a radiation source inside the body as close as possible to the cancer cells and then removing it between treatments.

high-energy photon therapy: A radiation therapy in which high-energy photons (units of light energy) penetrate deeply into tissues to attack tumors while imparting less radiation to superficial tissues, such as the skin.

high-grade lymphoma: A cancerous tumor of lymphoid tissue that grows and spreads quickly and has severe symptoms.

high-grade squamous intraepithelial lesion (HSIL): A precancerous condition in which there are abnormal cells of the uterine cervix.

high-risk cancer: A cancer that is likely to spread or come back.

homeopathic medicine: An alternative system of medicine based on the belief that a substance that causes particular symptoms in a healthy person can be used in minute doses to cure those symptoms in an ill person.

Hurthle cell neoplasm: A type of thyroid tumor that is uncommon and may be either benign or malignant.

hyper-: Excessive; above normal.

hyperalimentation: The intravenous feeding of nutrients to patients who cannot ingest or digest food through the alimentary tract.

hyperfractionation: The practice of giving smaller doses (fractions) of radiation more often than the standard radiation dose of once a day, resulting in fewer side effects.

hypernephroma: Kidney cancer that originates in the lining of the renal tubules in the kidney; it is the most common type of kidney cancer. (Also called renal cell cancer.)

hypersensitivity: An abnormal or excessive response by the immune system to a drug or other substance.

hyperuricemia: Presence of an excessive amount of uric acid in the blood, which is sometimes a side effect of anticancer drugs.

hypo-: Less than normal.

hypofractionation: The practice of giving larger doses (fractions) of radiation less often and over a shorter period of time than the standard radiation dose of once a day.

hypopharyngeal cancer: Cancer that originates in the bottom part of the throat (hypopharynx).

idiopathic pneumonia syndrome: A condition characterized by pneumonia-like symptoms, such as fever, chills, coughing, and breathing difficulties, with no obvious infection in the lung; it can occur after a stem cell transplant.

immature teratoma: A rare germ-cell tumor often containing different tissues, such as bone, hair, and muscle.

immunoglobulin: *See* antibody.

implantable pump: A small device that is implanted under the skin and that administers a steady dose of drugs.

incidence: The number of new cases of a disease diag-

nosed in a specific population during a specified period (usually a year).

incision: A cut or wound in body tissue, especially that made with a surgical instrument.

incisional biopsy: Surgical removal of a part of a lump or suspicious area for examination under a microscope.

incontinence: Inability to control the discharge of urine (urinary incontinence) or feces (fecal incontinence).

indolent: Slow to develop or progress.

indolent lymphoma: *See* low-grade lymphoma.

induction therapy: The initial treatment used in an effort to make subsequent treatments, such as surgery or radiotherapy, more effective and to evaluate the response to drugs or other agents.

infiltrating cancer: Cancer that has spread into nearby, healthy tissue. (Also called invasive cancer.)

intensification therapy: *See* consolidation therapy.

inter-: Between or among.

interstitial radiation therapy: Radiation treatment in which radioactive material sealed in needles, wires, seeds, or catheters is inserted into tissue at or near the tumor site.

intra-: Within, during, or between layers of.

intracranial tumor: A tumor situated in the brain.

intrahepatic infusion: The administration of drugs directly into the blood vessels of the liver.

intraluminal intubation and dilation: A procedure in which a tube (plastic or metal) is inserted through the mouth into the esophagus to keep it open; it is used especially during radiation therapy for esophageal cancer.

intramuscular (IM): Within or into muscle.

intraoperative radiation therapy (IORT): A procedure in which a concentrated beam of radiation is aimed directly at a tumor while it is exposed during surgery.

intraperitoneal (IP): Within the peritoneal (abdominal) cavity.

intraperitoneal chemotherapy: Treatment in which anticancer drugs are delivered directly into the peritoneal (abdominal) cavity through a thin tube.

intraperitoneal infusion: The administration of drugs and fluids directly into the peritoneal (abdominal) cavity through a thin tube.

intraperitoneal radiation therapy: Treatment in which a radioactive liquid is delivered directly into the peritoneal (abdominal) cavity through a thin tube.

intrathecal chemotherapy: Treatment in which anticancer drugs are delivered by injection directly into the fluid-filled space between the thin layers of tissue that cover the brain and spinal cord.

intravenous pyelogram (IVP): A series of X rays taken

of the kidneys, ureters, and bladder after intravenous administration of a dye that collects in and is excreted by the kidneys.

intraventricular infusion: The administration of a drug into the fluid-filled cavity within the heart or brain.

invasive cancer: *See* infiltrating cancer.

inverted papilloma: A tumor of the mucosal membrane of the nasal cavity, paranasal sinus, or urinary tract in which the epithelial cells grow downward into the underlying supportive tissue.

irradiation: The use of high-energy radiation to kill cancer cells and shrink tumors. (Also called radiation therapy.)

isolated hepatic perfusion: A procedure in which the liver's blood supply is temporarily separated from blood circulating throughout the rest of the body by the placement of a catheter into the artery that provides blood to the liver and the placement of a second catheter into the vein that takes blood away from the liver, so that high doses of anticancer drugs can be directed to the liver only.

isolated limb perfusion: A procedure in which a tourniquet is used to stop the flow of blood to and from a limb (arm or leg) temporarily so that high-dose anticancer drugs can be delivered directly to the limb where the cancer is situated.

isolated lung perfusion: A surgical procedure during which high-dose anticancer drugs are delivered directly to tumors in the lungs after separating the circulation of blood to the lungs from the circulation of blood through the rest of the body.

-itis: A suffix denoting inflammation or inflammatory disease.

J-pouch coloanal anastomosis: The surgical attachment of the colon to the anus after the removal of the rectum, performed by forming a J-shaped pouch from a 2- to 4-inch section of the colon as a replacement for the rectum.

jaundice: A condition in which the liver is not working properly or a bile duct is blocked, causing the skin and the whites of the eyes to yellow, the urine to darken, and the color of the stool to become lighter than normal.

juvenile myelomonocytic leukemia (JMML): A rare childhood cancer of the blood or bone marrow in which cancer cells spread into tissues such as the skin, lungs, and intestines.

Kahler disease: A cancer of plasma cells (immune system cells in bone marrow that produce antibodies).

keratoacanthoma: A quick-growing, rounded skin tumor that occurs on sun-exposed areas of the body, especially on the head and neck, and that tends to heal on its own.

Klatskin tumor: A cancer of the lining of the bile ducts in the liver at the junction where the left and right ducts meet; it is a type of cholangiocarcinoma.

large-cell carcinoma: The uncontrolled growth of large, cancerous cells of the lung.

late-stage cancer: A cancer that has been growing for a while and has spread to the lymph nodes or other parts of the body.

leiomyoma: *See* fibroid.

leukemia: A cancer of the blood or bone marrow that is characterized by an abnormal increase in the number of white blood cells in the tissues of the body and may also include an increase of those in the circulating blood; leukemias are classified according to the type of white blood cell most noticeably involved.

ligation: The surgical process of tying up a blood vessel to stop blood from reaching a tumor or part of the body.

light-emitting diode (LED) therapy: A therapy in which a special type of light is used to activate specific drugs that react when exposed to the light, enabling them to kill the cancer cells.

limited-stage small-cell lung cancer: Lung cancer in which cancer cells are found in one lung, only nearby lymph nodes, and the tissues between the lungs.

lipoma: A benign tumor consisting of fat cells.

localized cancer: Cancer that is confined to the original site without evidence of having spread.

locally advanced cancer: Cancer that has spread to nearby tissue or lymph nodes.

low-grade lymphoma: Cancer of immune system cells that grows and spreads slowly, inducing few symptoms. (Also called indolent lymphoma.)

low-grade squamous intraepithelial lesion (LSIL): Slight changes in the size and shape of the cells on the surface of the uterine cervix that are considered mild abnormalities caused by human papillomavirus (HPV) infection.

lower gastrointestinal (GI) series: A group of X rays taken of the colon and rectum following a barium enema; it is used to diagnose abnormalities in the large intestine.

lymph nodes: Glands that are located along the lymphatic system in many areas throughout the body and that filter impurities, such as cancer cells or bacteria, from the lymphatic fluid that flows through the nodes.

lymphoepithelioma: A cancer that originates in the tissues covering the nasopharynx (the upper part of the throat behind the nose).

lymphography: An X-ray study of lymphatic vessels and lymph nodes after injection of a special dye.

lymphoma: A malignant tumor of the lymph nodes or other lymphatic tissues.

lymphoscintigraphy: An imaging technique used in conjunction with a radioactive substance injected at the site of the tumor to identify the first draining lymph node near a tumor so that a physician can determine which lymph node to remove for examination.

Lynch syndrome: *See* hereditary nonpolyposis colon cancer (HNPCC).

lytic lesion: An area of bone that has been destroyed from a disease process, such as cancer.

magnetic resonance imaging (MRI): An imaging method using magnetism, radio waves, and a computer to produce images of organs and soft tissues; it provides spatial information about the size and shape of a tumor.

magnetic resonance perfusion imaging: A diagnostic technique that is used in conjunction with an injected dye to produce computerized images of blood flow through tissues; it is a special type of magnetic resonance imaging (MRI).

magnetic resonance spectroscopic imaging (MRSI): An imaging method that detects and measures activity at the cellular level, providing metabolic information; it is used in conjunction with magnetic resonance imaging (MRI).

magnetic-targeted carrier: A tiny bead containing iron and carbon particles that is attached to an anticancer drug and used to direct the drug to the tumor site with the use of a magnet outside the body, allowing a larger dose of the drug at the tumor site for a longer period of time, and protecting healthy tissue from the side effects of chemotherapy.

maintenance therapy: Treatment that is given to help a primary treatment continue working and to help keep cancer in remission.

malignant: Cancerous.

malignant ascites: An accumulation in the abdomen of fluid containing cancer cells.

malignant meningioma: A rare, fast-growing tumor that arises from the meninges (membranes that cover and protect the brain and spinal cord) and that may spread to other areas of the body.

malignant mesothelioma: A cancerous tumor of the lining of the lung and chest cavity (pleura) or lining of the abdomen (peritoneum); it is often caused by sustained exposure to airborne particles of asbestos.

malignant mixed Müllerian tumor (MMMT): A rare tumor containing carcinoma and sarcoma cells and often occurring in the uterus.

malignant peripheral nerve sheath tumor (MPNST): A soft-tissue tumor arising from a protective sheath (covering) around peripheral nerves (nerves outside the central nervous system).

malignant pleural effusion: A condition in which cancer, most often lung cancer, breast cancer, lymphoma, and leukemia, causes an abnormal accumulation of fluid in the lining of the lung and the wall of the chest cavity.

MALT: *See* mucosa-associated lymphoid tissue lymphoma.

Mammotome: A minimally invasive device used to perform a breast biopsy.

margin: The edge of the tissue removed in cancer surgery, which is examined for cancer cells to determine whether all the cancer has been removed.

marginal zone lymphoma (MZL): A slow-growing B-cell non-Hodgkin lymphoma that originates in the outer edges of lymph tissue.

mature T-cell lymphoma: A fast-growing non-Hodgkin lymphoma (malignant tumor of the lymphoid tissue) that originates in mature T lymphocytes.

mature teratoma: A benign germ-cell tumor often containing different tissues, such as bone, hair, and muscle.

maximum inspiratory pressure test (MIP test): A test in which a person inhales and exhales through a manometer, a device that measures the strength of the muscles used in breathing.

maximum tolerated dose: The highest dose of a drug or treatment that a person can tolerate before unacceptable side effects begin to occur.

mean survival time: The average time that patients in a clinical study stayed alive, beginning with the time of diagnosis or with the start of treatment.

median survival time: The length of time from diagnosis or start of treatment by which half of the patients with a specific disease have died.

medical nutrition therapy: Therapy in which appropriate foods or nutrients are used in the treatment of conditions such as diabetes, heart disease, and cancer, and which may include changes in a person's diet or intravenous or tube feeding.

medullary thyroid cancer: Cancer of the C cells of the thyroid, which make calcitonin (a hormone that helps maintain a healthy blood calcium level).

Merkel cell cancer: *See* trabecular cancer.

melanoma: A cancer that originates in pigmented tissues, such as the skin (in the form of a mole), in the eye, or in the intestines.

metaplastic carcinoma: A cancer that originates in cells that have changed into an abnormal form for that tissue; it is usually found in the alimentary or upper respiratory tract or in the breast.

metastasectomy: Surgical removal of one or more tumors that have formed from cells that have spread from the original (primary) tumor.

metastasize: To spread, especially cancer cells, from the original site in the body to another area of the body.

metronomic therapy: Low doses of anticancer drugs given continuously or frequently, usually in conjunction with other therapy methods.

mixed glioma: A brain tumor consisting of more than one type of cell.

modified radical mastectomy: Surgical removal of the breast, lymph nodes under the arm, the lining over the chest muscles, and sometimes part of the chest wall muscles.

molar pregnancy: A slow-growing tumor that originates in the cells (trophoblastic) that aid in embryo attachment to the uterus and in placenta formation after fertilization of an egg by a sperm; it is usually benign but can become invasive, as well as malignant (then called a choriocarcinoma).

molecular marker: A distinctive biological molecule found in the body that indicates a specific process, condition, or disease, and that may be used to determine the body's response to a treatment for that disease or condition.

MRI: *See* magnetic resonance imaging.

mucosa-associated lymphoid tissue (MALT) lymphoma: A cancer (non-Hodgkin lymphoma) that originates in B cells in mucosal tissue that are involved in antibody production.

Müllerian tumor: A rare cancer of the uterus, ovary, or Fallopian tubes.

multidisciplinary: Involving a number of different specialties (disciplines), especially in the approach to planning treatment and the team of experts who oversee that treatment.

neck dissection: Surgical removal of lymph nodes and other tissues in the neck.

necrosis: Death of living tissues.

negative axillary lymph node: A cancer-free lymph node in the armpit.

neoadjuvant therapy: Treatment given before the primary treatment to help the primary treatment, such as drugs given to shrink an inoperable tumor so that surgery is possible.

neoplasm: *See* tumor.

nephrectomy: Surgical removal of a kidney.

nephrotomogram: A series of X rays of the kidneys taken from different angles.

nephrotoxic: Poisonous to the kidney.

nephroureterectomy: Surgical removal of a kidney and its ureter.

nerve block: The injection of a local anesthetic around a nerve or into the spine to block pain.

nerve-sparing radical prostatectomy: Surgical removal of the prostate with an attempt at saving the nerves that help cause penile erections.

neuroendocrine carcinoma of the skin: *See* trabecular cancer.

neuroma: A tumor that originates in nerve cells.

neuropathy: An abnormal or degenerative condition of the nervous system that causes pain, tingling, numbness, swelling, or muscle weakness, usually beginning in the hands or feet and spreading to different parts of the body over time; physical injury, infection, toxic substances, disease (including cancer), or drugs (including anticancer drugs) may be the cause.

neurotoxic: Poisonous or damaging to the nervous system.

non-small-cell lung cancer: A group of lung cancers in which the cells, when viewed under a microscope, are not the small-cell type, and which include adenocarcinoma, large-cell carcinoma, and squamous cell carcinoma.

nonfunctioning tumor: A tumor occurring in the endocrine tissue that does not make hormones.

nonseminoma: A group of testicular cancers that begin in the cells that give rise to sperm (germ cells) and include choriocarcinoma, embryonal carcinoma, teratoma, and yolk sac carcinoma.

occult primary tumor: Cancer in which the original tumor site is unknown, and the metastases of which are mostly found in the head and neck.

ocular melanoma: A rare cancer of the eye occurring in the cells that produce the pigment melanin (melanocytes).

oligoastrocytoma: A brain tumor that is a type of mixed glioma (consists of more than one type of cell).

omentectomy: Surgical removal of all or part of the omentum (a fold of the lining of the abdomen).

open biopsy: A procedure in which tissues or lumps are removed through an incision in the skin to be examined by a pathologist.

open colectomy: Surgical removal of all or part of the colon through an incision in the wall of the abdomen.

operable: Referring to a condition that can be treated by surgery.

opportunistic infection: An infection caused by an organism that usually does not cause disease but can do so in people with weakened immune systems.

oral: Pertaining to the mouth.

osteosarcoma: Bone cancer, usually of the large bones of the arm or leg.

ostomy: An operation in which an artificial passage is created from an area inside the body to the outside for bodily elimination, such as in a colostomy, ileostomy, or urostomy.

ovarian ablation: Surgery, a drug treatment, or radiation therapy to prevent the functioning of the ovaries.

oxygen therapy: The administration of oxygen through a nose tube, mask, or tent.

Pancoast tumor: A type of lung cancer that forms at the very top (apex) of a lung and invades nearby tissues, such as the chest wall, ribs, and vertebrae.

papillary serous carcinoma: A fast-growing cancer that spreads rapidly and usually affects the uterus/endometrium, ovary, or peritoneum.

papillary thyroid cancer: A common type of slow-growing thyroid cancer that originates in the follicular cells in the thyroid.

papillary tumor: A mushroom-shaped tumor, the stem of which is attached to the inner lining (epithelial layer) of an organ.

papilledema: Swelling around the optic disk as a result of increased brain pressure, sometimes caused by a brain tumor.

paraganglioma: A rare tumor that arises from cells of the paraganglia and is usually found in the abdomen, thorax, or head or neck region.

parathyroidectomy: Surgical removal of one or more of the parathyroid glands.

parotidectomy: Surgical removal of all or part of the parotid gland (a salivary gland).

partial cystectomy: Surgical removal of part of the bladder.

partial hysterectomy: Surgical removal of the uterus only.

partial laryngectomy: Surgical removal of part of the larynx (voice box).

partial mastectomy: Surgical removal of a tumor of the breast, as well as some of the tissue around the tumor, the lining over the chest muscles below the tumor, and usually some of the lymph nodes under the arm. (Also called segmental mastectomy.)

partial nephrectomy: Surgical removal of part of a kidney or a kidney tumor.

partial oophorectomy: Surgical removal of part of one ovary or part of both ovaries.

partial remission: A decrease in the amount of cancer in the body or the size of a tumor as a result of treatment received.

partial vulvectomy: Surgical removal of part of the vulva.

pathologic fracture: A break in the bone due to a disease, especially the spread of cancer to the bone.

pathology report: A written report prepared by a pathologist describing the cells and tissues of a biopsy specimen after viewing under a microscope; it is used to help the primary physician make a diagnosis of a patient's condition.

patient advocate: A person who speaks on behalf of a patient to doctors, insurance companies, employers, case managers, or lawyers to protect the patient's rights and to help that patient resolve issues about health care, medical bills, and job discrimination as a result of the patient's medical condition.

patient-controlled analgesia (PCA): A method of pain relief in which a preset dose of pain medicine is automatically administered to the patient when that patient presses a button on a computerized pump, allowing pain relief as needed. The pump also monitors the amount of medicine the patient is receiving within a certain time period and limits that amount when needed to prohibit an overdose.

pelvic exenteration: Surgical removal of the lower colon, rectum, and bladder, as well as the cervix, vagina, ovaries, and nearby lymph nodes in women; then an opening is created through which urine and stool can pass out of the body.

pelvic lymphadenectomy: Surgical removal of lymph nodes in the pelvis for microscopic examination by a pathologist.

penectomy: Surgical removal of part or all of the penis.

percutaneous ethanol injection: An injection of ethanol (pure alcohol) through the skin directly into the tumor, using a very thin needle with the help of ultrasound or computed tomography visual guidance, to destroy cancer cells.

percutaneous transhepatic cholangiodrainage (PTCD): A procedure in which a stent is placed in the liver to drain bile and to relieve pressure in the bile ducts caused by a blockage; the bile may then drain through the stent into the small intestine or into a collection bag outside the body.

periampullary cancer: A cancer that occurs near the ampulla of Vater (the area where the pancreatic duct and the common bile duct from the liver join together and enter the small intestine).

perineal colostomy: An operation in which an artificial passage is created surgically to allow the colon to exit the body through the perineum (the area between the anus and the vulva in females and between the anus and the scrotum in males) after part of the colon has been removed.

perineal prostatectomy: Surgical removal of the prostate through an incision in the perineum (the area between the scrotum and the anus).

peripheral blood lymphocyte therapy: A treatment in which lymphocytes from a sibling donor are infused into a patient who is suffering from Epstein-Barr virus infection or overgrowth of white blood cells after an organ or bone marrow transplant.

peripheral venous catheter: A small, flexible tube inserted into a vein, usually in the back of the hand or forearm, taped in place and used to administer fluids into the body.

peritoneal cancer: A rare cancer that originates in the tissues that line the inside of the abdomen and cover the organs in the abdomen.

peritonitis: Inflammation of the peritoneum (the tissues that line the inside of the abdomen and cover the organs in the abdomen) as a result of infection, injury, or a disease.

photo-beam radiation: A radiation treatment that uses high-energy X rays to reach deep tumors.

photocoagulation: Sealing off blood vessels or destroying tissue with a high-energy beam of light.

photopheresis: A procedure in which blood is removed from the body so that it can be treated with ultraviolet light and drugs that become active when exposed to light, and then is returned to the body.

pineocytoma: A slow-growing brain tumor occurring in or near the pineal gland, which is near the center of the brain.

plaque radiotherapy: A type of radiation therapy used to treat eye tumors that involves sewing to the outside wall of the eye a thin piece of metal with radioactive seeds attached, leaving it there for several days, and then removing it at the end of treatment.

plasma cell myeloma: A cancer that originates in plasma cells (white blood cells that produce antibodies).

plasma cell tumor: A tumor that originates in plasma cells (white blood cells that produce antibodies); includes multiple myeloma, monoclonal gammopathy of undetermined significance (MGUS), and plasmacytoma.

plasmacytoma: A tumor that originates in plasma cells (white blood cells that produce antibodies) and may turn into multiple myeloma.

pleurectomy: Surgical removal of part of the pleura (the thin layer of tissues that covers, protects, and cushions the lungs).

pneumatic larynx: A device that uses air to produce sound to help a person whose larynx (voice box) has been removed to talk.

port: An implantable device that allows a medical profes-

sional direct access to an artery without having to put a needle into the artery every time treatment is given or blood is withdrawn.

positive axillary lymph node: A lymph node in the armpit area in which cancer cells are detected.

posterior pelvic exenteration: Surgical removal of the lower part of the bowel, rectum, cervix, uterus, ovaries, Fallopian tubes, and vagina; some pelvic lymph nodes may also be removed.

posterior urethral cancer: Cancer in the part of the urethra that connects to the bladder.

postremission therapy: Anticancer drugs given after remission induction therapy to kill any remaining cancer cells.

post-transplant lymphoproliferative disorder (PTLD): A condition in which a group of B-cell lymphomas occurs in a patient with a weakened immune system after an organ transplant; it is usually associated with patients who have also been infected with Epstein-Barr virus and may progress to non-Hodgkin lymphoma.

power of attorney: A legal document that gives one person the authority to make medical, legal, or financial decisions for another person; it may go into effect immediately or when that person is incapable of making those decisions.

precancerous: Pertaining to a condition that may become cancer.

precancerous dermatitis: A skin disease characterized by thickened or scaly patches on the skin, usually on sun-exposed areas, and often caused by prolonged exposure to arsenic.

precursor B-lymphoblastic leukemia: *See* B-cell acute lymphocytic leukemia.

preventive mastectomy: Surgical removal of one or both breasts to reduce the risk of developing breast cancer.

primary tumor: The original tumor.

primitive neuroectodermal tumor (PNET): A tumor that may develop in the brain or central nervous system (CNS-PNET), or in sites outside the brain such as the limbs, pelvis, and chest wall (peripheral PNET).

proctoscopy: Visual examination of the rectum by inserting a thin, tubelike instrument with a light and lens (a proctoscope) into the rectum.

proctosigmoidoscopy: Visual examination of the lower colon by inserting a thin, tubelike instrument with a light and lens (a sigmoidoscope) into the rectum.

prognosis: The most likely outcome of a disease, including the probability of recovery or recurrence.

progression-free survival: The length of time for which a patient's disease remains stable and does not progress both during and after treatment, often used in a clinical study or trial as a measure of how well a new treatment works.

prophylactic cranial irradiation: Radiation therapy to the head to prevent the spread of cancer to the brain.

prophylactic surgery: Surgical removal of a cancer-free organ or gland as a preventive step for a person with a high risk of developing cancer in that organ or gland.

prostate-specific antigen (PSA) bounce: A brief increase and then decrease in the blood level of PSA; an increased level of PSA occurs in men with disease or infection of the prostate, and that level may briefly rise and fall again one to three years after receiving radiation treatment for prostate cancer as a result of PSA being released from destroyed cancer cells or from normal prostate tissue exposed to the radiation treatment, not because the cancer has come back.

prostate-specific antigen (PSA) failure: An increase in the blood level of PSA after treatment with surgery or radiation for prostate cancer; it may indicate a recurrence of the cancer.

prosthesis: An artificial replacement for part of the body, such as a leg or an arm.

pruritus: Itching.

psoralen and ultraviolet A therapy (PUVA therapy): A type of photodynamic therapy in which psoralen (a drug that becomes active when exposed to light) is administered either by mouth or topically to the skin and then followed by ultraviolet A radiation to treat skin conditions such as psoriasis, vitiligo, and skin nodules of cutaneous T-cell lymphoma.

punch biopsy: Removal of a small cylinder of tissue, using a sharp, hollow instrument, for microscopic examination by a pathologist.

quadrantectomy: Surgical removal of approximately one-quarter of the breast—the quarter that contains the cancer.

quality of life: Degree of well-being and ability to perform daily activities.

radiation dermatitis: A painful skin condition in which the skin becomes red, itchy, and blistered as a side effect of radiation therapy.

radiation enteritis: A complication of radiation therapy to the abdomen, pelvis, or rectum in which the small intestine becomes inflamed, causing nausea, vomiting, abdominal pain and cramping, watery or bloody diarrhea, fatty stools, and weight loss.

radiation fibrosis: Scar tissue caused by radiation therapy.

radiation necrosis: Death of healthy tissue as a result of radiation therapy; this dead tissue may form at the site of an irradiated tumor months or even years after the radiation therapy has ended and may require surgery to be removed.

radiation surgery: A type of radiation therapy in which special equipment is used to position the patient so that a single large dose of radiation can accurately target a tumor; it is often used to treat brain tumors.

radiation therapy: *See* irradiation.

radical cystectomy: Surgical removal of the bladder and nearby tissues and organs.

radical hysterectomy: Surgical removal of the uterus, cervix, and part of the vagina; may also include removal of the ovaries, Fallopian tubes, and nearby lymph nodes.

radical local excision: Surgical removal of a tumor and a large area of surrounding normal tissue; nearby lymph nodes may also be removed.

radical lymph node dissection: Surgical removal of most or all of the lymph nodes that drain lymph from the area around a tumor for microscopic examination by a pathologist.

radical nephrectomy: Surgical removal of a kidney, the nearby adrenal gland and lymph nodes, and surrounding tissue.

radical perineal prostatectomy: Surgical removal of the prostate through an incision in the perineum (the area between the scrotum and the anus); nearby lymph nodes may also be removed through another incision in the wall of the abdomen.

radical retropubic prostatectomy: Surgical removal of the prostate and nearby lymph nodes through an incision in the wall of the abdomen.

radical vulvectomy: Surgical removal of the vulva and nearby lymph nodes.

radioimmunoguided surgery: Surgical removal of tumors that have been located using radioactive substances.

radiologic exam: An imaging procedure that uses radiation (such as X rays) to help diagnose certain cancers and other abnormalities.

radiology: The branch of medicine in which X rays, ultrasound, magnetic resonance imaging, and other imaging technologies are used to diagnose and sometimes treat certain diseases, such as cancer.

rectal reconstruction: Surgery in which the rectum is rebuilt using a section of the colon following the surgical removal of the rectum due to cancer or other diseases.

refractory cancer: Cancer that is resistant to treatment.

regional lymph node dissection: Surgical removal of some of the lymph nodes that drain lymph from the area around a tumor for microscopic examination by a pathologist.

regression: A decrease in the amount of cancer in the body or the size of a tumor.

remission: A reduction or cessation of any signs and symptoms of cancer, even though the cancer may still exist.

remission induction therapy: The initial treatment with anticancer drugs to bring about a reduction or cessation of signs and symptoms of cancer.

renal cell cancer: *See* hypernephroma.

resection: Surgical removal of tissue or part or all of an organ.

retropubic prostatectomy: Surgical removal of the prostate through an incision in the wall of the abdomen.

rhabdoid tumor: A malignant tumor found in either the kidney or the central nervous system.

risk factor: Something that increases the likelihood of developing a certain disease, such as family history, exposure to tobacco products or other cancer-causing agents, obesity, and age.

sarcoma: A malignant tumor of bone, cartilage, fat, muscle, blood vessels, or other connective or supportive tissue.

sarcomatoid carcinoma: Cancer that contains long spindle-shaped cells and that originates in the skin or in the lining or covering of internal organs. (Also called spindle cell cancer.)

scintimammography: A supplemental imaging technique that uses a radioactive substance (technetium 99) and a gamma camera to detect cancer cells in a breast with dense breast tissue or that has produced an abnormal mammogram.

segmental mastectomy: *See* partial mastectomy.

segmental resection: Surgical removal of part of an organ or gland.

seminal vesicle biopsy: Needle aspiration of fluid or tissue from the seminal vesicles (glands in the male reproductive tract that produce part of the semen) for microscopic examination by a pathologist.

seminoma: Cancer of the testicles that has the potential to spread to the bone, brain, liver, or lung.

senile keratosis: *See* actinic keratosis.

sestamibi scan: An imaging technique in which a radioactive substance (technetium bound to sestamibi) injected into a patient can be detected by a gamma camera when it collects in overactive parathyroid glands, cancer cells in the breast, or diseased heart muscle.

shave biopsy: Removal of a skin abnormality with a thin layer of surrounding skin for microscopic examination by a pathologist by using a small blade in such a way that stitches are not needed.

shunt: A passage that diverts a bodily fluid from one area of the body to another.

side-to-end coloanal anastomosis: The surgical attachment of the side of the colon to the anus after the removal of the rectum, by forming a small J-shaped pouch from a 2-inch section of the colon as a replacement for the rectum.

signet ring cell carcinoma: A highly malignant cancer containing cells that resemble signet rings and are usually found in the glandular cells that line the digestive organs.

skinning vulvectomy: Surgical removal of the top layer of skin of the vulva.

sleeve lobectomy: A lung-saving procedure in which a tumor in a central lobe of the lung is surgically removed along with a part of the main bronchus; then the ends of the bronchus are rejoined and remaining lobes are reattached to the bronchus.

small-cell lung cancer: A fast-growing cancer of the lung that can spread to other parts of the body.

smoldering myeloma: A slow-growing myeloma in which abnormal plasma cells produce too much of a specific protein (monoclonal antibody); this is an asymptomatic condition that could progress to fully developed multiple myeloma.

soft-tissue sarcoma: A malignant tumor that originates in the muscle, fat, fibrous tissue, blood vessels, or other supporting tissue of the body.

solar keratosis: *See* actinic keratosis.

solid tumor: A benign or malignant mass of tissue, usually free of any cysts or liquid areas; includes carcinomas, sarcomas, and lymphomas.

somatostatin receptor scintigraphy (SRS): An imaging technique in which a radioactive drug (octreotide) injected into a patient attaches to tumor cells, which can then be detected by a radiation-measuring device; a picture is then created that shows where the tumor cells are in the body.

spindle cell cancer: *See* sarcomatoid carcinoma.

spiral computed tomography (CT) scan: A series of detailed pictures of structures within the body, created by a computer linked to an X-ray machine that scans the body in a spiral path.

stromal tumor: A tumor that occurs in the supporting connective tissue of an organ.

subcutaneous port: A semipermanent device implanted just under the skin that allows a medical professional direct access to an artery without having to put a needle into the artery every time intravenous fluids or drugs need to be administered or blood samples need to be taken.

supraglottic laryngectomy: Surgical removal of the supraglottis (the part of the larynx that is above the vocal cords).

suprarenal glands: *See* adrenal glands.

syngeneic: Pertaining to individuals or tissues from those individuals containing identical genes, such as identical twins.

systemic therapy: Treatment that affects cells all over the body by traveling through the bloodstream.

T-cell depletion: Treatment that destroys T cells, especially from a donor's bone marrow graft, to reduce the risk of an immune reaction against the recipient's tissues.

T-cell lymphoma: Cancer of T-lymphocytes (cells of the lymph system).

terminal disease: An incurable disease that will lead to death.

thermal ablation: The removal, destruction, or severing of a diseased or damaged tissue, body part, or its function through the use of heat.

thermotherapy: The use of heat in the treatment of a disease.

third-line therapy: Treatment that is given after both an initial and a subsequent treatment fail or become ineffective.

three-dimensional conformal radiation therapy: A procedure in which a tumor is subjected to the highest possible dose of radiation while surrounding tissue is spared; accomplished by using a computer-generated three-dimensional picture of the tumor.

thrombectomy: Surgical removal of a thrombus (blood clot) from a blood vessel.

thrombolysis: Dissolving or breaking up a thrombus (blood clot), especially through the use of drugs.

thyroidectomy: Surgical removal of part or all of the thyroid.

time to progression: The length of time following diagnosis or treatment until the disease begins to get worse.

tissue flap reconstruction: Breast reconstruction using a flap of tissue surgically removed from another area of the body and formed into a new breast mound.

tomography: The process of creating a series of detailed pictures of structures within the body, by a computer linked to an X-ray machine.

tongue cancer: Cancer that originates in the tongue.

topical: Pertaining to the surface of the body.

topical chemotherapy: The application of anticancer drugs directly on the skin in the form of a lotion, an ointment, or a cream.

total-body irradiation: Radiation therapy to the whole body to kill cancer cells throughout the body and to destroy the bone marrow and immune system in preparation for bone marrow or stem cell transplantation.

total mastectomy: Surgical removal of the breast.

total nodal irradiation: Radiation therapy to the neck, chest, spleen, and lymph nodes under the arms, in the upper abdomen, and in the pelvic area.

total pancreatectomy: Surgical removal of the pancreas, as well as nearby lymph nodes, the common bile duct, the gallbladder, the spleen, and part of the stomach and small intestine.

total parenteral nutrition (TPN): The intravenous feeding of nutrients to patients who cannot ingest or digest food through the alimentary tract.

total skin electron beam radiation therapy (TSEB radiation therapy): Radiation therapy that directs electrons at the entire surface of the body, allowing the radiation into the outer layers of the skin but not penetrating deeper into the tissues or organs below the skin.

trabecular cancer: A rare cancer of the skin that may form on or just below the skin, especially in parts of the body exposed to the sun and in older people and those with weakened immune systems. (Also called Merkel cell cancer and neuroendocrine carcinoma of the skin.)

transperineal biopsy: Removal of a sample of tissue from the prostate, using a thin needle inserted through the skin between the scrotum and the rectum, for microscopic examination by a pathologist.

transrectal biopsy: Removal of a sample of tissue from the prostate, using a thin needle inserted through the rectum, for microscopic examination by a pathologist.

transsphenoidal surgery: Surgery in which part of the brain is accessed through the nose and the sphenoid bone (a bone at the base of the skull); this type of surgery is common when removing tumors of the pituitary gland.

transurethral biopsy: Removal of a sample of tissue from the prostate by inserting a thin tube with a cutting loop attachment through the urethra and into the prostate; the sample is then examined under a microscope by a pathologist.

transurethral resection of the prostate (TURP): Surgical removal of tissue from the prostate using an instrument inserted through the urethra.

treatment field: The area of the body at which the radiation beam is aimed during radiation therapy.

tubulovillous adenoma: An abnormal growth of tissue (polyp), in the colon, the gastrointestinal tract, or other parts of the body, that may become cancerous.

tumor: A new mass of tissue resulting from uncontrolled cell division and that serves no physiological function; it may be benign or malignant. (Also called neoplasm.)

tumor load: Pertaining to the size of a tumor, the number of cancer cells, or the amount of cancer in the body.

tumor volume: The amount of space taken up by a tumor.

ultrasound-guided biopsy: Surgical removal of a sample of tissue, using an ultrasound imaging device to locate and guide the removal of that tissue, for microscopic examination by a pathologist.

unilateral: Pertaining to one side of the body.

unilateral salpingo-oophorectomy: Surgical removal of the ovary and Fallopian tube on one side of the body.

unresectable gallbladder cancer: Gallbladder cancer that has spread to nearby areas, such as the lymph nodes, liver, stomach, pancreas, and intestine, so that it cannot be surgically removed.

unsealed internal radiation therapy: Radiation therapy in which a radioactive substance that has not been sealed in a container is injected into the body or swallowed.

upper endoscopy: *See* gastroscopy.

upper GI series: *See* esophagram.

urinary diversion: A surgical procedure to create an alternative passage for urine to exit the body; it may include redirecting urine into the colon, draining the bladder through the use of catheters, or making an incision in the abdomen and collecting urine in a bag outside the body.

vaginectomy: Surgical removal of part or all of the vagina.

ventilator: A machine that helps a patient breathe.

video-assisted resection: Surgery in which a video camera projects and enlarges the surgical field onto a television screen, allowing the surgeon an enhanced view of the surgical field.

villous adenoma: An abnormal growth of tissue (polyp) in the colon, the gastrointestinal tract, or other parts of the body that may become cancerous.

visual pathway glioma: A tumor that occurs along the optic nerve (the nerve that sends messages from the eye to the brain).

wedge resection: Surgical removal of a triangle-shaped piece of tissue or a tumor with some of the normal tissue around it.

Whipple procedure: Surgical removal of the head of the pancreas, the duodenum, part of the stomach, and other nearby tissues to treat pancreatic cancer.

whole genome association study (WGA study): A study in which the deoxyribonucleic acid (DNA) of people with a disease or medical condition is compared to the DNA of people without it in an effort to discover the genes that are involved in the disease and to aid medical professionals in the prevention, diagnosis, and treatment of the disease.

wide local excision: Surgical removal of the cancer along with healthy tissue around it.

X-ray therapy: Radiation therapy that uses X rays to shrink tumors and kill cancer cells.

▶ Bibliography

General Studies and Reference Works

Altman, Roberta, and Michael J. Sarg. *The Cancer Dictionary*. New York: Facts On File, 1994.

American Cancer Society. *Quick Facts on Advanced Cancer*. Atlanta: Author, 2008.

Bloch, Annette, and Richard Bloch. *Fighting Cancer: A Step-by-Step Guide to Helping Yourself Fight Cancer*. Kansas City, Mo.: R. A. Bloch Cancer Foundation, 1990.

_____. *Guide for Cancer Supporters: Step-by-Step Ways to Help a Relative or Friend Fight Cancer*. Kansas City, Mo.: R. A. Bloch Cancer Foundation, 1995.

Bognar, David, and Walter Cronkite. *Cancer, Increasing Your Odds for Survival: A Resource Guide for Integrating Mainstream, Alternative and Complementary Therapies*. Alameda, Calif.: Hunter House, 1998.

Brownworth, Victoria A., ed. *Coming Out of Cancer: Writings from the Lesbian Cancer Epidemic*. Seattle: Seal Press, 2000.

Cancercare. *A Helping Hand: The Resource Guide for People with Cancer*. New York: Author, 2008.

Epps, Roselyn Payne, and Susan Cobb Stewart, eds. *The American Medical Women's Association Guide to Cancer and Pain Management*. New York: Dell, 1996.

Fischer, William L. *How to Fight Cancer and Win: Scientific Guidelines and Documented Facts for the Successful Treatment and Prevention of Cancer and Other Health Related Problems*. Baltimore, Md.: Agora Health Books, 1992.

Friedberg, Errol C. *Cancer Answers: Encouraging Answers to Twenty-five Questions You Were Always Afraid to Ask*. New York: W. H. Freeman, 1992.

Getz, Kenneth, and Deborah Borfitz. *Informed Consent: The Consumer's Guide to the Risks and Benefits of Volunteering for Clinical Trials*. Boston: CenterWatch, 2002.

Haylock, Pamela J., and Carol P. Curtiss. *Cancer Doesn't Have to Hurt: How to Conquer the Pain Caused by Cancer and Cancer Treatment*. Alameda, Calif.: Hunter House, 1997.

Kneece, Judy C. *Helping Your Mate Face Breast Cancer: Tips for Becoming an Effective Support Partner*. North Charleston, S.C.: Educare, 2001.

Moritz, Cynthia. *About Cancer*. Syracuse, N.Y.: New Readers Press, 1994.

Oster, Nancy, Lucy Thomas, and Darol Joseff. *Making Informed Medical Decisions: Where to Look and How to Use What You Find*. Foreword by Susan Love. Sebastopol, Calif.: Patient-Centered Guides, 2000.

Schimmel, Selma R., with Barry Fox. *Cancer Talk: Voices of Hope and Endurance from "The Group Room," the World's Largest Cancer Support Group*. New York: Broadway, 1999.

Schine, Gary L., and Ellen B. Berlinsky. *Cancer Cure: The Complete Guide to Finding and Getting the Best Care There Is*. New York: Kensington, 1996.

Souhami, Robert, and Jeffrey Tobias. *Cancer and Its Management*. Malden, Mass.: Blackwell Science, 2005.

Zakarian, Beverly, and Ezra M. Greenspan. *The Activist Cancer Patient: How to Take Charge of Your Treatment*. Hoboken, N.J.: John Wiley and Sons, 1996.

Abdominal Cancers

Abbruzzese, James, and Ben Ebrahimi. *Myths and Facts About Pancreatic Cancer: What You Need to Know*. Melville, N.Y.: PRR, 2002.

Alschuler, Lise N., and Karolyn A. Gazella, eds. *Alternative Medicine Magazine's Definitive Guide to Cancer: An Integrative Approach to Prevention, Treatment, and Healing*. Berkeley, Calif.: Celestial Arts, 2007.

American Cancer Society. *Quickfacts Pancreatic Cancer*. Atlanta: Author, 2008.

Brunschwig, Alexander. *Radical Surgery in Advanced Abdominal Cancer*. Chicago: University of Chicago Press, 1947.

Cameron, John L. *Pancreatic Cancer*. Hamilton, Ont.: BC Decker, 2001.

Cohen, Isaac, O.M.D. *Breast Cancer: Beyond Convention: The World's Foremost Authorities on Complementary and Alternative Medicine Offer Advice on Healing*. New York: Atria, 2003.

Henderson, Bill. *Cancer-Free: Your Guide to Gentle, Non-toxic Healing*. 2d ed. Bangor, Maine: Booklocker, 2007.

Icon Health Publications. *The Official Patient's Sourcebook on Pancreatic Cancer: A Revised and Updated Directory for the Internet Age*. San Diego, Calif.: Author, 2002.

Morra, Marion, and Eve Potts. *Choices: Realistic Alternatives in Cancer Treatment*. New York: Avon, 1987.

Murray, Michael. *Encyclopedia of Natural Medicine*. 2d ed. Roseville, Calif.: Prima, 1998.

_____. *How to Prevent and Treat Cancer with Natural Medicine*. New York: Riverhead Trade, 2003.

O'Reilly, Eileen, and Joanne Frankel Kelvin. *One Hundred Questions and Answers About Pancreatic Cancer*. Sudbury, Mass.: Jones and Bartlett, 2002.

Pierce, Tanya Harter. *Outsmart Your Cancer: Alternative Non-toxic Treatments That Work.* Stateline, Nev.: Thoughtworks, 2004.

Rains, Calvin E., Sr. *My Journey with Pancreatic Cancer.* Bloomington, Ind.: AuthorHouse, 2006.

Reber, Howard, ed. *Pancreatic Cancer: Pathogenesis, Diagnosis, and Treatment.* Totowa, N.J.: Humana, 1998.

Riess, H., A. Goerke, and H. Oettle. *Pancreatic Cancer.* Berlin: Springer, 2007.

Rossman, Martin L. *Fighting Cancer from Within: How to Use the Power of Your Mind for Healing.* New York: Holt, 2003.

Smith, Tom. *Coping with Bowel Cancer.* London: Sheldon Press, 2006.

Von Hoff, Daniel D., Douglas B. Evans, and Ralph H. Hruban. *Pancreatic Cancer.* Sudbury, Mass.: Jones and Bartlett, 2005.

Bone Cancers

American Cancer Society. *Quick FACTS Bone Metastasis.* Atlanta: Author, 2008.

Body, Jean-Jac. *Tumor Bone Diseases and Osteoporosis in Cancer Patients: Pathophysiology, Diagnosis, and Therapy.* New York: Informa Healthcare, 2000.

Davies, Andrew. *Cancer-Related Bone Pain.* New York: Oxford University Press, 2007.

Orr, Tamra. *Frequently Asked Questions About Bone Cancer.* New York: Rosen Publishing Group, 2007.

Shaffer, Marianne. *Bone Marrow Transplants: A Guide for Cancer Patients and Their Families.* Blue Ridge Summit, Pa.: Taylor Trade Publishing, 1994.

Singh, Gurmit, and Shafaat A. Rabbani. *Bone Metastasis: Cancer Drug Discovery and Development.* Totowa, N.J.: Humana Press, 2005.

Brain Cancers

Ali-Osman, Francis. *Brain Tumors: Contemporary Cancer Research.* Totowa, N.J.: Humana, 2005.

Black, Peter. *Living with a Brain Tumor: Dr. Peter Black's Guide to Taking Control of Your Treatment.* New York: Holt, 2006.

Raizer, Jeffrey J., and Lauren E. Abrey. *Brain Metastases: Cancer Treatment and Research.* New York: Springer, 2007.

Sawaya, R., W. K. A. Yung, Franco DeMonte, and Mark R. Gilbert. *Tumors of the Brain and Spine.* New York: Springer, 2007.

Zeltzer, Paul M. *Brain Tumors: Leaving the Garden of Eden—A Survival Guide to Diagnosis, Learning the Basics, Getting Organized, and Finding Your Medical Team.* Encino, Calif.: Shilysca Press, 2004.

Breast Cancers

American Cancer Society. *Breast Cancer Clear and Simple.* Atlanta: Author, 2007.

Batt, Sharon. *Patient No More: The Politics of Breast Cancer.* Charlottetown, P.E.I.: Gynergy, 1994.

Burt, Jeannie, and Gwen White. *Lymphedema: A Breast Cancer Patient's Guide to Prevention and Healing.* Alameda, Calif.: Hunter House, 2005.

Chang, Alice F., with Karen Mang Spruill. *A Survivor's Guide to Breast Cancer.* Oakland, Calif.: New Harbinger, 2000.

Eisenpreis, Bettijane. *Coping: A Young Woman's Guide to Breast Cancer Prevention.* New York: Rosen, 1996.

Elk, Ronit. *Breast Cancer for Dummies.* Hoboken, N.J.: Wiley, 2003.

Friedewald, Vincent E., Aman U. Buzdar, and Michael Bokulich. *Ask the Doctor: Breast Cancer.* Kansas City, Mo.: Andrews and McMeel, 1997.

Haber, Sandra, Catherine Acuff, and Lauren Ayers. *Breast Cancer: A Psychological Treatment Manual.* New York: Springer, 1995.

Hirshaut, Yashar, and Peter I. Pressman. *Breast Cancer: The Complete Guide.* New York: Bantam, 2000.

Jacobson, Nora. *Cleavage Technology, Controversy, and the Ironies of the Man-made Breast.* Piscataway, N.J.: Rutgers University Press, 2000.

Kneece, Judy C. *Finding A Lump in Your Breast: Where to Go . . . What to Do.* North Charleston, S.C.: Educare, 1996.

_____. *Your Breast Cancer Treatment Handbook: Your Guide to Understanding the Disease, Treatments, Emotions, and Recovery from Breast Cancer.* West Columbia, S.C.: Educare, 2004.

Lange, Vladimir. *Be a Survivor: Your Guide to Breast Cancer Treatment.* Atlanta: Lange, 2007.

Leopold, Ellen. *A Darker Ribbon: A Twentieth-Century Story of Breast Cancer, Women, and Their Doctors.* Boston: Beacon Press, 2000.

Link, John. *Take Charge of Your Breast Cancer: A Guide to Getting the Best Possible Treatment.* New York: Holt, 2002.

Love, Susan M. *Dr. Susan Love's Breast Book.* 4th ed. New York: Da Capo Lifelong Books, 2005.

McTiernan, Anne, Julie Gralow, and Lisa Talbott. *Breast Fitness: An Optimal Exercise and Health Plan for Reducing Your Risk of Breast Cancer.* New York: St. Martin's Griffin, 2001.

Maslin, Anna, ed. *Breast Cancer: Sharing the Decision.* New York: Oxford University Press, 1999.

Mayer, Musa. *Examining Myself: One Woman's Story of Breast Cancer Treatment and Recovery.* London: Faber and Faber, 1993.

Olivotto, Ivo, Karen Gelmon, and Urve Kuusk. *Intelligent Patient Guide to Breast Cancer*. Seattle: Gordon Soules, 2001.

Raz, Hilda, ed. *Living on the Margins: Women Writers on Breast Cancer*. New York: Persea Books, 2000.

Shockney, Lillie. *Breast Cancer Survivor's Club: A Nurse's Experience*. Loveland, Colo.: Real Health Books, 2001.

Steligo, Kathy. *The Breast Reconstruction Guidebook: Issues and Answers from Research to Recovery*. San Carlos, Calif.: Carlo Press, 2005.

Stumm, Diane, P.T. *Recovering from Breast Surgery: Exercises to Strengthen Your Body and Relieve Pain*. Alameda, Calif.: Hunter House, 1995.

Cancer Screening and Testing Procedures

Finkel, Madelon L. *Understanding the Mammography Controversy: Science, Politics, and Breast Cancer Screening*. Westport, Conn.: Praeger, 2005.

International Agency for Research on Cancer. *IARC Handbooks on Cancer Prevention: Cervix Cancer Screening*. Geneva: World Health Organization, 2005.

Morrison, Patrick J., Shirley V. Hodgson, and Neva E. Haites. *Familial Breast and Ovarian Cancer: Genetics, Screening and Management*. Cambridge, England: Cambridge University Press, 2005.

Parvin, Elizabeth. *Screening for Breast Cancer*. New York: Oxford University Press, 2007.

Reintgen, Douglas S., and Robert A. Clark. *Cancer Screening*. St. Louis, Mo.: Mosby-Year Book, 1996.

Thompson, Ian M., Jr., Martin I. Resnick, and Eric A. Klein. *Prostate Cancer Screening*. Totowa, N.J.: Humana, 2001.

World Health Organization. *Cervical Cancer Screening in Developing Countries*. Geneva: Author, 2002.

Cervical, Ovarian, and Uterine Cancers

Conner, Kristine, and Lauren Langford. *Ovarian Cancer*. Sebastopol, Calif.: Patient-Centered Guides, 2003.

Dizon, Don S. *One Hundred Questions and Answers About Cervical Cancer*. Sudbury, Mass.: Jones and Bartlett, 2008.

Fuller, Arlan F., Jr., Robert H. Young, and Michael V. Seiden. *Uterine Cancer*. Hamilton, Ont.: BC Decker, 2004.

Luesley, David M., Frank Lawton, and Andrew Berchuck. *Uterine Cancer*. New York: Informa Healthcare, 2005.

Piver, M. Steven, Gamal Abbakh, and Harriet Phillips. *Myths and Facts About Ovarian Cancer: What You Need to Know*. 2d ed. Melville, N.Y.: PRR, 2000.

Rohan, Thomas E., and Keerti V. Shah. *Cervical Cancer: From Etiology to Prevention*. New York: Springer, 2004.

Sheen, Barbara. *Diseases and Disorders: Ovarian Cancer*. Farmington Hills, Mich.: Lucent, 2005.

Chemotherapy

Bruning, Nancy. *Coping with Chemotherapy: Compassionate Advice and Authoritative Information from a Chemotherapy Survivor*. Rev. ed. New York: Avery, 2002.

Chu, Edward, and Vincent T. DeVita, Jr. *Physician's Cancer Chemotherapy Drug Manual 2008*. Sudbury, Mass.: Jones and Bartlett, 2008.

Cukier, Daniel. *Coping with Chemotherapy and Radiation Therapy*. New York: McGraw-Hill, 2004.

Dodd, Marilyn J. *Managing the Side Effects of Chemotherapy and Radiation Therapy*. San Francisco: University of California, 2001.

Fischer, David S., Henry J. Durivage, M. Tish Knobf, and Nancy Beaulieu. *The Cancer Chemotherapy Handbook*. 6th ed. Philadelphia: Mosby, 2003.

Geier, Mary Alice. *Cancer, What's It Doing in My Life? A Personal Journal of the First Two Years of Chemotherapy in the Career of a Cancer Patient*. Pasadena, Calif.: Hope Publishing House, 1997.

Lyss, Alan P., Humberto Fagundes, and Patricia Corrigan. *Chemotherapy and Radiation for Dummies*. Hoboken, N.J.: Wiley, 2005.

McKay, Judith. *The Chemotherapy and Radiation Therapy Survival Guide*. Oakland, Calif.: New Harbinger, 1998.

Moss, Ralph W. *Questioning Chemotherapy*. Lanham, Md.: Equinox Press, 1995.

Naparstek, Belleruth. *Health Journeys: A Meditation to Help You with Radiation Therapy*. Akron, Ohio: Health Journeys, 1999.

Perry, Michael C. *The Chemotherapy Source Book*. Philadelphia: Lippincott Williams and Wilkins, 2007.

Polovich, Martha, Julie M. White, and Linda O. Kelleher. *Chemotherapy and Biotherapy Guidelines and Recommendations for Practice*. 2d ed. Pittsburgh: Oncology Nursing Society, 2005.

Raftopoulous, Harry, and Erin O'Driscoll. *Exercises for Chemotherapy Patients*. Long Island City, N.Y.: Hatherleigh Press, 2003.

Skeel, Roland T. *Handbook of Cancer Chemotherapy*. Philadelphia: Lippincott Williams and Wilkins, 2007.

Children and Cancer

Ackermann, Adrienne, and Abigail Ackermann. *Our Mom Has Cancer*. Atlanta: American Cancer Society, 2002.

Blake, Claire, Eliza Blanchard, and Kathy Parkinson. *Paper Chain*. Santa Fe, N.M.: Health Press, 1998.

Brack, Pat, with Ben Brack. *Moms Don't Get Sick*. Pierre, S.D.: Melius, 1990.

Buscaglia, Leo. *The Fall of Freddie the Leaf.* Thorofare, N.J.: Slack, 2002.

Carney, Karen L. *What Is Cancer Anyway? Explaining Cancer to Children of All Ages.* Wethersfield, Conn.: Dragonfly, 1998.

Harpham, Wendy S. *When a Parent Has Cancer: A Guide to Caring for Your Children.* New York: Harper, 2004.

Janes-Hodder, Honna, and Nancy Keene. *Childhood Cancer: A Parent's Guide to Solid Tumor Cancers.* Sebastopol, Calif.: Patient Center Guides, 2002.

Jones, Susan. *Until We Meet Again.* Illustrated by Shirley Antak. Minneapolis: 50-50 Publishing, 2007.

Karu, Tim. *Henry and the White Wolf.* Illustrated by Tyler Karu. New York: Workman, 2000.

Keene, Nancy, Wendy Hobbie, and Kathy Ruccione. *Childhood Cancer Survivors: A Practical Guide to Your Future.* Sebastopol, Calif.: O'Reilly Media, 2006.

Kohlenberg, Sherry. *Sammy's Mommy Has Cancer.* Illustrated by Lauri Crow. Washington, D.C.: Magination Press, 1993.

Krishner, Trudy. *Kathy's Hats: A Story of Hope.* Illustrated by Nadine Bernard Westcott. Morton Grove, Ill.: Albert Whitman, 1992.

Martin, Kim. *H is for Hair Fairy: An Alphabet of Encouragement and Insight for Kids—and Kids at Heart!—with Cancer.* Illustrated by Wend Broomhower. Victoria, B.C.: Trafford, 2005.

Mills, Joyce C.. *Gentle Willow: A Story for Children About Dying.* Illustrated by Cary Pillo. Washington, D.C.: Magination Press, 2003.

Mundy, Michaelene. *Sad Isn't Bad: A Good-Grief Guidebook for Kids Dealing with Loss.* Illustrated by R. W. Alley. St. Meinrad, Ind.: Abbey Press, 1998.

Murray, Lisa, and Billy Howard. *Angels and Monsters.* Atlanta: American Cancer Society, 2002.

Pennebaker, Ruth. *Both Sides Now.* New York: Laurel Leaf, 2002.

Richmond, Christina. *Chemo Girl: Saving the World One Treatment at a Time.* Sudbury, Mass.: Jones and Bartlett, 1996.

Schulz, Charles M. *Why, Charlie Brown, Why? A Story About What Happens When a Friend Is Very Ill.* New York: Ballantine Books, 2002.

Schweibert, Pat, and Chuck DeKlyen. *Tear Soup.* Illustrated by Taylor Bills. Portland, Ore.: Grief Watch, 2005.

Silverman, Janis. *Help Me Say Goodbye: Activities for Helping Kids Cope When a Special Person Dies.* Minneapolis: Fairview Press, 1999.

Speltz, Ann. *The Year My Mother Was Bald.* Illustrated by Kate Sternberg. Washington, D.C.: Magination Press, 2002.

Torrey, Lisa. *Michael's Mommy Has Breast Cancer.* Illustrated by Barbara W. Watler. Tallahassee, Fla.: Hibiscus Press, 1999.

Colon and Rectal Cancers

Adrouny, A. Richard. *Understanding Colon Cancer.* Jackson: University Press of Mississippi, 2002.

American Cancer Society. *American Cancer Society's Complete Guide to Colorectal Cancer.* Atlanta: Author, 2005.

Bub, David, Susannah Rose, and Douglas Wong. *One Hundred Questions and Answers About Colorectal Cancer.* Sudbury, Mass.: Jones and Bartlett, 2002.

Cassidy, Jim, Patrick Johnston, and Eric Van Cutsem, eds. *Colorectal Cancer.* New York: Informa Healthcare, 2006.

Donehower, Ross C. *Colon Cancer 2007: Johns Hopkins White Papers.* Baltimore, Md.: Johns Hopkins Medicine, 2007.

Holen, Kyle. *Dx/Rx: Colorectal Cancer.* Sudbury, Mass.: Jones and Bartlett, 2007.

Johnston, Lorraine. *Colon and Rectal Cancer: A Comprehensive Guide for Patients and Families.* Sebastopol, Calif.: Patient-Centered Guides, 2000.

Lange, Vladimir. *Be a Survivor: Colorectal Cancer Treatment Guide.* Atlanta: Lange Productions, 2006.

Larson, Carol Ann, and Kathleen Ogle. *Positive Options for Colorectal Cancer: Self-Help and Treatment.* Alameda, Calif.: Hunter House, 2005.

Pochapin, Mark Bennett. *What Your Doctor May Not Tell You About Colorectal Cancer: New Tests, New Treatments, New Hope.* New York: Grand Central, 2005.

Rozen, Paul, Graham Young, Bernard Levin, and Stephen J. Spann, eds. *Colorectal Cancer in Clinical Practice: Prevention, Early Detection and Management.* Florence, Ky.: Taylor and Francis, 2002.

Scholefield, John, Herand Abcarian, Tim Maughan, and Axel Grothey, eds. *Challenges in Colorectal Cancer.* Malden, Mass.: Wiley-Blackwell, 2008.

Smith, Tom. *Coping with Bowel Cancer.* London: Sheldon Press, 2006.

Coping and Survivorship

Anderson, Greg. *Fifty Essential Things to Do When the Doctor Says It's Cancer.* New York: Plume, 1993.

Armstrong, Lance. *It's Not About the Bike: My Journey Back to Life.* New York: Putnam, 2000.

Canfield, Jack. *Chicken Soup for the Breast Cancer Survivor's Soul: Stories to Inspire, Support, and Heal.* Deerfield Beach, Fla.: HCI, 2006.

Clifford, Christine. *Not Now—I'm Having a No Hair Day.* Minneapolis: University of Minnesota Press, 2003.

Cohen, Deborah A., with Robert M. Gelfand. *Just Get Me Through This! The Practical Guide to Breast Cancer*. New York: Kensington, 2000.

Cousins, Norman. *Head First: The Biology of Hope and the Healing Power of the Human Spirit*. New York: Penguin, 1990.

Dunstone, Carol, and Ann Bennett. *Trilogy: How to Help the Mind, Body, and Spirit Survive Mouth, Head, and Neck Cancer*. Bloomington, Ind.: AuthorHouse, 2006.

Goleman, Daniel, and Joel Gurin. *Mind/Body Medicine: How to Use Your Mind for Better Health*. Yonkers, N.Y.: Consumer Reports, 1995.

Gottlieb, Bert. *The Men's Club: How to Lose Your Prostate Without Losing Your Sense of Humor*. Oxnard, Calif.: Pathfinder, 2000.

Granet, Roger. *Surviving Cancer Emotionally: Learning How to Heal*. New York: Wiley, 2001.

Halverstadt, Amy, and Andrea Leonard. *Essential Exercises for Breast Cancer Survivors* . Boston: Harvard Common Press, 2000.

Harpham, Wendy Schlessel. *After Cancer: A Guide to Your New Life*. New York: W. W. Norton, 1994.

Harwell, Amy, with Kristine Tomasik. *When Your Friend Gets Cancer: How You Can Help*. Wheaton, Ill.: Shaw, 1987.

Holland, Jimmie C., and Sheldon Lewis. *The Human Side of Cancer: Living with Hope, Coping with Uncertainty*. New York: HarperCollins, 2000.

Hope, Lori. *Help Me Live: Twenty Things People with Cancer Want You to Know*. Berkeley, Calif.: Celestial Arts, 2005.

Kahane, Deborah Hobler. *No Less a Woman: Femininity, Sexuality, and Breast Cancer*. Alameda, Calif.: Hunter House, 1995.

Korda, Michael. *Man to Man: Surviving Prostate Cancer*. New York: Vintage, 1997.

McCoy, Linda P. *Twenty-Something and Breast Cancer*. Sedona, Ariz.: In Print, 1995.

Marchetto, Marisa Acocella. *Cancer Vixen*. New York: Knopf, 2006.

Pesmen, Curtis. *The Colon Cancer Survivors' Guide: Living Stronger, Longer*. Suffern, N.Y.: Tatra Press, 2005.

Phillips, Robert H., and Paula Goldstein. *Coping with Breast Cancer: A Practical Guide to Understanding, Treating, and Living with Breast Cancer*. New York: Avery, 1998.

Ratner, Elaine. *The Feisty Woman's Breast Cancer Book*. Alameda, Calif.: Hunter House, 1999.

Rollin, Betty. *First, You Cry*. New York: Harper, 1976.

Seligman, Linda. *Promoting a Fighting Spirit: Psychotherapy for Cancer Patients, Survivors, and Their Families*. Hoboken, N.J.: Jossey-Bass, 1996.

Soffa, Virginia M. *The Journey Beyond Breast Cancer: From the Personal to the Political—Taking an Active Role in the Prevention, Diagnosis, and Your Own Healing*. Rochester, Vt.: Healing Arts Press, 1994.

Walker, Laura Jensen. *Thanks for the Mammogram!: Fighting Cancer with Faith, Hope, and a Healthy Dose of Laughter*. Grand Rapids, Mich.: Revell, 2006.

Weiss, Marisa C., and Ellen Weiss. *Living Beyond Breast Cancer: A Survivor's Guide for When Treatment Ends and the Rest of Your Life Begins*. New York: Crown, 1997.

Endocrine Cancers

Arnold, Andrew. *Endocrine Neoplasms*. New York: Springer, 1997.

Horwitz, Kathryn B. *Endocrine Aspects of Cancer*. Chevy Chase, Md.: Endocrine Society, 1993.

Santen, Richard J., and Andrea Manni. *Diagnosis and Management of Endocrine-Related Tumors*. New York: Springer, 1984.

Head, Neck, and Oral Cancers

Ahuja, A. T., R. M. Evans, A. D. King, and C. A. van Hasselt. *Imaging of Head and Neck Cancer*. San Francisco: Greenwich Medical Media, 2003.

Baert, A. L., and Robert Hermans. *Head and Neck Cancer Imaging*. New York: Springer, 2006.

Brockstein, Bruce, and Gregory Masters. *Head and Neck Cancer*. New York: Springer, 2003.

Ensley, John Frederick, Silvio Gutkind, John A. Jacobs, and Scott Lippman. *Head and Neck Cancer: Emerging Perspectives*. San Diego: Academic Press, 2002.

Hong, Waun Ki, and Randal S. Weber. *Head and Neck Cancer: Basic and Clinical Aspects*. New York: Springer, 1995.

Leupold, Nancy E. *Meeting the Challenges of Oral and Head and Neck Cancer: A Survivor's Guide*. San Diego: Plural, 2008.

Silverman, Sol, and American Cancer Society. *Oral Cancer*. Hamilton, Ont.: BC Decker, 2003.

Stafford, Nicholas, and John Waldron. *Management of Oral Cancer*. New York: Oxford University Press, 1990.

Werner, Jochen A., and R. Kim Davis. *Metastases in Head and Neck Cancer*. Berlin: Springer, 2005.

Leukemias, Lymphomas, and Myelomas

Adler, Elizabeth M. *Living with Lymphoma: A Patient's Guide*. Baltimore, Md.: Johns Hopkins University Press, 2005.

Ball, Edward D. *One Hundred Questions and Answers About Leukemia*. Sudbury, Mass.: Jones and Bartlett, 2002.

Bashey, Asad, and James W. Huston. *One Hundred Questions and Answers About Myeloma.* Sudbury, Mass.: Jones and Bartlett, 2004.

Burke, John, and Manish A. Shah. *Dx/Rx: Leukemia.* Sudbury, Mass.: Jones and Bartlett, 2004.

Holman, Peter, Jodi Garrett, and William D. Jansen. *One Hundred Questions and Answers About Lymphoma.* Sudbury, Mass.: Jones and Bartlett, 2003.

Icon Health Publications. *The Official Patient's Sourcebook on Adult Non-Hodgkin's Lymphoma: A Revised and Updated Directory for the Internet Age.* San Diego, Calif.: Author, 2002.

Johnston, Lorraine. *Non-Hodgkin's Lymphomas: Making Sense of Diagnosis, Treatment, and Options.* Sebastopol, Calif.: Patient-Centered Guides, 1999.

Lackritz, Barbara. *Adult Leukemia: A Comprehensive Guide for Patients and Families.* Sebastopol, Calif.: Patient-Centered Guides, 2001.

Leonard, John P., and Morton Coleman, eds. *Hodgkin's and Non-Hodgkin's Lymphoma.* New York: Springer, 2006.

Marcus, Robert, John W. Sweetenham, and Michael E. Williams. *Lymphoma: Pathology, Diagnosis, and Treatment.* Cambridge, England: Cambridge University Press: 2007.

Mauch, Peter M., et al., eds. *Non-Hodgkin's Lymphomas: A Self-Study Program.* Philadelphia: Lippincott Williams and Wilkins, 2003.

Mughal, Tariq, John M. Goldman, and Sabena Mughal. *Understanding Leukemias, Lymphomas, and Myelomas.* New York: Informa Healthcare, 2005.

Parker, James N., and Philip M. Parker. *The Official Patient's Sourcebook on Adult Acute Myeloid Leukemia.* San Diego, Calif.: Icon Health Publications, 2002.

Tanner, Jerome E. *Myeloma.* New York: Chelsea House, 2008.

Lung Cancers

Henschke, Claudia I., Peggy McCarthy, and Sarah Wernick. *Lung Cancer: Myths, Facts, Choices—and Hope.* New York: W. W. Norton, 2003.

Johnston, Lorraine. *Lung Cancer: Making Sense of Diagnosis, Treatment, and Options.* Sebastopol, Calif.: Patient-Centered Guides, 2001.

Parles, Karen, and Joan H. Schiller. *One Hundred Questions and Answers About Lung Cancer.* Sudbury, Mass.: Jones and Bartlett, 2002.

Roth, Jack A., James D. Cox, and Waun Ki Hong. *Lung Cancer.* Malden, Mass.: Blackwell, 1998.

Scott, Walter. *Lung Cancer: A Guide to Diagnosis and Treatment.* Omaha, Neb.: Addicus Books, 2000.

Nutrition and Cancer

Budwig, Johanna. *Flax Oil as a True Aid Against Arthritis, Heart Infarction, Cancer, and Other Diseases.* Ferndale, Wash.: Apple, 1996.

Ghosh, Kris, Linda Carson, and Elyse Cohen. *Betty Crocker's Living with Cancer Cookbook.* Minneapolis: Betty Crocker, 2001.

Keane, Maureen, and Daniella Chace. *What to Eat if You Have Cancer: A Guide to Adding Nutritional Therapy to Your Treatment Plan.* Lincolnwood, Ill.: NTC Publishing Group, 1996.

Keim, Rachel, with Ginny Smith. *What to Eat Now: The Cancer Lifeline Cookbook.* Seattle: Sasquatch Books, 1996.

Quillin, Patrick. *Beating Cancer with Nutrition: Clinically Proven and Easy-to-Follow Strategies to Dramatically Improve Your Quality and Quantity of Life and Chances.* Tulsa, Okla.: Nutrition Times Press, 1998.

Reuben, Carolyn. *Antioxidants: Your Complete Guide— Fight Cancer and Heart Disease, Improve Your Memory, and Slow the Aging Process.* Roseville, Calif.: Prima Lifestyles, 1994.

Ricketts, David. *Eat to Beat Prostate Cancer Cookbook.* New York: Harry A. Abrams, 2006.

Sanders, Buffy. *The Prostate Diet Cookbook: Cancer-Fighting Foods for a Healthy Prostate.* Gig Harbor, Wash.: Harbor Press, 2001.

Weihofen, Donna, with Christina Marino. *The Cancer Survival Cookbook: Two Hundred Quick and Easy Recipes with Helpful Eating Hints.* New York: John Wiley and Sons, 1997.

Prostate and Testicular Cancers

Dattoli, Michael J. *Surviving Prostate Cancer Without Surgery: The New Gold Standard Treatment That Can Save Your Life and Lifestyle.* Sarasota, Fla.: Seneca House Press, 2005.

Grimm, Peter. *The Prostate Cancer Treatment Book.* New York: McGraw-Hill, 2003.

Icon Health Publications. *The Official Patient's Sourcebook on Testicular Cancer: A Revised and Updated Directory for the Internet Age.* San Diego, Calif.: Author, 2002.

Johanson, Paula. *Frequently Asked Questions About Testicular Cancer.* New York: Rosen Publishing Group, 2007.

Lange, Paul H. *Prostate Cancer for Dummies.* Hoboken, N.J.: Wiley, 2003.

Marks, Sheldon. *Prostate and Cancer: A Family Guide to Diagnosis, Treatment, and Survival.* 3d ed. Cambridge, Mass.: Da Capo Press, 1999.

Oesterling, Joseph. *The ABC's of Prostate Cancer: The Book That Could Save Your Life.* Ann Arbor, Mich.: J. W. Edwards, 1997.

Rous, Stephen N. *The Prostate Book: Sound Advice on Symptoms and Treatment.* New York: W. W. Norton, 1995.

Strum, Stephen. *A Primer on Prostate Cancer: The Empowered Patient's Guide.* Hollywood, Fla.: Life Extension Media, 2002.

Torrey, E. Fuller. *Surviving Prostate Cancer: What You Need to Know to Make Informed Decisions.* New Haven, Conn.: Yale University Press, 2008.

Walsh, Patrick C. *Dr. Patrick Walsh's Guide to Surviving Prostate Cancer.* New York: Grand Central, 2002.

Skin Cancers

Buckmaster, Majorie L. *Skin Cancer.* New York: Benchmark Books, 2007.

Kenet, Barney J., and Patricia Lawler. *Saving Your Skin: Prevention, Early Detection, and Treatment of Melanoma and Other Skin Cancers.* New York: Four Walls Eight Windows, 1998.

McClay, Edward F., Mary-Eileen T. McClay, and Jodie Smith. *One Hundred Questions and Answers About Melanoma and Other Skin Cancers.* Sudbury, Mass.: Jones and Bartlett, 2003.

Schofield, Jill R., and William A. Robinson. *What You Really Need to Know About Moles and Melanoma.* Baltimore, Md.: Johns Hopkins University Press, 2000.

Schwartz, Robert A. *Skin Cancer.* Malden, Mass.: Wiley-Blackwell, 2008.

Indexes

▶ Category List

Chemotherapy and other drugs

Complementary and alternative therapies

Diseases, symptoms, and conditions

Social and personal issues

▶ Index

A page number or range in boldface type indicates that an entire entry devoted to that topic appears in the set. Compounds are listed under their main root (hence, 4-Aminobiphenyl appears under "A").